3.99

CW01465298

CALCUTTA YOGA

CALCUTTA YOGA

How Modern Yoga Travelled
to the World from the Streets
of Calcutta

JEROME ARMSTRONG

MACMILLAN

First published 2020 by Macmillan
an imprint of Pan Macmillan Publishing India Private Limited
707, Kailash Building,
26, K. G. Marg, New Delhi – 110 001
www.panmacmillan.co.in

Pan Macmillan, 6 Briset St, Farringdon, London EC1M 5NR
Associated companies throughout the world
www.panmacmillan.com

ISBN 978-93-89109-30-6

Copyright © Jerome Armstrong 2020

All rights reserved. No part of this publication may be reproduced, stored in or introduced into a retrieval system, or transmitted, in any form, or by any means (electronic, mechanical, photocopying, recording or otherwise) without the prior written permission of the publisher. Any person who does any unauthorized act in relation to this publication may be liable to criminal prosecution and civil claims for damages.

The views expressed in this book are the author's own and the facts reported by him have been verified by the publisher to the extent possible. The publisher hereby disclaims any liability to any party for loss, damages or disruptions caused by the same.

1 3 5 7 9 8 6 4 2

This book is sold subject to the condition that it shall not, by way of trade or otherwise, be lent, re-sold, hired out, or otherwise circulated without the publisher's prior consent in any form of binding or cover other than that in which it is published and without a similar condition including this condition being imposed on the subsequent purchaser.

Typeset in Dante MT Std by R. Ajith Kumar, New Delhi
Printed and bound in India by Gopsons Papers Ltd

For Chitralekha Shalom and Pavitra Shekhar;
without them I would not have started.
Claudia Guggenbühl and Arup Sen Gupta;
without them I could not have started.
And for Mataji (Swamini Guru Priyananda),
whose enduring spirit, I hope, pervades this book.

CONTENTS

The Ghosh and Bose "Yoga Family"

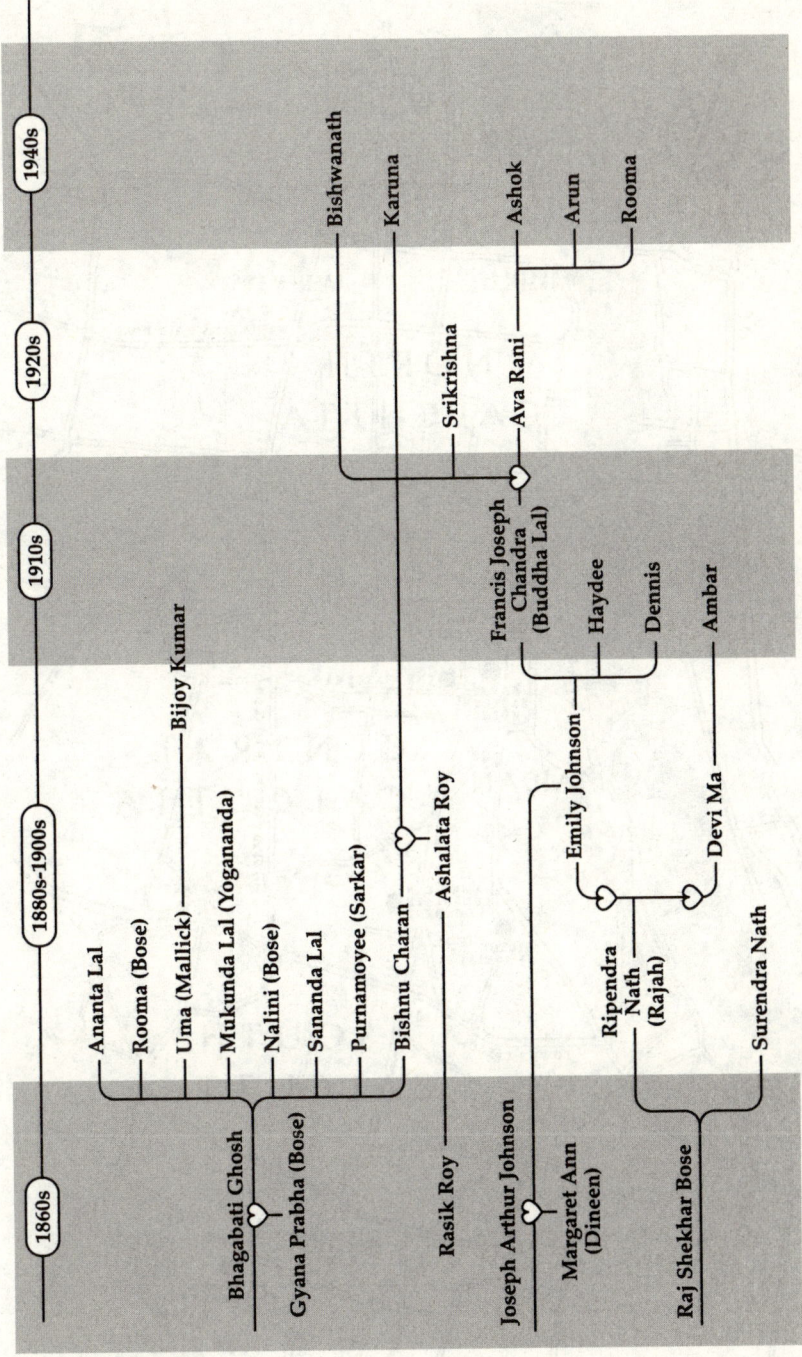

Circa 1970s, Arun is wedded to Swapna; Karuna to Jibananda Ghosh; Bishwanath to Anjana; Ashoka to Chitralekha; Rooma to Shibnath De. Of their children, Muktamala (1976 to Bishwanath & Anjana) and Pavitra Shekhar (1976 to Ashok & Chitralekha) are among a dozen in the current generation; most also teach yoga or bodybuilding.

Calcutta, India

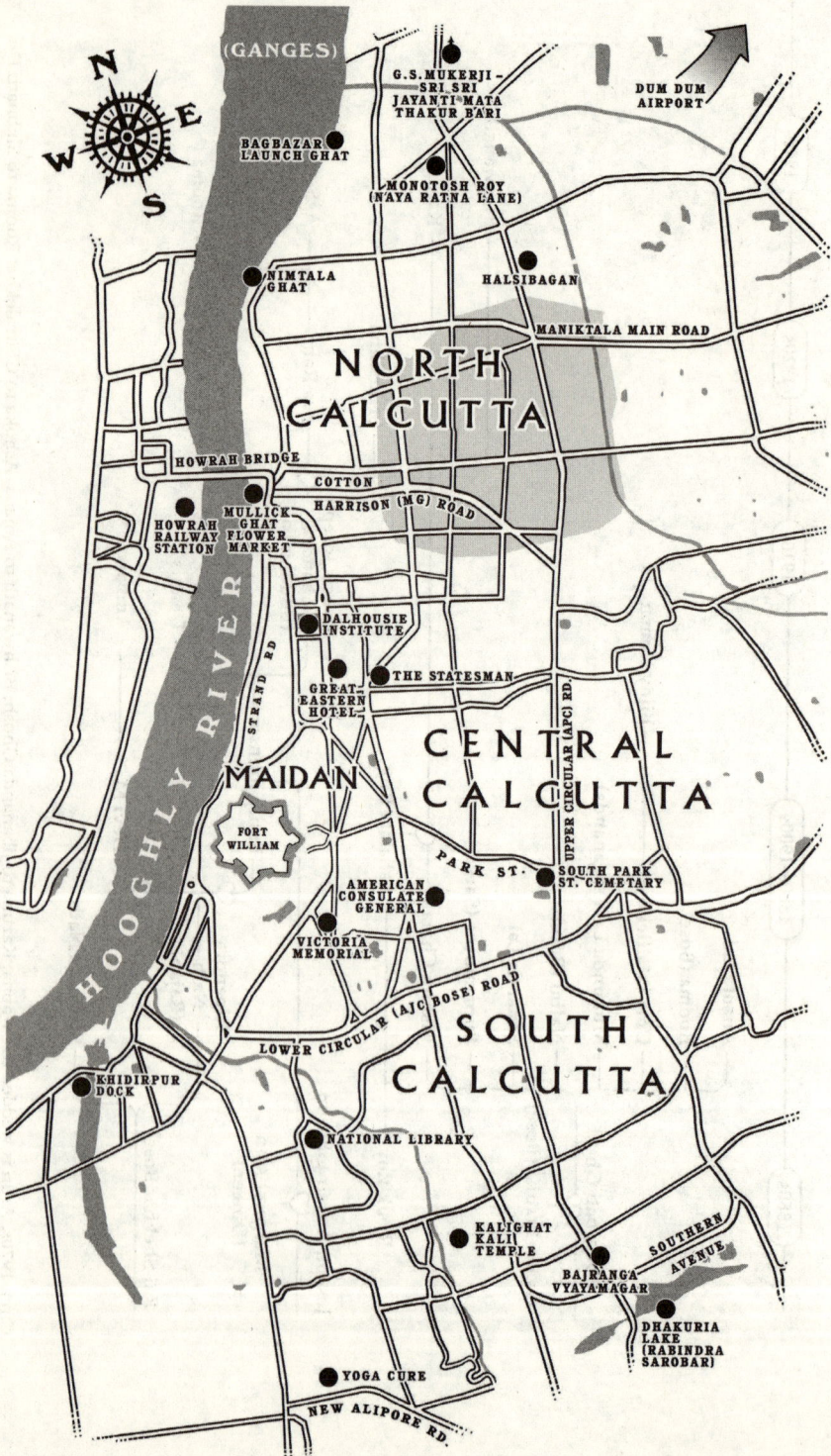

(GANGES)

N W E S (compass)

DUM DUM AIRPORT

G.S.MUKERJI —
SRI SRI
JAYANTI MATA
THAKUR BARI

BAGBAZAR
LAUNCH GHAT

MONOTOSH ROY
(NAYA RATNA LANE)

NIMTALA
GHAT

HALSIBAGAN

MANIKTALA MAIN ROAD

NORTH CALCUTTA

HOWRAH BRIDGE

COTTON

HARRISON (MG) ROAD

HOWRAH
RAILWAY
STATION

MULLICK
GHAT
FLOWER
MARKET

STRAND RD

DALHOUSIE
INSTITUTE

THE STATESMAN

GREAT
EASTERN
HOTEL

CENTRAL CALCUTTA

UPPER CIRCULAR (APC) RD.

MAIDAN

FORT
WILLIAM

PARK ST.

SOUTH PARK
ST. CEMETARY

AMERICAN
CONSULATE
GENERAL

VICTORIA
MEMORIAL

HOOGHLY RIVER

LOWER CIRCULAR (AJC BOSE) ROAD

SOUTH CALCUTTA

KHIDIRPUR
DOCK

NATIONAL LIBRARY

KALIGHAT
KALI
TEMPLE

BAJRANGA
VYAYAMAGAR

SOUTHERN
AVENUE

DHAKURIA
LAKE
(RABINDRA
SAROBAR)

YOGA CURE

NEW ALIPORE RD.

North Calcutta

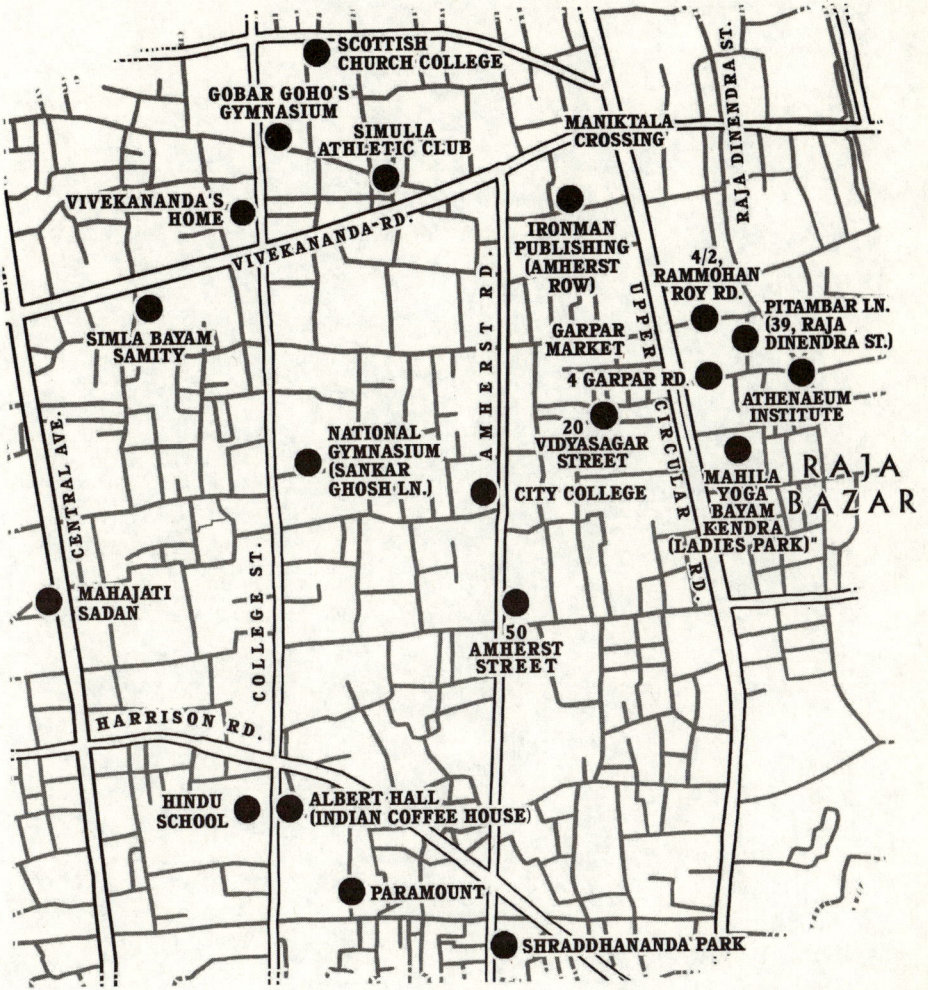

North Calcutta

Map labels:
- SCOTTISH CHURCH COLLEGE
- GOBAR GOHO'S GYMNASIUM
- SIMULIA ATHLETIC CLUB
- MANIKTALA CROSSING
- RAJA DINENDRA ST.
- VIVEKANANDA'S HOME
- VIVEKANANDA-RD.
- IRONMAN PUBLISHING (AMHERST ROW)
- 4/2, RAMMOHAN ROY RD.
- PITAMBAR LN. (39, RAJA DINENDRA ST.)
- SIMLA BAYAM SAMITY
- AMHERST RD.
- GARPAR MARKET
- 4 GARPAR RD.
- ATHENAEUM INSTITUTE
- CENTRAL AVE.
- NATIONAL GYMNASIUM (SANKAR GHOSH LN.)
- 20 VIDYASAGAR STREET
- CITY COLLEGE
- UPPER CIRCULAR RD.
- MAHILA YOGA BAYAM KENDRA (LADIES PARK)"
- RAJA BAZAR
- COLLEGE ST.
- MAHAJATI SADAN
- 50 AMHERST STREET
- HARRISON RD.
- HINDU SCHOOL
- ALBERT HALL (INDIAN COFFEE HOUSE)
- PARAMOUNT
- SHRADDHANANDA PARK

PREFACE

The name I knew.
What drew me in, what made me linger,
was a desire to know what was missing, forgotten.

It was a wintry day in November 2013. I travelled from my home and across the Potomac River to one of the Smithsonian buildings in Washington DC. On display in the gallery were materials tracking the historical roots of yoga as it morphed from its classical practice within India into a modern worldwide cultural phenomenon.

I closely examined the documents and photographs on display and purchased a commemorative book: *Yoga: The Art of Transformation*. In a chapter on the origins of yoga asana practice was a full-page photo of Buddha Bose. Beneath the photo was a caption:

> Buddha Bose, a student of yoga master Bishnu Ghosh, shows his skills at a yoga exercise demonstration, London, ca. 1930s.

The photo of Buddha was phenomenal; he was performing a difficult abdominal muscle control posture.

After admiring the photo, my attention was drawn to the lack of attendant details. There was no mention of a photographer, location or even a date; only the decade the photo was taken featured. And nothing about Buddha Bose was included elsewhere in the book.

He forgot the world.
And the world forgot him.[1]

Few have heard the name Buddha Lal Bose. Even fewer have heard his story. In March 2014, after locating a copy of the hard-to-find Volume 1 of *Key to the Kingdom of Health through Yoga* (1939) written by Buddha, I wondered about the whereabouts of Volume 2. I thought, 'Well, someone must have already found out what happened; why it wasn't published.' A search revealed little information.

I found a 1938 newspaper article which described the performance of eighty-four asanas by Buddha Bose in London and Washington DC; a 1939 issue of *Ken* magazine out of New York included four photographs of Buddha, in postures that were not included in Volume 1. But that was about all. More than seventy-five years had passed since Volume 1 was published, which led me to conclude that the story of Buddha Bose's life had not yet been told.

This book tells the story of what happened to him: the forgotten yogi of the twentieth century and his life inside the yoga family of Calcutta.

I knew I would write this book when I uncovered a lone copy of Buddha's unpublished manuscript – an entire album titled 'Yoga Asanas'. Buddha had brought the nearly finished manuscript from Calcutta to London in 1938 and left it there to be published. But his personal ordeal and the world affairs of the forties put things on hold. Indefinitely. What had happened to the manuscript and photos next was a mystery.

In London, the manuscript was placed in a family trunk and forgotten. Four decades later, two young sisters pulled it out and attempted to get into the 'funny shapes' made by 'Uncle Buddha'. They soon tired and returned it to the trunk. Two more decades and another generation went by before the belongings of the London house were sold off.

Later in the research, I encountered another possibility. An American man, by the name of Edward Groth, was a yoga student of Buddha's in the 1930s, while he worked at the American Consulate in Calcutta. Groth was an avid photographer, and may have taken the photographs of Buddha found within the manuscript, and brought it back with him to the states when he retired.

Whatever the case, the manuscript went missing, only to reemerge at an estate sale in San Francisco.

In 2003, an art collector of specialty prints from the 1930s won a bid for the manuscript, paying $11,000. He prized its pristine condition and only once showed it publicly, at the Association of International Photography Art Dealers Fair in March of 2011. I discovered this through a lone online review, praising the collection of photographs as one of 'the best' booths at the fair. The article contained this gem of a clue, written by Emma Allen:

And most mysterious and charming of all, a series of instructional yoga photos depicting the 20th century master 'Buddha Bose' in various improbable poses. Wall text enigmatically explained that the gleaming, well-oiled Bose made the series for his 'Uncle Edward'.

'Who is Uncle Edward?' was the first question that popped into my mind. Then came the second, 'Is this the missing Volume 2 from Buddha Bose?'

With this article I had something tangible. I needed to find the art collector. The author of the article provided clues, explaining that the San Francisco collector displayed 'nostalgic silver gelatin photographs' from the past and the gallery was 'moving soon to New York'. The article was a few years old, though; and I couldn't locate the collector in San Francisco or New York. When I finally tracked him down through a web-archived page, I contacted him via email.

He replied, 'I am deep in the Colorado mountains … next week I will tell you more about the Buddha Bose thesis I own and its ninety asana photographs and detailed descriptions. It's quite amazing.'

A couple of months later, in July of 2014, after many more emails back and forth, I ventured to Connecticut to view the manuscript. It was complete and had never been published. Signed by Buddha Bose on 15 July 1938, it contained dozens of intermediate and advanced asanas not included in Volume 1.

Michael Shapiro, the owner, asked why I wanted access to the manuscript.

I replied simply, 'To share it with others.'

He responded, 'I've been waiting fifteen years for someone to show up and say that to me.'

He agreed to allow it to be published but requested that I seek out Buddha's living family and learn the history of the manuscript. Little did I realize that this was like being given a map and sent out on a global treasure hunt; the mystery quickly turned into an adventure!

Through Bose's family members in London and Calcutta, I uncovered the story of Buddha's father, a magician. In India, I went deep into the Himalayas to meet a ninety-two-year-old *swamini* known as Mataji, who was Buddha's friend and disciple. And in Calcutta, I became friends with an exemplary former yoga assistant and the daughter-in-law of Buddha, who shared photos and memories and translated materials from Bengali.

The journey to research this story led to interviews with about fifty of his relatives and former students, travels throughout India and the Himalayas, the cities of Colombo, Yangon, Bangkok, Tokyo, London, Zürich, Washington DC and Los Angeles.

German and Japanese writings by the students of Bishnu Ghosh and Buddha Bose were found and translated into English. Trips to the Library of Congress in DC, the National Library in Calcutta, and the Cambridge and London libraries in England filled in further details.

Over and over again, I returned to Calcutta, drawn specifically to the Bengali neighbourhoods of north Calcutta, where streets with multiple names led to winding and intimate alleyways. In this city, whose heyday was a century ago, I searched for individuals who would share a story, a house where relatives still lived or a venue where important events once occurred.

I dug up and stumbled upon photographs, letters, books and magazines within the city's libraries or in old homes. Most were written in English or Bengali, worm-eaten and crumbling from old age. When I uncovered something, it was like finding a treasure.

As I was drawn further into the history, filling in the gaps of Buddha's life, I got to know Bishnu and Yogananda's family too. It was their family – the Ghosh family – that Buddha had married into, and their house where Buddha Bose lived and raised his family.

I even moved into that very house, which is still standing in a north Calcutta neighbourhood, to study at Ghosh's Yoga College. I learned the one-on-one therapeutic model of yoga, passed down for three generations, from Bishnu Ghosh's marvellous granddaughter, Muktamala.

In time, the history of north Calcutta became clearer to me. I began to understand how the Bengali–English linguistic cultural interaction shaped the philosophical and religious minds of Buddha Bose, Bishnu Ghosh and Yogananda. I realized how Calcutta met a tragic fate through economic stagnation, war, famine and communal fighting. The steady march of modernism had shoved aside a culture steeped in spiritual practice in favour of overpopulated urban drudgery.

It was not just the city of Calcutta that changed in the forties. Buddha, Bishnu and Yogananda each encountered a personal tragedy in that fateful decade. The trio met life's darkest moments and rose out of those depths to bring yoga to the world. I found out what happened to Buddha, why he disappeared and what happened next.

In the history of modern yoga, the name Yogananda is one of the most famous, and his brother, Bishnu Charan Ghosh, is one of the most influential. Through family, fame and their teachings, Buddha Bose's life was intertwined with the two; yet he is rarely mentioned in history books. He was at the heart of Calcutta's yoga family, helping bring yoga to the world in the twentieth century. He was poised to popularize hatha yoga on a global scale as a modern, spiritually inclined form of exercise. He was a disciple of the Ghosh brothers, Bishnu and Yogananda.

Bishnu Ghosh was among India's vanguard in bringing classical hatha yoga out of the ashrams and hermitages, where it was taught only to *sannyasis*, and into India's crowded twentieth-century cities with the goal of providing a 'yoga cure' for ailments and diseases. Bishnu laid the groundwork for the emergence of the gymnasium and bodybuilding practice that integrated strength building with yoga in the forties. He developed the technique of alternating effort and rest – asana and savasana – that informs Bikram yoga, and many 'hot yoga' styles that set Calcutta yoga apart from other Indian yoga traditions. As a *bayamacharya* (teacher of exercise), he was known for his circus, which mixed performances of feats of strength with physical culture.

Yogananda (born Mukunda Lal Ghosh) had immense cultural influence in America and the West for three decades. An exponent of kriya yoga, he also taught Yogoda, a physical practice that mixes *bayam* (exercise movements) with asanas and meditation. He advocated a peaceful vegetarian lifestyle and presented a philosophy of self-realization through meditation. His book *Autobiography of a Yogi* became one of the top-selling spiritual books of all time. His impact on the Western world's modern spiritual lifestyle and culture is difficult to overstate.

Both of the brothers were Buddha Bose's teachers, one in physical exercise and the other in spirituality. Together, the trio toured south India in 1935. Then Buddha and Bishnu went to Europe and America in 1938–39 on a world tour, where Buddha performed 'India's physical culture system' of eighty-four yoga asanas. The two stayed in California for a while, teaching Yogananda's disciples the asanas of hatha yoga.

Upon returning to Calcutta, Buddha published his 1939 book, *Key to the Kingdom of Health through Yoga* (Volume I). The book reached his Calcutta students and made its way to foreign students in London, New York and Los Angeles. By all indications, Buddha appeared to be on the verge of becoming one of the world's first transnational modern yoga asana teachers. He then disappeared, and no further mention of him was made outside of India.

Much of who Buddha, Bishnu and Yogananda became was derived from their parents. Their yoga family began four generations ago, with magicians on the British stage, *kriyaban* meditating householders and gymnasiums in Calcutta. Familial traits such as stage performance, an energy-based worldview and the maintenance of a daily physical practice were passed down over generations. These formed the foundation of later endeavours by Buddha, Bishnu and Yogananda, who developed modern yoga in Calcutta and then brought its message and practices to the world through tours. All of this set the stage for the next generation – their children, students and disciples – as Calcutta's yoga reached Europe, Japan, Thailand and America.

The story begins with Rajah, the father of Buddha, the magician of British stage fame.

PART ONE

MAGICIAN OF BRITISH
STAGE FAME

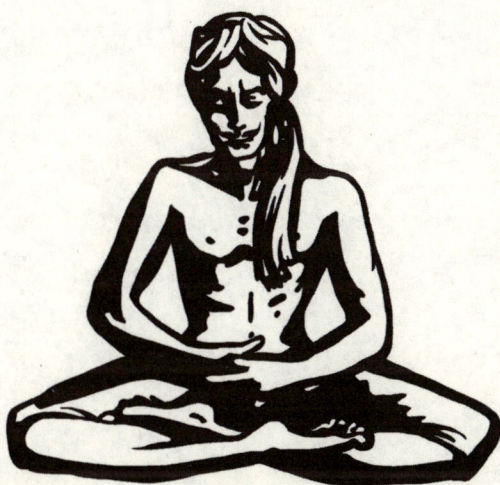

PART ONE

MAGICIAN OF BRITISH STAGE FAME

1

RAJAH THE MAGICIAN

It starts with only a name – Rajah – and a story from his descendants that he had gone to England as a magician around the turn of the twentieth century.[1] Like his son Buddha, documenting Rajah's story uncovers a lost figure of history, except the story of Rajah is even further obscured by time. Slowly though, moving from family anecdotes to English and Bengali writings, from old Calcutta magic magazines to London newspapers from the turn of the century, a portrayal of Rajah the Magician emerges.[2]

Rajah Bose was born in 1885 and given the name Ripendra Nath.[3] His father was Raj Shekhar Bose. Magic entered the boy's life while the family lived in Pakokku, Burma, a port city near the capital Mandalay and along the Irrawaddy River. Ripendra became friends with Po Htike, the grandson of a magician at Pakokku, and through this Burmese family Ripendra was 'initiated into the art of deception'. The ancient practice of magic 'took deep root'. In 1895, when Ripendra was ten, the family moved to Calcutta, India. He 'rigged out a small show' as entertainment for friends at school and visitors to the family home.[4]

In 1903, the great showman and escape artist, Harry Houdini, performed magical escapes and feats to great acclaim in London. His fame quickly spread throughout the world, including the colonial outpost in Calcutta. English periodicals raved about the stage shows, especially the 'magical performances in London'. The 'acts became more and more sophisticated, and the props increasingly complex'[5]. It was the height of the stage magician era. At the age of twenty-two, Ripendra, enthralled by the milieu of magic and the fame of magicians in London, left India and travelled to England. His father, Raj

Shekhar Bose, who had accumulated wealth in Burma, paid for the passage. On 8 September 1907, Ripendra arrived in England by boat.[6] He began classes at the University of Leeds, in subjects such as leatherwork and organic chemistry.[7] He also started giving performances before the other students. With 'encouragements from the Professors and fellow students', he decided to act on his 'desire to go on the stage'.[8] During his second year at Leeds, his schoolwork began to suffer with 'at least two fails recorded'.[9] Since 'his shows were much in request', he abandoned school and vocational classwork in favour of his passion: a career as a stage magician.

In 1909, England was a difficult and competitive place to make it on the professional stage, especially for an unknown artist of Indian origin. Rajah became 'the first Indian accredited by the Variety Artists' to appear in the British music halls and variety theatres as a conjurer and animal mimic 'on the same terms and rank as any European professor of the art'.[10] A journalist would later write that 'when performing, Rajah drew his audience into the illusions, weaving a story that left audience members feeling that they were part of a magic event and not just spectators at a magic show'.[11] Years later, Rajah recalled that he would become so focused on each moment that even the simplest trick could come alive. His ability to create an intense presence within a shared moment with an audience was the real magic and the key to his success.

In London, Rajah was one of the 'yogic magicians of the mystical East' who appealed to the 'esoteric audience's thirst for stories'. A 'sea-change in attitudes towards the Indian magician on the British and International stage' had taken place, with a fascination towards the Oriental and 'new Indian modes of performance' that 'were later taken up by Western performers'.[12] The performances 'emphasized magical powers and were full of fortune-seekers, sorcerers, and miracle workers'.[13]

In 1910, Rajah's stage act was featured in 'The Blue Pearl', a stage fantasy of seven extravagantly produced scenes created by Harry Sears, a young American vaudeville magician at the height of his career. 'The Blue Pearl' was subtitled 'The Quest of World's Desire', and contained 'a story of Indian life told in the pantomime' through 'the theft by a Rajah of a great blue pearl from the image of the god Shiva'.[14]

Rajah joined a horse, camel, scantily clad female assistants holding snakes and an additional forty-five others in the wide-ranging show. He also performed an iconic rope trick brought to the West from India.[15] The trick, like Jack and the

Beanstalk, held universal appeal; it portrayed the ability to escape the earth's hold to an abode in the sky.[16]

Rajah had mixed feelings about this opportunity. He appreciated the exposure, but did not like the stereotype of performing an Indian trick, portrayed as the Hindu or Oriental magician.[17] With a move that would change everything, Rajah decided to set out on his own with a different stage partner.

2

OF BRITISH STAGE FAME

Rajah's new stagehand was the 'bewitching damsel Emily Johnson'. The lore about her from the Bose family was plentiful. Descendants in Calcutta claimed 'Amy', as the niece of the Archbishop of Canterbury. London descendants claimed 'Emma', with her aristocratic background, as the daughter of a respected Yorkshire mill owner with considerable wealth. She used 'Emily' to sign documents, went by 'Emmie' at times and carried three different last names over the course of her life. She went so far as to use her magic skills on her travel documents, making a decade conveniently disappear from her age. There was a mysterious air about the woman and a bit of non-conformist impracticality. (Not once did she provide an answer to the question of occupation on immigration documents). Curiously, she had no middle name.[1]

Rajah and Emily met while at Leeds, and it was there that they first partnered on the stage. Afterward, she was the only true partner in his magic shows, and when she was absent from Rajah's shows, he would perform alone or with an entourage. While at Leeds, 'it didn't take long for Rajah to attract the attention of Emily. The glamour of the stage, the dark complexion and the wily charms of the orient proved too bewitching. Emily became smitten, and was happy to be sawn in half twice nightly.'[2]

She might have come from a conservative, respected and well-off London family, but her sense of adventure was radical for its time. In the first decade of the 1900s, Emily fit a prototype of the emergent suffragette movement that campaigned for equal rights for women: highly educated, young, aristocratic or professional; working to become equal politically. Emily had 'really upset the apple cart when she fraternized and eventually fell in love with a gentleman from Calcutta'. After his time on the stage with the American magician Sears, Rajah and Emily began their solo act.[3]

In February and March of 1911, Rajah was on the bill at the London Coliseum. In April, he was at the Alhambra, and in September, their show was presented at the Hippodrome. The Hippodrome, which opened in 1900, is known today as the Hippodrome Casino, but the historic great hall of old is still intact. The venue hosted Houdini in 1904, when he performed the *Mirror* handcuff escape challenge. Then, in 1911, it hosted Rajah and Emily. The show of the duo 'tops the bill at the Hippodrome', declared one review. The 'Hindoo illusionist' and his 'lady assistant' had officially arrived.[4]

Performing at these London venues was a big deal for Rajah and Emily. Rajah had reached for the fame of Houdini, his idol, and now performed on that same stage with Emily. Their performance brought with it the 'Egyptian Dancing' theme which had been prevalent in Rajah's show with Sears. Rajah performed 'the whole gamut of the conjurer's tricks, old and new, with the exception that he did them better' said one reviewer. He went on:

He imitates with striking realism the noise of things animate and inanimate, babies and gramophones, for instance, and gives a striking vocal impression of a battle royal between a couple of infuriated tigers.

Every interaction on stage with Emily was dramatic:

He is hooded and cloaked and duly placed in a cage, every side of which is visible to the audience. Curtains are drawn upon him for the space of a second or two, and, lo! He is seen making his way from the back of the auditorium while in his place in the cage stands his lady assistant.[5]

Rajah and Emily displayed the special demonstrable powers of magic with an air of modernity, leaving their audiences in awe of their flair on the stage. They were socially accepted as performers and members of society. They embraced the contemporary role of the modern stage magician, the British conjurer.

Rajah the stage magician dressed formally, in light-coloured suits and slacks instead of sorcerer-like robes – a significant step away from India's street magician yogi with his portrayal of *siddhis* (powers), or the medieval robed Magi who performed sorcery on the stage. Emily wore black on stage, topped with a wide-brimmed black hat.

Rajah had reached the British stage and paved the way for British-Indian magicians, but his fame faded quickly. Today, when one searches for Indian magicians of the past, one will not find Rajah Bose. Instead, P. C. Sorcar tops the list. Sorcar, also from Calcutta, is recognized as the 'father of Indian Magic' in the modern era.[6] Regardless, decades before the worldwide acclaim for Sorcar, Rajah was on the British stage and hailed as Calcutta's top magician.[7] He was, for a short time, India's Great Master of Magic, but was soon erased from history.

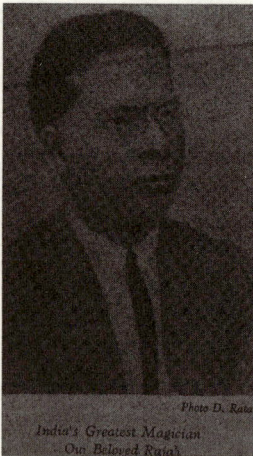

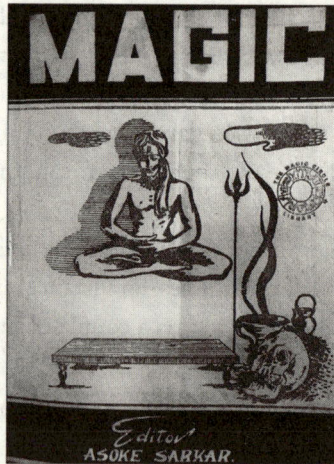

Left: Rajah Bose (*Source: Magic magazine*); Right: PC Sorcar, *Indian Magic*

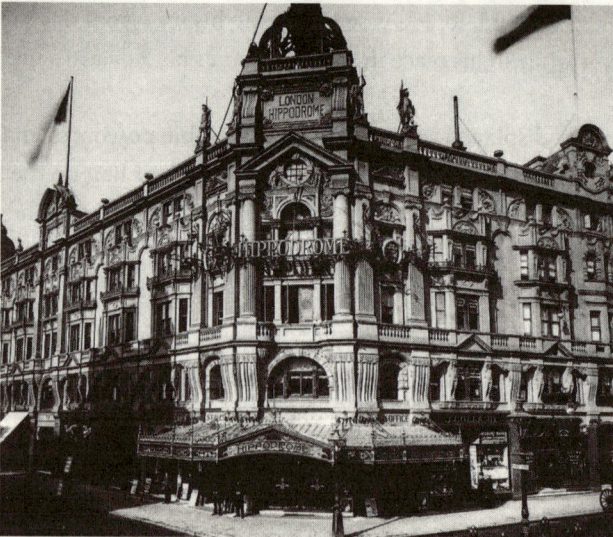

Hippodrome (London) (*Source: Wikimedia commons*)

3

COLOMBO, CEYLON, 20 SEPTEMBER 1912

Rajah and Emily performed alongside the era's top acts at all the top venues, but the Spring of 1911 was climactic due to another pressing matter:

> It came as no surprise when her mother and father of such high standing disowned her as she continued her relationship with Rajah, and inevitably fell in love. Sadly, her very slight figure was to bloom, as she had fallen pregnant.[1]

When Emily became pregnant, there was no record of Rajah and Emily having a registration for marriage, nor did they share the same address.[2] That April, the London census recorded Ripendra Bose, aged 26, living at 7 Manchester Street, Southampton; with many foreign room-mates who were also fledgling performers. Four months later, when Emily gave birth to Haydee on 14 August 1911, the couple provided the address of 19 Danville Road.

Neither Rajah nor Emily were prepared for a child, nor did they understand how this would mark the end of their career on the British stage. The interracial mix in their show challenged cultural norms of the time, and their unwed relationship had scandalous implications. Rajah may have been removed from the magician's guild to which he belonged and faced discrimination. With the birth of a child, Emily's father of 'high standing' made life difficult for both of them.

The following year Emily became pregnant with their second child, and the couple decided to leave Britain for Calcutta, bringing their magic duo to the Bengal region of India. They travelled by an ocean vessel named the *SS Derflinger*. On this particular voyage in 1912, before they had reached Ceylon and the Indian Ocean, Emily gave birth to her second child. The couple had left London while she was in her last trimester of pregnancy and, since the voyage to Calcutta by boat was quite long, Buddha Bose was born at sea with the given name Francis Joseph Chandra Bose. It was a Christian name given by his mother, paired with Chandra, a Bose family middle name selected by his father.

Even though his official birth certificate listed 20 September, the birth date Buddha would provide throughout his life was 10 August. He would later say he was 'born on the deck' of the boat.[3] It is possible he was born on the earlier date and then registered later at the Colombo port, or perhaps the date just got mixed up later on.

Over the final ten days of the voyage, they crossed the Indian Ocean and the Bay of Bengal before entering the mouth of the Ganges River and arriving at the Port of Calcutta.

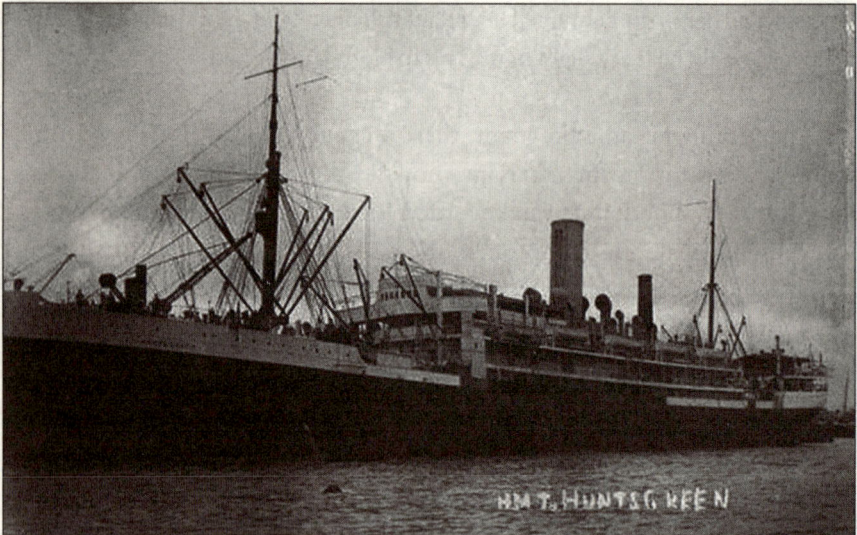

SS Derflinger (*Source: Wikimedia Commons*)

4

RAJAH'S RETURN

Then, the steamer rounded the great muddy bend called Garden Reach, and there
it was – newer than New York, richer than Rome, more populous than either –
revealing itself with a sweeping panorama that took your breath away.[1]
– Calcutta, circa 1850

It was early October and Durga Puja – the biggest Hindu festival in Bengal – was about to begin. In those days, it was common for stage feats and all sorts of demonstrations to be held in the neighbourhood pandals, which were set up throughout the city during the week-long celebration. A magic show would be certain to gain maximum exposure.

Rajah returned to India having performed on the British stage alongside other greats like Houdini, and that gave him a claim to fame. One piece of family lore was that Rajah began his career on the stage in London as an assistant to Houdini, but Houdini had left London prior to Rajah's arrival. One Calcutta reviewer wrote, 'Rajah Bose was unquestionably the king of all the magicians who appeared in the first two decades of the twentieth century.' Rajah was even able to enthrall those in his audience who frowned at his 'nativeness' and to 'make them bow down to his skill'.[2] This was perhaps the highest compliment Rajah could receive: to stand as an equal with the British.

His mystique was complicated by the fact that Rajah had brought a British woman as his assistant back with him, and they had come with children. This framed Rajah in a radical and non-conformist light that only a magician could pull off.

Before leaving Calcutta for England in 1907, Rajah had been in an arranged marriage with a Bengali girl. The couple had no children, but his Bengali wife was living in a north Calcutta house where he too was expected to live. Upon his return to Calcutta in 1912, his plan was to carry on living two lives, with neither family knowing about the other, even while both were in Calcutta.

When Rajah, Emily and the children arrived at Calcutta's Kidderpore dock in 1912, they debarked and rode a carriage into Central Calcutta, along Strand Road, to reach Waterloo Street, home of the renowned Great Eastern Hotel. Rajah promptly put up Emily, Haydee (the oldest, a girl) and Buddha at the hotel. They would stay there alone, without him.

5

THE GREAT EASTERN HOTEL

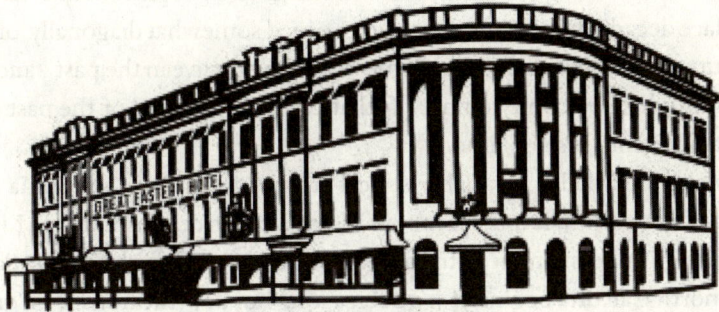

Great Eastern Hotel

'In those days,' wrote the magician John Booth,
'the Great Eastern was a very famous address.'[1]

The Great Eastern Hotel was a colonial architecture, located in the heart of the British part of the city. It is Asia's oldest luxury hotel and was referred to in its heyday as 'the Jewel of the East'. This was at a time when Calcutta was a stronghold of British colonialism, and the Chowringhee Road mansions gave it the name 'city of palaces'.[2]

Occasionally, while researching in Calcutta, I book a room at the Great Eastern. Until about 2010, the hotel was in disrepair, but it has since undergone renovation. Still, much of the original layout and structure remains intact from the time when Emily and her children lived there. Its circular iron staircase, the Great Hall and the lily pond garden are left as reminders.

Each morning, an English breakfast is served next to the hotel's lily pond and garden. I land a seat next to the water and gaze at the lilies. After breakfast, I catch a yellow taxi or an Uber car. Or I take the metro – the underground city transit that runs north to south.

I go north and exit at Girish Park, a few blocks from the heart of where the yoga proponents lived – where I've entered the family homes of Vivekananda, Yogananda, Mahendranath and the others who brought yoga to the modern world. While central Calcutta is populated with large, iconic buildings, the northern part of the city is differentiated   by its urban intimacy and liveliness.

As I step into north Calcutta, it feels like I've time-travelled to a distant place. Walking through its streets, the buildings and people hint at events that took place decades prior. The alleyways proceed somewhat diagonally, offering shortcuts off the crowded street. Some say, 'Bengalis live in the past', and since the past is what I've come to find, I feel at ease.[3] Knowledge of the past places me in a different sense of time.

Towards nightfall, I invariably set off from Garpar Road or Sukia Street and walk by the Bose family home on Vidyasagar Street. From there I'll walk south along Amherst Street or the alleyways nearby and reach College Square, where north Calcutta begins. If it's been a long hot day (the norm), I'll quench my thirst at Paramount, a small sherbet joint next to the Mahabodhi Society, with drinks named 'Daab Sherbet' and 'Cocoa Malai'. Opened a century ago, it was once a meeting place for nationalist revolutionaries. Its marble-top tables complement the cool drinks made of fruits, curd, coconut water and essence. Revived, I continue the walk to the Great Eastern Hotel.

Along this route, from north Calcutta to central Calcutta, to the Great Eastern Hotel, Rajah travelled every morning during the fall of 1912. I am retracing his path.

6

THE REVEAL

It was autumn, 1912. The monsoon and humid temperatures of summer had passed, making it easier for Emily to adjust to the climate of Calcutta. The central part of the city was probably also comforting to her because of its London esque/ish feel. But more significant for Rajah was that this location set his English wife and their children apart from his life with the Bengali family.

After dropping off Emily and the children at the Great Eastern, Rajah ventured into north Calcutta. It was just a four-kilometre ride to the home where his father and his Bengali wife were staying, but it was a world apart.

Each morning, Rajah hired a hackney carriage to take him back from his home in north Calcutta to the Great Eastern Hotel. There, he would spend the day with his family at the hotel, sometimes outside on the grounds near the lily pool. In the evenings he would return to his home.

The home in north Calcutta was a large, four-storey duplex with a central corridor. It was also the home of Rajah's father, Raj Shekhar. Before long, Rajah's 'daily excursions aroused suspicion', and Raj 'made it a point to follow his son'.[1]

Raj Shekhar watched Rajah 'go into a hotel room' at the Great Eastern and spied, watching as his son brought a woman and two children outside, by the hotel's lily pond. He did not say anything to his son at the time. But later, after Rajah was gone, Raj went to the hotel room and knocked on the door.

When Emily answered the door, he said, 'Please do not get annoyed, but may I ask, who is the person who came into your room?'

Looking quizzically at the old man, Emily answered, 'He is my husband.'

Upon hearing this, all Raj Shekhar could muster was, 'I am sorry,' as he backed away and left for his home.[2]

Whatever Rajah's long-term plan could have been, his father intervened to resolve the deceptive situation. Rajah would no longer be able to lead one British life and one Bengali life.

Raj Shekhar scolded his son, 'That is my daughter-in-law, those are my grandchildren, and you have kept them in a hotel room? Go and bring her home right now.' Even as adults, Bengalis are still the children of their parents, so Rajah agreed to his father's wishes. He brought Emily and the two children, Buddha and Haydee, into the world of the Bengali family.

Since he left them alone each evening, Emily must have wondered where Rajah's home was located and what the living conditions were like. But she had not known of his second wife, the one he had married before going to Britain, until this day. Buddha would later say, 'I cannot say anything wrong about my mother. She was from a different culture and the Indian culture is different from hers. My father had to accept both the ladies as his wives.'[3]

Emily and the children left the Great Eastern and the two families resided together in north Calcutta. Somehow it worked, or seemed to, as Rajah returned to the stage with Emily and a sense of normalcy ensued.

Just a few months after their return to Calcutta, 'for an unbroken period of 30 days in December of 1912', Rajah and Emily began to perform daily shows at the Kohinoor Theater in North Calcutta. Their show was 'as big and extensive as that of any European Illusionists'.[4] Then, from Calcutta they took the train to Dacca (present-day Dhaka), which was part of Bengal at the time. An old promotional clipping described their advance:

> As the people of Dacca awoke in the morning, their confused and drowsy eyes were amazed to see the most sensational posters displayed throughout the town, proclaiming that the 'Greatest Magician of the Orient, Rajah, and the Queen of Witch, Miss Emily, are Coming Shortly with their Party'. The thought in the minds of hundreds of men and women that morning was, Rajah? Who is he? Before that day, none of them had heard the name, but all of them were soon happy to learn that Rajah was actually Indian (Bengalese), the Magician Rajah Bose.[5]

The climax of the performance in Dacca was an illusionist act. It was similar to 'The Artist's Dream', a stage illusion, in which a woman steps out of a picture painted by the magician. The theme was first created by David Devant and performed at the Egyptian Hall in Piccadilly, London, during the 1890s. Rajah and Emily called it 'Return of She':

> After a brief introduction, Rajah took on the persona of a French artist whose fiancé had died a premature death, dressing himself on stage with loose garments and a wig, moustache, and beard. The curtains then opened, revealing an artist's studio. Rajah, as the artist, stands before an unfinished piece of sculpture on which he has been working. It is clearly a representation of his lost fiancé. After working on it briefly, he gives in to the desire to see his lost love as he remembers her, and he goes to a cabinet on the stage and retrieves a beautiful dress, which he places on the unfinished statue. He then places a veil over the face of the sculpture, and, as he sits down and contemplates the likeness of his lost love, he falls asleep. Suddenly, though, he awakens and finds that the statue had turned into a living being – the fiancée that he had lost long before.[6]

To perform this as David Devant did with 'The Artist's Dream', Rajah would have Emily concealed behind the curtain hangings. From there, she would emerge to replace the sculpture and become the long lost fiancée, alive again. Rajah added a twist:

> But at this point a monstrous masked demon appears from the wings and hypnotizes the artist, who is then ordered to enter the cabinet from which he had removed the dress. The demon then approaches the woman and drags her to the front of the stage. He then rips the mask from his face, revealing that the demon is the artist himself![7]

The ending represented the subterfuge of replacement – how the two mixed identities included duplicitous actions. From there, the act could be viewed entirely as a subconscious reflection of their shared reality.

It was in Calcutta on 16 May 1914, that two sons were born. One was born to Rajah's Bengali wife, her first, and he was named Ambar. The other was born to Emily, a son named Dennis, her third child. Rajah was the father of both. It was the simultaneous birth that apparently broke Emily's will to stay with

Rajah. 'My mother could not stand the fact that my father kept a relationship with the other lady,' Buddha recounted, 'and so she decided to go back to London.'[8] Neither woman would ever bear another child of Rajah's.

Emily decided to return to England and sought out help from her parents to do so. Despite 'the disavowal of her father' over her unwed relationship with Rajah during the previous years, she wrote to him, pleading that he finance her return to England, along with three children in tow.

His stunning rebuke came as a two-pence coin in the envelope, and a note, 'I care tuppence for you.' Her father, Joseph Arthur Johnson, had disowned her. Though Emily desperately wanted to return to London, she was stuck in Calcutta for another year and a half.

According to both the English and Indian sides of the family, it was Rajah's father who finally resolved the dilemma.

He told Emily, 'Since you have decided, I will not stop you. You go but keep some remembrance with me.'

Emily asked, 'What remembrance?'

He replied, 'You have got three children; keep at least one child with me.'

A deal was struck. Raj Shekhar would arrange the fare, but on the condition that one of the grandchildren be left behind with the Calcutta family. Which child stayed would be Emily's choice. Emily could not refuse the offer and was forced to choose a child to abandon.

In 1916, Emily boarded the City of Karachi steamship, which returned her to London on 6 February. On the incoming passenger list under 'Mrs. Emmie Bose' were Dennis (one and a half years) and Haydee (four and a half). Her son Francis (Buddha), two and a half years old, had been left behind in Calcutta. Emily said to her grandchildren in England decades later that 'it was something she regretted to her dying day'. There was resentment from the ancestors on the English side, passed on by Emily, who 'tearfully regretted leaving Francis'. The fateful decision fell entirely on the grandfather as 'it was her father-in-law that asked her to leave one child behind'.[9]

Buddha later recounted the resolution:

Mother thought, the eldest child is a daughter and I cannot keep her here. She was worried about in what condition she would be raised. So she decided not to leave the daughter. And when the grandfather asked her to leave behind the younger child, she refused as he was only months old. I was the lucky or unlucky one, who was left behind here.[10]

In the garden at the Great Eastern Hotel, the showy flower of the water lily blossoms and floats effortlessly top the water. But after just a few days, the colour fades, the petals wilt and fall into submersion. Underwater, the stalks curl up and the petals turn in. The once fragrant lily transforms into seedpods. The seeds can be sown; but it's not a necessity – the lily is a rhizome. In dormancy it will remain, until awakened for the next growth cycle. Then, from its mass of roots below, a new generation of stems emerge, and again the lily blossoms.

7

YOUR NAME IS BUDDHA

Filling in the early years of Buddha's life – after his mother left, but before he met the Ghosh family – requires some assistance and digging into. Chitralekha Shalom is among the first I get to know in this process. She had married into the family and worked by Buddha's side at the Yoga Cure Institute in New Alipore (south Calcutta), from the mid-1970s until 1982. She taught yoga to the women while Buddha taught the men. 'If history could be re-written,' Chitralekha tells me one day, 'I would make Rajah and Emily stay back in England.' Their time on the stage in London together was full of fame and romance, but like the fleeting lily above the water, fame did not last.

I ask Chitralekha, 'Did Buddha ever talk about the difficulty of his childhood?'[1]

She replies, 'Baba used to tell me his stories in snatches, randomly, not in one sitting. I remember these sessions would take place only when we were alone.' The two would sit 'alone under the *jamrul* tree in front of the small office room' where Baba, as she called Buddha, shared his memories and confided in her. Buddha was a private person. Even those who knew him well cannot recall him talking about his own life.

Then I meet Mataji (Swamini Guru Priyananda), a 92-year-old *swamini*, who called Buddha her *guruji*. Now she lives the life of a *sannyasini*, splitting her time between the ashram near Ahmedabad and the foothills of the Himalayas.[2] I visit Mataji in Mussoorie, the cool hill station where she lives during the hot summer months. Chitralekha, who has not seen Mataji in over thirty years, is there too, and together they answer questions about Buddha's upbringing and the difficulties he encountered in his youth.[3]

'When you listen to his life story, you wonder what gave him courage to go on,' remarks Mataji.

I ask, 'Did he remember his British mother, from that young age?'

'Yes,' she replies. 'In Central Calcutta, whenever he saw a white woman in a frock he would run to her shouting, "Mama, Mama!"' He 'would only keep crying and not eat properly; he would cry only for mama'. This continued until his Bengali stepmother decided it was her duty to give him the love of a mother. She 'took him in her lap and said, "I am your Mama. No one has named you yet. Let me name you. Your name is Buddha."' Gradually, 'he accepted the Bengali mother as his real mother'.

Buddha would tell of how 'he'd grown up listening to stories of *Ramayana* and *Mahabharata* at home and was very attracted to gods and goddesses and scriptures.'[2]

His father, Rajah, called it 'all rubbish', and would shout, 'There are no gods!' and then insist Buddha had 'no table manners' and should 'sit with the dog'.

'And so he had to sit with the dog and have his food,' Mataji explains. She reflects on Buddha retelling the events with 'tears in his eyes'.

'You are a foreigner's child,' his father told him.

It was true, Chitralekha explains of Buddha. 'He was British-fair, and his skin pigmentation stood out among the darker Indians wherever he went. The colour became a stigma, as in those days most Hindu Indians considered anyone outside their particular caste as rejects or *mleccha*.'[4] When young Buddha went to a friend's place he was made to stand outside the house. If he requested water, the tumbler 'would be thrown in the dustbin after he drank'. It was a difficult situation for him, 'but luckily, the new mother was all love and care'.

PART TWO

MOTHER, A SCHOOL
FOR BOYS

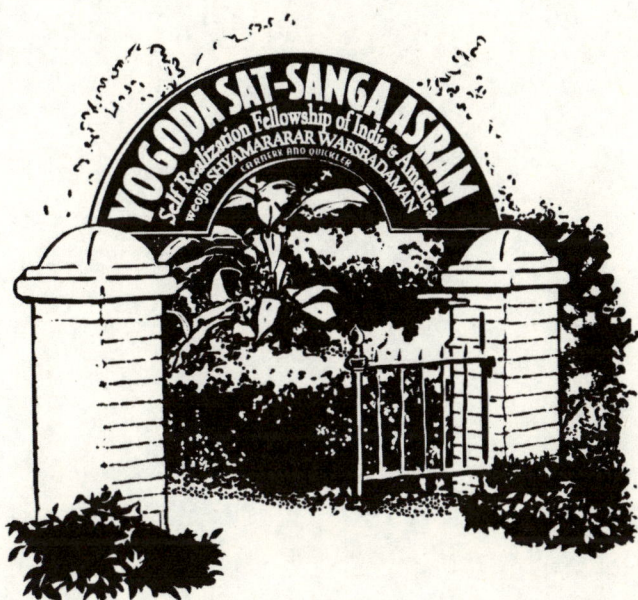

8

KALI MA

My biggest problem was this, I had no idea who or what was a mother. I still do not know what a mother is and so, talking about a mother seems an assumption.[1]
– Bishnu Ghosh

In the early 1880s, Bhagabati Ghosh arrived in Calcutta from rural Bengal and married Gyana Prabha Bose, who was from Serampore, about 40 miles outside of Calcutta.[2] The Ghoshs started their family in Rangoon, Burma, where Bhagabati was a British railway administrator. After a decade in Burma, they moved back to India as a well-salaried, but otherwise ordinary family. At that time, in the early 1890s, Bhagabati was secular in his beliefs, a non-believer in anything mystical. After a supernatural experience, Bhagabati dramatically turned towards the practice of Kriya yoga,[3] and thereafter his occupational lifestyle was augmented with a daily Kriya practice involving pranayama techniques. Gyana was a traditional Hindu mother and devotee of Kali with her daily bhakti (devotional) practice; she too became a *kriyaban*. It is not a stretch to say that their children had a congenital inclination to practise Kriya yoga.

In 1893, Gyana became pregnant with Mukunda Lal (who later became Yogananda).[4] When Bishnu Charan was born on 24 June 1903, Mukunda Lal was nine years old.[5] Like Buddha Bose, both of the Ghosh boys would have to confront the loss of their mother at a young age. Soon after Bishnu's birth, the family gathered at 50 Amherst Street in north Calcutta; for what was supposed to be a celebration of the wedding of Bishnu's eldest brother, Ananta Lal. But it was deep into the rainy season and Gyana contracted cholera. Bishnu was less than a year old.[6] Too young to remember, he would tell 'the story as I heard it from others', how within a few hours, the celebration turned to mourning.

Bishnu asked, 'In all this havoc and tragedy where was I? What did I feel? Nothing. No memory at all!'[7]

The Ghosh and Bose boys were all impacted by the loss of their mothers during their childhoods. For Bishnu, the loss meant never having a memory of his mother, and his lack manifested physically. He was ill and in poor health when he was young. Sananda Lal, his elder brother, wrote of Bishnu, 'His health suffered because he could not have Mother's nourishing milk nor her loving care. Consequently, he was frail.'[8] For Buddha, there came a period when he was 'withdrawn and did not show his emotions freely and honestly to people around him'. And though Buddha was 'highly influenced by the thinking pattern of his father', it was the maternal instinct of his Bengali stepmother that helped him to 'never give up'.[9] For Mukunda (Yogananda), who had an ordinary upbringing until the age of ten (with the exception of his psychic abilities manifesting every now and then), the visceral event resulted in a radical plan of action.

In *Autobiography of a Yogi*, Yogananda recounted the events surrounding the loss of his mother: 'The rent left in the family fabric by Mother's death was irreparable.'[10] Thirty years later, he said, 'I studied Yoga in my childhood days ... but it was not until I was profoundly moved by the death of my mother when I was a young man that I brought my powers to their full pitch.'[11] The event thrust his otherworldly desires and manifestations to the forefront. Though his name did not formally change for another dozen years, upon his mother's death, Mukunda became Yogananda in spirit as he chose the path of the sannyasi.

For a time, Yogananda returned with his father to Bareilly, a city in the north Indian state of Uttar Pradesh. There, he met a cousin 'fresh from a period of travel in the holy hills'. After Yogananda 'listened eagerly to his tales about the high mountain abode of yogis and swamis', he felt the impulse to 'run away to the Himalayas'. This was a manifestation of his desire to get beyond the physical realm, free of the pain of his loss. 'Intense pangs of longing for God assailed me. I felt powerfully drawn to the Himalayas.'[12]

Yogananda told his boyhood friend, Satyananda, 'I was completely set within, that I would leave and become a *sadhu*. I wanted to properly see my brothers and sisters one last time. When I saw my baby brother Bishnu by the stairs on the way to the second floor, I just could not hold back my tears at all.'[13]

The family lived in Bareilly for another year. Then in the spring of 1906, they moved to Chittagong in eastern Bengal. They lived in Chittagong for a year and then moved back to Calcutta, where Gyana's death had occurred in 1907. They rented and eventually purchased a house at 4 Garpar Road.

Once he arrived and was living in Calcutta, Yogananda tried to reconcile his mother's death, leaving 'no stone unturned in his spiritual investigations'. It was said that whenever Yogananda 'heard that a saint was in the area, he sought him out'. Yogananda visited the Nimtala Ghat along the Howrah River, where his mother's body had been cremated. 'In the stark atmosphere of death, he contemplated the uselessness of attachment to the impermanent body and its ceaseless demands.' One time, Yogananda even brought 'a matted-haired ascetic, dressed in a dark red cloth' with red eyes, into the family home.[14]

In 'his attic room' upstairs, Yogananda had placed 'a human skull and two human bones'. The skull 'had a vermilion mark like the *sadhu's'* on the forehead and the bones were 'placed crosswise', resting on a wooden stand. His ritualistic experiments were short-lived. Yogananda's younger brother Sananda Lal, was so frightened by the scene that he told their father. Once Bhagabati found out, he 'explained the harm that could come' from these sorts of 'degenerate offshoots' of tantric practice.[15]

Two years prior, in 1905, a sage had moved into 50 Amherst Street and begun to live on the top floor.[16] The sage began using three floors for a school called the Morton Institution of Education, but on the top floor he held spiritual lessons in the evenings for anyone who happened to attend. Soon after Yogananda found out about this, he brought his brother Sananda along with him to the lessons. Upon their visit to the schoolhouse, an apprehensive Sananda told Yogananda, 'Our mother died in this house.' Yogananda consoled him by replying, 'A great sage lives here now.' The sage was Mahendranath.

The brothers would climb the stairs to the fourth-floor meditation room where Mahendranath would ask them to sit down with him and meditate. They remained 'quietly behind him or at his side in the room, absorbed in the aura of devotion that saturated the atmosphere'.[17] Summoning their courage, Sananda and Yogananda requested that Mahendranath call their 'mother from the astral world to appear'. Mahendranath initially resisted. Then, on a subsequent visit, as they sat in meditation, Mahendranath told them to 'look behind you and see who is standing in the doorway'. The two boys did so; and a 'vision of her form' spoke to them, saying she remembered and watched over them.[18]

As their relationship developed, 'on many occasions', Mahendranath would take Yogananda 'to visit Dakshineswar'. They would travel to the Kali temple there, about three miles north of Calcutta on the banks of the Howrah

River, where Sri Ramakrishna once lived.[19] They would meditate together and
Yogananda would observe Mahendranath 'talking' with 'Divine Mother' Kali.
Yogananda felt no such connection. Instead, he felt only the 'bitter separation'
of death 'as the measure of all anguish'.[20]

One evening at his home, 'Divine Mother' put the young boy at peace. The
period of reconciliation with his mother's death culminated in the development
of a deep connection with the mother goddess through devotional practice.

Having experienced love from the 'universal mother' Kali, both destroyer
and creator, he returned to 50 Amherst the following day, 'climbing the staircase
in the house of poignant memories', to reach 'the fourth-floor room' of
Mahendranath. With Mahendranath, Yogananda worshipped her 'in the form
of Goddess Kali'.[21]

As he grew older, Yogananda's 'meditations deepened' and his spirituality
'outgrew reverence for images of worship'; he experienced an 'awakened'
form of realization.

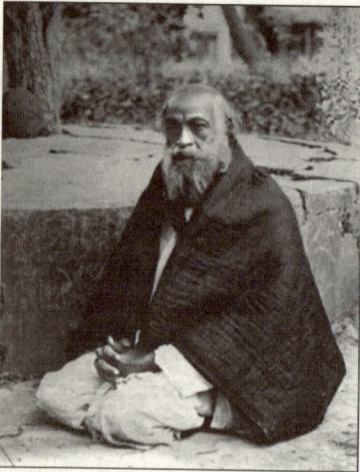
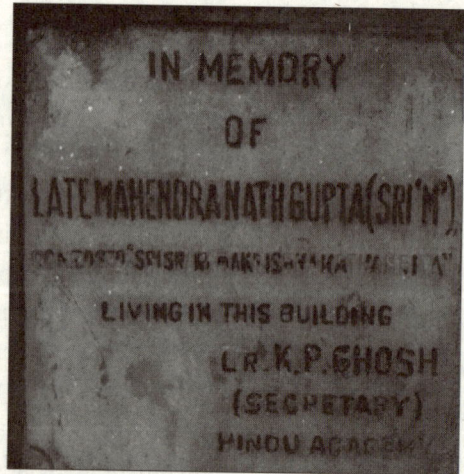

Left: Mahendranath (Sri M), circa 1920. Right: Plaque at 50 Amherst St, 2017.

9

50 AMHERST STREET

I feel eerily drawn to visit the house at 50 Amherst Street. Not because it is the place of Gyana's death, but because of a spiritual pull I feel from it. Whenever I walk from Ghosh's Yoga College to College Square, passing by the large vacant house, the gates always seemed to be locked. One evening, as I gaze towards the four storey red-brick building, I notice a white plaque near the front gate, which I have never seen before, embedded in the red-brick wall. The plaque is marble, and the black ink inside the engraving has been washed out. In the twilight it is difficult to make out the text. I find a nearby knick-knack shop where I purchase a black felt-tip marker. I go back, turn on my phone flashlight and trace the words. It reads, 'In Memory of Sri Mahendranath Gupta (Sri "M")'.

The next day, Sunday, I walk by 50 Amherst and am met with a surprise. The gates are open and there is a swarm of activity inside. I walk in, locate the office and politely ask permission to go upstairs. After a few moments, an elderly man takes down a set of keys from a hook above the desk. He motions for me to walk beside him and heads up the stairs. The place is old and dilapidated. As I walk up the staircase to the top floor, I drag my hand along its wooden rails and slip back a century in time. I recall Yogananda 'descending the long stairway' and being 'overwhelmed with memories'. Once his 'family home', these 'hallowed walls', he wrote, had borne 'silent witness' to the greatest tragedy in his life and the 'final healing'!

I look into the small shrine on the top floor, then peer out over the veranda, though there is no longer a 'roof-garden' or anything green at all. Today it's a bare concrete rooftop under a covering of winter smog. I look out over the buildings of this neighbourhood and make out where the Ghosh and Bose houses are, alongside other notable north Calcutta locations. It's mostly asphalt and concrete now; nothing like those days.

Standing there, I ask myself, 'Why am I here?' It has been so long since these events occurred; over a century now. What is it that draws me to these places? The research is here, but I want more than just to learn the story. I want to feel the presence of what once lived and breathed in these places. To make a subtle connection, stand where they once stood and live where they once lived. Whatever the drive is, I'm searching for the connection in a tangible way.

It is this drive that leaves me reflecting on the loss of Gyana. Losing their mother shaped the lives of Bishnu and Mukunda – who would become Yogananda about a decade after his mother's death – tremendously. Without this loss, it's questionable whether the young Mukunda would ever have felt the urge to become connected to an astral archetypal mother. The event severed his ties to his personality and physicality, and it developed his interconnected spirituality. The death, in a way, is the beginning of what he becomes.

A friend of his asked Bishnu once about his mother:

'Do you want to know what I wrote about her?' Bishnu did not wait for my reply but opened his red diary and started reading from it. He hardly read a few lines when his eyes got watery and his voice choked with emotions.

We sat in silence for some time then he started to read again when he came back to normal. It happened again – his voice choked off and tears rolled down his cheeks. I said, 'Let it be, Bishnuda. I shall read it on my own.' He replied, 'No, please let me read some more. I love reading about my mother.'

And so it continued; he would read a few lines and stop and then start again. This way he completed the chapter on his mother. At the end I could see he was exhausted and sweating, as if he had journeyed a long way. I left the house at Rammohan Roy Road with a heavy heart that night. I constantly saw a small, sickly motherless child's tearful face. This was a pitiful void inside his heart.[1]

Themes of abandonment, detachment and loss were frequent in the 1965 article 'From the Past' where Bishnu wrote, 'My life's beginning itself was a problem.' When saying this, he was not referring to his own problem but rather that of his father, since at the age of fifty-two, Bhagabati was suddenly without a wife. He 'had no idea what to do with me', Bishnu wrote, handing him over to the maid.[2]

Bishnu recollected the experience in a Bengali poem (the title translates as 'Longing') about the 'confusion' he felt waiting for his mother to return. He 'refused to be soothed by a maid's lullaby', not accepting her as a substitute for his mother. 'Toys galore you give me through the maid – none will be spared as I thrash them dead. I shall punch her, sock her, give her no peace – for I only want my own mother, please.'[3]

Aside from the maid named Jhima, his elder brothers and sisters helped raise Bishnu. Later, Yogananda took a more important role in Bishnu's life, and under his physical and spiritual guidance, Bishnu 'was fully cured of his debility'.[4] After this healing mentorship, their bond was inseparable. Bishnu followed his elder brother 'like a shadow during childhood' and from him, 'learned about physical culture, *yoga-bayam* and character building'.

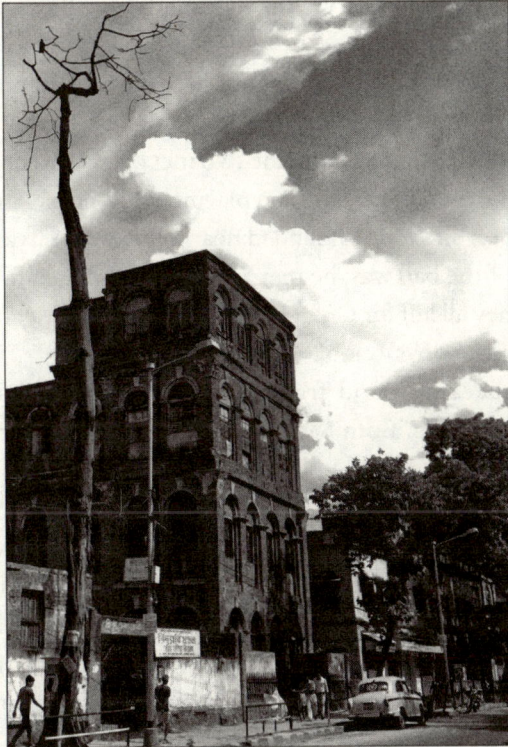

50 Amherst St, Calcutta, 2017

10

SADHANA MANDIR

Mukunda went through a transitional period 'in his youth' before taking the name of Swami Yogananda, as his drive to escape and meditate alone was gradually replaced with a desire to serve and teach others. Even in the more tranquil moments of youth, Yogananda was drawn to young friends who shared his spiritual thirst.

Manomohan Mazumdar, who would become Swami Satyananda, lived across the street from 4 Garpar Road.[1] The story goes: Shortly after the Ghosh family returned to Calcutta in 1906, the two met over a soccer ball. Yogananda and some other boys were kicking and playing with the ball on the street, and the ball was low on air. When it landed near the feet of Satyananda, he asked who the owner of the ball was; he met Yogananda and then filled the ball with air. Afterward, they all left for Greer Park to play their daily games. Satyananda became a part of the boys' 'club'.[2]

Satyananda became good friends with the middle Ghosh brothers, Yogananda and Sananda. Both Satyananda and Sananda shared Yogananda's early thirst for meditation.

While the three of them were walking 'along the railroad track on the east of Upper Circular Road' one evening, Yogananda's thoughts were elsewhere. Sananda wrote, 'The last rays of the setting sun had beautifully colored the western sky.' Instead of an acknowledgement, Yogananda remarked, 'Just imagine right now the saints in the Himalayas are meditating in their caves. I feel the entrancing beauty of the holy mountains drawing me, let us follow the footsteps of the ascetics.'[3] Encouraged by Yogananda, the two other boys 'dug a cave for meditation in the embankment of the pond' near their home; a 'grotto' made to look 'like those used by Himalayan yogis'.[4]

In 1906, Yogananda and Satyananda informally received 'the preliminary kriya' techniques from the *kriyaban*, Bhagabati Ghosh.[5] Sananda wrote that Yogananda 'had learned from father' the introductory techniques of Kriya yoga that included *Maha Mudra* and *Jyoti Mudra*.[6] Bhagabati, 'who was a disciple of Lahiri Mahasaya', but 'not permitted to initiate', was making an attempt to placate the boys' thirst for spiritual practice and keep his son at home.[7]

Nevertheless, Yogananda's desire to 'escape to the Himalayas' continued, and an attempt was finally made. Upon hearing his friends approach the Garpar Road house one night, Yogananda 'hastily tied together a blanket, a pair of sandals, Lahiri Mahasaya's picture, a copy of the *Bhagavad Gita*, a string of prayer beads, and two loincloths'. He then tossed the bundle out his third-story window' to the ground below and 'ran down the steps'. Thus they began their escape to the Himalayas.[8]

The boys made progress for a few days. They hopped onto a northbound train from Howrah station, using European dress as camouflage, and had a timetable of train connections for their attempted escapade 'to holy Rishikesh' and the Himalayas.[9] They made it as far as Haridwar, when they were detained by railway officials who had received a telegram from their worried families. A day later his eldest brother, Ananta Lal, arrived to take Yogananda back to Calcutta.

Upon returning home, Bhagabati 'touchingly requested me to curb my roving feet until, at least, the completion of my high school studies', wrote Yogananda.[10] Bhagabati also arranged 'for a saintly pundit, Swami Kebalananda, to come regularly to the house' as a 'Sanskrit tutor', hoping to satisfy his son's 'spiritual yearnings by instructions from a learned philosopher'. Kebalananda, then a householder, was known by the title of 'Shastri Mahasaya', because of his 'authority on the ancient *shastras*'.[11] He was also a *kriyaban*, a disciple of Lahiri Mahasaya of Benares. His stories of Lahiri Mahasaya kept Yogananda rapt. 'Within a few days' of encountering the new teacher, Yogananda discovered that Kebalananda was not only 'well versed in the scriptures, he was a yogi'.[12] Thereafter, Yogananda 'sought every opportunity to forsake prosaic grammar and to talk of yoga and Lahiri Mahasaya' with Kebalananda.[13] They were able to discuss 'meditative practices and experiences'.[14]

Then, in 1907, Yogananda and 'his best friend Satyananda' were 'formally initiated into Kriya yoga by Shastri Mahasaya (Kebalananda)'.[15]

With Kebalananda as their spiritual guide, the boys' 'desire for *sadhana*, or meditation, doubled'.[16] They meditated together on the ground floor of the 4 Garpar Road home. At this point, in 1908, Tulsi Narayan Bose became friends with Yogananda.[17] Bishnu, now about six years old, had a playful and mischievous relationship with Yogananda. Bishnu, along 'with his little friends, used to wait outside the room', playing in the enclosed open-sky courtyard. When Yogananda and his friends 'finished their meditation and came out of the room, Bishnu would tease them', asking Tulsi and Yogananda, 'Did you find God after your meditation?' Yogananda, an agitated older brother, replied, 'Bishnu you don't know anything of this meditation, why are you teasing us?'[18]

Eventually the group of boys decided to find a more permanent place for their meditation. At first, they congregated inside a palm-thatched mud hut across the Maniktala canal from their Garpar home, 'at Bagmari, in the Kankurgachi area of Calcutta'. They called the ashram Sadhana Mandir, a 'temple of spiritual discipline'.[19] The site had been found by a boy named Pulin Bihari Das. Pulin was 'physically strong' and later ran an akhara.[20] Bishnu wrote that it was Pulin who showed him the 'arm and chest muscle movement' first and that he 'learned to do them quite well' under Pulin's guidance.[21] About a year later, in 1909, the ashram was relocated to a building near the back of Tulsi Bose's home.

Yogananda spent his formative years as a youth at the home of Tulsi Bose, at 17/1 Pitambar Bhattacharya Lane. Next door, where a small library was housed and the first school for boys was built, a small ashram formed, which allowed the boys more solitude than the 4 Garpar Road home. The family's Sanskrit tutor, Swami Kebalananda, also began teaching the boys at this location. They learned the Vedic treatises such as the *Yoga-Shastra*, *Sutras* and the *Bhagavad Gita*, along with 'pranayama life energy control, and how the life and consciousness in deep yoga meditation are withdrawn from senses, nerves, and spine into the *sushumna*, or astral spine, with its spiritual centers of divine awakening'. The 'saintly Sanskrit tutor enhanced his students' understanding' and quelled Yogananda's impulse for flight towards the Himalayas.[22]

After graduating from high school in 1909, with his father's reluctant blessing, Yogananda left Calcutta to live in an ashram in the ancient holy city of Benares. His mother, Gyana, had been from Serampore, where a highly respected *kriyaban*, Sriyukteswar, lived for part of the year. Sriyukteswar was in Benares at the time, so Bhagabati asked him to be on the lookout for the young Yogananda. The ultimate connection in Benares between Sriyukteswar and Yogananda resulted in a guru and disciple relationship. Sriyukteswar settled the wanderlust of the young aspirant, and for the next five years Yogananda went to college and practised Kriya yoga with the continued support of his father.

First Yogananda attended Scottish Church College and then Serampore College. It was 'in a history class' at Scottish Church College that he met Basu Kumar Bagchi. Like Yogananda, Basu was initiated into Kriya yoga by Kebalananda. Basu would later become Swami Dhirananda under Sriyukteswar. The three of them – Dhirananda, Yogananda and Satyananda – became 'the trio' who lived as sannyasins.

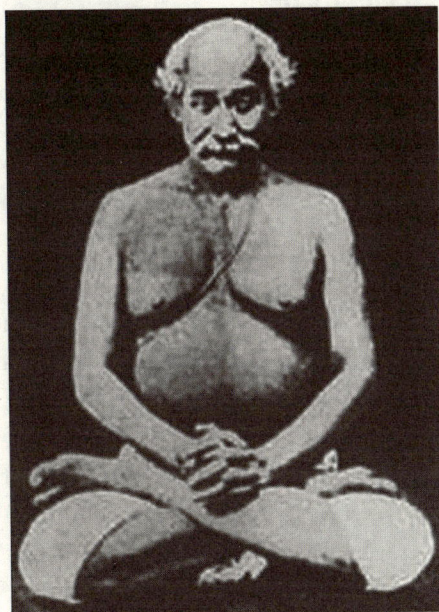

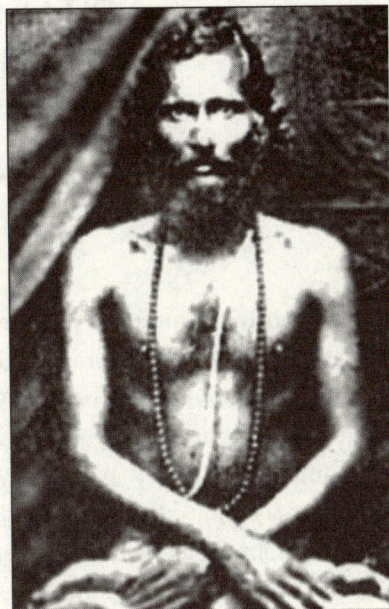

Shyama Charan Lahiri (Mahasaya, 1828-1895);
Ashutosh Chatterjee (Kebalananda, 1863-1931).

11

PITAMBAR LANE

You are sitting on the bed where Sriyukteswar would sleep
when he stayed in Calcutta.
– Hassi Mukherjee (Bose)

I am in north Calcutta, the Garpar Road area, where many of the scenes from *Autobiography of a Yogi* transpired in the first few decades of the twentieth century. The book was written seventy years ago, but surprisingly, many of the places remain intact.[1]

I am looking for where Yogananda and his friends moved their Sadhana Mandir once they'd become friends with Tulsi Bose. It is where they formed Saraswat Library, and where their school for boys was located for a brief time. All I know is it is where 'a little alleyway to the property opened onto Garpar Road'.[2] It changed names and locations, so I'm depending on my research guide, Arup Sen Gupta, to find it.

We wander around without any luck until he asks just the right person. I ask him how he knew who to ask.

'I saw that the elderly man was carrying a couple of books,' he said with a grin, 'so I knew he was a reader, and might know the location.' The man, who had just returned from a different library, leads us down Garpar Road, then a few turns along alleyways to the destination, which has a small plaque on the door announcing this as the home of Tulsi Narayan Bose, 'Boyhood friend of Paramahansa Yogananda'. Arup and I knock on the door, and it opens.

What happens next is one of the strangest moments that occured while writing this book. The woman who opens the door looks grandmotherly, with a smile across her face. I don't know who she is. When our eyes meet, though, it feels like I step into a body from some time in the past, and I am looking into her eyes as if I know her.

A feeling like 'I have returned' comes over me.

She, in turn, looks surprised, with a look like, 'Oh, you again', which I interpret to mean, 'I can't believe you've returned.'

I can't explain or see anything beyond that, as it all happens in a fleeting moment. Her English is limited, but Arup asks her about it in Bengali. She confirms that she feels the same sense of knowing, and asks if I have been there previously. I haven't; this is my first time. I leave my shoes at the door and tour the house.

Her name is Hassi Mukherjee, and she's the daughter of Tulsi Bose. She was born just after Yogananda visited and stayed at their home in 1936.

'My grandfather, Harinarayan Bose, told Yogananda that he should treat this house as if it is his own home,' she says.[3]

I ask, 'Who was your grandfather's guru?'

'My grandfather's guru was Shyama Charan Lahiri Mahasaya.'

Yogananda had said, while she was still in the womb, 'This child will be a girl, and will be very devoted. Her name, Hassi, means "laughter" and is confirmed by her "happy" disposition.'[4]

'Did you know Buddha Bose personally?' I ask.

'Yes, I knew Buddha well enough. He would come here to this house and have sweets with us,' Hassi explains. 'I used to go to their house when the college was established and the yoga centre was started.' She proceeds to tell me of the marriages and longstanding relations between the families.

Many photos of Tulsi with Sriyukteswar, Yogananda and others cover the walls. There are photos of Kebalananda, the Sanskrit teacher of Yogananda and Tulsi, along with photos of her grandfather, who 'was Swami Vivekananda's friend. They studied together in Scottish Church College. Both of them would often sit in *dhyana* (absorbed meditation) in this very house.'

Upstairs, there is a puja room with all sorts of artifacts, including a *trishula* (trident) that is said to have been passed down from Babaji to Lahiri, Sriyukteswar and then Yogananda. Hassi has me sit on a bed and then begins to tell stories, with Arup translating them from Bengali. She recounts stories of her husband, Devi Mukherjee's travels as a disciple of Yogananda. Later I will pick up a copy of his book *Shaped by Saints*, which details his travels throughout India.

Hassi then says something that makes Arup smile, and he turns to me with a sly grin, 'You are sitting on the bed where Sriyukteswar would sleep when staying in Calcutta ... the same bed was used by Yogananda from the time he was a youth, even before he became a monk.

When he returned to India as an adult, he would often come and stay here due to problems about property-related matters at his home.'

I learn a bit more about the people in the photographs. As I point them out, she relates stories of the visitors – some she'd witnessed as a child; others she had been told about by her father. The position of the chairs around the main downstairs room, around twenty of them, welcomes one to sit amidst the silence, where those before have meditated. Here, Hassi explains a vision of a blue Krishna that appeared before her grandfather and Vivekananda.

'Yogananda', when he returned to India, 'preferred staying with us'. So many saintly people from years past have meditated in the house.[5] Each subsequent visit to Calcutta, I go by the house. Sometimes Hassi is there, other times just the caretaker. I find the entire place, at Pitambar Bhattacharya Lane, to be one of the most peaceful locations in Calcutta.

12

SCHOOL FOR BOYS

Bhagabati had been a stern disciplinarian with the children while Gyana was alive but developed a softer side after her death. He had done well financially, but his mentality towards money was formed from having to work to pay off debt in his youth, leading him to view prosperity with a sort of equilibrium. When Bishnu questioned why he 'did not use a horse carriage' to go to work, instead taking the Upper Circular Road trolley to the Sealdah railway station, Bhagabati replied, 'I do not wish to spoil my children by flaunting a wealthy style of living.' However, perhaps taking pity on his motherless children, he became softer and 'allowed some liberty' for their requests. His children recalled that 'the first word' for any type of expenditure would be 'no', from which they would need to plead and bargain to get further with him. Yogananda reflected, 'If I could bolster up my numerous requests with one or two good arguments, he invariably put the coveted goal within my reach, whether it were a vacation trip or a new motorcycle.'[1]

The motorcycle – a 901 Triumph – was outfitted with a carriage seat to the side, and was Yogananda's favoured mode of transportation. It was operational for over two decades. It caused quite a stir to see 'the ochre-outfitted *sannyasi* youths driving' around on it, creating an 'elated excitement in the neighbourhood'. Many persons had the opportunity to 'ride the vehicle'.[2] After his graduation from Serampore College, Yogananda's family attempted to have him marry, but he resisted, and instead formally became a sannyasi under Sriyukteswar in 1915. He was initiated into the spiritual order and given the name 'Swami Yogananda Giri'. Mukunda wanted a name 'with the word yoga' in it, in order that 'the ideals of yoga would be constantly evident even in his name'.[3] The name 'Giri' (mountain) was of the same 'branch of the Swami order' as Sriyukteswar.[4]

Yogananda was not sure what to do next at this point in his life. In what is portrayed as a rash decision, he left for Japan during the rainy summer months of 1916. For the voyage by boat, he shaved and cut his hair, and used his given name Mukunda. It had been hastily arranged that Yogananda go there to 'study agriculture'.[5] He had wanted to go to America for his PhD but could not due to the ongoing First World War; limited visas were available for travel abroad. So he went to Japan; 'perhaps there he would be able to obtain a visa to the West'.[6] The plan did not work out, and feeling culturally uneasy in Japan, he returned to Calcutta after a few weeks, just after Ananta Lal, the eldest brother, died of typhoid fever (the same illness which took their mother at Ananta's wedding).

Yogananda was again confronted with family death, and again contemplated abandonment of the world, but Sriyukteswar asked him to consider how he could be of service. The question provoked and impressed Yogananda so much that he decided to change his course. Bhagabati also wanted to change the course of Yogananda's life, arranging a railway executive position for him 'at 2000 rupees a month'.[7] When he refused, Bhagabati lamented that Yogananda 'took me near the roof of happiness but when I had almost reached there, he pulled the ladder of his life from beneath me and I fell shattered to the floor'. Yogananda replied that instead he was 'starting a great school', to which Bhagabati replied: 'Seeing is believing.'[8]

Yogananda was already at work on the idea. Alongside Dhirananda and Satyananda, he wanted to start a religious school for boys in accordance with the ancient yogic system of spiritual education. In November 1916, the Pitambar Lane ashram at Tulsi's home was restarted as a school for boys, funded by Bhagabati. Bishnu was the first student.[9] Yogananda transitioned into a more settled role as a teacher and taught a small group of neighbourhood children balanced educational lessons, with spiritual practices as a main feature of their education.

From the very beginning, Yogananda, Dhirananda and Satyananda looked for sources of funding beyond Bhagabati. They found Sri Nandi, the maharajah of Kasimbazar, who was well known for donating to advance causes that helped children, including schools. The school began its relationship with him 'one late evening in November, 1916'. 'Yogananda drafted a letter' with his two friends saying that they would set up 'a residential Ashram-school for the young children'. When the maharajah opened the letter, he 'sparkled with excitement', saying, 'Oh, Swamiji, what a coincidence, I too have been planning to establish a school of similar nature for some time now. Give me your plans in detail.' Later, the trio presented the plans and invited the maharajah to visit.

'When Maharajah Manindra Chandra Nandi first visited Yogananda's tiny shack of an ashram in the slums of Calcutta', the thirteen-year-old boy 'Bishnu Charan was there, dressed as a child-*brahmachari* to welcome the Maharajah'.[10] Their plan claimed that moral and spiritual values were lacking in ordinary instruction, and made the case for an educational system that combined the formal curriculum, which emphasized intellectual development, with a spiritual focus.[11] After the school's proposal was accepted, the maharajah funded both the land and the operating expenses.

Bishnu gave a slightly different account of these events:

At around 3 a.m. Swami Yogananda woke up Basuda (Dhirananda) and made him write down the school's ideals and the method of teaching. Basu Kumar (Dhirananda) went to read this aloud to Maharajah Manindra the next morning. The Maharajah was getting his shave done when good-looking, ochre-robed Basuda stood in front of him. The Maharajah was delighted to see him and asked what brought him here. Basuda replied by reading aloud the draft that had been prepared the night before.

When he was just halfway through, the Maharajah shouted, asked him to stop and then exclaimed, 'You are God-sent. Only last night I was dreaming of establishing such a school with these ideals. I am coming to your ashram tomorrow to meet your guru and the ashram boys.'

The next morning the Maharajah came to visit us at the Pitambar Bhattacharya Lane ashram. Khirod and I welcomed him and sang some *stotra*. Then he declared that he gives permission to establish such a school in Dihika.[12]

Sriyukteswar led the inauguration for the school on 22 March 1917, a date he had chosen in accordance with astrological considerations.[13] In its first year, it was located in a small village named Dihika, outside of Calcutta. The 'brahmacharya school was founded at the courthouse of Manindra Chandra Nandi, the Maharajah of the Dihika village near Burnpur', recalled Bishnu Ghosh.[14] It was named 'The School of Divinity'. Lessons in 'yoga, pranayama, and *jyoti darshan* [divine light initiation]' were given to the students by Yogananda, and once the school was moved to Dihika, 'this part of the education stepped up further', to include Hatha yoga.[15]

13

DIHIKA AND RANCHI HATHA YOGA

The Dihika ashram sat atop a small hill, an abode of tranquility. Quite picturesque, it overlooked the winding Damodar River. A nearby railroad bridge was backed by a hilltop 'seen far in the distance'. The school day started at dawn, with boys in yellow robes reciting Sanskrit and chanting devotional songs. There were just seven students, one of whom was Bishnu, who were introduced to yogic exercises and techniques that Bishnu later used as muscle control.[1] In Dihika, Yogananda began his experimentation with various vegetarian dishes, a trait he would later continue in America. The evening concluded with meditation and spiritual discourse. The schedule, even from the beginning, included daily yogic exercises, which were done alongside other outdoor games.

Satyananda and Bishnu have provided accounts of the Hatha yoga practice in Dihika during 1917. Satyananda recalled that 'at the wishes of the patron', an expert 'Hatha yogi named Alokananda Brahmachari came to the school and made preparations for teaching many different kinds of yogasanas'. Satyananda noted Alokananda 'was quiet and reserved at first', but with Yogananda's 'touchstone effect, he too became cheery and upbeat'.[2] Bishnu mentioned another yogi, Swami Kapilananda, as the main teacher. It may have been that Kapilananda implemented the 'preparations for teaching' done by Alokananda, so that the two worked together.[3] What exactly they taught was not detailed, but Bishnu's account showed it was thorough:

I was in 8th standard then and I, along with 7–8 other boys, were sent to this school. The others who went with me were Satyananda Ji's brother Khirod, Basuda's brother Bhishma and others. The Maharajah had brought in a Hatha yogi, Swami Kapilananda, to teach us yoga and pranayam. Prior to this we had taken lessons from Swami Yogananda on yoga, pranayam and *jyoti darshan*. With the advent of Swami Kapilananda, this part of the education stepped up further. Needless to say I was a keen student and soon learned asana, *dhauti*, pranayam, mudra, *nauli*, *uddiyana*, *basti*, etc. I just enjoyed practising all of this for no particular reason; although I do remember I soon got rid of my tonsil problems and fevers.[4]

These were all components of a 'classical' style of Hatha yoga, derived from texts or manuals available from around the fourteenth to seventeenth century at the earliest, such as the *Hatha Yoga Pradipika*, *Gheranda Samhita* and *Shiva Samhita*, to name the three most prominent. The instructions centred on postures, breathing and purification techniques, such as cleansing the internal organs.

As the first year neared its end, Bishnu 'returned home for a few days' during the rainy season and 'in the meantime all the boys succumbed to malaria, all except Swami Yogananda'.[5] The following year, in 1918, the maharajah of Kasimbazar decided to transfer the school to a drier climate; where he could observe its growth more closely. Yogananda acquiesced and moved the fast-growing group to Ranchi, a small town in Bihar, about 200 miles from Calcutta. Although at first the group did not want to leave the Ganges riverside, it was a very beneficial move since the climate of Ranchi was one of the healthiest in India. The site was composed of 25 acres, with a large bathing pond.[6]

In its new home, the Ranchi School for Boys, or Ranchi Brahmacharya Vidyalaya, grew to over hundred students and included regular academic study, Yogoda and *brahmacharya* (sustained vitality) training, agricultural and industrial work, night school and village-cooperation in its activities. It was a moral and non-sectarian religious training center for an all-round education.[7] The inclusion of the term 'brahmacharya' within the name of the school signified that it was in accordance with the educational ideals of the rishis and their forest ashrams, which previously had taken in and raised youth. Yogananda further explained that their school included the name 'brahmacharya' in reference to the first stage of the Vedic plan for life: that of the celibate student. This, he explained, was followed by the stages of being a householder, then a hermit, and finally, a wanderer, 'free from all earthly concerns, a *sannyasi*'.

Bishnu enrolled in the first session at the Ranchi Brahmacharya Vidyalaya, and found the climate very healthy.[8] However, the growth of the school lessened the intimacy between Bishnu and his elder brother. Bishnu 'studied at the Ranchi school for a few months' and then 'returned home' to 4 Garpar Road. Choosing not to stay for long at Ranchi, he wrote, perhaps trivially, that he 'longed for his non-vegetarian food'.[9] Bishnu's introduction to Hatha yoga had been established, and it had improved his health, setting him on a course to radically develop and transform his body through physical culture.

14

VIVEKANANDA AND YOGANANDA

Forget you were born a Hindu, and don't be an American.
Take the best of them both.[1]
– Sriyukteswar

In 1920, Yogananda left for America. While standing inside the food storehouse at the Ranchi school, he had a vision of himself in the West. He had been sent an invitation to participate in the 'Congress for Religious Liberals' in Boston, which was secured with an endorsement from the principal of City College, the same Brahmo Samaj school where Bishnu would begin Physical Culture a couple of years later.[2] Yogananda was influenced by his guru Sriyukteswar, who had extensive knowledge of the Holy Bible and seamlessly integrated ideals from Christianity into Hinduism.

There were not many swamis in the US when Yogananda arrived in Boston.[3] An estimate of 'the Hindu Swamis and Yogis' in America numbered 'about 25 or 30' out of an Indian population of around 3,000.[4] On the voyage he shaved his beard, which he felt allowed other passengers to not feel so alienated next to the robed and long-haired swami.[5]

From a historical vantage point, it is impossible to look at Yogananda's travels without the context of Swami Vivekananda, who had previously forged a path to the West that made it appealing for Yogananda to bring his message to America and Europe. Though he never met Vivekananda, he viewed himself as the successor to Vivekananda's legacy.

Vivekananda was a disciple of Ramakrishna, the same saint who Mahendranath (Sri M) followed. In 1893, Swami Vivekananda had given a speech in Chicago, during the World's Fair, with a central message of commonality in humanity.

The speech would go on to become a historical event; symbolising universality. Most of Vivekananda's American speeches were given in the Midwest to northeastern belt of the country. His topic of worldwide fellowship of humanity reached those who had an understanding of the writings of the transcendentalist, Ralph Waldo Emerson, the poet Walt Whitman and other free thinkers who were looking for alternative forms of spirituality.

The narrative themes of Vivekananda's speeches during the late 1890s were similar to those of Yogananda's speeches after he arrived in America in the early 1920s. Terms from both Christianity and Hinduism were easily integrated, giving their messages a pluralistic sense of shared faith and helping them fit into the predominantly Christian culture. Looking back into their formative younger years, one realizes how their unique messages had been shaped by their surroundings and the similarity of their upbringing.

The two Swamis were cut from the same cloth. Although a generation apart, they had grown up just three blocks away from each other in the same north Calcutta neighbourhood; they had similar educational backgrounds. Like many middle to upper class children in the British capital of the East, they had parents who pushed them towards Western ideals of European history, philosophy and logic. Even though their parents raised them hoping that they would use their education to succeed in the industrial world, both of the two future Swamis had mystical visions during their childhood.

Education had a profound impact on the lives of Vivekananda and Yogananda, contributing to their assimilative world view. Mid-nineteenth century reforms in Calcutta were aimed at uplifting the educational standards of Bengalis, with a strong focus on learning English over the next few generations. Alongside the industrialization of India, which brought moderate wealth to India's middle class, a culturally educated group called the *bhadralok* emerged. They knew English, but did not have power in the traditional sense of class like the Brahmins did. Instead, the families used their knowledge to gain power.

Both Vivekananda and Yogananda attended Scottish Church College, where English-speaking teachers educated the Bengali youth. The Scotsmen who taught these young Calcuttans were familiar with the transcendentalist writings of Ralph Waldo Emerson and the early Oriental translations of Indian Sanskrit texts. The teachers exposed their students to the Christian religion and a Western perspective, which the students were coaxed to reconcile with their Hindu upbringing.[6] The resulting universal outlook was an integration of the two worlds. On one side, they were reared in a culture that embodied the non-rational and the sublime, along with the necessity of spiritual engagement. On the other side, for the purpose of future employment, they were educated in logic, reason and the sciences. Their professors and the culture would force them to reconcile the traditional with the modern.

Once both Vivekananda and Yogananda had mystical experiences, a natural, personally grounded synthesis emerged. Their early English education and exposure to Christianity laid the foundation, which enabled them to integrate Western culture, converse in a shared religious language and make it easier for Americans and Europeans to accept the Indian spiritual world view.

While studying at Scottish Church College, Yogananda gave his 'first public speech at the Atheneum Institution'. His topic was how those 'who meditate in Himalayan caves to realize the source of all happiness' lay in opposition to the 'gratificationof the senses', which only produced 'the alternates of temporary pleasure and subsequent sorrow'.[7] Just a handful of years later, when he left for the United States, his boyhood friends Dhirananda, Satyananda and Tulsi Bose worked with him to write the book *Science of Religion*.[8] Yogananda took this with him when he spoke at the International Congress of Religious Liberals. With the book, Yogananda 'tried to make people understand that religion is universal and one', and that everyone shares the aspiration of 'attaining bliss'. It was a very similar message to Vivekananda's, with the additional practices of '*japa* (repetition of mantra), *puja* (worship), *dharana* (tranquility), and *dhyana* (meditation)'. The difference was the practice that Yogananda brought for 'the seeker', the practice of *kriya pranayam*.[9]

An excerpt from a speech about common themes between Vivekananda and Yogananda (in his magazine) shows that Yogananda approved of being portrayed as Vivekananda's successor. In the speech, Dr Omar Garrison said:

> Swami Vivekananda ... taught no particular religion. He taught to love humanity. Many Swamis are in America who are vastly learned and I have learned many things from many of them. But the second man who made India glorified in the eyes of America is Swami Yogananda. I went to Swami Yogananda with a skeptical mind. But he gave me not religion, not philosophy, but unconditional love.[10]

The main difference between Yogananda and Vivekananda was that while the latter was only in America and Europe for about three years and reached very few persons, Yogananda was in America long enough for three generations to be exposed to his message. Yogananda thoroughly Americanized his message, which can be seen in his speech 'Increasing Awareness', given fifteen years after he arrived:

> First find out what you want; ask divine aid to direct you to right action, whereby your want will be fulfilled; then retire within yourself. Act according to the inner direction that you receive; you will find what you want. When the mind is calm, how quickly, how smoothly, how beautifully will you perceive everything. Success in everything will come to pass in a short time, for Cosmic power can be proved by the application of the right law.
>
> Last of all, don't concentrate without; don't do things in a haphazard way. Start everything from within, no matter what it is, whether writing or anything else. Pick up the more important things and do them with all your heart. Cultivate the habit in this life of picking up more worthwhile things.[11]

And then in his writings about practising his technique of Yogoda:

> The last great scientific method is to magnetize and to send the current around the brain and spinal column, and thereby secure one year's health by twenty minutes of this practice ... with the awakened brain cells from intelligent Beings whom you have kept uneducated, vibrant with the joy of God, all knowledge can be had in this life; Eternity realized now; AWAKE!

The proclamations were entirely in English, without any hint of Sanskrit or linguistic hurdles, and conversational in tone. They spoke to an audience interested in an inner world, which was accessible to them if they followed his directions.

Yogananda only wrote about Vivekananda in his *Autobiography* once, stating merely that 'Swami Vivekananda was the chief disciple of the Christlike master Sri Ramakrishna'. In the text, a story called 'Your Teacher Will Come Later' from Mr E. E. Dickerson, a devotee of Yogananda's, was told. It is as close to a presumed divine succession as one could get.[12] Dickerson had met and heard Swami Vivekananda in 1893 in Chicago, and was told personally, 'Your teacher will come later, he will give you a silver cup.' Dickerson kept the 'prophecy' a secret. Then, during a Christmas celebration in 1936 where Yogananda passed out gifts he had brought back from India, he presented Dickerson with a silver cup. Yogananda, Dickerson surmised, had followed Vivekananda 'to America' for himself 'and other past-life disciples'.[13]

Like Vivekananda before him, Yogananda drew upon the socio-cultural educational sources within Calcutta to present a vision of yoga to the world, in order to be relevant to the religious condition at a time when Christianity was prevalent. The universal message is echoed in the common refrain that anyone can practise yoga today.

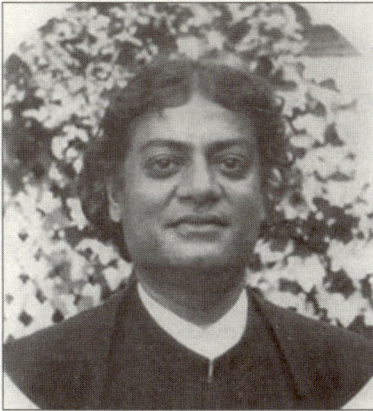

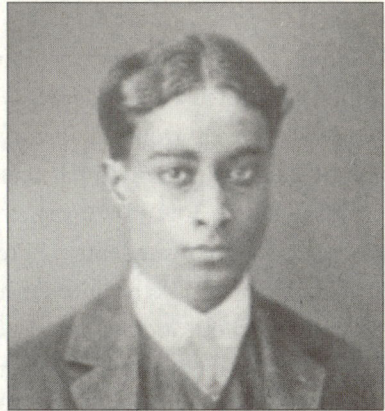

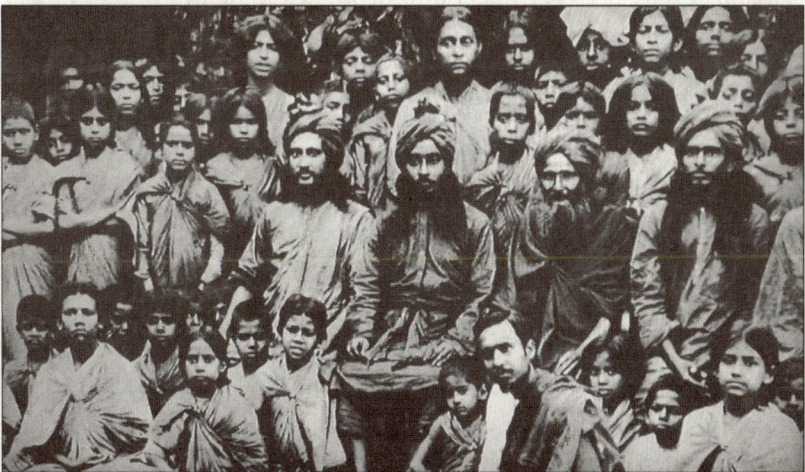

Top: Swami Vivekananda, Swami Yogananda.
Bottom: Ranchi School for Boys, 1920. (*Source: Wikimedia Commons*)

15

SCOTTISH CHURCH COLLEGE

Scottish Church College was founded on 13 July 1830. I visit on 13 July, now celebrated as Founders Day. After talking about the school's history for a while with a group of history professors, I go to the library to view some of their collections. In particular, I look at a couple of anthologies that were done for the 100and 150-year commemorations, which have articles and listings of prominent students. There are articles on Vivekananda but nothing about Yogananda. I ask the librarian about it, and she confirms that Yogananda attended the school and that it must be some sort of mistake. She would have to check why he is not listed among the prominent students. I am not surprised. It would be a stretch to even call it an oversight, given how understated Yogananda's presence is throughout Calcutta. Coming from America where few know of Vivekananda, I can see how Calcutta is the exact opposite, though the reversal of roles is surprising at first.

Today, Vivekananda is celebrated everywhere in Calcutta.[1] There are statues, parks and signs throughout the city, commemorating his name and teachings. His books and pamphlets are in every shop. The main street that runs by his house is named Vivekananda Road. His photo can be found hanging on the walls of houses, usually at a position near a shrine or a room for puja. This is not so for Yogananda.

I become aware of this the first moment I arrive in Calcutta. The plane lands at 4 a.m., and before proceeding to my hotel, I figure that taking a cab for a glimpse of the famous house where Yogananda grew up would be a pretty short order. I quickly find out that you can't get into a taxi, say '4 Garpar Road'[b] or 'Yogananda's home' and be able to arrive at the house in north Calcutta if you're relying on the driver to know where it is located.

There are no statues of Yogananda in Calcutta. You will not find his books among the many booksellers, and very few even know of him. Over the summer months, while I am away from Calcutta, this point is made yet again. Arup Sen Gupta, my research assistant in the city, mails me a copy of *The Telegraph*, which nowadays is the main daily English newspaper of Calcutta. The article begins:

> Most Bengalis would be familiar with Garpar Road as the birthplace of Satyajit Ray and the residence of Jatayu, a detective fiction writer, rather than the childhood home of Paramahansa Yogananda.[2]

A scandal had erupted when some fanatical people died of self-starvation – they had photos of various saints, including Yogananda, on the walls of their home. Detectives had been deployed to research the writings of Yogananda, not knowing what to make of the claims that there was some sort of association between the deeds of these two persons who had starved themselves to death and Yogananda's teachings.[3] It was almost comical, with the Calcutta police replying that their 'sleuths were trying to understand the teachings', and Calcutta journalists purchasing copies of *Autobiography of a Yogi* (one of the bestselling books on spirituality in America during the twentieth century) in order to learn about this person named Yogananda.

Yogananda is probably the most influential yogi from India to live in the United States during the twentieth century. That claim is attributed to the three generations he interacted with through his teachings – from musical icons, Elvis Presley and George Harrison of the Beatles to Steve Jobs, who gifted iPods with the *Autobiography of a Yogi* pre-downloaded. From 1920 until his death, thousands and thousands of people were influenced by direct interactions with Yogananda. Many more thereafter were touched by the teachings that reached them through his book. In his hometown of Calcutta, he is hardly known today.

When Yogananda left India in 1920, his impact on Buddha Bose's life had not yet occurred. Even for Bishnu, more was yet to come. These influential experiences would have to wait until Yogananda's return to India. During the 1920s, all three led vastly different lives. Buddha was in school, Bishnu immersed in physical culture training and Yogananda abroad in America. Later on, Buddha and Bishnu would come together, and in 1935 the three of them would unite.

Given Buddha's position at his father's home, he couldn't have imagined in 1920 that such a scenario was in his future. The physical status Bishnu would achieve could only be a dream. For Yogananda, it was not imagination or a dream at this point, but a vision of America that set it all in motion.

PART THREE

PHYSICAL CULTURE
AND *BAYAM*

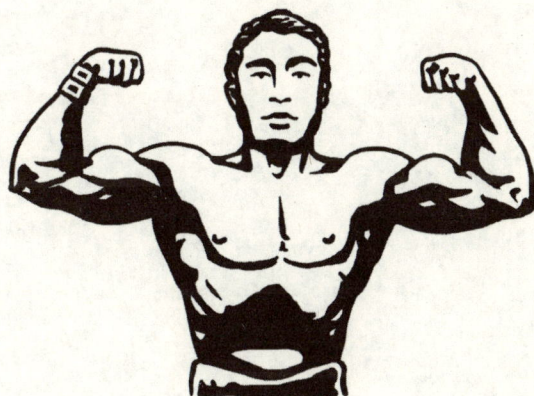

16

FAMILY AND PRACTICE

Above all be strong, be manly.
— Swami Vivekananda

In India, physical culture dates back centuries in dietary matters, lifestyle and exercise training. The traditional outdoor akhara that was used for physical exercise in the tradition of *kushti* (wrestling), done in a dirt pit, dates back at least to the Mughal Empire period, if not before. Exercises like using weighted stones (*nalls*) and notched logs (*santals*) for strength building, swinging clubs (*gadas* and mace) for rotational flexibility and doing leg exercises were all commonplace.[1] *Bayam* is the Bengali term to describe exercises that are typically freehand and dynamic.[2] By all accounts, this practice seems to have occurred daily within the Ghosh family.

As Bishnu came of age, he recalled his father Bhagabati and elder brothers, Yogananda and Sananda, practising different exercises using weights and freehand techniques. He wrote in *Bayam Charcha*:

From the time I became aware of my surroundings I often saw my father doing ten rounds of *dand*, ten rounds of *baithak*, and 10 rounds of swinging a small club.[3] Then he would sit, doing pranayam for an hour and practising *mahamudra*. I saw my Mejda, Paramhansa Yoganandaji, sit in *dhyana* doing pranayam in the middle of the night and then in the morning do *dand-baithak* and exercises with Sandow's grip dumbbells. Chotda practised on the parallel bar, and performed *dand-baithak* and swinging clubs; he did wrestling but did not do any yoga or pranayam.[4]

The combination exercise mentioned, *dand-baithak*, formed 'the core of a wrestler training program', not unlike push-ups with a modern squat.[5] It is this resemblance, 'similar to certain aspects from *surya namaskar*', that lead some to portray it as a precursor within historical yogic texts. Within this context, each *dand* represented a bodily bend, which was performed during a tantric prostration among certain lineages. However, the more recent dand-baithak were fitness-based, originating from within wrestling traditions.[6]

The mention of 'Sandow's grip dumbbells' is a testament to the fad in Calcutta at the time. Eugen Sandow's arrival in Calcutta in 1903 was a larger-than-life event and contributed to India taking up weightlifting. A popular framework among European scholars was that Sandow propelled the spindly Bengali weakling to bulk up physically, though this was probably a glorification that enhanced Sandow's reputation more than it reflected the reality in Bengal.[7]

Sandow did sell a lot of barbells and dumbbells in Calcutta, as alluded to in Yogananda's description of having them as a youth. The use of the barbell was controversial at first, due to the discussion of whether it was helpful or not. But the allure of the bicep, both in showmanship and photographical representation, ensured its adoption.

When Bishnu was 'about 12 or 13 years of age' in 1915, his home tutor 'brought along a young boy' of the same age in order for Bishnu 'to train him in *bayam* and wrestling'. The boy's name was Moni Sanyal, and he would be Bishnu's first student. While this was the beginning of his *bayam* focus, it wasn't until after Bishnu returned from Ranchi in 1918 that the first of 'three incidents, one after another' pushed Bishnu 'towards *bayam*' and physical culture.[8]

His older brother Sananda (Chotda) played a pivotal role in the first incident. Bishnu had gone to Nagpur, capital of the western state of Maharashtra, where the family of Sananda's wife Parul Lata resided. A few days after he arrived, Bishnu found Sananda 'applying oil all over his body after his *bayam* practice in the morning'. The younger brother wrote:

> I too, took off my clothes and started massaging oil onto my skinny body. Chotda looked at me and said, 'How can you live with this sparrow-like body? Are you not ashamed to stand bare-bodied with this physique?' Of course I was ashamed of my skinny self and decided to build my body. I took my first lessons of *dand-baithak* from him.

Bishnu stayed with him for a month, practising *bayam* 'zealously' and when he returned home to Calcutta, he 'continued in equal earnestness'.[9]

17

BISHNU AND BUDDHA'S FRIENDSHIP

Bengal (in India) and Burma were both parts of the British Empire. Travel between the colonial capitals of Calcutta and Rangoon was done on a British passenger steamer, which also went to Penang and Singapore.[1] The Burmese physical culturist Walter Chit Tun had been involved with independence activities in Burma that were brought there by Gandhi and other Indian National leaders. By 1920, a nationalist agitation had become prominent in Burma and Chit Tun's involvement in resistance efforts led him to relocate to Calcutta, where he operated out of his home on Creek Row.

Bishnu's introduction to Chit Tun was the 'second incident' impacting Bishnu's physical culture career. In 1922, while Bishnu was studying at Scottish Church College, a friend of his stopped by to tell him that he 'had missed a beautiful display of muscle movement by an Anglo-Burmese boy named Chit Tun'. A few days later, Bishnu learned that Chit Tun was to perform again at a university function. Years later he recalled the event:

On that day I quietly stood next to the gate. I was a small, slightly built person so no one took notice of me. Soon a phaeton car arrived and three handsome, well-dressed young men got out at the gate. Their physique was spellbinding. I just followed them into the campus building and got as far as the wings of the stage. Soon, there was a call for Chit Tun to appear on the stage, bare-bodied in his underwear. This incident happened 35 years ago but I distinctly remember it today, as I was thrilled to see his incredible muscles. They were beyond my imagination. I got the chance to enter the stage with him and sat quite close, to observe every move he made. Every ripple of his muscles was met with wild clapping from the audience and brought the house down. At the end, he showed *nauli* and the crowd was spellbound.[2] But I was amazed because I thought I can do this much better than him, and yet the crowd is awestruck![3]

When Bishnu saw Chit Tun perform muscle control, 'the art was ... unknown in Bengal'. Chit Tun popularised the technique in Calcutta in the early 1920s. But soon, Bishnu would also become acclaimed for his abilities, having learned 'muscle controlling' from Swami Kapilananda while at Yogananda's school for boys in Dihika.[4] Though *nauli* and *uddiyana* would not have been taught under the title of 'muscle control' by the Hatha yogis, they were well-known techniques for those trained in classical Hatha yoga.[5] The *Hatha Yoga Pradipika* gives a full description of the technique of nauli, which is prescribed so one can 'increase the fire element in the body'. The *Gheranda Samhita* mentions nauli as a 'cleansing technique' within the section on purification.[6] To perform the practice, 'lean forward, protrude the abdomen and rotate (the muscles) from right to left with speed. This is called *nauli* by the *siddhas*. Nauli is foremost among the Hatha yoga practices.'[7]

After the show, Bishnu found his friend who had told him about Chit Tun. 'Yes, I saw an amazing body, much like Sandow's, but what stunned everyone was his *nauli*, and I can do that better. Do you want to see?' Bishnu recalled taking off the clothes covering his torso to show his friend nauli right then and there. His friend was dumbstruck and responded, 'I did not know you could do this! Develop your body and show this art – you will soon become famous.'

Up to this point in time, Bishnu did not have the 'advantage of using the college gym', and 'practised *bayam* only at home'.[8] Bishnu's friend Kalinath later told him, 'I shall take you to Rajen Guha Thakurta and he will be so happy to teach you *bayam*.' This started the '*bayam* journey' for Bishnu, and Thakurta became Bishnu's teacher at City College.[9] He practised in earnest 'on parallel bars and other devices in the evenings, and wrestling and *dand-baithak* in the mornings after oil massage'.[10]

Bishnu was thin in his youth, and his body was somewhat 'sickly' until he took up *bayam*, but he still performed well in athletics. (Some jokingly referred back to the days of the 'thin body' Bishnu.)[11] Sprightly and adept at 'jumping, running, and high jumps', which 'were naturally easy' for him given his lightness, he started doing stunts such as jumping from heights:

One day Mejda (Swami Yogananda) ran to catch me for some reason. I slipped into the room on the road and by the time he was in the room I was on the balcony. Mejda came to the balcony and said, 'Now where will you go?' I got up on the railing; Mejda started shouting, 'Aye! Aye!' even before he finished saying, I had already jumped down on the street and disappeared from sight. Mejda complained that night to Baba, and Baba said, 'This is his normal practice, he does it every day.' Mejda was left dumbfounded.[12]

At the 4 Garpar Road house, the jump from the balcony to the street is a good 20 feet!

Bishnu had begun a personal daily exercise regime in 1921, when he was nineteen years old, and began formal training in 1922 at City College under Thakurta. By 1923, he began to teach others.

The end of the nineteenth century in Calcutta was a period when the adoption of a sedentary lifestyle by the Bengalis contributed to an overall decline in health. City College was formed during an intensive effort to spread English education throughout Bengal, while also including exercise. The school's system bore the same influence as the National Gymnasium (in which Swami Vivekananda had participated as a youth), placing a deliberate focus on integrating physical development with intellectual value. When Bishnu attended the gymnasium, of which nothing remains today, it was located in the central courtyard of the school.

In 1922, just a month prior to the start of his training, the Calcutta University Student's Welfare Committee had conducted a thorough medical test of all its students. Bishnu's weight was 68 pounds, his chest measured 25 inches, and his height was 4 feet and 6 inches.[13] The regimented training with Thakurta at the City College gymnasium proved to be quite effective. In a matter of months, he wrote that his chest measurement was 'up to 34 inches with his weight increasing to 100 pounds'. His height had increased to 5 feet.[14]

In 1923, a 'third incident' impacted Bishnu and 'changed the whole course' of his life. An annual physical culture exhibition was held 'just before the *puja* holidays' at City College. Professor Thakurta told Bishnu, 'You will have to participate in this exhibition!'

Bishnu later recalled meeting this command with excitement and nerves:

I could not believe my ears! Me at the *bayam* exhibition? With my skinny limbs? The people would shoo me out in the first moment! But this was my professor's orders and I was shaking with apprehension and at the same time madly hoping I could depend on my *nauli*, *uddiyana*, and other skills I would hone up for the occasion. But big and huge students objected to my participation and made it clear to the professor that it would lower their prestige. However, I found the professor got more determined that I must participate in the exhibition.

Bishnu naturally took to the stage. 'I showed my muscle movements and I can still hear the resounding claps I received. The people shouted from the gallery – "it was worth the eight *annas* spent".' Once he had 'performed the muscle control' exercises of nauli and uddiyana under 'gas lights shown from below with reflectors', he came on stage 'dressed like a clown' and took part in all the performances, such as 'parallel bar and ring acrobatics', creating a 'storm in the audience'. As he performed, Bishnu heard someone shout, 'Did I not tell you, it is the same boy who has come back as a clown? He is the best performer.' Though it was his first performance, he won a silver medal that day. Bishnu later recalled:

I was stupefied! Thank God I was in a clown's dress or else everyone would have been witness to my highly emotional expressions that day. Lalbabu must have given such silver medals to many such students but it was like *manna* from heaven for me that day. I cried the whole night, tears of emotion. That silver medal gave me the incentive to proceed in this path for the last 40 years.[15]

This was not a one-time act; Bishnu 'became famous as a clown' during the early 1920s.[16]

As he took up *bayam*, combat sports and feats of strength, Bishnu had two qualities that he felt propelled him to succeed: 'determination to finish a job' and a desire for praise. He candidly stated, 'I paid full attention to anything I did so that I would be loved and praised.'[17] Alongside Thakurta, Bishnu participated in boxing, wrestling and jiu-jitsu matches, *lathi-khela* (stick fighting) and lifting tonnage. They performed in Calcutta at Seller's Circus and Gemini Circus, and at events in the villages throughout Bengal.[18] The troupe organized demonstrations either for charity or to raise funds for the City College akhara (gymnasium) managed by Thakurta.[19]

Around this time, in the early 1920s, Bishnu and Buddha were about to become friends. Rajah Bose's house, where Buddha and the family lived, was just across

Upper Circular Road, a short distance from the Ghosh family home. Bishnu would see Buddha pass by in the morning on the way to school. 'I wished to speak to Buddha, and every day thought I must wait for the right moment. My eagerness to be friends with him just grew day by day', reflected Bishnu.

He watched Buddha 'walking past holding on to his books tightly', and noticed how he 'never let his gaze stray from his path'. Bishnu attributed this character to Buddha's Bengali mother. 'Truly a *devi*, she named Francis as "Buddha".'[20] Bishnu remembered:

I knew he was magician Rajah Bose's son through his foreign wife and that the boy's name was Francis Joseph Bose. I knew his mother got sick and went off to England with her other two kids – one daughter and a son – and left him in the care of Rajah Bose's Bengali wife.[21]

Every morning, Bishnu would pick up heavy barbells on the footpath, kick iron balls from one side of the road to the other, practise high jump, pole vault, etc., on the road, which eventually caught Buddha's attention and they 'finally became friends'.[22] With a nine-year age gap between them, Buddha 'eagerly watched' the actions of Bishnu, who took him under his wing, becoming a sort of older brother.[23] Buddha began training in physical culture at City College with Bishnu, riding pillion on his cycle every evening to practise *bayam*, 'then gradually he started with dand, then baithak, spring pulling, dumbbells, etc.'.

Even after Bishnu was admitted to Shibpur Civil Engineering College, he would 'cycle to the City College for … *bayam* practice' each evening. Buddha would accompany him, and afterwards Bishnu would 'help him with his studies'.[24]

Around the same time, Rajah Bose had 'just started a mica business in Giridih', a rural area of Bengal. For the time being, he 'had given his magic show tools and apparatuses to Buddha's youngest maternal uncle'. The uncle, whose stage name was Master Picklu, kept Buddha and Bishnu 'as his assistants'. They combined muscle control with magic. 'Bishnu would put on a *Bayam* display for intermission.' During that period, 'Buddha and I became very close,' wrote Bishnu.[25] Buddha went so far as to refer to Bishnu as 'mama', the affectionate term for 'uncle' in India.

But their friendship was interrupted when Buddha left Calcutta suddenly 'to live with his father in Giridih', where he was put to work.[26] For five years the two did not see each other. Occasionally, Bishnu would stop by Buddha's house 'to make enquiries', but Buddha was not there.[27]

Under his Bengali stepmother's guidance, young Buddha had chosen 'Ma Durga with a smiling face' over 'Ma Kali with her tongue out' or 'Shiva standing with a *trishul* (trident)' for a personal god. His mother advised him 'to hide the picture as his father would get angry if he saw Buddha worshipping'. Then one morning, 'he was caught by his father when he was wearing the loincloth'.

Rajah shouted, 'What are you doing? Throw off everything. There are no gods.'

Buddha replied, 'Ma Durga is mine, you cannot touch her!' Rajah said, 'Your stepmother has spoiled you.'

'Don't call her my stepmother, she is my real mother.'[28]

It was this sort of incident which led Rajah to decide that Buddha needed to be toughened up with manual labour in rural Bengal.

Bishnu remained close to his teacher, Professor Thakurta, and in 1926, they formed the All Bengal Physical Culture Association, which continued to put up performances at circuses and shows in Calcutta and throughout Bengal. After completing his college undergraduate degree, Bishnu got married to Ashalata Roy. They had their first child in 1928, a girl named Ava Rani.

In 1929, Bishnu began running his own gymnasium, named 'Ghosh's College of Physical Education', at 4 Garpar Road.[29] Bishnu started to compile photographs of himself and his top students, which would eventually include Buddha, for a publication. This group included Moni Roy, a favourite of Bishnu's, and grew to include others. But, it was not until the shocking death of a student named Noni, one of Bishnu's very first students, that Bishnu and Buddha were ultimately reunited.

FOR

"MUSCLEPOSE"

PHOTOGRAPHS OF YOUR OWN

Come to—

S. GHOSE & BROS.

4; GURPAR ROAD, CALCUTTA.

Phone B. B. 31

Because Mr. Bisnu Ghose is the Director here.

—Genuine Muscle Pose Photographs on post cards of various Indian Atheletes can be had of us at a very low price.

Our Portrait paintings are as good as, if not better than, the photographs taken by us.

GHOSH'S GYMNASIUM

4, Gurpar Road, Calcutta.

Phone B. B. 3132.

Come—

Young and old, there is a different exercise for each of you—an experienced trainer can only rightly select them. Wrong method of exercise is worse than no exercise.

Just as you should know the right path if you want to go to a place, so also you must know the proper way of exercise to attain certain amount of development.

Physical Deformities, Dispepsia. Asthma and other Nervous Diseases at all ages are cured in not time.

——— TAKE THIS BOOK FROM US ———

"BARBELL EXERCISE & MUSCLE CONTROL"

BY

SEN GUPTA & GHOSH.

PRICE Rs. 4 ONLY.

IMPERIAL

Ghosh's advertisement for the first gymnasium at 4 Garpar Road, 1923

(*Source: National Library, Calcutta*)

18

JIU-JITSU AND FEATS OF STRENGTH

I enjoyed showing my skills after signing a risk-bond paper –
took a two-ton roller on my chest, held back a running car,
pulled a cow cart full of people with my chest, muscle movement ...
and jiu-jitsu, of course.[1]
– Bishnu Ghosh

Jiu-jitsu swept through Bengal in the 1920s, capturing the focus of Bengali youth.[2] The family most often credited with popularising jiu-jitsu in India was the Tagores. In his lecture 'The Spirit of Japan', given after he returned from Japan in 1916, Rathindranath Tagore effusively praised the country's culture and practice.[3] He recollected that his 'father had brought a jiu-jitsu expert from Japan. We took lessons from him in order to prepare ourselves to fight the British! Had not the spirit and training of judo helped the Japanese to win the war?' Tagore was referring to Japan's victory over Russia in 1905, which led to resounding the slogan 'Asia is one' leaving an impression on Tagore about the potential power of countries when combined with physical practice.

For Tagore and the generation coming of age in the first quarter of the century, jiu-jitsu became an icon of Asian nationalism. As Japan had been able to thwart the onward march of Western imperialism, it inspired Bengalis, seeking their own way out from under British rule. Pratyay Banerjee wrote in *Tagore & Judo*, 'Thus this nationalistic impulse played an important part in fostering Japanese martial art. Tagore's admiration for this traditional Japanese art and game was quite evident in his writing.' The strength of jiu-jitsu practice, he remarked, is in its 'possibility of developing self-discipline and spirituality among the learners'.[4]

Bishnu Ghosh picked up the practice of jiu-jitsu as it became popular in the 1920s and then taught others. City College built a jiu-jitsu ring in its gymnasium, which was where Bishnu excelled at it 'pretty quickly', having already been a wrestler. 'I practised there to my heart's content', and jiu-jitsu training 'taught me new punches and tricks I could use in my wrestling'.[5] Bishnu explained other personal benefits stating, 'jiu-jitsu gave me a lot of self-confidence'.[6] Integrating martial arts into his training was for strength-building. It was a process that Bishnu emphasised to his students throughout his teaching career. The first emphasis was conditioning and strength-building through *bayam* and activities such as wrestling and jiu-jitsu, then muscle control, and finally, feats of strength.

Buddha wrote of learning 'the art of jiu-jitsu' from Bishnu, who was 'a past master in these arts'. He was 'perhaps the best trainer here in Bengal' with 'hundreds of students for these arts'.

Bishnu's most famous student was Ghulam Hussain, whose alias was the Great Gama of India, an Indian wrestler who achieved worldwide fame. The Great Gama was crowned wrestling World Champion in London in 1910; in 1916, he was presented with the Silver Mace from the Prince of Wales. Afterwards, he was in Calcutta, where he encountered Bishnu, who wrote:

Gama, the world famous wrestler was in Calcutta. One day a man came to me and when I asked him the reason he said Gama had heard from the police commissioner that I knew jiu-jitsu. Gama wanted to meet me. I was thrilled. He wanted to see my jiu-jitsu performance. I went to this house opposite Jorasanko police station and found a huge man reading the Koran. He was dressed in a white *lungi* and appeared a great personality. I was introduced to him as soon as he finished reading the Koran.

Gama said in Hindi, 'Babuji I have been invited to Japan to participate in a fight, but they insist on jiu-jitsu art of wrestling. I do not know jiu-jitsu. I wish to know the various tricks.' I replied in Hindi, 'I will show you if you stand up.' Then I showed him a few techniques after which he commented, 'These are very dangerous techniques. I will not go to Japan unless they agree to wrestle Indian style, not jiu-jitsu style.'

I wonder how many can claim to have shown Gama some jiu-jitsu tricks and techniques? I hold this experience as one of the greatest moments in my life. I even bought some jiu-jitsu books for Gama and gave those to him.

Jiu-jitsu students of Bishnu were the first to go abroad to teach and perform, long before bodybuilders or yoga experts. An early student of Bishnu's, named Sukumar Bose (no relation to Buddha), was sent by Bishnu 'on deputation to Japan to learn the art of jiu-jitsu'. In Japan, Sukumar taught at 'a Judo College' and then 'worked as a physical instructor in Manchuria for a year', before returning to Calcutta.[7]

Before he left for Japan, Sukumar asked Bishnu 'not to teach anyone his specialty – taking 30 men riding in cow cart on his stomach'. Sukumar told him, 'No matter how strong that person's stomach muscles may be, this is a very dangerous act. They have no idea.'[8] However, another student named Shusil Kumar Chakrabarty, or Noni, 'knew about it and persisted continuously' that Bishnu 'teach him the trick'.[9] Bishnu 'refused many times but finally had to give in to his constant nagging'. He regretted it soon thereafter.

At a performance for a Calcutta Municipal Corporation administrator, 'Noni was supposed to perform the roller passing' and the 'passing of a cow cart over his stomach'. Unexpectedly, Noni 'hurt himself during the first act' when a large steel roller used to flatten roads and earth gave him a muscle cramp. It was 'nothing serious', but he hid it from Bishnu. During the second act, Noni 'was unable to harden his stomach when the cow cart was passing over his stomach', and Bishnu 'noticed his stomach was too low down during the act'.[10]

A little later 'Noni whispered, "Bishtuda please let us go home as soon as possible,"' admitting he had lied.

Bishnu got very angry, 'Why did you lie to me earlier?'

Noni replied, 'If I had told you the truth would you have let me do the act?'

It proved to be Noni's last act. He was in extreme pain, and Bishnu 'sped out in his Red Buick' to the hospital. The road was empty and Bishnu 'increased the speed, but Noni's screams could be heard above the sound of the engine'. The doctors 'could not operate', since there was 'much internal bleeding inside his stomach', as well as a damaged spleen and liver. 'They stitched him up quickly, gave a morphine injection, and let him lie in peace.'

An hour later, Noni 'opened his eyes, called out Bishnu's name and then he closed his eyes forever'. The death of Noni 'was a severe blow' to Bishnu. He recalled, 'I could not close my eyes for a month after his passing away. He was always there in front of my eyes.'[11]

It was a recognition of how dangerous these feats were, if the breath was not used to contract the muscles properly. 'It was a game of life and death', said Bishnu.[12] In all of the photos taken of Bishnu with his students performing these feats, he hovers over them, willing them cautiously and unwilling fatal mistakes.

After the accident, Bishnu took a voyage to Chunar, an ancient city on the banks of the Ganges near Benares, in order to get away from it all. There, Bishnu found, 'God sent someone else to help me forget the tragic death of Noni – Buddha. I had gone to Chunar to forget and here I met Buddha once again.'[13]

19

THE BLUE PEARL, 28 MAY 1931

Bishnu and Buddha reunited in 1928 after Bishnu's daughter Ava Rani was born. Buddha was fifteen. Bishnu was in the final year of his law studies when his infant daughter, Ava Rani, fell very sick and Bishnu decided to take his family to Chunar, a city along the Ganges River.

'We were to drive along the Grand Trunk Road and since the town of Giridih was on the way, I decided to stop there overnight, and meet Buddha once more,' wrote Bishnu. Upon their meeting, Bishnu thought it was a difficult situation for Buddha. 'He had gotten thin, and was without shoes or slippers', but after the initial discomfort of his situation passed, he enjoyed the company of his 'Bishtu Mama', the nickname for Bishnu, and Buddha 'reverted to his old ways'. The next morning, while Bishnu was to proceed to Churnar, Buddha broke down and cried his heart out. Bishnu insisting on knowing the reason, but Buddha would not say anything. Bishnu gave Buddha his Chunar address and told him, 'Fine, if you cannot say it then write it and let me know at this address.'[1]

A few months later, another voyage led them to meet again. Bishnu rode his motorcycle with a friend 'to a workshop in the town of Kulti, in order to see Buddha', who was working there, in rural Bengal:

By the time we reached Buddha it was quite late in the night and Buddha had finished his dinner. We told him we too had our dinner on the way, so we spent the night chatting. Next morning I took both of them on my bike and sped back to Calcutta – again another hundred and a half mile stretch.[2]

Bishnu had talked with his father Bhagabati, and arranged for Buddha to move into the Ghosh family home in Calcutta. Years later, Buddha told others, 'I owe everything' to Bhagabati for the welcome into 4 Garpar Road.[3] In 1929, when Buddha returned to Calcutta, he enrolled in Calcutta Academy on Amherst Road to finish school while he lived with Bishnu's family. The next year, in 1930, Buddha wrote a four-page letter to his younger brother Dennis, with a return address of '4 Garpar Road, c/o, Babu, Bishnu Charan Ghosh'.

Buddha's father, Rajah, had recently visited Europe and London. Rajah had not travelled abroad for at least a decade when he returned to London in 1929 and performed several solo magic acts. While in London, Rajah spent time with Haydee and Dennis. The children were living with their mother outside of London. Emily's brother (Arthur Denin Johnson) had helped her for a period, but died early in 1926. And sometime prior to 1928, Emily had begun a relationship with a man by the name of Charles Hopkins, who became the stepfather of Haydee and Dennis.[4] For Buddha, Charles came to be known as Uncle, serving as a father figure and a benefactor of sorts, who later funded the manuscript and photo album of Buddha performing asanas (as described in the Preface).[5]

Dennis, in London, did not get along with his new stepfather at all. Just as Buddha did not get along with his father in Calcutta. Instead, they idolised each other's fathers. It was quite mixed up. Buddha was very gracious to Uncle Hopkins, whom Dennis abhorred. And Rajah made a favourable impression on Dennis, and this instigated Buddha's fury with his younger brother, for having enjoyed Rajah's visit.

When Rajah returned to the stage in London in 1929, eighteen years had passed since he and Emily had performed at the Coliseum and Hippodrome. His shows were no longer the big splash that they were during the heyday of the 1900s, when stage magician shows were all the rage. *The Magician Monthly* from London reported in a brief note that Rajah 'showed us some of the latest things from India'. Another headline, a bit more enthusiastic, read, 'For the First Time in the World, Rajah Bose exhibited the magical fantasy, "Theft of the Blue Pearl" in London' on 18 July 1929.[6]

This was an obvious play upon the performance he had done with the American Harry Sears in 1911, titled 'Blue Pearl'. The stage trick dealt mainly with the theft of a great blue pearl from the image of the god Shiva. The article went on to say Rajah was 'notable' and 'very interesting' in his performance, but he failed to capture wide attention, as he had done twenty years earlier, when Emily, his 'bewitching damsel', was by his side.

Rajah returned to Calcutta, and on 15 November 1931, a magicians' conference was held in the Bowbazar part of north Calcutta at Sradhananda

Park. 'All of the leading magicians of the time took part', including Rajah, coming out of retirement to perform one of his most popular acts, 'The Barrel Illusion'. At the end of the night, he was awarded 'Best Magician of the Evening'. Following the 1931 magicians' conference, he became the president of Calcutta's Wizard's Club, which, at the time, was 'the premier and leading magicians association in India'.[7] The performance at Sradhananda Park was the last recorded magic show by Rajah Bose.[8]

Buddha took to the stage at the same time his father was stepping down. And, by the time Rajah returned to Calcutta, Buddha was no longer at work in the Bengal countryside, nor living in the Bose family home in Calcutta. Instead, while Rajah was away, Buddha had taken the opportunity to move into 4 Garpar Road.

In Buddha, Bishnu Ghosh saw a handsome personality who would be his disciple. With ardor and earnestness, Buddha put all his anger, angst and hatred into this new craft: his body. He was praised, given respect and admiration by Bishnu and the other students who congregated with them at the akhara. On the stage, he was applauded and awarded for his muscle control exercises or, as they would later be named, yoga asanas. Fans would sing praises of his beautiful, fair-skinned body and his handsome personality. Buddha had become like his father: a star of the stage, admired by the crowd of onlookers.

I read Buddha's letter and feel a sense/levelling of humility for myself and anyone who would seek to place him on a pedestal. He was oh so human, a seventeen-year-old, but with more than your average level of anger-management issues when it came to dealing with his father. Already deep into my research, this letter serves as a reminder of how we create wonderful pictures of our heroes in our minds, forgetting that they are human too.

I am also taken by how the letter indicates that the young boys were on opposites sides of the same dilemma. Both had tremendous resentment for the father figures they lived with, while idolising the other from across the ocean. Both brothers were looking for the other to validate their negative feelings regarding their family issues; however, both had highly different perspectives on the situation. Dennis must have been shocked by all this when he received this letter from his elder brother, marked by the fact that this was the one letter Dennis kept, and it was passed on to successive generations.

c/o, Babu, Bishnu Charan Ghosh.
4, Gurpar Road
Calcutta
23rd May 1931.

My dear Brother,

I knew that inspite of my request to mother not to share my letters to you, she will share it. But I don't mind it for your knowing my ins and outs, what I was — I was. I have wiped away my past and have become perhaps good as you are. I don't think you won't feel it a shame to call me your elder brother. I am worthy of it now I think. I also knew that if you go through my ~~letter~~ your fond memories for your father will vanish like the soap bubbles vanishing in the air and your blood will rise to boiling and will feel miserable for missing a chance of ~~avenging~~ avenging your-self on behalf of your brother. The chance may or may not come again — for opportunity never comes twice. He had spoken all false. He told you that he trained me to think kindly of my mother. Oh! God! Did I not write mother that he often called me a Bastard? How can I

Pages 70–73: Letter by Buddha Bose (Calcutta) to Dennis Bose (London), 1931.
Courtesy of Susan Barrett (Bose).

form a good idea of my mother — whom I have never seen and whom my Father often abuses with filthy languages. Please ask mother to excuse me ignorant as I was I have sinned to think mother otherwise than a loving mother.

Dear brother please learn to excuse — there is a pleasure ∙ in it, which ‸you must have never enjoyed. ‸I can twist my father's neck in between my two fingers. Still I excuse him — I do not want to spoil my hands on such a rouge

Let me thank our ‸uncle father Hopkins for offering me with his food and shelter and I thank you also for inviting me ‸with too your company — But I cant go now — because that will hamper my studies. I want to stand before you as your worthy elder brother whom you will be proud to introduce to your friends. When you have waited all these years you can want wait another couple of years too. But not like before — we much smell, touch and talk with each other through the medium of letters.

You have got a wrong impression about me. I was never a sports-man — I never played anything or joined the sports, thus I was trained by my father; father used to thrash me if I went out of doors and joined the foot-ball or

hocky teams. A strange man he is — Don't you know
that he him himself never joined any sport? Only these
few months that I am taking physical exercises
scientific and new novel methods of muscle control
and also the art of "ju-jut-su", from my uncle
who is a past master in these arts and perhaps
the best trainer here in Bengal. He has got
hundreds of students for these arts to learn.
Soon I will send you some photographs of his
worthy pupils peoples. He gives me hope that I will
be his masterpiece work. You dont know how
have improved in these few months.

My uncle may soon go to England to be
a Barister. He says he will take me with him
positively. I am trying to send you the photograph
of my full body soon.

Father knows nothing of these my happy
news that I have got a hearty welcome from
you all. Let me convey to you one happy news
I stood first in my last examination. Also
first in mathamatics, second in English and
second in Bengali and in other additional

subjects I have done very & good too. Hope you
appreciate me, For after two years gap in my
~~Studies~~ student carrier it is a difficult job to do.
    Meore in my next letter. Love to you all.
        Yours affectionately.
        Francis Joseph Bose

P.S
    Tell to uncle Carli
    that I will give the
    reply of his letter in
    the next mail.
        Yours Reporter

20

BETWEEN TWO TRAMS

What I was, I was. I have wiped away the past.
– Buddha Bose, 1931

Buddha was aware that a change had occurred when writing the letter to his younger brother Dennis. Regardless of the physical practice he was engaged in, the letter implied a change deeper than a purely physical one. He was establishing a sense of self-worth. And while the letter portrayed the entangled relationship between father and son, it pointed towards something else at work in Buddha's life. A new and important figure was emerging: his teacher, Bishnu Ghosh. The juxtaposition of past anger and future hope was laid bare in the letter. Buddha was a young man, right at the beginning of his training with Bishnu, and was already expecting great things.

Once he began training with Bishnu, Buddha developed much in the way of self-confidence, and was able to direct the anger previously aimed at his father towards something useful. Bishnu, who had a knack for finding latent potential in students, trained them to excel. Buddha's practice and expertise in muscle control took off. It was, Bishnu wrote of Buddha, his 'ardent endeavour' that 'lifted him above the common level'.[1]

Buddha had been doing 'physical exercises, scientific and novel methods of muscle control' for a few months at the time. His adoration of Bishnu was obvious in his letter to Dennis. 'I will send some photographs of his worthy pupils. He gives me hope that I will be his masterpiece work. You don't know how I improved in these few months.' From both Bishnu and Buddha's writing at the time, one can sense something special was occurring. Buddha, with a 'natural love for a symmetrical body' was being 'fostered by the encouraging words' of Bishnu and therefore, Buddha's 'progress was rapid'.[2] Like his father,

Buddha was a natural on stage. Within six months of learning muscle control techniques, Buddha was already on the stage, having been 'invited to give a demonstration before a large audience in Calcutta', while still just sixteen years old.[3]

One of the changes Buddha made during this time was dropping his given Christian name, Francis Joseph Chandra. He still went by Francis with the family in London, but in Calcutta, he went so far as to take the Ghosh middle name of Lal. The back and forth continued in official documents until 1938, when he adopted the name Buddha Bose for good.[4] At the same time Buddha re-entered his life, Bishnu's wife, Ashalata, gave birth to a son, Sriman Srikrishna Ghosh. His nickname would be Gublu. Even with a son, Bishnu wrote years later, Buddha was, 'My dearest. I loved Buddha from the bottom of my heart. I have often felt Gublu knew this and so, it has left me with a hurt feeling.'[5]

Moving into 4 Garpar Road, Buddha became Bishnu's sidekick, including travelling as a daredevil duo. Much of Bishnu's life consisted of dangerous extracurricular activities, and now Buddha joined in. Gradually, Bishnu's activities took on more flair, to the point of being deathdefying, especially while riding a motorcycle.[6]

Perhaps weightlifting created an intensity, both in body and mind, which spilled over into dangerously competitive events. Or perhaps his motivation was similar to his elder brother Yogananda – the appeal of being closer to the afterlife, the supernatural and their deceased mother. His brother Sananda commented once that, 'Whenever Bishnu goes out our hearts flutter dangerously, wondering when will he return. And when he does, he comes home with blood splattered all over him. And yet, he is completely unconcerned.'[7]

Whatever the reason, riding motorcycles, along with all sorts of insane stunts and long road trips, became Bishnu's youthful passion. 'I have travelled to different countries, villages, towns in the last forty years doing my *bayam* exhibition,' wrote Bishnu. 'Some of those experiences still shine in my mind and some have been obliterated.' The lasting ones were those which included travels by train and motorcycles. Bishnu writes that he was 'crazy about driving on wheels from an early age.'[8] A daredevil, his 'many tricks of cycling on Circular Road' and elsewhere were dangerous. One time, riding double with Buddha, Bishnu recalled:

Swiftly turning the face of the bike backward when driving in full speed was my best act. One day after performing such a dangerous act on the road, with Buddha in tow, I reached home to find the famous wrestler Gobar Babu waiting. He said, 'I was sitting in the first compartment of the tram when I saw you speed between two trams. I was shaking with fear and closed my eyes; when I dared to open my eyes I was sure it was the end of you. But there were you alive and riding! But please do not do such dangerous acts anymore.'[9]

The north Calcutta wrestler Gobar Goho, who had gone to wrestle in America during the 1920s, had little effect on dispelling the stunts or the racing of Bishnu.

A crash did happen while Buddha was riding pillion (on the back seat), but it was not serious for Buddha or Bishnu. When others rode pillion on his Ariel motorcycle, Bishnu would warn them 'not to get scared and try to jump off or cling', as that would put him off balance. 'One day we decided to race all the way to Giridih and Buddha, as usual, was my partner,' Bishnu wrote. What followed was a string of stunts at daredevil speed.[10] Soon after, Buddha began riding on his own, along with a number of others who followed Bishnu's lead, as he was 'probably the first one in Calcutta to show acts on a running motorcycle'. It is not surprising that the performance of yoga asanas requiring balance (headstand, handstand, etc.) atop the moving motorcycle became one of their specialties.

Bishnu was in a few other 'major accidents'. The first resulted in a head injury, the second to his knee. 'Once I was acting smart, riding hands-free only holding on to the fork when one wheel fell into a pit. I fell crashing and hurt my right knee; I tried to put a brave face, which was ashen by then, trying to stand up but I could not. My knee hurt terribly, a little later I limped and dragged the cycle home and I was bedridden for a long time. Ever since then my right knee has not been normal.' And deaths occasionally occurred.

'Once, in Calcutta I showed Apurbo Da some of Lalit Roy's ring acts on the street; even Buddha and I had serious injuries while doing those acts. Apurbo returned to his hometown in Allahabad and tried to do the same act in his show. He crashed, hurt his head badly and passed away after seven hours of unconsciousness. Such deaths have hurt me immensely, no doubt, but I did not stop loving my bike; I still do.'[11]

21

THE GYMNASIUM

The first students of Bishnu were displayed inside the 1930 book, *Muscle Control and Barbell Exercises*. Photographs showed Buddha doing 'isolation of the abdominal muscles' and the 'obliquus abdominis'. His control was striking and it depicts a more intricate form of the practice than what Bishnu or others performed. During the period when the book was published, abdominal muscle control had become a fad among physical culture proponents throughout India.

Half of the book, titled 'Barbell Exercises', was written by Bishnu's collaborator, Keshub Sen Gupta. It mostly followed the order and content provided in a previously published book, also titled *Barbell Exercises*, by Walter Chit Tun. Chit Tun had written his *Barbell Exercises* in 1926. Before that, he had impressed upon Bishnu the performance of muscle control. The exercises, which included barbells, are from European influence, but Chit Tun did not indicate where he had learned muscle control. His knowledge could have come from his home country of Burma, or it could have come from the German strongman named Max Sick, professionally known as 'Maxick'.

The other half, 'Muscle Control', was authored by Bishnu. This followed Maxick's work, specifically a 1911 publication titled *Muscle Control*. The mimicking pattern can be readily seen within the first few pages of each of the two sections. For example, the instructions given for 'relaxation' by Maxick: 'Allow each muscle to drop as you think of it, but care must be exercised that, while doing so, you do not contract other muscles which you have already relaxed.'[1] Bishnu's 'relaxation' instructions: 'Allow your muscles to droop one by one ... guard yourself against contracting any muscle already relaxed when trying to relax another.'[2]

The most noticeable piece of information in Bishnu's book was an advertisement at the end, which promoted a 'different exercise' for each person.

This individual method became a defining characteristic for Bishnu. He learned the method under his teacher, Professor Thakurta, at the City College gymnasium. The central tenet of Bishnu, as a physical culture teacher, was to customise the exercise for the individual and for the latter to do the exercise correctly. Bishnu was very particular that one needed to train in this manner for development to occur. He referred to this as the 'proper way of exercise', explaining that one should first develop the muscles, and then, in the second stage, undergo muscle control to make the muscles shapely and increase one's power.

In the 'Come, young and old' announcement, however, Bishnu was beginning to speak openly to those with all sorts of physical ailments, not just the bodybuilders. It was the first indication of what is now called 'Therapeutic Yoga' in Calcutta. However, in 1930, Bishnu was calling it exercise, not yet yoga. That transition would occur over a couple of decades at least, alongside wider societal changes in Bengal.

The basis of physical culture, as taught by Bishnu Ghosh, was daily practice. In the 1930 preface he wrote, 'When you find time to sleep, to take your bath, to take your meals, you can easily find time for a little exercise, which is no less important than any other dire necessity of life.' Daily practice was introduced to him by his father Bhagabati; again during his days at Yogananda's school in Dihika and Ranchi; and again under Rajen Thakurta at City College. Throughout, daily practice was synonymous with *bayam*. So much so, that later in his life, Bishnu was the editor of three different magazines, each containing the word *bayam* in the title (Bishnu is often addressed in these magazines as 'Bayamacharya').[3] *Bayam* comprises free-hand exercises similar to yoga, but it is more movement-based and dynamic.

One of the earliest books expounding on *bayam* dates back to 1874. It is a book titled *Bayam Shikshak* (The Physical Instructor) by Shyama Charan Ghosh (unrelated to Bishnu Ghosh). The book includes forty free-hand exercises 'classified into three categories of *ugra* (extreme), *mridu* (mild), and *mishra* (mixed)'. These exercises were commonly used by wrestlers, to warm up and by the peasantry of Bengal, being a common feature of village life throughout the nineteenth century.[4] The book shows that *bayam* was already a feature of Bengali life. Now, in the urban setting of Calcutta, it was becoming more organized and influenced by Western ideas of exercise through the urban gymnasiums – the modernised akharas.

In the eighteenth and nineteenth centuries, Bengali families migrated from the villages to the city, changing their lifestyle. In Calcutta at the time, Bengali people 'were becoming conscious of the merits of exercise ... because of their affinity with the English lifestyle'.[5] One ramification of this was the growth of public physical facilities like the Calcutta Cricket Club, which traces its origin to around 1792; the Calcutta Rowing Club, established in 1858; and the Calcutta Football Club and Dalhousie Athletic Club, established in 1872. Outside the UK, these are some of the oldest clubs in the world.[6] The club culture became the institutional format for 'the growth of physical culture'. In the process, 'a distinct locus of sporting activity was created, in which the involvement of the public mattered'.[7]

In the first part of the twentieth century, the Calcutta gymnasium played a significant role in the development of modern yoga, providing a training ground where indigenous *bayam* free-hand movements became intermingled with classical Hatha yoga postures. However, the nationalistic nature of the gymnasiums in Calcutta cannot be ignored. From the perspective of the British, 'the genesis of the terrorist movement in Bengal can be traced to the establishments of *akharas* in the metropolitan city of Calcutta'.[8] From the perspective of Bengal, these establishments were an impetus for independence.

The East India Company had a presence in India dating back to the 1600s. The Company maintained a militarised expansionist mission to extract riches from India. On the night of 20 June 1756, an event known as 'Black Hole' occurred in Calcutta, which changed everything. According to the British narration of the event, in a small single room, 146 British soldiers were confined for a day, after which only 23 came out alive. The accuracy of the claims was disputed by Bengalis, but an incensed tabloid press and populace in London demanded an increase of the British force that already occupied and ruled India.

The governing class in England, 'the masters of the masters of India', thought of itself as enlightened. It had superior technology, and through 'British skill and science, was ready to usher mankind into a golden age'. Victorian-era England did not share the conquest-minded world view of the East India Company. Rather than the subjection of native peoples, 'their lofty opinion of Empire' sought elevation of native peoples.[9]

By the beginning of the nineteenth century, reform efforts were underway, led by Christian missionaries, to educate Bengalis by teaching them English and the British way of life. During this process of cultural assimilation, Hindu College and School were established in 1817–18, near College Square where north Calcutta begins. A few decades later, an intellectual and cultural 'Bengali Renaissance' ensued, which included social and education reform.

Bishnu's book was dedicated to Young Bengal, one of the first organizations to emerge, emphasising free will, free thought and rebelling against religious traditions. Their modern thinking was closely aligned with the quasi-religious Brahmo Samaj movement, which relegated religious belief behind other social necessities such as education. While most members of Brahmo Samaj adhered to universalism, others rooted their desired reforms within a nationalist perspective, which later became accompanied by martial physical training.[10]

22

NATIONAL *BAYAM*

The idea of a training system that required a gymnasium in the city was the brainchild of Akshay Kumar Dutta of Brahmo Samaj and the Bengal Renaissance, 'and it took its course from 1848 onward'. Dutta stressed 'the scientific importance of exercise, physique, physical culture among the youth force of the then Bengal ... It was a collective effort on the part of the nineteenth-century educated and cultured elites' to instill a physical practice both for men and youth.[1]

The 1857 rebellion by Indians may have failed to overthrow British rule, but a decade later socio-cultural nationalism emerged in response to the cultural domination, the so-called 'Britishness in the colonies'.[2] In 1866, the Bengali intellectual, Rajnarayan Bose, called for the revival of national gymnastics exercises.[3]

In order to resist British cultural colonialism, the founders of the Chaitra Mela (early spring gathering), funded by the Tagore family, advocated a revival of indigenous ideals and practices of Bengali culture in 1867. The Tagore family was one of the first in India to become involved with the promotion of physical exercise at their palatial home of Jorasanko Thakurbari in north Calcutta. There, a *bayamgar* (gymnasium) was built for 'a regular practice of gymnastics', inspiring other like-minded efforts.[4] Called the Hindu Mela in its second year, the effort sought to re-popularize Bangla folklore, literature, music, poetry and nationalistic songs. And physical culture – at the gymnasium – took a central role.

The concept of a gymnasium had been brought to India from Europe. It was a 'distinctive colonial public sphere' where the English 'kept themselves fit through exercise'. Up to the period of the Hindu Mela, this public space had not undergone a critical 'systematic exploration of its actual imbrications in the ideologies and practices of imperial rule'.[5] The process of cultural assimilation would be turned on its head. From the Hindu Mela, where 'young men showed off their newly developed bodies', the Calcutta gymnasium and the Bengal circus emerged, through which physical culture became a component of the daily practice of Bengalis.[6] Though the Hindu Mela was not regarded as having a political agenda, Mitra himself organized a National Association, and under it a National Circus and a National Gymnasium, in 1868. The National Gymnasium of Calcutta, founded by Nabagopal Mitra, stood out among the early Bengali gymnasiums; Swami Vivekananda was among its early students. The National Gymnasium was located across the street from Vidyasagar College in north Calcutta; students at Mitra's gymnasium integrated systems of European-style exercises with Indian indigenous traditions.

The National Circus was short-lived, but the Mitra effort at including physical feats in the circus was followed by Priyanath Bose and the Great Bengal Circus, founded in 1887:

> Professor Bose's circus had magic shows, short stick acts, sword fighting, Hatha yoga, fire act, being buried alive, etc., as part of the performances. The crowds were incredibly massive at the Eden grounds. People came from far away regions of the country to watch his shows – the audience used to be swayed by the patriotic fervor and would feel a sense of pride just to be there. Money was the least criteria in Bose's shows, the people felt grateful and proud to be a part of the national performance. It used to be a nationalist craze.[7]

At the start of the Great Bengal Circus, Priyanath Bose 'would call on the audience to practice *bayam* for their own and their country's health'.[8] Vivekananda remarked that the Bengali circus was more than just a source of amusement. It also served as a school for physical instruction, 'where a Bengali could see how they could excel in the field of physical strength and stamina by the training and cultivation of nerves and muscles'.[9]

Bose brought in animals and troupes for all types of feats, including acrobatics and a 'boneless man' who 'tied himself up into knots that seemed impossible to undo'.[10] The schools in Calcutta became engaged with the promotion, arranging 'circus shows for their students to enhance their interest in physical culture and gymnastics'.[11]

The National Gymnasium emphasized physical exercises and introduced modern equipment to Calcutta residents. Gymnastic bars and trapeze were purchased in 1869 and the gymnasium employed a British trainer of European-style gymnastics. This was followed up in Calcutta during the 1870s, when European-style gymnasiums were included in government schools and colleges as part of educational policy. In 1879, one of the most prominent gymnasiums, at the Hindu College (Presidency University) and School, 'started offering gymnastics classes'. It was equipped with parallel and horizontal bars, so the students could 'train as soldiers'.[12]

The gymnasium created a space where indigenous traditions such as *bayam*, dand-baithak and various weighted exercises could be integrated with imported exercises like gymnastics and calisthenics, which were popularized internationally via imported English manuals and texts. In turn, Bengalis began to publish exercise books such as *Bayam Sikshak* (1874) and others.

The influence of the Mela, however, was short-lived. Economic security played a role. In North Calcutta, some Bengalis benefited from British capital circulating throughout Calcutta. They were a new form of elite due to their educational advances.[13] However, the benefits of well-paid employment were scarce even for the well-educated, and their advancement only grew so far. The number of educated Bengalis increased by the thousands, but 'the job market was overcrowded' which resulted in a crisis.[14] Newspapers like *Amrita Bazar Patrika* led the intellectual vanguard of Calcutta and voiced the frustration in print, while others in north Calcutta became more martial. Political nationalism became more prominent and insurgent acts of violence against British rule increased.

23

YOUNG BENGAL

In the early decades of the twentieth century, those aligned with the Bengali bodybuilding society *Anushilan Samiti*, advocated the use of violence as a means for ending colonial rule in India. Within the north Calcutta Garpar-Maniktala area, the Jugantar movement emerged under the leadership of Sri Aurobindo Ghosh among others.[1] It started under the guise of a fitness club but took young teenagers in and turned them into revolutionaries. Sri Aurobindo, who was 'jailed by the British for plotting a *sannyasi* revolt against the empire', combined his yogic spiritual impulse with nationalistic efforts.[2] Violence emerged in Calcutta, with assassinations and underground groups creating chaos. The akharas and gymnasiums served as a means of physical strength building, as well as a cover for their political organizational efforts.[3]

As the Bengalis' organizational ability grew, the colonialist Lord Curzon and other British rulers countered the emergent threat to their hegemony with an attempt to partition Bengal in 1905. The Swadeshi movement, which was both a boycott of British goods and a promotion of indigenous goods, emerged in protest to the partition. It provoked and became springboard for Indian nationalism as a whole, and for subsequent Hindu and Muslim animation along communal lines. Swadeshi succeeded and Bengal was eventually reunited in 1911, but not without divisive societal ramifications becoming embedded into the communities. While the communal differences receded into the background, Indians in general hardened their demands. 'In the wake of the *Swadeshi* movement', the 'anti-colonial revolutionary organizations' flourished.[4]

The British responded by moving the colonial capital from Calcutta to New Delhi in 1912. The British crackdown on the insurgency within Calcutta was brutal. Freedom-fighters and revolutionaries were persecuted and served long jail sentences. Violence had less appeal in the 1920s and intellectuals fled during that time. Sri Aurobindo Ghosh, once an influential leader of Indian independence in Calcutta, left politics altogether to focus exclusively on spiritual practice. Still, fiery nationalism remained in Bengal. Subhas Chandra Bose, who served as Calcutta's mayor and the leader of the National Congress, advocated violence when necessary.[5] This conflicted with the idea of ahimsa (non-violence), a tenet within the Swadeshi movement, which Mahatma Gandhi carried forward.

Bishnu's good friend and neighbour Nilmoni Das, a bodybuilder known as the 'Ironman', ran a competing neighbourhood gym and was said to have known 'that many freedom fighters would practise body-building from his charts and he liked this idea. This is how he indirectly supported the freedom fighters.'[6] However, there was no indication that Bishnu Ghosh was active or involved in the independence effort, as supporting Indian nationalism wasn't one of his father's priorities. Many of his clientele were British colonialists such as Stanley Jackson, who was the governor of Bengal from 1927 to 1932, and his successor John Anderson, who served from 1932 to 1934. Bishnu wrote:

> Sir Hassan Surabardi was also very fond of me and once we were invited to hold a show in his house. Present were Sir Stanley Jackson, Governor of Bengal and his wife. They were completely fascinated by Buddha's performance and in fact, Lady Jackson hugged and petted Buddha. Sir Hassan started his yoga lessons from Buddha right from that day.[7]

On another occasion Bishnu wrote:

> The Maharajah of Santosh had a tree planting ceremony and invited the Bengal Governor, Sir John Anderson. He had also arranged for me and my students to hold a show in his honor. My eldest son, late Srikrishna was just 3 years old then. The main attractions in the show were Buddha, Moni Roy and Srikrishna.[8]

This should not to present Bishnu as the equivalent of a babu to the Englishman. Obnoxious colonialists were too common in his eyes; he saw himself as equal to any Englishman.[9] In fact, Bishnu did not mind confrontations with the colonialists, even if it were sparked by something trivial, such as a bit of road rage: 'We were finally in Calcutta, and on the way home I had a little tiff with an Englishman on the road – I won.'

Recalling another confrontation, Bishnu went on:

We were an object of ridicule and hatred in the eyes of the English people those days; no wonder we too had developed a similar attitude towards them. They would not leave any chance of humiliating or insulting us. Once while travelling, I remember an Englishman put up his shoe-clad feet right towards my face. I picked up a pair of slippers and shoes with my big toes and put up my feet in front of his face. He put down his feet – so did I. He had met his match.[10]

Bishnu loved to compete, and his approach to physical culture was one of professionalism rather than insurgency. It is an alternative 'trajectory' of physical culture, one not solely about nationalism but instead 'a preoccupation with bodybuilding and feats of strength', which ultimately led to the inclusion of Hatha yoga.[11]

For Bishnu and his students, physical culture and feats of strength were a sport, and his students were professionals with rehearsed performances. Strongman feats were part of the lore of Bengal and India as a whole, but 'a tension' arose 'in the physical culture movement' between the amateur and the professional. With Bishnu, the emphasis upon physique and demonstrating muscle control on the stage moved to the forefront, a departure from the way Indian feats of strength and stage performances had been done in the past. An entirely new system was brought forth, which focused on the outward form, printed photographs and the integration of European methods (barbells and other equipment). Bishnu assimilated these with the yogic techniques of breath and contraction and relaxation techniques he had learned as a youth at the Dihika ashram. Soon, this would also impact the formation of a modern yoga system.[12]

Bishnu's dedication of *Muscle Control* to Young Bengal reflected the idea upon which City College – where he learned physical culture – had been formed. The College was 'famous for the influence of *Brahmo Samaj*' and its advocation of education alongside physical culture within Bengal society. The dedication 'was for the younger generation',[13] aimed at developing 'the strength and power in the Bengali youth'.[14]

Figuratively, Bishnu's physical activities drew inspiration from nationalist pride, but it was not overt (nor was it for his brother Yogananda).[15]

Bishnu was much more interested in the professional, educational and physical side than in recruiting or espousing for political independence. Bishnu's nationalism was more along the lines of taking pride when Bengalis took on Europeans and defeated them, whatever the contest happened to be. The victory was seen as a conquest, and it strengthened their cultural consciousness. 'Middle class Bengalis made several efforts to combat this imperial stereotype in the sporting fields' of cricket and football.[16] Wrestling was also particularly formative in this regard, as was boxing. Then too, Hatha yoga, with which they one-upped the West by being the modern originators of 'the world's oldest physical culture system'.

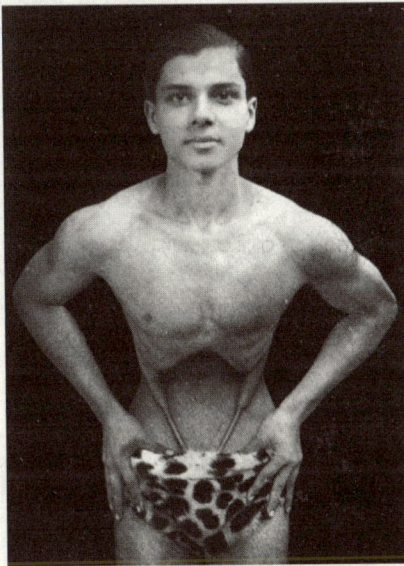

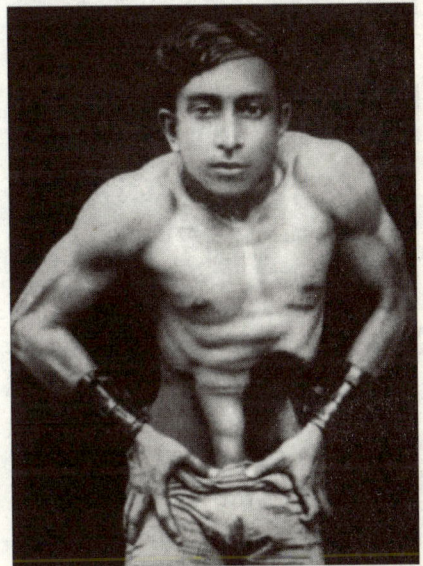

Left: Buddha Lal Bose. Right: Bijoy Kumar Mullick.
Source: Muscle Control (Calcutta, 1930)

BARBELL EXERCISE
by Keshub Ch. Sen Gupta B.A.

MUSCLE CONTROL
by Bishnu Charan Ghosh B.Sc.

1930

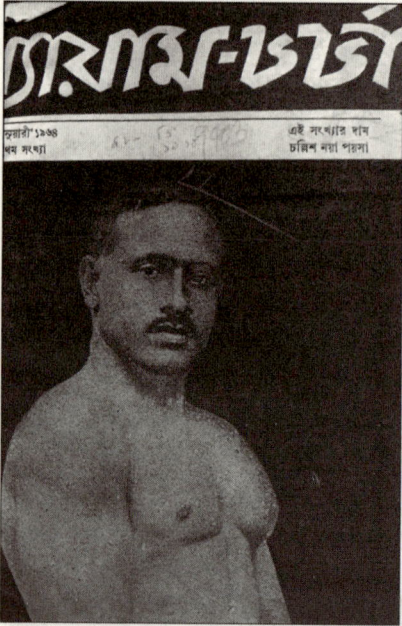

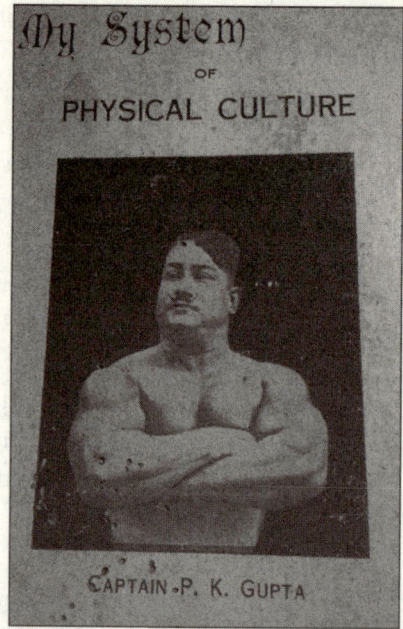

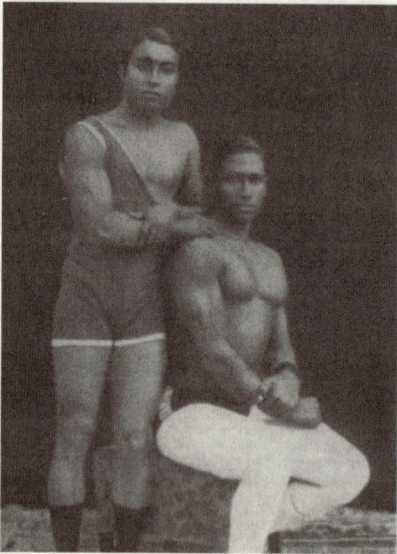

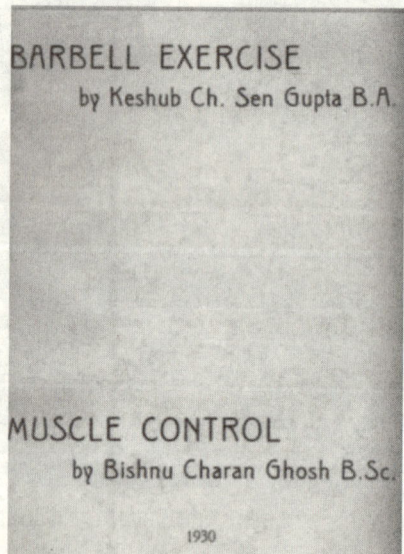

Clockwise from top left: R.N. Thakurta; P.K. Gupta; Bishnu Ghosh (standing)
and Keshub Sen Gupta.

Source: Bayam Charcha; My System (1929); Barbell Exercise & Muscle Control (1930).

24

OBSCURITY OF HATHA YOGA

During the 1920s, yoga asanas still belonged in the realm of sannyasis and those free from societal responsibilities. Asanas were restricted to those who had been initiated, usually families who had inherited the practices and who kept them secret.[1] This perspective can be seen in the encounter between Surendranath Dasgupta and the yogi Yogendra.

In 1922, Yogendra, a Hatha yogi, returned to India after living in the United States for two years. By chance, he met the Bengali Sanskrit professor Dasgupta, as they were both enroute from London to Calcutta, and they discussed how 'not much was known about the history of yoga'. Thereafter, Yogendra visited Dasgupta in Chittagong for advice on how to paramedicalize the yoga asanas. 'The two discussed the philosophical background of yoga' and Yogendra learned 'the history of yoga' from Dasgupta.[2] During the visit, 'Yogendra demonstrated some yogic acts, *dhauti*, *neti* etc., many asanas, many impossible positions and postures and created a commotion among the professors' because 'at that time no one knew that Yoga could be practised by ordinary men'.[3]

This conflict was also apparent in the teachings of P. K. Gupta, who was a contemporary of Bishnu's teacher, R. N. Guha Thakurta. Gupta, like Thakurta, promoted a daily regime men of exercises and bodybuilding. He became known as the 'Indian Sandow' (after the European strongman Eugen Sandow) for his promotion of physical culture. In 1927, Gupta authored a book titled *My System of Physical Culture*, which profoundly influenced Calcutta's physical culture clubs and organizations. His motto, taken from Latin, was *Mens sana in corpore sano*, which translates to 'a sound mind in a sound body'. The contents include physiological and physical explanations of *bayam*, followed by descriptions of free-hand exercises and 'exercises for athletes with weights'. In the chapter on the 'utility of physical culture', the text explained that there were 'three phases of physical culture', which were 'physical, mental, and spiritual', foreshadowing the 'body, mind, spirit' trinity that would become part of the US counter-culture fifty years later.[4]

My System of Physical Culture provided a glimpse into the mentality of the times, with a nearly militant focus on achieving physical perfection to match mental perfection. Against the backdrop of the colonial setting, Gupta, a nationalist Calcutta University lecturer, was inspired to 'improve the degenerated physical condition of the educated Bengalis' through a revival of physical culture. Near the end of the book was a succinct description of Hatha yoga as it related to the physical culture movement, able to 'cure most of the cases' by enabling 'physical well-being' rather than by 'medicine and doctor'.

Gupta confirmed the word-of-mouth lineage of yoga cure, but thought it too fringe to be widely suitable. He knew many 'so called pranayam experts' and from a physiological viewpoint, 'the system of pranayam' in Hatha yoga was 'suitable to the yogis, and to their peculiar and irregular habits', but 'not that of the *'Greehis'* (family men)'.[5] Other historians in Calcutta confirmed this orientation. 'The common man used to be terrified of practising yoga' in India.[6] For the most part, Hatha yoga practice 'was completely confined within the ashrams of the yogis and saints'.[7]

Within the text of Bishnu's *Muscle Control* (1930), there was only one mention of asana practice. Describing one of his first students, Moni Roy, Bishnu wrote, 'his peacock asana [*mayurasana*] balancing on two fingers is really wonderful'.[8] Doing asanas as exercise, one was more likely to be called a gymnast than a yogi.

Outside Calcutta, when B. K. S. Iyengar started learning yoga in Mysore in the 1930s, he expressed a similar sentiment. 'In those days there were hardly any yoga teachers and we could count them on our finger-tips', wrote Iyengar. 'The subject of yoga was spread only among a few selected people. This greatest art of India was sometimes ridiculed.'[9]

The 'early yogis' had 'started awakening Yoga from its "sleep of exclusiveness" in the 1920s'.[10] Among these giants in the 1930s were Swami Sivananda of Rishikesh, Krishnamacharya of Mysore, Yogendra from Santa Cruz and Devananda from Lahore. In Eastern India, yoga began to emerge in the 1930s 'as entertainment in bodybuilding shows by B. C. Ghosh', wrote Claudia Guggenbühl in 2003.[11]

I first introduce myself to Claudia via email in 2014, to tell her about the overlap between our research. I tell her that my interest in the origin of Calcutta Yoga had begun with the unlikely discovery of Buddha Bose's unpublished work. His manual is not just an enigma but a missing link. Claudia replies:

> How lucky you were to find the totality of the asanas Buddha Bose and Ghosh toured with – I never saw any of them! But I did write the entire history of Ghosh's Yoga College in Calcutta (as far as I could unearth it); it's all part of a 250 page 'book' which I wrote nearly 10 years ago, but which never got published.[12]

The outline of her unpublished 2003 book, *Yoga in Calcutta*, includes chapter titles, such as 'The Yoga Empire of Calcutta' and 'The Legacy of Bengal's Iron Man', with a range of topics such as the life of Buddha Bose, Bishwanath Ghosh and Bikram Choudhury while at Ghosh's Yoga College. Another chapter is on yoga therapy, and another links yoga and bodybuilding in Calcutta titled 'Yoga for a Strong Independent India'.

She has documentation stemming from three years of research and interviews with over sixty persons in Calcutta and other places in India. Her research spans a large arc of time, from the 1920s into the 1970s. Her argument though, much like others that have since covered the same territory, lacks a deep textual example of the transition from nationalistic bodybuilding and indigenous exercise (*bayam*) to modern yoga. What Claudia is missing in her research is a student of Bishnu Ghosh's who embodied this link: Buddha Bose.

Claudia concludes that 'towards the end of the 1920s, Bishnu Charan Ghosh began to turn bodybuilding into a stage show', and that 'he travelled with a troupe of students to the villages of Bengal to attract more men into the new cult of the body (and the ideals of Vivekananda connected with it)'. Then, 'in the '30s he suddenly added yoga exercises in his shows as intermediate elements to increase the attractiveness of the performance'. Unfortunately, she writes, 'I wasn't able to determine exactly how Bishnu Charan came up with the idea of bringing yoga to the stage.' She adds, 'The obvious presumption is that Yogananda's influence was present.'[13] Though that is partly the case (Yogananda and Bishnu did both contribute), Buddha Bose is the key. His unpublished *Yoga Asanas* album proves to be the missing link.

25

BUDDHA BEGINS HATHA YOGA

I was best in abdominal control but [Buddha Bose]
has surpassed by far his trainer in his wonderful abdominal control.[1]
– Bishnu Ghosh

Bishnu and his top students 'spent their youth pursuing Western styles of exercise, practising and doing research on them'.[2] Though they had learned about muscle control from books by European strongmen, the link between these practices and their yogic heritage had not been explored until Buddha Bose became intrigued with the heritage and began asana practice.

In 1932, the famous boxer, Madhu Mazumdar, returned from a tour in America and was about to hold a show at Shraddhananda Park in Calcutta. The park was a famous venue for shows and pujas. Just a year prior, Buddha's father, Rajah, had performed in a magicians' conference there. Buddha wanted to attend Mazumdar's show and asked Bishnu to come along. This would be Buddha's first introduction to Hatha yoga. Thirty-five years later, Buddha remarked, 'The day is a clear picture to me even today.' On reaching the park, Buddha 'saw a village boy from rural Bengal doing some yoga-*bayam*' postures of *dhanurasana, bhujangasana, vrischikasana, sarvangasana,* etc., and had a startling revelation 'that this was our heritage'. Up to this point he had 'been practising the Western exercises' such as *uddiyana* and *dhauti* 'without knowing these were indigenously Indian'.[3]

Coming to realize the exercises were not imported but rather indigenous, he remarked, 'The West had borrowed these from us. That day I felt my chest expand ten times with pride.' A great impression was made on Buddha who told Bishnu, 'Now that is India's physical culture system.'

Buddha entreated his teacher, 'Allow us to learn yoga-*bayam* and show the world India's true creation.'[4]

Bishnu, not missing a beat, replied, 'Oh, you want to learn Hatha yoga?'[5]

Of course, Bishnu knew the practices already, having learned yoga asanas in his youth.[6] He was just as eager as his student to reintroduce them. According to Buddha, 'a few days later', Bishnu had already acquired writings and the book 'by Swami Kuvalayananda on yoga from Bombay'. Right away, they were 'totally immersed in the yoga books and asana practice'.[7] Buddha remarked, 'Bishnu always urged me to improve my own body and to take up the ancient Yoga system of body culture, assuring me that if I did so I would have a better body than his own.'[8]

'India has a position in the world of *bayam* (exercises),' wrote Buddha, 'I knew we would not only excel in the field of yoga-*bayam*, but scientific research would prove its benefits.'[9] For Buddha, the encounter encouraged an ongoing transformation of the practice, in an effort to make it transhistorical and transnational. He began integrating disparate traditions, which included modern writings, neighbourhood teachers and Sanskrit vernacular sources.

Much of the content in Kuvalayananda's book was in earlier issues of his magazine, *Yoga Mimansa*. The magazine was widespread throughout India, Europe and America, and featured the same abdominal techniques which Buddha and Bishnu practised as 'muscle control', including *nauli*, uddiyana and other variations. The exercises were a unique form of classical Hatha yoga performed for intestinal and glandular purification. *Yoga Mimansa* intersected the yoga exercises with modern science. It included detailed descriptions of these and other yogic techniques, and had both a 'scientific' and a 'semi-scientific' section. This made it the first para-medical exploration of yoga.

Buddha encompassed more classical yogic techniques as the 1930s progressed. Influences like *Yoga Mimansa*, with its exposition of classical yogic abdominal postures, became more relevant as he expanded his practice of muscle control to an extensive practice of yogic asanas. Eventually he realized the novelty of combining multiple asanas with muscle control in a performance.

From 1931 to 1935, Buddha also transitioned from being a student to becoming a teacher himself, mostly for foreigners and the colonial elite. The aspirations which Buddha wrote about in his letter came into fruition as he began to travel and perform abroad.

26

BODY PERFECTION COMPETITION

I find Buddha, along a corridor, inside the d'Orsay museum in Paris. It's L'Age
d'airain, The Age of Bronze, a life-size sculpture by Auguste
Rodin. I couldn't place it when I'd first seen it in Calcutta, inside Bishnu's first
floor room at 4/2 Rammohan Roy. There, on the top row, in the corner, was
Buddha Bose. He's standing, with his head cocked up over his shoulder, one arm
raised, and wearing nothing but a leaf to hide his privy, everything else exposed
in a frontal nude pose. Buddha's body is
'Most Beautiful' in the pose; he'd won the contest to prove it.

Bishnu and Buddha went to London by boat in the summer of 1932.[1] The two were fairly young: Bishnu was twenty-nine years old and Buddha nineteen. Bishnu's trip was paid for by his father Bhagabati, who provided travel stipends to his children; Buddha's was paid for by his Uncle Hopkins. Unlike their later and more notable travels, the trail of their '32 voyage to London was sparsely written about.'[2]

Bishnu and Buddha had different reasons for travelling to London. Bishnu's motives were written about the previous year in the letter Buddha sent to his brother Dennis: 'My Uncle [Bishnu] may soon go to England to be a barrister. He says he will take me with him positively.'

Bishnu may have been looking into possibilities for work in London or more schooling. In his passport, he listed his profession as 'Probationer Lawyer'. It also noted a 'visible distinguishing mark', a 'scar on right side of forehead', from, of course, motorcycle exploits.[3]

In London, Buddha went 'to meet his English mother'.[4] It had been sixteen years since he last saw her. Chitralekha, Buddha's former daughter-in-law, wrote of his attempt to tell her the story, saying, 'It must have been an intensely emotional moment in his life because *Baba* (Buddha) stopped relating anything further that day to me; he was choked with emotions.'

Emily and 'Uncle Edward' Hopkins lived in Brixton at Effra Mansions, outside London. Buddha would tell others that his father encouraged him to go to London (showing some sort of reconciliation), but he 'was dreaming of an Indian mother. He kept wondering how he would greet her ... should he shake hands or what?' When they met for the first time since she'd left him as a toddler, Buddha saw she looked British, and turned away. 'No, this cannot be my mother,' he thought. Then his mother came to him and said, 'I know you are my neglected child,' and touched him. At this moment, Buddha recalled, 'I knew what a real mother was.'[5]

The meeting provided closure on a painful part of his personal life, as his relationships with his mother, brother and sister were restored. Buddha also met his stepfather, 'Uncle Edward' on this trip.

For Bishnu, the biographical record states he 'went to England in 1932 for further studies on physical culture'. There was no indication of him pursuing a law career.[6] They may have visited popular physical cultural gymnasiums and met with other physical culturists of the time. For instance, the popular *Health and Strength* magazine headquarters were located in London. Photographs of Bishnu and his students would soon appear in the magazine.

In 1933, Bishnu travelled to Burma, taking a large group of physical culturists and other performers. With an eye on the Burmese performances, Bishnu had trained a young Bengali swimmer, Prafulla Ghosh, to break the world record of continuous time in a pool in Calcutta. 'Now my troupe and I are taking Prafulla Ghosh to Rangoon where he is scheduled to swim for 50 hours straight.'[7] Also part of the troupe were his nephew Bijoy Kumar Mullick and Buddha Bose.

In a short biography about the event, Bijoy included the fact he had earned the name 'The Mystic Muscle Controller' from the mayor of Rangoon who 'presented him with a gold wrist watch for his wonderful feats'.[8] Buddha also mentioned the Burma trip, saying he had 'been awarded several gold medals' for having given exhibitions.[9]

In May 1935, *The Calcutta Municipal Gazette* showcased a five-page article with photographs titled 'What Physical Culture Has Made of Them'.[10] Buddha, Bishnu, Bijoy and Keshub Sen Gupta (the co-author of *Muscle Control and Barbell Exercises*), along with fifteen others, most of them students of Bishnu, were

featured. They were 'widely known in the Physical Culture world', including
Moni Roy, 'The Finest Gymnast of India'.[11] Along with the two pages of
photographs were biographies of Buddha and Bishnu. Buddha's, twice the
length of the others, read in part:

> BUDDHA BOSE: He has appeared in the Matriculation examination this
> year from the Calcutta Academy. He was the finest specimen in the 'Body
> Beautiful' Competition held on the 4th December, 1934, at the Corinthian ...
> Dr. B. C. Law has presented him with a Sunbeam Motor Cycle. He
> entertained His Excellency Sir John Anderson, the Governor of Bengal,
> several times last year and tore in his presence three and a half packets of
> cards packed together and obtained from him a certificate of appreciation.[12]

There were several narrative themes in this biography that would be
repeated over time, by Buddha or on his behalf. In particular, the 'most beautiful
body' competition would become a staple in their publicity and certainly a
claim to fame. It was included in the first paragraph of Bishnu's introduction
to Buddha's 1938 book, *Key to the Kingdom of Health through Yoga*, Volume 1: 'In
a Body Perfection Competition held in India, Buddha Bose, out of more than
200 entrants, was unanimously selected by the judges as possessing the most
symmetrical and perfectly developed body.'[13]

Some would refer to this period as a 'cult' to develop 'India's most perfectly
developed man'.[14] *A Muscle Cult* (1930) and *A Quest For the Perfect Physique* (1936)
were the titles of books by the Indian K.V. Iyer, right alongside *Suryanamaskar*
(1937).[15] Buddha echoed the sentiment:

> I have seen hundreds of physical culturists with mighty muscles, sports
> men of great efficiency, powerful wrestlers, champion swimmers and
> clever boxers with immense powers of endurance and have respected the
> determination and ability which produce their skill. Personally, I have been
> more interested in well-balanced bodies with fairly developed muscles,
> having the bloom of youth and beauty and tinge of power in them, and I
> feel that there are many persons who will agree with me in this.[16]

Another repeated theme in the biography was Buddha's performances of
strongman feats. These included steel rod-bending with the throat and tearing
a deck of cards. Bishnu wrote that Buddha 'amazed me, and the public as well
by tearing two and a half packets of cards' in half with his bare hands. Five

years later, this particular feat of strength, which used an iron-like grip with a slight twist of the deck, had increased to 'three and a half packets of cards'.[17]

Despite Buddha's occupation changing from 'student' to 'physical instructor' between 1932 and 1935, he was not yet seen as a man. The *Gazette's* biography described Buddha as 'the first boy' with isolated control of 'the Obliques Abdomines', and also 'the first boy' who 'demonstrated rod-bending by throat'. Buddha was younger not only in age but also in appearance and demeanor.

The *Gazette's* language reflected the period's colonialism. It was obvious that Buddha, by way of Bishnu's prodding, directed his services to the colonial Europeans in Calcutta, and a class of wealthy Indians, known as babus. The well-known clients were also known for their extravagant spending, like gifting a Sunbeam motorcycle to their physical instructor!

SOME CALCUTTA ATHLETES

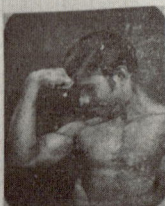 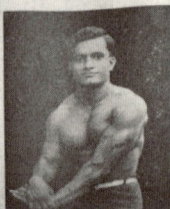 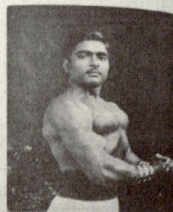

RANJIT BOSE   NANU BOSE   LALIT ROY

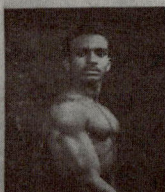 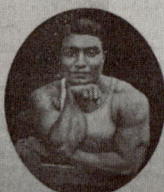 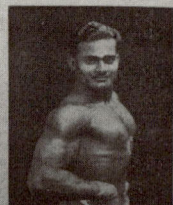

KAMAKHYA GANGULY   BISHNU GHOSH   MONI ROY

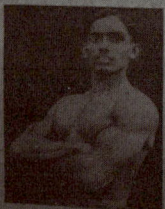 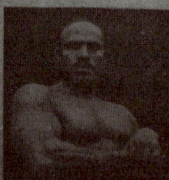 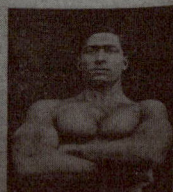

SUSHIL MUKHERJEE   J. K. SHIR   KISHARI SEN-GUPTA

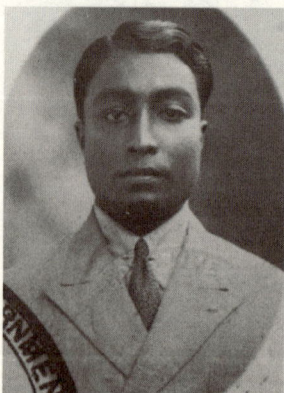 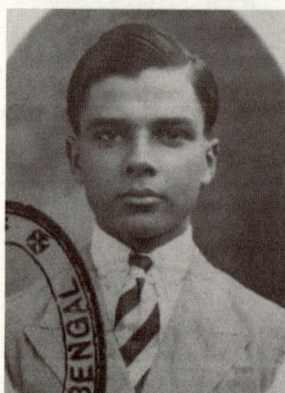

Top: Bishnu Ghosh surrounded by students and contemporaries, 1935.
Lower left: Bishnu Charan Ghosh. Lower right: Buddha Lal Bose, 1932.
Source: Calcutta Municipal Gazette; British Library (London).

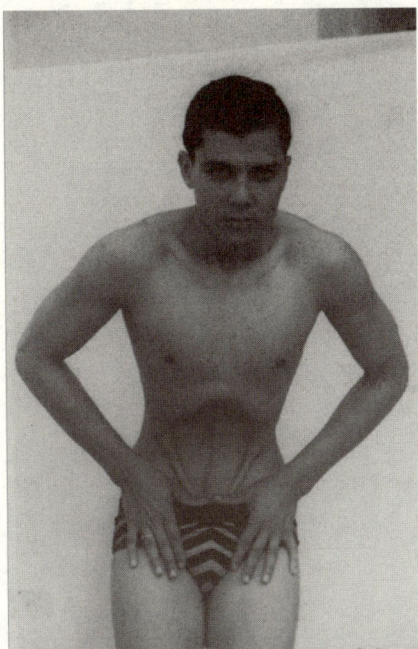

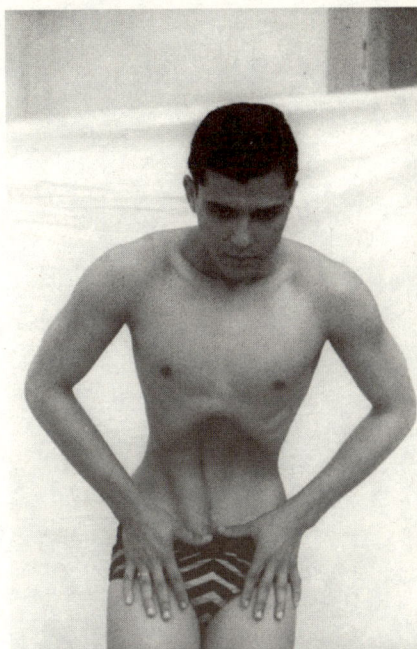

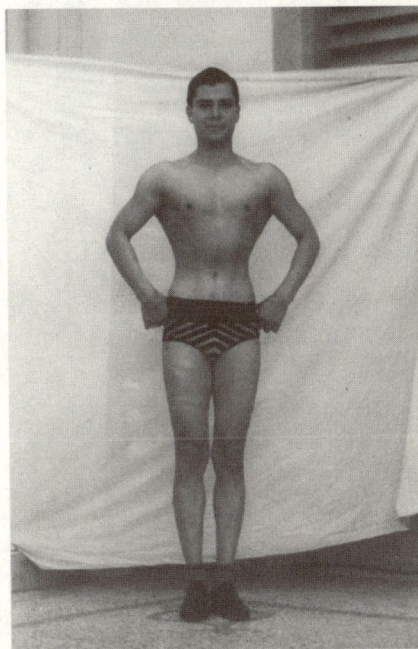

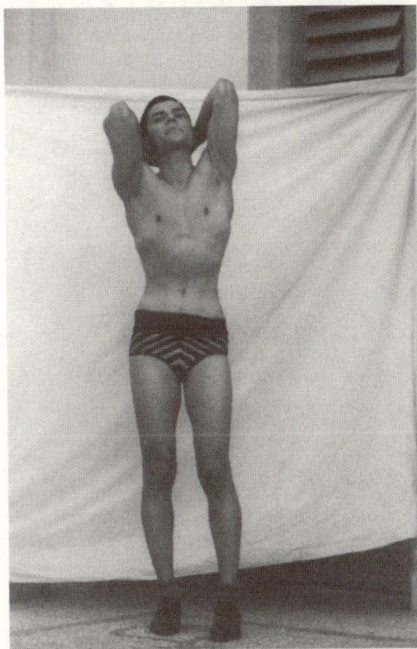

Buddha Bose as Most Beautiful Body, 1932. Theos Bernard Papers.

Courtesy of the Bancroft Library (Berkeley, CA).

PART FOUR

THE PHYSICAL–SPIRITUAL SYNTHESIS

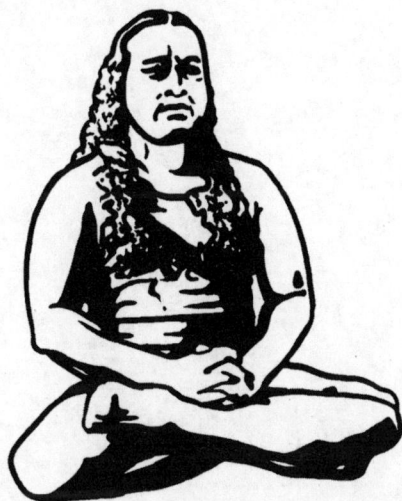

PART FOUR

THE PHYSICAL-SPIRITUAL SYNTHESIS

27

YOGODA AND HATHA YOGA

In a 1935 photo spread printed in the *Calcutta Municipal Gazette*, Bishnu was in the centre of the page, while his students surrounded him. Underneath his photo, the caption read, he 'who needs no introduction'. By this time, Bishnu was well known in Calcutta for his physical feats of strength and muscle control. A short biography followed:

> BISHNU GHOSH: The founder and physical director of Ghosh's College of Physical Education at 4/2, Rammohan Roy Road, Calcutta. He is a Science Graduate and a Bachelor of Law of the University of Calcutta. He learned the art of muscle control from his elder brother Swami Yogananda, A.B., who has been in the U.S.A. for the past 14 years teaching people the art of physical culture through 'Hatha Yoga'. Ghosh has trained hundreds of boys during the last few years.[1]

In 1934, Bhagabati Ghosh had bought the house at 4/2 Rammohan Roy Road.[2] One street over from their home at 4 Garpar Road, the new home was almost directly behind the other. Soon after, Bishnu relocated 'Ghosh's College of Physical Education' to this larger property. Bishnu's biography in the *Gazette* mentioned one important person – 'his elder brother Swami Yogananda' – even though, when it was written in May 1935, Yogananda's return to Calcutta had not yet been finalized. Bishnu had already begun the promotion of Yogananda's eventual homecoming. Also striking was how willingly Bishnu adapted the meaning of Hatha yoga to represent what Yogananda was teaching in America. It may have been the first appropriation of Hatha yoga. Yogananda, and later Bishnu and Buddha, would adjust and adapt Hatha yoga to fit the spiritual and physical exercise needs of the people they encountered and taught in the spirit of pragmatism. Bishnu read the pamphlets which Yogananda published in America and noted the much-used term 'Yogoda' to describe his popular system. However, the term would not make as much sense to a reader in Calcutta as the 'art of physical culture through Hatha yoga'.

The origins of Yogoda are mysterious. In his 1946 *Autobiography*, Yogananda mentioned that he 'had discovered in 1916' the principles of 'a unique system of physical development'. He started to call these physical exercises Yogoda while he was in the USA. According to Yogananda, the word Yogoda was derived from combining 'yoga' with the morpheme 'da', which means 'impart' or 'that which gives'.[3] Later, when someone argued with Yogananda that yoga did not have an 'o' at the end, and his title should be 'Yogada' in order to signify yoga, he brushed it off with the simple response, 'For us it's fine.'[4]

When Yogananda described Yogoda in the early 1920s, he reasoned that the body 'could be recharged through the direct agency of human will', the 'prime mover'. The practice of Yogoda would 'renew' one's 'bodily tissue' without 'burdensome apparatus or mechanical exercises'. The mental focus of willing is the body's 'life force'. It was 'centred in man's medulla oblongata' and could be 'consciously and instantly recharged' from an 'unlimited supply of cosmic energy'.[5]

At a glance, Yogoda did not seem to be based 'on the principles' of either classical 'Hatha yoga or early twentieth century postural yoga'. Some exercises were based on physical culture, including swinging and trunk twisting exercises, but 'using one's hands to stimulate the medulla oblongata is something else entirely'.[6] Within a broader perspective of modern yoga asana practice, which included dynamic movement, it fit perfectly.[7]

As for the Western physical culture influence, different muscle exercises had been impressed upon Yogananda in his youth. The Athenaeum Institution 'had a wrestling gymnasium on Garpar Road', which he had attended. Yogananda would give 'sideline advice' to help a 'wrestler gain the advantage' in a match. 'The coaching he was doing was coming spontaneously to his mind', so he asked to wrestle as well. They thought he was too small, but the wrestlers 'agreed to teach him' anyway. Later, he brought friends and taught them a 'special set of muscular exercises'.[8]

Satyananda mentioned that 'a book on physiology written by a German author' (most likely J.P. Müller) 'fell into Yogananda's hands' around 1915.[9] The techniques provided by Müller were widespread around the globe and the book went through many imprints after its first edition in 1904.[10] Its information concerning 'muscle-building techniques' was what Yogananda was looking for and they 'helped substantially to shape the Yogoda techniques'.[11] The exercises were similar to Yogoda and followed a similar format, but the Muller exercises did not employ progressive muscle relaxation like Yogoda, with its alternation of tension and relaxation ('Tense with will; relax with feel' was the 'motto all through the exercises').[12] The format of relaxation given by Max Sick (in *Muscle Control*) was compatible with the relaxation instructions laid down by Yogananda for his Yogoda exercises.[13]

However, Yogananda was also said to have integrated the progressive 'tense, stretch and relax' system based on the observation of cats. Yogananda had tried 'all kinds of muscle pumping exercises to develop and improve the strength of his body', but he thought, 'there must be some better way of exercising'. He observed how 'immediately upon rising ... the cat stretched its body' which gave Yogananda the idea of tensing exercises. Each morning and evening, he began to stretch, himself in this way and discovered that he 'felt so much more life' in his body after the stretch Later on, it became the first Yogoda lessons.[14]

At its most basic level, Yogoda employed tension with a particular body point in mind, along with a mental push. This was followed by using the will to relax; with a feeling of awareness and expansion of the mind.

Yogananda showed an aptitude for innovation in his ability to create a unique system for wider appeal. From the Kriya yoga practices, he incorporated mental concentration, including sounds and visualisations. From Hatha yoga, certain postures were modified. Common free-hand exercises, both indigenous and European, were also included to create a popular sequence.

In America, the Yogoda exercises eventually became a complete set of physical exercises that worked on different parts of the body in a systematic way. They were later called Energization Exercises. During his extensive tours of the United States, the Yogoda exercises, which he had first taught at the Ranchi School for Boys, served as an introductory practice for Americans. This system taught focus and introduced an internal physical-mental practice. After this was assimilated, Yogananda went on to teach the more subtle techniques of Kriya yoga, both individually and later to groups.

An early disciple of Yogananda, Oliver Black, first met Yogananda in 1931. Black was a self-described 'hypochondriac' who 'took aspirins for headaches, and laxative pills, and probably would have taken tranquilizers if they'd had them'.[15] Yogananda 'set me straight', Black said:

He changed the whole direction of my life. Haphazardly, I had studied the yoga physical exercise – Hatha yoga. I had listened to all the wise men from the East who came through Detroit, for whenever they lectured I was in the audience. They all said the same thing: 'Go within; learn to meditate.' But they never told me how. I'm an American and I was impatient for results. I wanted them right way. Yogananda taught me that important things aren't achieved overnight.

'You have to do the work,' Yogananda told him, which begins with the physical. Asked to describe the 'formula' that Yogananda taught him, Black snorted and replied, 'Shortcuts, again. Everybody wants a shortcut. There aren't any.'[16] He provided a pragmatic example, stating that 'yoga isn't a religion' but 'a science' and that the 'law of cause and effect applies' to its practice. 'It's a fact.'

By stretching the nerves you lessen the tension. Yoga is for everybody, not just a few rare individuals. It helps adolescents with posture, complexion and growing problems; it definitely helps them overcome teenage inferiority complexes. Older people get all the benefits of calisthenics without any of the drawbacks. We can do all these exercises if we're taught properly.

The key to the practice, Black said, was 'to learn how to breathe correctly', something which 'yogis knew 5,000 years ago'. Even as he reached his mid-seventies, he still felt the practices were necessary. 'I stand on my head every day, and always do a combination of at least six to seven exercises daily. I meditate, in lotus posture, and I find the shoulder stand as invigorating as a cocktail – without the stick.'[17]

28

YOGODA AT RANCHI

'We are arriving at Ranchi in a half an hour,' I jot down in my journal. 'From the train station, we'll walk straight out about a half a mile to the entrance of the Ranchi School for Boys founded by Yogananda.'

Along with me are Pavitra Shekhar Bose (the grandson of Buddha and great grandson of Bishnu), Ida Jo and Scott Lamps. Ida and Scott are American yoga teachers.

After a cold night on the train, we all just want to move. None of us have any idea what to expect once we reach the place. I've done very little research on it, other than knowing generally where it is, and of course, its significance. We invited Pavitra to come along with us, and even though Yogananda was his great uncle, he too was unfamiliar with the place.

I had found references to other travellers who had made pilgrimages to Ranchi, mostly through groups led by Swami Kriyananda of America and other followers of Yogananda. I half-expected to find a couple of old shacks, and perhaps a guardsman or two on the grounds.

When we arrive, the entrance is open. We step into the Ranchi school, Yogoda Satsanga, and are greeted with wonderful blooming flowers – roses of many colors and perfumed jasmine. Deciduous palms and trees line a clean gravel walkway. After a week in the urban blight of Calcutta, it is an amazing sight to behold. But there isn't much time to take it in. Instead, what catches my eye is a man doing movements in front of a large, white, octagonal marble temple. It seems odd, sort of like tai chi, but more upright and not as refined in movement. A few steps in, the path opens onto a large grassy field where about thirty persons are performing the same exercises.

'Yogoda!' I realize. This is the first time I have encountered individuals

doing the practice. With its smooth bodily flows, it seems more similar to
the movements of Daoist qigong, or viewed from a postural-movement yoga
perspective, one of the first dynamic yoga asana practices developed within
modern India.

We drop our overnight bags to the side of the clearing and join in the
movements on the well-manicured lawn facing the newly built temple.
It has been one hundred years and the Yogoda exercises are still practised
every morning on the Ranchi ashram grounds at 7.30 a.m. After finishing
the exercises, the people head inside a large hall, leaving their shoes outside.
We follow. No one stops us. In fact, no one even bothers to notice us. It is
apparently just pure acceptance of whatever physical manifestations show up
in this place! The group is mostly Indian, with about a dozen persons standing
out as monks, dressed in long orange robes. We go inside the meditation hall,
meditate for an hour with various chants and intervals of silence, and then
it is over. Pavitra stays in the hall for a longer meditation, while I wander the
grounds looking for the past.

In Ranchi, and previously for a year in Dihika, Yogananda first applied the
Yogoda techniques to students. The boys at the school responded 'wonderfully
to this training', wrote Yogananda. With it, they were able to develop 'the
ability to shift the life energy from one part of the body to another part'.
This translated into being able to hold yoga postures and the ability 'to sit
in perfect poise in difficult body postures. They performed feats of strength
and endurance which many adults could not equal.'[1] Swami Pranabananda of
Benares, the 'saint with two bodies', visited Ranchi to view 'the picturesque
outdoor classes, held under the trees, and saw in the evening that young boys
were sitting motionless for hours in yoga meditation'. Yogananda wrote, 'it is
not a novelty' to see the boys 'sitting for an hour or more in unbroken poise,
the unwinking gaze directed to the spiritual eye'.[2]

When Yogananda left for America in 1920, he remained in contact with the
Ranchi school through letters. In the early 1930s, 'the patron of the Ranchi
school', the elder maharajah of Kasimbazar, had 'left for the afterworld'.
An 'anxiety set in on the work and operations of the Ranchi Brahmacharya
Vidyalaya because of financial lack'.

His boyhood friend Satyananda, diligently ran the school, and wrote of
Yogananda in early 1935, 'fifteen years had passed, and there was no sign of him

coming home'. The stress overcame Satyananda at one point, and he took leave to 'recuperate away from the ashram'. When he had recovered and returned, an 'unexpected letter' arrived from London in July of 1935.

Yogananda wrote, 'Though it may be unbelievable, it is true. I am in London and will be seeing the land of India very soon.'[3]

Eighty years later, Ida, Scott and I fill our afternoon at Ranchi sitting on the manicured lawn beside the temple. We work on editing the recently discovered 1938 Buddha Bose album, which we would publish a few months later, as well as composing a beginners' class of postures. At 4 p.m. we head over to one of the original buildings for tea, under a silent air of observance, then reboard the train for Calcutta.

We arrive the next morning at the Howrah Railway station. This is the same station in Calcutta where a 1935 photo shows Yogananda being welcomed by his family and others upon returning to his homeland, fifteen years after he had left for America. Photos and a video of the event show an immensely proud younger brother Bishnu, who stands beside Yogananda, eagerly welcoming his brother home.

29

YOGANANDA FROM AMERICA

It had been fifteen years since Yogananda took the month-long voyage from his homeland to America via the ocean liner named City of Sparta. He had been so eager to go that he took the first passenger boat available from Calcutta after the close of the First World War.[1] He arrived in America on 19 September 1920 but did not have immediate widespread success. He brought along his book *Science of Religion*, which he described as 'not speculative, but practical, even when dealing with the utmost reaches of metaphysics' and which 'offered a clue to the universe'.[2] He began teaching classes, at first for free. He relied upon a lump sum of money he had brought with him, additional funds sent by family and other financial support 'by collections, and classes later on'.[3]

Yogananda modelled his first years after Vivekananda and had moderate success on the East Coast while living in Boston. He went on multi-city tours that were focused on a unified religious message. A 'generous check' from his father supported him during the first three years, and afterwards, he integrated into the capitalistic system, charging membership fees and establishing a presence with his teachings.[4] When he started to take in funds he must have believed it would be quite a bit of money, because in August of 1923 he wrote a letter to his father stating that he was elated that he could 'make a fortune and then return to India', according to British officials.[5]

He taught an introductory practice of his muscle-will system of physical perfection, Yogoda. His first office was located at 30 Huntington Avenue in Boston, and he lived in the home of a middle-aged couple, named Mildred and Dr Lewis, who were among his first devotees. A few years later, he brought over his boyhood friend Dhirananda, who proceeded to produce written material for their Yogoda Satsanga organization.[6] The early written teachings were 'practical methods for all around culture' which were 'suited to the spirit of the modern age of realism'. The new materials also secured another revenue stream.[7]

The British Consulate began to surveil Yogananda's activities as early as 1923, when they intercepted a letter he had written to his father, Bhagabati.[8] Yogananda was 'careful to avoid reference to political questions'. Still, the Washington DC British Embassy made the unfounded claim that Yogananda had 'seditious tendencies', because he was the 'recipient' of information that the British had spied upon and was 'reputed to be an agent of Gandhi'. Rather than having 'openly preached any revolutionary doctrines', the British consulate stated, 'his notoriety being mainly due to the way in which he obtains money from audiences attracted by his mysticism'.[9] The investigation turned up nothing, except for sarcasm. 'Yogananda is not doing much good for India as his compatriots are either laughing at him or disgusted,' said one British official. If Yogananda 'became too interested in politics, his fellow countrymen of the agitator variety will soon ask him to subscribe to revolutionary funds'.[10]

Yogananda stood out in crowds, and as the *Washington Post* wrote, he was 'undoubtedly effective by reason of the strong contrast of the brilliant robe and the dark flowing hair'.[11] He integrated mainstream Christianity into his teachings by highlighting mystical quotations from the New Testament.[12] His initial appeal was aimed at the very spiritually inclined, including those who were wealthy and influential, as in the case of Luther Burbank, the famous botanist who lived in California.

Yogananda relocated to Los Angeles in 1925, where he laid down an organizational church presence and founded the Mt. Washington Education Center. Around this time, a magazine called *East-West* began circulating,[13] published by Yogananda with the symbol of the lotus to signify 'the single spiritual eye of meditation'.[14] Early on, the maga zine was mostly promotional in focus, with pleas for 'monthly donation pledges', and testimonials from 'prominent Yogoda students'.[15]

Praise of Yogoda overflowed from the testimonials in *East-West* magazine. One stated, 'I know now how to draw the unlimited storehouse of Cosmic Energy.'[16] Another explained that it took just 'one lesson' to be healed from four years of insomnia and went on to give advice 'to those who have not found the key to life and its so-called mysteries, I beg you will not miss this opportunity'.[17] The little politics *East-West* provided were covert, such as a universalist quote by the socialist Eugene V. Debs, a former populist candidate for president,[18] or the inclusion of writings from the spiritual side of Mahatma Gandhi's message.[19] Photos of Yogananda from this period, the 'roaring 20s' in America, show a more flamboyant side. He wore the attire of a businessman at times and owned nice cars. An accumulation of wealth was visible as he travelled the promotional circuit.

By 1926, Yogananda had renewed his passport twice. He applied again and was 'authorized' to travel abroad to places, including Europe and India, for an 'indefinite' length of stay.[20] However, nothing would come to fruition from these early plans.

An early high point for Yogananda came in January 1927, when he was in Washington DC for a series of talks and a meeting with the president. The *Washington Herald* of DC stated, 'crowds are flocking to hear Swami Yogananda' and his 'remarkable series of twelve public lectures at Washington Auditorium', in which his audiences each night have increased.[21] One claim said there were 'audiences numbering five thousand persons'.[22] The British Consulate wrote that the 'Swami's only reference to political matters [in the speeches] was to invoke a blessing upon the British and all "good" governments'.[23]

The British Intelligence Bureau in New Delhi picked up on the meeting between Yogananda and President Coolidge when it was reported in the Indian newspaper *Hindustan Times*, and asked 'whether this newspaper report [was] correct'. The clerks clearly expected the claim to be false since they included the postscript, 'The British Embassy in Washington may be amused!' The New Delhi British officials probably were not amused when they learned that yes, Yogananda was presented to President Coolidge by the Second Secretary of the British Embassy, John Balfour. It was said to be 'the first time that a Swami has been received officially by a President' of the United States.[24] Yogananda declared his interest in America 'because it is a very powerful factor in the world and because its people are desirous of improving themselves in every way'.[25] Yogananda pressed two issues in his interview with Coolidge: vegetarianism and world peace.

Of Coolidge, Yogananda said, 'I found him looking in good health,' and felt that he 'required health and calmness in order to discharge his many important duties'.[26] Even so, Yogananda advised the President 'to follow a vegetarian diet'.[27] In his talk with President Coolidge, the Swami said, 'It is only spiritual understanding between nations that can bring lasting peace.'[28]

To which Coolidge replied simply, 'This is very true.'[29]

While in Florida in 1928, Yogananda, was embroiled in a mini scandal involving lessons which provoked reactionary mindsets. Once again, the British Information Office followed the coverage, which lasted into 1929. In Florida, the chief of police stated that Yogananda was 'notified that he must not give any more lectures in Miami' due to complaints from husbands. The Miami city manager explained the situation to the British Consul in a letter. 'Unfortunately he is what is considered in this part of the country, a colored man.' And given the publicity of the case, 'and a strong public sentiment against a colored person acting in the capacity of teacher to white women', the manager 'considered that the Swami was in great danger of suffering bodily harm from the populace, if he attempted to give any more lectures'. [30]

This was a low point for Yogananda, who agreed to stop lecturing but wanted 'to clear his name and reputation' and 'blamed the local press for stirring up trouble' in Miami'. [31]

The notorious Hearst publications claimed he was making '\$35 each from more than 200 Miami women for instruction of a love cult'. Yogananda responded, 'I am not a love cult member,' and vowed to 'stay and fight it out'. Then, more craziness emerged when the police official who interviewed Yogananda reported that the latter tried to hypnotize him.

Yogananda eventually left Miami, calling it a 'crucifixion', and went to New York, where he continued to battle through the media. He published a lengthy article with the title, 'Yellow Journalism Versus Truth'. The scrum with the media was uncharacteristic of the style and type of Yogananda's writings. Even while battling 'misconceptions', Yogananda's other articles stayed on his message that 'Practice is Essential' and 'Truth Not Eastern Nor Western'. [32]

After New York, Yogananda seemingly tired of the US and left for Cuba, and then later, Mexico. The time he spent in Chapala, Mexico, seemed magical in his poem 'Ode to Lake Chapala'. [33] A photo showed Yogananda on a boat on Lake Chapala, outside Guadalajara, and he wrote, 'The Mexican people are spiritually inclined.' [34] He was successful in establishing a centre for 'a staunch Yogoda student of Mexico City' and was presented by the British Legation to Portes Gil, the president of Mexico, a meeting similar to the one he had at the White House in 1927.

A few months later, he tried to return to the US, but had trouble crossing the border. He had been issued a passport which was good until July 1929, and 'valid for travelling to the United Kingdom and other European countries, but this endorsement was canceled' by the UK officials in New York City. [35] He was detained for being 'unable to secure documents required' by the immigration officials.

Yogananda gained reentry, but the lawyer working on his behalf was told that, because he had 'claimed the right to come to the US as a professor' or teacher, he would need to prove he had 'been acting as a professor' or teacher for 'two years immediately preceding the date of his application for admission'.[36] Yogananda knew this particular issue might come up again if he left the US; his ability to return was not certain. Nevertheless, the 1929 November/December issue of *East-West* printed a notice for an upcoming 'visit to India, combined with a trip around the world'. The issue stated, 'if enough members' committed to the voyage, Yogananda would 'lead the party' in September of 1930. However, just as the issue was reaching the Yogoda Satsanga members, the Wall Street Crash began on 24 October 1929. Yogananda himself, 'in order to support the work' of his Church, 'had to invest' in the stock market, and was caught up in some of the losses, along with his supporters.[37]

In the mid-thirties, when he was able to get the funding, mostly from a wealthy new disciple named James Lynn, he finally left the US for India. He had desired to return to India for so long, especially to see his family, Sriyukteswar, the Ranchi school and his friends.

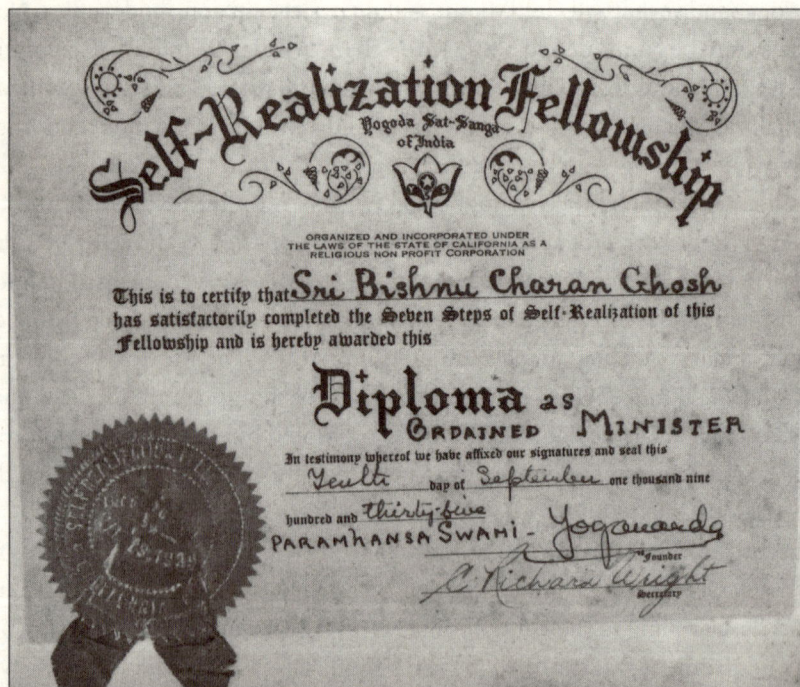

Bishnu Charan Ghosh, SRF Diploma, 1935.
Courtesy of Ghosh's Yoga College.

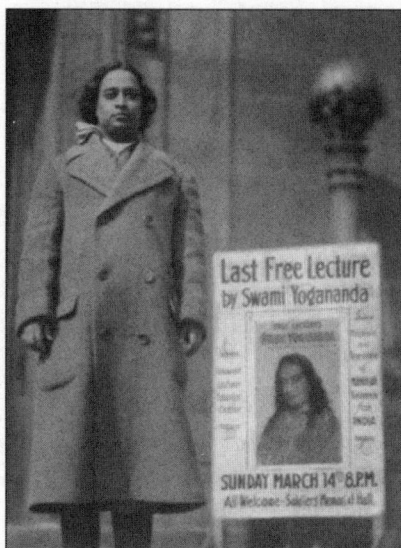

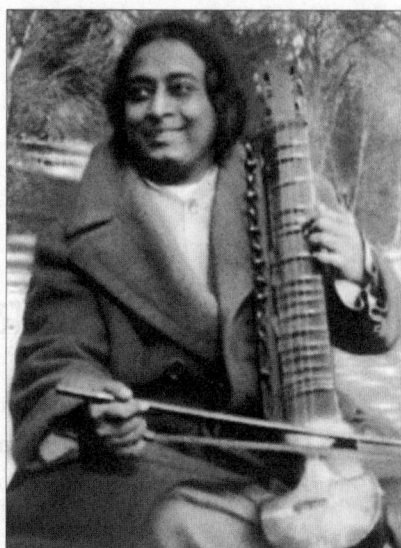

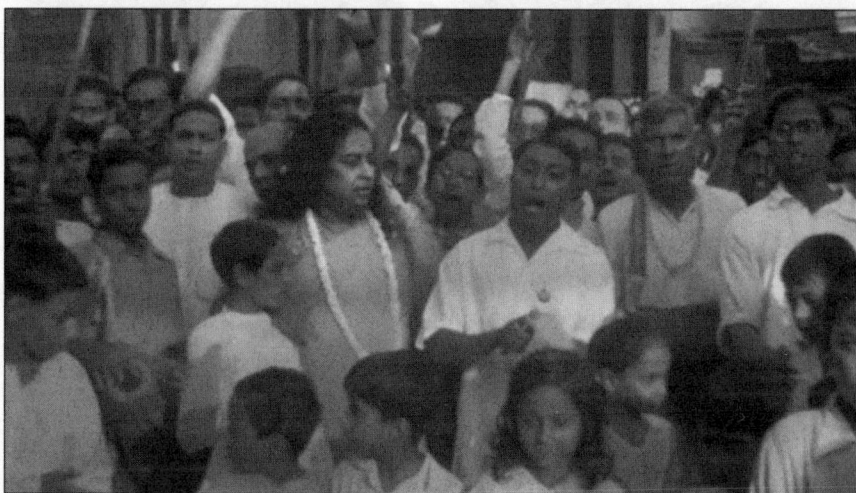

Clockwise from top left: Yogananda in Boston (circa 1921); Yogananda in America (1922); Yogananda with Bishnu & Ghosh children (Howrah Station, Calcutta, 1935).

Source: Wikimedia commons; courtesy of Ghosh's Yoga College.

30

PHYSICAL–SPIRITUAL SYNTHESIS

My brother Bishnu Charan is taking charge of physical culture and
myself taking charge of the spiritual side.[1]
– Yogananda

In the September of 1935, Yogananda was met by a throng of visitors at the Howrah railway station, across the river from Calcutta. Upon his arrival, he wrote that he 'found such an immense crowd assembled to greet him that for a while he was unable to dismount from the train'. He attributed it to 'London publicity', writing to his disciples, 'whatever goes in London, goes to India'. Since the important newspapers had provided a summary of his London lectures, he was 'now known all over India'.[2] The maharajah of Kasimbazar and Bishnu led the reception committee. Yogananda's 'welcome home' was also Bishnu's reintroduction to his brother.

When Yogananda had left Calcutta in 1920, Bishnu was a self-proclaimed '90 pound weakling'. Now, not only had he radically reshaped his body, but also 'made a mark in the domain of physical culture' and gained a reputation as one of the best trainers in Calcutta.[3] The 2015 movie *Awake* showed Yogananda walking alongside a beaming Bishnu with a group of children in front them. These included Bishnu's two young children, Ava Rani and Srikrishna.

After his arrival at Howrah station, Yogananda went to the new Ghosh family home at 4 Rammohan Roy Road in a Rolls Royce borrowed from the maharajah.[4] The entourage was adorned with garlands and included 'a line of automobiles and motorcycles', accompanied by the 'sound of drums and conch shells'.[5]

Just a few days after his arrival, Yogananda performed a group initiation into Kriya yoga for his family and close friends. In order to accommodate more people than could fit inside the family home, 'an outdoor lecture hall was created in the garden area on the north side' of the house. A 'canopy was hung and fabric was draped on all four sides', forming a gathering space on the lawn.[6] The 'enclosed hall' was on a portion 'of Bishnu's large open-air gymnasium in the north section of the compound' of his father's house.

Yogananda had the devotees sit 'on a large carpet that had been spread in the improvised hall', and his brother Sananda, who had been initiated by Sriyukteswar, 'demonstrated the technique' of Kriya for the new initiates.[7] Then Yogananda 'bestowed the sacred *diksha* (initiation)' on the devotees. This 'American-style session of giving Kriya yoga' was quite different than what had usually been a secret and one-on-one practice. This new Kriya yoga initiation included demonstrations by Yogananda, 'showing the technique personally and individually to everyone'. When asked about whether 'mass initiation' can 'produce the same result' as 'the secret affair between guru and disciple with its deep connection', Yogananda responded that it was necessary 'to throw the net far and wide, so that at least a couple of big fishes can be caught'.[8]

Bishnu was initiated into Kriya yoga with the others on 12 September 1935, certifying him as having 'completed the Seven Steps to Self-Realization' within the fellowship. He was now an 'Ordained Minister'. His certificate was signed by the founder, 'Paramhansa Swami Yogananda', and the secretary, Richard Wright. For Bishnu, the event was profound, a moment he would recall as when his elder brother became 'my *diksha* guru'.[9]

One week later, in a letter addressed from 'Ghosh's College of Physical Education' back to his disciples in America, Yogananda praised his brother Bishnu, who was taught the yoga exercises at his Ranchi school and now had '400 strong athletes' as his students. He remarked, 'I daresay you've never seen such prime of youth, as if their bodies were made in a factory.' And he was excited about having health and spiritual centres across India. 'We are going to do unprecedented work here,' he wrote.[10]

When Yogananda went back to India, his initial focus was on starting a Calcutta centre for his organization and getting the Ranchi school on good financial footing. However, once he arrived, Yogananda become so enamoured with Bishnu that he started to focus on how they could work together and combine their physical and spiritual training. The brothers quickly focused on how compatible their teachings were, at least theoretically. Bishnu saw Yogananda's 'widespread and immense influence' and Yogananda 'was also quite taken' by Bishnu's 'accomplished students of physical culture at his health and fitness centre'. Yogananda 'began to think that these physically fit youth and their leader Bishnu Charan would be able to bring new life into the work of Yogoda Satsanga in India'.[11] One practice was physically based, the other spiritually based. The idea resembled Vivekananda's proclamation for Bengalis, and Indians in general, to get spiritually, intellectually and physically stronger as a nation; they should study both the *Bhagavad Gita* and pump barbells.

Bishnu and Yogananda went straight ahead with the plan of combining the practices: 'We are shortly opening an extensive institution for the scientific physical training of all castes and creeds in Calcutta. After that, my plan is to open up health and spiritual centers all over Bengal and the principal provinces of India,' Yogananda told a reporter.[12]

Within a month of his return, a 'citizens' meeting' was organized for Yogananda to show 'appreciation of his services to country's cause'. The *Amrita Bazar Patrika*, one of the oldest daily newspapers in South Asia, described his reception and stated, 'In spite of inclement weather the Albert Hall was packed to suffocation on Saturday evening when a public reception was accorded to Swami Yogananda on his return to India from America after fifteen years of work there.'[13]

Albert Hall was built in 1888, and from 1890 until 1944, served as a theatre in Calcutta where large public events could be held. The 'main room of the venue' was of respectable size and held about 200 persons when packed.[14] In the mid-1940s, Albert Hall was renovated, and became known as the Coffee House. Located within the College Square area of Calcutta, the Coffee House holds a vivid role in Calcutta's more recent cultural history, though its older past is largely forgotten. Patriots held intellectual debates there during the nationalist period in the forties, and then later, avant-garde literary movements in the sixties were hatched over coffee and cigarettes (the latter is why Arup, my research guide, liked to arrange meetings for me there).[15]

The meetings held by Yogananda at Albert Hall in the thirties were 'spiritually eloquent', with speeches that 'mesmerized the entire crowd'.[16] During the first meeting, 'the venue was completely full with an audience eager to see and hear' Yogananda.[17] A few weeks after he reunited with his Guru Sriyukteswar in Serampore, Yogananda again spoke at Albert Hall in Calcutta.[18] 'Sriyukteswar consented to sit beside me on the platform', wrote Yogananda. He would glance towards his guru 'from time to time' during the address and recalled detecting 'a pleased twinkle in his eyes'.[19]

Yogananda brought along his nephew, Hare Krishna (a son of Sananda), for one of the meetings. During his lecture many devotees asked Yogananda to show them something so they could know God. They wanted a supernatural display, but Yogananda demurred. However, 'after repeated requests', Yogananda said, 'OK, I will show you something.' Yogananda had the 200 persons gathered in the hall clasp their hands together, fingers interlocked. He then told them 'to think of God, and concentrate on the brow point, between the eyebrows'. Yogananda counted from one to ten and 'everyone found their hands were locked. Nobody could separate their hands.' Then, after some time, Yogananda said, '*Om, shanti, shanti*, and everybody's hands came out.' Yogananda then explained that he had done it 'only for them to have faith in God'.[20] Yogananda lectured in English. He 'pushed aside the microphone' and faced the audience directly 'with a deeply resonating voice, powerful language and incomparable mannerisms and gestures'.[21] Those in Calcutta 'were able to catch a glimpse of the magic by which Swamiji had gained the endless praise and admiration of thousands and thousands' in America. Yogananda's initial talk was attended by dignitaries, such as Maharajah Santosh and the former mayor of Calcutta, Santosh Basu, who performed the introductions.[22]

The speech was 'highly lauded by newspapers and journals' and 'praise spread throughout the city'. Yogananda's 'presence caused a considerable stir in the minds and hearts of the people of Calcutta'.[23] In his speech he revealed his plans with Bishnu, 'I conceived the idea of starting *Brahmacharya* schools, health centers, which impart to men, women, and children of the world an all-around education of the full development of body, mind and soul. My mission of health and all-around uplift being not confined to the fancy-frozen boundaries of one nationality, I was divinely ordained to America.'[24]

'I pointed out to America that she was over-active and had a tendency towards being a colossal automaton and I also admitted that India had a tendency of being too calm and too religious.'[25] 'Now, having finished my work to my satisfaction in America, I have come to teach my practical health system and teachings' of Kriya yoga 'here in India'. Back in Calcutta, Yogananda told his fellow Indians, 'Yogoda is the modern and ancient system of body, mind and soul culture.'[26] Since Yogananda had successfully branded the term in America, he set out to do the same in India.

Reception To Yogananda

CITIZENS' MEETING

—oOo—

Appreciation Of His Services To Country's Cause

In spite of inclement weather the Albert Hall was packed to suffocation on Saturday evening when a public reception was accorded to Swami Yogananda on his return to India from America after fifteen years of work there. Raja Sir Manmathanath Ray Chaudhury of Santosh presided.

SEND YOUR BOY
TO
RANCHI BRAHMACHARYA VIDYALAYA

SWAMI YOGANANDA

Press release of Yogananda and Ranchi School.
Source: Amrita Bazar Patrika, Calcutta, 1935.

31

YOGODA AND MUSCLE CONTROL

In *Muscle Control*, Bishnu described how to employ the use of 'contraction' and 'relaxation of the body' during bodybuilding exercises. For example, one should 'contract all muscles simultaneously', then examine the body to 'find out if there is any muscle left uncontracted … one should feel the thrill of relaxation'. He stressed that for 'a well-developed body', one should relax progressively. 'Begin with the calf and the thigh and then gradually work upward', while making sure not to contract 'any muscle already relaxed when trying to relax another'. Contraction and relaxation complemented each other, and 'the first thing that should be kept in mind is that perfect relaxation of muscles is as good as hardest contraction to build up muscles'.[1]

Similarly, Yogananda had focused on the muscles when he had introduced Yogoda to America in the twenties. Under the headline 'Muscle Coordination', the 'remedy for all ills', he said, was 'the exercise of muscle will, or the concentration of the mind and will upon each muscle of the body individually, exercising them and bringing about a harmonious working of each in coordination with the others'. Regarding concentration, Yogananda clarified, 'I mean the focusing of mental energy on one point.'[2] Yogananda was also keen to place the concept in an age-old tradition, stating that this specific art of concentration had been 'known in India for 5,000 years'. Just ten minutes a day 'develops the muscles of his pupils by willpower alone'. It was a physical and spiritual system which used meditation and concentration to 'recharge the body battery' with a 'spiritualization of the body'.[3]

Bishnu and Yogananda's goal of spreading their system across India depended upon getting financiers. Bishnu had been able to gain assistance from a wealthy supporter, Yugal Kishor Birla, who was 'so impressed with Bishnu's work he purchased land and built a large gymnasium' for Bishnu in Ballygunge, a neighbourhood in south Calcutta.[4] The supporter was overjoyed that 'Bishnu Charan had made the discipline of high-level physical culture available for Bengali Hindu youths'. With the north Indian merchant's help, 'Bishnu Charan was able to found large centers for physical culture at the Jadavpur College, Banaras Hindu University and the Kangri Guru-Kula Ashram in Haridwar', with the instructors being 'graduates of Bishnu Charan's school'.[5] While in Benares, Bishnu took Yogananda to meet with Moni Roy, a student he had placed there as the director of Physical Education.[6]

Everything seemed to be in line, but their attempts to get financing from millionaire supporters in 'wealthy Marwari circles' failed. Bishnu put the onus on Yogananda for 'not being able to stop his heart from beating' in order to impress 'Kishor Birla and quite a few other wealthy Sheth' that had come together 'at Bishnu Charan's insistent effort'. They had wanted to see Yogananda demonstrate this 'extraordinary and inhuman ability'.[7] Yogananda's guru, Sriyukteswar, had frowned upon Yogananda's involvement with Bishnu and for having performances, 'particularly in wealthy Marwari circles'. This may have played a part in his inability to follow through.[8]

The two brothers may not have been determined enough when it came down to more practical matters. In America, Yogananda taught that using weights was useless and that 'dumbbells have been relegated to the woodpile, because they are not a natural means of exercise'. Simply exerting 'complete control of muscles by will power' yielded full results, stating that 'and when a seven-year-old child learns it he can carry a 200 pound man'.[9] While Yogananda was teaching this in America, Bishnu was in Calcutta using weights and co-authoring a book of barbell exercises. One biographer wrote that after Sriyukteswar died, Yogananda became 'more introverted than usual' and 'the vision he had of working with Bishnu Charan gradually faded and eventually disappeared'. As a 'remnant of that idea', they eventually selected 'a master of physical culture' from Bishnu's center to 'teach all sorts of athletic arts' at the Ranchi School for boys.[10]

In the fall of 1935, an advertisement was placed in a Calcutta newspaper atop a photo of Yogananda, with the headline 'Send Your Boy to Ranchi Brahmacharya Vidyalaya'. Just above the address to apply for a prospectus at the Yogoda Satsanga Headquarters (Lahiri Mahasaya Mission):

SPECIAL! Unique bodybuilding training will be conducted by famous physical culture experts of Bengal.[11]

All of the feats – both spiritual and physical – performed by Yogananda, Bishnu and his students were presented as Yogoda. In Ranchi that September, Yogananda noticed that 'a large conference of *rajas*' had assembled a 'huge *pandal*' (an open air tent-like structure). He 'expressed the wish to hold a public lecture' at the space in order 'to raise funds for the school'. He was granted a time to make this happen. Alongside his speech, 'an added attraction was to be a physical culture demonstration by Bishnu and his students'.[12] Tickets were sold and handbills distributed. 'The notices proclaimed that Swami Yogananda, recently returned from America, would lecture on Hindu religion. And that there would also be an extraordinary gymnastic demonstration by Bishnu Ghosh, nationally known physical culture director, and his students.' Shortly thereafter, Yogananda lectured 'under the auspices' of Calcutta University, where he had had his experience with Mahendranath, and where he had earned a bachelor of Arts degree for the Indian Philosophical Congress. With 'European officials' in attendance, 'Yogananda and his brother Bishnu and nephew Bijoy and Mr Buddha Bose gave wonderful demonstrations of Yogoda feats and physical culture feats.'[13] Both events wound up being a success and set the formula for what they would repeat on a tour of south India.

32

MYSORE PALACE

Though Yogananda wanted BKS Iyengar to demonstrate the asanas abroad, it was Buddha Bose, Bishnu's student, who would perform all of the Hatha yoga asanas before Western audiences in a few years time. The Mysore meeting of the founders of the most popular asana-based systems of modern yoga inspired Buddha and Bishnu to make the voyage to America.

Yogananda wrote in *Autobiography of a Yogi* that, in November of 1935, he was able to stay as a guest of the state of Mysore and the Krishna Raja Wadiyar IV, in order to visit the 'enlightened and progressive realm' of the maharajah of Mysore.[1] Among those with Yogananda were his brother Bishnu, his nephew Bijoy Kumar Mullick and Buddha Bose. A woman from Ohio, Ettie Bletsch, and Richard Wright, Yogananda's secretary, were also there, as they had come over from America to help with tour logistics.

For the south Indian performances, Yogananda had a particular format in mind: a combination of his spiritual teachings alongside a physical performance, all grouped together and called Yogoda. Bishnu combined feats of strength and muscle control. The 'real tour in India has begun,' wrote Yogananda.[2]

First the group went to Bangalore for three days of performances. Thousands came out to 'listen to the Swami', with hundreds 'joining his classes'. One of the events was held at Chetty Town Hall and attended by a crowd of 3,000. The physical performance included 'demonstrations of "Yogoda", the action of will in the muscles, by the Swami's brother Bishnu Charan, and his two students'. Yogananda spoke and performed, drawing a 'glowing picture' of America and sharing his thoughts on 'the mutual benefits that could flow from exchange of the best features in the East and West'.[3] He talked about 'the action of will power and magnetism' and included an example for those who could 'accurately tune in with him'.

Yogananda, 'arousing the energy in their bodies', ordered for their hands to become clasped together, which they did, 'as if shackled by ropes'. This was the same demonstration he had given at Albert Hall in Calcutta, but this time, when he ordered them to release, all did 'except one man who was ailing' from conditions of the heart and stomach. Upon request, Yogananda used his hands to parlay 'soothing vibrations', and the pain vanished from the man whose hands thereafter unclasped. Yogananda explained that he 'merely served as a channel for the flow of the Cosmic Energy from God which has the power of healing'.[4] He gave *darshan*, utilized pranayam, and 'the rare yogic feats done by his disciples (Bishnu Charan, Buddha Bose and Bijoy Kumar Mullick) ... opened the eyes of many to the latent powers in man and how they can become patent'.[5]

After three days, the entire crew went to Mysore by train. Their first performance was at the maharajah's college on 18 November, and then at the Town Hall of Mysore on 20 November. Both events were met with 'wild acclamation and appreciation of his lecture and healings'.[6] In Mysore, Yogananda gave a talk titled 'Art of Living' during a meeting on 'spiritual utilitarianism'. Swami Vasananda thanked the maharajah for 'inviting the Swami (Yogananda) to the State of Mysore, as Swami Vivekananda, 40 years ago, was invited by the Mysore State'.[7] For two weeks, the group stayed at the Mysore Palace. 'Busy day and night,' Yogananda wrote, 'we are literally "idolized" here'.[8]

'They were invited by the Maharajah of Mysore for dinner,' Omkar Mullick tells me.[9]

By chance, while in Calcutta, I receive a message from Kavya Dutta, whose father, Omkar Mullick, was the son of Bijoy Kumar Mullick. Little has been written about Bijoy, and I am thankful for the invitation. The photo of Bijoy performing *nauli* is breathtaking, and I had heard from others that he became a kirtan singer, somehow integrating it with his strongman feats. Omkar goes on:

> After dinner at the Mysore Palace, the Maharajah told Swami Yogananda to show the powers of yoga as they were all yogis. Paramhansa said, 'Of course we can.' The Maharajah asked, 'What will you do?'
>
> Swami Yogananda called his twenty-seven-year-old nephew Bijoy Mullick to him and asked him to lie down on the ground. The nephew, my father, did what his uncle asked him to do. Then Paramhansa asked the Maharajah, 'How many servants do you have here right now?' The Maharajah replied,

'About 26 or 27.' Swami Yogananda told the Maharajah to call all of them into the room. So all the attendants were lined up in the room.

Now, the dining table was big enough to seat a minimum of 50 guests, and it had a marble table top. Swamiji asked the servants to pick up the marble table top and place it on Bijoy Mullick. The Maharajah was astounded and said, 'What are you doing? It weighs about 4 or 5 tons, the man will be crushed immediately!'

Bijoy, my father, understood he had to go into *kumbhaka*; he used to pass a three and a half ton roller on his chest. The table top was placed on Bijoy's chest and Paramhansa asked all those present to stand on the marble table top. My father realized he was in *kumbhaka*, but for how long could he stay?

His lungs would burst after a few seconds if he did not release his breath and then he would be crushed. This is where Paramhansa activated his will force. He came and stood at the my father's head and said, 'You release everything and start singing *Bhojo Hari Radha Krishna*.' My father started his *kirtan* of *Bhojo Hari Radha Krishna*.

Anyone else would have died, but my father kept on singing because his guru was standing at his head. When he finished, the people got off and the marble slab was removed. The Maharajah was so impressed he took off his gold chain and presented it to my father as token of appreciation.[10]

'Do you still have the gold chain?' I ask.

Omkar replies, 'That gold is lost – I have lost all things.'

I ask, 'What was this *kirtan*, *Bhojo Hari Radha Krishna*?' To my delight, Mukul Dutta, the *yogacharya* taught by Bishnu in the sixties, who is accompanying me for the interview, breaks out into a rendition of the song with Omkar.

Afterwards, I ask about *kumbhaka*, the retention of breath, and how Bijoy had been able to sing while holding his breath?

'When my father was singing he was not holding his breath,' Omkar replies. 'Naturally when you hold your breath you cannot pronounce anything. It is physiology. This was actually a spiritual thing. It was the spiritual power of Paramhansa Yogananda.'

I wonder aloud if this was the impetus for Bijoy to begin singing kirtan with such a passion?

'Yes,' he replies, 'when he came back from Mysore he was totally changed. He became a singer, left being a bodybuilder' and 'started singing all of Yogananda's Krishna songs.'

We look at photos. One in particular shows the honoured guests seated outside the Mysore Palace: Yogananda with Bishnu, Buddha and Bijoy. A group of men are standing behind them, whom I do not recognize. 'That person,' Omkar tells me, pointing to the man standing behind Yogananda, 'is B. K. S. Iyengar.'

The same Maharajah of Mysore who invited Yogananda and the others to Mysore also supported Tirumalai Krishnamacharya, the architect of yoga *vinyasa*, which combined breathing with a dynamic movement of yoga asanas. Many of his disciples, and those who practise 'flow yoga' variations, now refer to Krishnamacharya as the 'father of modern yoga'.

Krishnamacharya's *yogashala*, the Sanskrit Pathshala, opened in 1933. His two most famous early students, B. K. S. Iyengar (born in 1918) and Pattabhi Jois (born in 1915), were also in Mysore during the 1935 Yogoda tour of south India. Iyengar had joined Krishnamacharya in 1934 in order to improve his own health through yoga practice. Iyengar later said that the period was a turning point in his life. He stayed in Mysore until 1936 before moving to Pune to teach yoga asanas.

Krishnamacharya often had Iyengar and other students give yoga demonstrations at the maharajah's court in Mysore. Iyengar learned more by being an 'on-the-spot performer in demonstrations' than from his lessons, commonly being 'called on to illustrate poses for many eminent guests of the Maharajah'.[11]

Iyengar saw the talk and performance given by Yogananda and company, and observed that 'this had little in common with the asanas that Krishnamacharya had learned' or what 'he taught in the Sanskrit college'. But 'the eminence', Yogananda, 'nevertheless called it yoga'. The 'encounter burst open Iyengar's world'.[12]

One evening, Iyengar and other students were sternly called by Krishnamacharya to perform before Yogananda. 'Each student was asked to do certain asanas in turns.' Iyengar was told 'to perform *hanu-manasana*', the splits. He pleaded with Krishnamacharya, since he had just joined a year earlier with the sole desire 'to learn and practice a few asanas to gain my health'.[13] He whispered to Krishnamacharya, 'I don't know the asana.' Krishnamacharya commanded him, 'Place one leg forward and one leg backward and sit on the floor with straight legs.'[14]

The guru persisted and Iyengar recalled, 'I could not escape. I had to do it, and I did.'[15] 'I surrendered to his wishes and performed the asana, but with a tear in my hamstrings which took years to heal.'[16]

While 'watching the young contortionist', Yogananda 'was overcome with awe'. He singled out Iyengar and asked whether he 'would accompany him to America'. Iyengar felt the stirring desire to leave for America, but 'his guardian refused to let him go'.[17] Iyengar sensed that he was being trained 'in a yoga of "physical culture", something associated more closely with wrestling and gymnastics'. Through the 'divine bearing of the yogi Yogananda' he sensed 'inaccessible worlds', in which the 'secrets of Tibet had been withheld' by Krishnamacharya.[18]

Years later, Iyengar recalled the incident in a different light. In *Astadala Yogamala*, he stated that when Yogananda 'tried to tempt him to accompany him to America', he had refused on his own, though 'the episode left its imprint' on him and 'one day there could be a possibility to go to the West'. Years later, when the opportunity approached him, he 'did not take it as a surprise'.[19] Much later, in 1982, he recounted Yogananda saying, 'What a superb structural movement and control on the body you have got. Come with me … I will give you all facilities.' Though still a beginner, and only sixteen years of age, Iyengar said he had declined. 'I have only one guru, my guru is Krishnamacharya, I cannot have two gurus,' he told Yogananda. 'I am sorry, I will not come and your offer does not tempt me at all.'[20] Then again, in a different time and place, Iyengar stated that it was his guru who told him he could not go with Yogananda, and said, maybe 'the next time'[21] on 'his next visit'.[22]

Soon after the incident, Krishnamacharya asked Iyengar 'to run classes at the *yogashala* whenever he stayed home'.[23] The following year, in 1936, Iyengar went on his first multi-city performance tour alongside Krishnamacharya.[24] From 1937 onwards, stage performance, alongside teaching in Pune, became a lifelong craft.

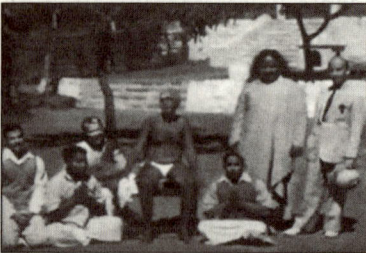
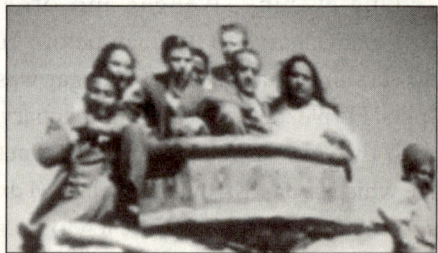

Left: Entourage at Sri Ramana Ashram, 1936. From left: Buddha Bose, Bishnu Ghosh, Ettie Bletch, Ramana Maharshi, Bijoy Mullick, Yogananda, Paul Brunton.
Right: Entourage (same) touring atop an elephant in Mysore, India, 1936.
Courtesy of Bijoy Mullick family.

33

YOGANANDA AND BUDDHA

*Buddha was transformed in this phase of his life. From a person who had
no problem letting the world accept him for what he was, to someone really
conscious of himself ... he wanted to take on something transformational ...
Maybe it was a journey that was meant to be taken by him, all alone!*[1]

Buddha Bose was twenty-two when Yogananda returned to Calcutta. He
often dressed in a Westernized suit and tie, since he was under various
religious and secular influences. His former daughter-inlaw, Chitralekha, 'found
his religious or philosophical thought process' to be 'very encompassing, liberal,
logical, practical and scientific'. She 'loved it', as it was very much like 'that of
Brahmoism'. His stepmother was Hindu, and he grew up learning those religious
stories. But his father had no respect for religious beliefs. Whatever religious
inclination Buddha had at this point in his life, his outward expression of it
was restrained, and his public clothing was not of traditional Bengali attire.

A video taken with 'the great Maharshi' at the foot of Arunachala Hill in
Tamil Nadu on 29 November 1935, captured the more Western expressions
of Buddha. Towards the end of the clip, the trio of Buddha, Bishnu and Bijoy
Kumar Mullick made their way between Yogananda, Paul Brunton and Ramana
Maharshi.[2] In the silent, short, black and white film, Bishnu and Bijoy were
dressed in the traditional Indian dhoti, seated in front, in a cross-legged position.
Buddha, dressed in European slacks and jacket, was off to the side, sitting on
his heels. Bishnu and Bijoy bowed forward with hands clasped, while Buddha
looked over, seeming unsure of what to do with himself. His hands were placed
on his lap until the end, when he made a small gesture, inclining his body. He
was clearly more secular and detached than the others.[3]

Buddha may have taken part in the family-and-friends Kriya and Yogoda initiation, but he did not become an ordained minister at this time, as Bishnu did. However, Buddha did have a spiritual moment with Yogananda.

When they arrived back in Calcutta from south India, a students home for Kriya yoga was established near City College. New initiates were told they 'should regularly visit the Calcutta Yogoda Satsanga centre', known as the 'Inner Circle' where 'they could learn everything about the path and its spirituality'. Yogananda loved to play the harmonium while the group chanted there. 'He sang Bengali songs and American divine songs also. You can just imagine what a wonderful voice I heard when he was only forty-three years old', recalled one relative.[4]

At the students home in Calcutta, 'the ex-students of Ranchi Vidyalaya clustered together' within what Yogananda would call a 'beehive' of activity, comprising kirtan and throngs of bhakti:

> There on Saturday nights in the gatherings I have sung and danced [as did Sri Chaitanya and his disciples]; and at the end of the dance I have let my body go into rigid ecstasy. I feel I am swimming in the ecstasy while I dance, then all becomes light and my body falls lifeless to the ground. Sometimes I watch my lifeless form on the ground swimming in God; and sometimes I see the Ocean of Happiness in which the body is no more. Sing to yourself the song you like and you will get *bhakti samadhi*, which God Loves also from his devotees. As the women of America are very spiritual and given to loving God, so are the boys here. I have extremely enjoyed my ecstasies with them when all or most of the boys and men would become God-stricken with me on these occasions.[5]

Buddha attended an evening meeting there, during which Yogananda 'delivered a brilliant discourse on Kriya yoga', followed by a chant, 'Om Krishna, Om Christ' with arms raised. Yogananda called the devotional verses 'Cosmic Chants' and explained that each one 'had been composed to satisfy a special need of mind or life'. Through their practice, the 'various moods and inner desires could be strengthened or changed by the repetition of one particular chant suitable for that purpose'.[6]

Buddha Bose, normally reserved and suave, participated in the chant 'Om Krishna, Om Christ', but Yogananda noticed that Buddha had not raised his hands. So, while increasing the tempo, Yogananda started to chant: '"Buddha, *tumi hath tolo*" (Buddha, raise your hands) alternating with "Om Krishna,

Om Christ" in the same voice.' The chanting reached such a crescendo that 'Buddha Bose was mesmerized and willingly participated with arms raised'. 'The chanting came to a halt with Yogananda smiling to Buddha Bose.' Buddha was 'so utterly thrilled' that he came again to the next meeting, 'but on that day, to his dismay, there was no chanting'. Afterwards, he asked Yogananda about it, who replied that 'the chanting was performed the day before to make him understand the inherent power of chanting'. For Buddha, 'the vibrations of the chanting lingered in his mind for ten more days'.[7]

PART FIVE

TRAVELS TO THE GOLDEN BEACH

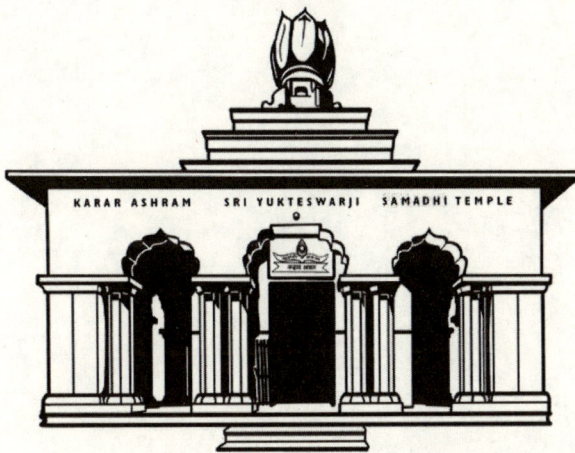

34

YOGANANDA IN INDIA

In late January 1936, Yogananda and a group of family members piled into a Ford and drove throughout northern India. Yogananda had brought the black Sedan Ford from America. The model had just been introduced in 1935: the Model 48, a four-door convertible with a V8 engine and a large trunk. Yogananda called it 'The Pride of Detroit'. They drove along the Grand Trunk Road, which stretched from Calcutta to New Delhi and beyond. Bishnu, who would go afar and then 'speed back to Calcutta' on the open road, wrote, 'riding on the Grand Trunk road was great in those days'.

The group consisted of Yogananda, his brothers Bishnu and Sananda and their families. Three adults would ride in the front seat, with three adults and two children in the back. Yogananda felt Bishnu was 'a spendthrift' and would instead trust his brother Sananda with managing funds while they travelled.[1] Similarly, he wished to keep Bishnu from getting behind the wheel, preferring that Sananda or Richard Wright, his personal secretary, drove.

Sananda once wrote of leaving Ranchi with Bishnu. The 'fiercely competitive' Bishnu had a tendency to 'drive recklessly', according to his brothers. Yogananda had not allowed Bishnu to drive the Ford, but was not in the car at the time, so Sananda relented to the 'brooding' Bishnu and his desire to drive. Letting him 'take the wheel', Sananda quickly realized, was a mistake. 'As we turned off Grand Trunk Road to cross the Bally Bridge', another car, driven by a European, overtook them 'with a rush of speed'. Bishnu was irate and 'immediately took up the chase', with 'repeated reckless attempts' to overtake the car and barely missed collisions 'with oncoming cars'. Finally, 'at the intersection of Maniktala and Upper Circular Road', just around the corner from home, Bishnu 'got his opportunity'. He passed the car and hurled 'a look of determined defiance and triumph at the driver'. The others all 'heaved a sigh of relief'. Later, Yogananda was 'justly angry' when he was told of the incident.[2]

As the family-filled Ford approached Benares, Richard Wright wrote in his diary:

We rode in the Ford across the very low Ganges on a creaking pontoon bridge, crawling snakelike through the crowds and over narrow, twisting lanes, passing the site on the river bank where Yoganandaji pointed out to me as the meeting place of Babaji and Sriyukteswar. Alighting from the car a short time later, we walked some distance through the thickening smoke of the *sadhus'* fires and over the slippery sands.[3]

Still in Benares, they visited a student of Bishnu's before going to the Vishwanath Temple and Lahiri Mahasaya's home. A main objective of Yogananda's visit to India, he wrote, was 'to collect the material for his new book on the lives of some of India's spiritual Masters', which 'will be published as soon as possible after his return to America'.[4]

A photo of the group was taken in Agra during a visit to the Taj Mahal. After which they travelled to Brindavan, to visit Swami Keshabananda and ancient temples, and then to Delhi. Afterwards, they went to the places of Yogananda's childhood, like Meerut, Bareilly and Gorakhpur (his birthplace), before they returned to Calcutta. Since they only went where a car could take them, they did not go into the Himalayas.

During this return trip to Calcutta, Yogananda left Wright behind in Ranchi for a few days, one of the only breaks between the two for any considerable amount of time. While in India, Wright wrote letters from his own perspective as a Western disciple.

In Ranchi, he lamented and apologized for his infrequent entries, writing:

[It has] been no easy task for me to adapt my awkwardness to the many strange ways and customs, and added to this the fact that I require at least two hours to scribble a letter, two hours that are might impossible when Swamiji is laboring and continuously calling: 'Mr Wright, Mr Wright.'

Even with the demand on his time, Wright noted that he served Yogananda 'all too briefly and stingily' when 'India's charms are everlastingly beckoning and enticing me by a come here, and look, and feel'.

Some of his most eloquent letters were written at this moment, when he was alone in Ranchi; 'feeling lonely' and 'a bit relaxed', watching as 'the ghostly, yellow light flickers from one of those old-fashioned kerosene (coal oil) lamps, casting weird, eerie shadows on the white walls of my little den at the Ranchi Ashram or newly acquired India Temple'. He wrote about taking a stroll around the ashram and that 'one's thoughts can go far astray in this soothing atmosphere; this calmness is as conducive of meandering thoughts as a trip-around-the-world'. He went on:

> I can sit here under the spell of this lamp and the calmness and coolness of the night and travel mentally to our night at the Pyramids, our night at the Dead Sea, our dip in the Sea of Galilee, our camel ride on the fringe of the desert, our pause at the Birth Manger of Christ, our dawn right out of Jerusalem, our elephant ride, our stroll through Sir Walter Scott's Abbotsford, or Robert Burns's cottage, or St Peter's in Rome, St. Mark's in Venice, or St. Paul's in London, our sojourn with Gandhi, our many visits with Swami Sriyukteswarji, and so on and on, endlessly happy.[5]

Then, speaking directly to his American audience:

> I'm tossing around in the entrancing lap of the East, and hope I'm making you envious; envious enough to make you want us to return so that we may share our experiences with you.[6]

In a subsequent letter, Wright enticed his American audience further:

> It would be of some interest perhaps to tell you of the wonderful meditations we had on Saturday evenings with the ex-students of Ranchi. On these particular Saturday nights, friends and devotees used to gather from all over Calcutta, sit cross-legged at Swamiji's feet (the harmonium in front of him) many young men and old men drinking in every word he uttered and really diving in with his chanting. This spirit didn't last only one hour but everyone was sitting with rapt attention chanting and meditating all night long and not just a few hours. I am deeply indebted to Swamiji for the privilege of having been taken into such an atmosphere.[7]

In late February 1936, Yogananda went to the Kumbha Mela in Allahabad, having found 'the *mela* dates in a Bengali almanac'. He hoped he would be fortunate enough to behold 'the blessed sight of Babaji'. While there, he met other earthly saints, but not Babaji. After a few weeks, he returned to Calcutta, where an urgent telegram awaited him. 'Come to Puri ashram at once.' In 1906, Sriyukteswar had established an seashore ashram in the quiet town of Puri, where he was residing at this time.

The telegram had been sent on 8 March, and in the early hours of 9 March, Sriyukteswar died. Yogananda arrived by train that very morning, but missed his guru's death. He 'conducted the solemn rites on 10 March. Sriyukteswar was buried with the ancient rituals of the swamis in the garden' of Karar Ashram in Puri, facing east.[8]

Once Yogananda returned to Calcutta, he reflected on the days with his teacher. Swami Sriyukteswar used to shift from Serampore to his seaside hermitage in Puri during the hot Bengali summers, and Yogananda spent many months there, at the feet of his guru. He told his friends who had gathered of an experience he had in Puri during his youth when he was in a deep practice of Kriya.

One afternoon, when Yogananda had been sitting in meditation for hours, 'he heard the voice' of Sriyukteswar, who then 'touched him on the forehead and chest'. Yogananda 'lost all physical consciousness. It seemed that he had become one with the Infinite. The waves of the ocean far away – he could see everything. He saw that he pervaded everything. This was an incredible, indescribable experience', with 'no knowledge of the amount of time that had passed while he was in this state'. Once Sriyukteswar 'again touched his forehead and chest', Yogananda returned to his normal state. Filled with 'devotion and gratitude' he prostrated before Sriyukteswar, and then heard the stern order, 'Go quickly and sweep the veranda. Then we must take a walk by the seaside.' Even in 1936, when Yogananda recounted the event to those assembled, 'he could still not hide his heartbrokenness of that time', to be assigned something so mundane. 'Who knows,' surmised Dasgupta, 'perhaps this was the type of discipline he needed. Perhaps this type of dry physical task was assigned so that this ecstatically prone child of humanity would not float away with the buoyancy of Divine Ecstasy and forget the mundane.'[9]

35

CLAUDIA, ARUP AND DURGA PUJA

A decade previous to my own fieldwork, Claudia Guggenbühl researched yoga in Calcutta between 2003 and 2005. It was groundbreaking. She found the roots of modern yoga in Calcutta to be tied up with bodybuilding and muscle performance, before it turned towards therapeutic yoga. The formulation of modern asana-based yoga has happened much more recently than it has been portrayed.

A longtime Kriya yoga meditator, Claudia had been the translator for a Kriya yogi, named Swami Dhirananda (a different Swami than the friend of Yogananda). Dhirananda was from Calcutta, but he taught in Europe and introduced Claudia to Calcutta. In 2002, after completion of graduate studies in Switzerland, she joined a Zürich University group researching the history of yoga in Calcutta, sponsored by the Swiss National Fund for Scientific Research. The project's title was 'Yoga between Switzerland and India: the hermeneutics of an encounter'; with this Claudia began her field research in Calcutta.

During her time in Calcutta, she worked with a research assistant, an artist named Arup Sen Gupta. Arup and Claudia, both about forty years old, began a relationship. Six months later, they shared the wild, week-long Hindu celebration of Durga Puja, which consumes Calcutta, and within a year, she was pregnant.

Claudia couldn't imagine trying to raise a child in Calcutta. She planned to return to Europe, but Arup in his condition of dependency could only live in Calcutta. As a single, full-time working mother, she taught yoga in Thalwil (a village near Zürich, Switzerland) and gave lectures in Indian philosophy all over Switzerland, but she was not able to publish the nearly completed book.

In 2005 Claudia went from nearly ready to release her groundbreaking yoga research to devoting her energies towards raising her child.

Claudia and I email about this subject at all hours of the day. It is as if I am speaking to my alter ego. In the beginning, much of the time it seems like I am following in her footsteps, doing what she has already attempted. It has been a decade since she finished her research and her work, having left it all behind, 90 per cent complete. Since I am to go to Calcutta in a few months for the first time, her unpublished research is a boon.

In February 2015, I attend a PhD conference in the Swiss Alps, just miles away from her home, where she lives alone with her ten-year-old daughter. For three days we talk Calcutta Yoga, but for her the topic is inseparable from her life. It is a bit difficult for her, no doubt, my rekindling the past. I stir up all of her old memories, rummaging through the past. She shares with me the turn of events that led her to Calcutta.

She explains her relationship with Arup, a slight German accent under her English, 'I feared it would probably be impossible, but I clung to hope.' Hearing Claudia recount her story, I of course think of Emily and Rajah, in London and then Calcutta. Rajah falls in love with his stage assistant, but it doesn't work out. Now here I am, encountering a modern-day relationship with the same patterns.

Claudia's book *Yoga in Calcutta* has still not been published. The lone work she was able to finish from that period was a rehabilitative book on the Calcuttan scholar Surendranath Dasgupta, and his tangled mentorship with Mircea Eliade.[1] (After falling in love with Maitreyi Devi, his teacher's daughter, Eliade was ostracized from the family and the two lovers separated for life.)

There are many levels to love, relationships and their entanglements, but the inherent repetitive cycle is too obvious to deny. There are cards in this deck being played, shuffled and replayed again. Only the players are changing.

Learning about what she uncovered in her research is fascinating, but also difficult for Claudia to rummage through. Since her book was never published, an unresolved feeling remains. Before I leave Zürich, Claudia puts me in touch with Arup, whom she thinks will agree to also be my research assistant during my first trip to Calcutta in the coming months.

Arup is talented but tragic as well. He exemplifies a well-rounded Calcutta intellectual scholar and lover of music, books and poetry. He is a trained sculptor, under Mira Mukherjee, one of the leading sculptors of India at the time. Arup also leads a Dionysus-like life that seems to require alcohol and chain smoking in order to continue.

To really describe Arup, one can imagine a caricature from *The Autobiography of an Unknown Indian* by Nirad Chaudhuri. The book describes a particular sort of Indian-British mind that is cultivated in Calcutta. Arup's access to the Bengali world of North Calcutta is unique, but so is his understanding of the Western mind. With nearly every question, I turn to Arup, and he always has an answer ready or is able to explain a situation, giving me insight into the foreign context of my research. And for any potential source of interview, all I need is a telephone number, never an email. Arup does everything over the phone. He is not online, nor will he text message with his old flip phone.

By the time Arup begins assisting my research, he is nearing the end of his professional life. Not because of his age, but his habits. As the typical American, I constantly want to do as much as I can, as fast as possible, and this mentality, the opposite of Calcutta's lifestyle, wears on him. During the first year of research and interviews, which includes half a dozen trips to Calcutta, Arup is able to familiarize me with the city, which is no easy task.

At the tail end of my first year of research, Arup and I map out a week-long trip to Orissa. We plan to visit historical archaeological sites and temples related to yoga, as well as an ashram in Puri. It is the first voyage I will make with Arup outside of Calcutta, and likely his last.

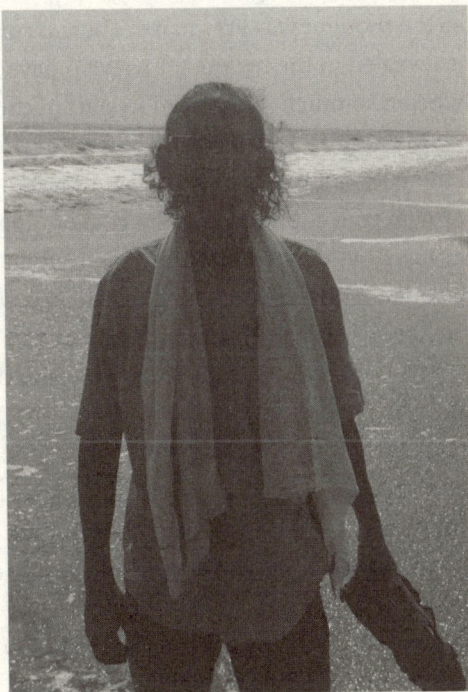

Arup Sen Gupta, Puri golden beach, 2015.

36

TEMPLE OF THE SUN AND SIXTY-FOUR YOGINIS

'I am really about done with all of the research. I may come back here again in March, if the events line up to make that happen. But for now, I feel finished.'

I write this after a visit to Puri, in Orissa, towards the end of a year of research. In hindsight, I was only about one-quarter through just the research, so the thought was very naive. There is something else at work though, which is revealed in the next line I write: 'I have the story now in my head, and I've written so much, I just need to start putting it all together.'

My approach to the work and the entire research project is that of a miner. I mine for knowledge, with an approach to interviews and research as a means of data collection towards the goal of digging deep enough to figure it all out in my head. Once I feel I have arrived, in some semblance or another, I will be done with the book. To a certain extent, I reach that state of mind in Puri.

Yet it is also an apparent motive of mine to be a traveller, mapping out the terrain where these individuals – Bishnu, Buddha and Yogananda – lived and walked. I'm on a voyage to the same places these historical characters travelled, places where I can feel they still linger today. That comes to a head for me in Puri, where I experience something else I've been searching for all along: a connection to their practice.

I arrange for Arup to make the trip to Orissa and Puri with me. It is surprising how difficult it is for him to leave his entrenched habits in Calcutta. We arrive at the airport, and he has no ID with him. He hasn't flown in over a decade. His response of 'Just to Orissa, why!' doesn't cut it with the door guards. A train arrives in Puri each morning from Calcutta. I now wish we'd gone that route, taking the overnight voyage and avoiding the hassles of the airport.

Once we arrive in Puri, the driver who picks us up insists on honking his horn at every single thing that moves on or along the side of the road. He follows each honk with a glance at his watch. I finally get him to stop this ten-second-interval habit by telling him that if he honks more than once a minute, Arup is going to drive and he will get no tip. Arup gives me a sideways glance at that statement; he is in no condition to drive. Besides, he is more annoyed by the glancing at the time; but with the driver now untrained of his habits, we continue on.

In the state of Orissa, we plan to go to a few places associated historically with the roots of yoga. We begin by visiting temples and cave ruins, and then an ashram. First we stay in Konark, located on the shores of the Bay of Bengal, where an ancient Sun Temple stands. I am intrigued by the fact that Carl Jung and Francis Yeats-Brown came away with exactly opposite experiences from their visits to these temple ruins.

Yeats-Brown and Jung had followed along with 'the oriental wave' that brought European and American 'scholars into the cultural landscape of India in the 1930s'. Jung, after falling ill in Calcutta, felt his health return while he was here along the coast. Viewing the Sun Temple, he saw the sculptures, with their assimilation of the erotic within religious schemes, as 'a necessary function of life, before one embarked on the higher plane of spiritualism'. For this, the place gained his critical praise.[1]

Yeats-Brown could not make that bridge, and found the Black Pagoda 'stupendous, unforgettable'. He wrote of the Sun God traditions that still 'haunt the place' when the 'tantric gurus come here for their rites' during the dark moon. 'Circles are formed in which the female energies of the gods are invoked by various rituals which are never consummated', the 'vital energies' are reabsorbed and re-manifested instead 'on the astral plane'.[2] Yeats-Brown sought out the physical side of Hatha yoga, but saw nothing of its roots in the strands of tantra where 'lust is deified'.[3] Jung beckoned those ethereal spirits and the dark unknown.

When Jung had a 'near-death experience' a decade later, he floated out of his body above 'the globe of earth' and then observed, 'far below', a 'tremendous dark block of stone floating in space'. He remembered having 'seen similar stones on the coast of the Gulf of Bengal', referring to the temples. 'An entrance led into a small antechamber,' he wrote. 'To the right of the entrance, a black Hindu sat silently in lotus posture upon a stone bench. He wore a white gown … I knew that he expected me.'[4]

Arup wants to visit these temple grounds too. He especially wants to take me to an ashram that was set off from the Sun Temple, a place where those with leprosy would come to be cured. According to the legend, a son of Krishna, named Samba, was told by a sage to worship the Sun God in order to cure his ailment. The original Konark temple, dating to the ninth century, was attributed as the location for his penance, which included yogic postures.[5]

Upon our arrival to Konark, Arup spends the first day and night reeling from alcohol withdrawal; unbeknownst to me, he quit the day prior to our journey. I walk all over the coastal area and return late in the day to find Arup lying on the couch. He usually wears a back brace for his lower lumbar, due to a deterioration of the spine, and it's lying on the table. I pick it up and imagine having to wear one of these things all the time, the pain.

He hasn't eaten dinner, or breakfast or lunch for that matter. The Indian breads, dishes and Chinese rice that I'd ordered before I'd left that morning sit untouched. On the way back from the Sun Temple, I'd picked up a bag of masala snacks and a bag of fresh fruit from a vendor. The fruit in season is small yellow bananas, a green/orange citrus and apples delivered from Kashmir. I shine them up, then place an apple on the table in front of the couch where he is sleeping. I just sit there and look at him.

I wish he could just transform himself right now. I wonder what is holding him back from giving up cigarettes and alcohol. He certainly has wonderful things to live for: a mother, a girlfriend and a ten-year-old daughter living in Europe. I think he has to make a transformative decision, right now, that changes everything from here going forward. A decision that takes back what has been stuck in habitual form for decades, stuck like these massive Surya temples that worship the life-giving power of the sun in our lives, carved into stone. The decision, like the temples, is about celebrating life by living as purely as possible while at the same time holding personal transformation close. I mention this all to myself as Arup lies silently on the couch, like I am willing it into his mind. But I am aware his mind belongs to his body.

I relax for the evening, listening to a 'Chill Watts' YouTube music clip. 'You can really, honestly, transmute pain into a form of play,' I hear Alan Watts say, amidst the ambient tune. Pain is 'a form of weird far-out sensations'.

I wonder, how does that get transformed? Alan Watts continues:

So long as you fail to see the inner unity of the opposites. So long as you fall for the idea that you are nothing more than this particular life, than this particular ego. Which came from nowhere and is going no-where. While you remain under that illusion, you don't see your identity with everything else which exists.

I'm asking Arup to go somewhere that no one I know has gone, certainly not myself.

The next morning, still at Konark, I awake just past 3 a.m. and set out for the temple half an hour later. It's still dark; few people are awake. I befriend a dog on the way out of the hotel who walks along with me in the dark morning. We head out to the temple. Through the tourist bazaar, I notice waves of emotion moving through me. A general notion of fear; it's dark and I am going into places where I could be… 'What nonsense!' I then think. But it's interesting to watch this travel through my thoughts. I breathe it out, letting it go.

India has made a promotional tourist map for people to travel throughout the country, and I notice on a painted map that this is one of the dozen or so spots that are highlighted – places to avoid. It has become the worst sort of tourist trap. No one is inside the ticket counter at the far end of what must be over fifty stalls on both sides of a long aisle, leading to the temple entrance. It is like a gauntlet of successive pitches, trying to exchange money for factory trinkets. After I walk around the outside of the temple and its environs, I come back by the ticket counter again. It's 5 a.m. They are awake and tell me to come back at 6.

I walk with the dog, wondering whether to make a venture through the woods to the sea, but he turns and goes over to the place I was the night before. I follow.

There is a large horizontal black rock, a 20-foot-long slab, with nine planetary gods. Early every morning the stone and its carvings are thoroughly washed in ritual. Vedic astrology has nine planets in its most recent conception, and each has a representation carved in the stone. Surya (Sun), Chandra (Moon),

Mangal (Mars), Budha (Mercury), Brihaspati (Jupiter), Shukra (Venus), Shani (Saturn), Rahu (North Lunar Node) and Ketu (South Lunar Node). There were originally only seven, but in order to incorporate predictive eclipse patterns, they included the moon nodes, first Rahu and then Ketu.

As I watch the priests wash the black chlorite stone figurines, I eye that a nearby outdoor tea stand is open, with a fire burning. I walk over, sit down to gain some warmth and am handed chai in a clay earthen vessel. I don't really care for chai at all, especially in the morning, but accept what's given. Next to me, a person lights up a cigar of ganja, which he asks me to take. Chai and ganja, not exactly what I expected when I walked over here at 6 a.m. to practice Sun salutations with the rising sun. I'm obliged now to stay a bit longer, and notice that the dog has left.

The few locals sitting with me query a few typical questions I've been asked many times here now.

'The United States,' I answer when they ask where I'm from.

Sometimes this is met with an 'ah' that understands but not here. 'Where?' I change the name, seeing what will click. 'USA' usually works.

Or 'America', without fail.

And then the conversation turns to where I am staying. I answer, 'The Tourism Hotel', ITC or ITDC or whatever the acronym is. I spell it out a few ways, seeing whether they know it. They don't.

'How much?' They want to know what I pay in rupees to stay here per night and how many rupees is it in my amount, the dollar. I tell them the sum is 3,600 rupees per night. The exchange rate is 65 rupees to 1 dollar. It's less than $50, but they nod in disbelief, and mumble something that probably means 'Holy shit!' Perhaps what's running through their mind is that the chai is 10 rupees, they pay 10 rupees for a rolled cigarette and it's free to sleep outside.

I give the chaiwala a 50-rupee note and make signals to buy a round for the persons here with me. After I linger long enough, I walk over to pay the temple fee and gain entrance before all the shops open. A guide insists on trailing me, asking if I want a photograph standing next to each of the figurines; I finally pay him to leave.

I stop before the carved rock figurines, see *supta vajrasana*, the diamond pose, and get Jung's point. How, 'in the mental makeup of the most spiritual you discern the traits of the living primitive, and in the melancholy eyes of the illiterate half-naked villager you divine an unconscious knowledge of spiritual truths'. It is the way of a civilization 'without suppression, without violence, without rationalism'. Instead, side by side, the two polar opposites exist, a more simpatico relationship among the forces, rather than antagonistic swings to the opposite. I want to live with that duality, but I can't avoid having the same disgust that Yeats-Brown had with this place, for altogether different root expressions.

When they were here, the 'isolated sites' could be pondered for hours at a time. Now it's just another spot overrun with tourism. In order to protect the remainder of stone carvings, trees have been planted to block the salt-laden breeze from the sea; they also block the view. There's no longer a sunrise to see from the Temple of the Sun.

An hour or two later, I head back for the hotel. I meet Arup at the gate outside and he is clean, showered and dressed in all white, shining. He has come out the other side. He looks serene, cooled off; I feel hot already.

I know where he wants to go. He's going to find the lepers ashram that he visited a few decades earlier; he'd felt something there. He wants to wash away something in his life and start over. But between that eventful encounter he'd had years ago, around 1980 and now, the thirteenth Century Chariot of the Sun God Temple has become a UNESCO World Heritage monument; it is placed squarely on the Indian and international tourist map. I know what he will encounter, the temple glutted with cheap consumerism and various petty schemers. I know too, the lepers ashram is not there, perhaps moved to a more remote area; perhaps just completely gone. I meet his eyes and nod my head, letting him pass by to find out for himself. I head into our room to eat leftovers before going to the extensive collection of fallen sculptures at the Konark Archaeological Museum next door to the hotel. As I view the collection, which extends outside to include hundreds more just lying about on the ground, the tantric postures of the sculptures is fairly obvious as to how similar they are to Hatha yoga. We don't yet have the historical text to firmly link the two, but it is inductive.

When I meet back up with Arup later that day, he doesn't talk about what he's found. He'd left dressed in white, but now he has put on his old clothes and returned to his habits: a cigarette and a drink. When I ask about the lepers ashram, he shrugs it off, smiles, and we laugh, sadly. The following morning, we leave for the inland temple of sixty-four yoginis.

Little is known of its tantric origins.[6] The stone-carved figurines, in a circular outdoor temple, perform a variety of postures using parts of their body, along with hand mudras. It was a bodily practice which tapped into a divine energetic movement, with mantra and pranayama. This particular yogini temple, like the others which survive in India, is round and open to the sky, connected to the patterns of earth, moon and sun. In places like this, practitioners created a blissful dance that spiritually merged their identity, as portrayed in the six rock carvings. The carvings do not look like Hatha yoga exactly, but it's probable that these were precursors to at least some of the Hatha practices of mantra, asana, pranayama and mudra. Matsyendranath, whom tradition claims as 'the first teacher of Hatha yoga' after Shiva,[7] was closely connected with the Yogini Kaula school within the tantra tradition of Bengal.[8]

Afterward, Arup and I visit the caves of Udayagiri and Khandagiri, where Buddhist and Jain recluses meditated in solitude 2,000 years ago. The guide tells us that various Hatha yoga postures emerged here among the yogis as a sort of therapeutic cure, first among themselves in their seclusion from outside help, and then when they were visited by ailing persons who asked for a cure.

The next day, we head to the ancient holy city of Puri. The beach strip of this old city caters to crowds of Indian visitors. During the hippy days of India in the late 1960s, Puri emerged as a sort of Goa of the east coast of India.

That phase has long passed, and now it's mostly a religious site for Hindus. The enormous twelfth century Jagannath temple and Govardhan Math, both Hindu institutions of major pilgrimatic importance for Indians, are located in Puri. The place where we are going is much less well-known, named Karar Ashram' – it is one of the few places deeply associated with Yogananda that is not owned by SRF.[9]

37

YOGANANDA RETURNS TO AMERICA

After the death of Sriyukteswar, Yogananda felt pulled between 'two fires' – of service and solitude; his charge of students in American and the longing for caves and river banks to be alone in meditation. Writing to Saint Lynn, his disciple, he said, 'We are puppets dancing with strings of emotions and habits on the stage of time.'

Yogananda bemoaned 'the dilemma of financing the organization and being 'a prisoner of duties'.

'I wonder,' he wrote, 'if the mighty wind would sweep away all my spiritual karmic duties and let me go free in the woodlands of India.' He sought 'to roam by the Ganges and in the Himalayas' but instead was 'grievously answered' with the 'bondage of work and responsibility'.[1]

Yogananda, who had put on weight while in India, was also weighed down by the task of settling organizational legal issues, as well as the pressing issue of ownership and use of the Ghosh homes. With two houses and three brothers, he had initially wanted to persuade his family members to transfer the ownership of the house at 4 Garpar Road to his spiritual organization, but Sananda and Bishnu resisted, which caused some conflict.[2] Their father Bhagabati had spent a considerable amount of money to help get the Ranchi School for Boys on solid financial footing. Yogananda was also thwarted in another attempt to purchase a nearby house.[3]

Though their collaboration with the hopes of nationwide spiritual–physical synthesis did not pan out, Yogananda and Bishnu were able to form a system at the school in Ranchi. From May to June, 'in sultry Calcutta', Yogananda organized 'a scientific gymnasium with apparatus and Yogoda exercises' for the Ranchi school, with 'a wonderful athlete in charge'.[4]

The athlete was Sri Krishna Kali Bandyopadhyay, a student of Bishnu's who was appointed as the 'director of physical education at the Ranchi centre'. But, between the two brothers, nothing notable was made beyond that partnership effort.

The other outstanding issue was the impending return to the United States, which had become complicated. At the end of June 1936, Yogananda and Richard Wright left Calcutta for Bombay. Once there, Yogananda made the decision that he must return to Calcutta one last time. He left Wright in the moderate climate of Bombay, just before the monsoon was expected to burst. Somewhat abandoned, and with some time on his own, Wright found Bombay 'rather appealing' with its 'blue of the night', like a 'fresh sea zephyr kissing the leaves and cavorting in our room in ecstasy under the fan'.[5]

When Yogananda returned to Bombay in August, the group left for London. 'On his way back' to America, Yogananda had 'plans to lecture and hold classes in London, and to visit both Mussolini and Hitler'.[6] This was reiterated by Yogananda in Calcutta; 'I propose to interview Signor Mussolini and Herr Hitler on my return trip to America.' His organization was 'non-sectarian and non-political', but with the world war looming, he wanted to make an attempt.[7] Yogananda clearly misunderstood the ultimate direction of Hitler and Mussolini. The interviews did not happen.[8] Instead, Yogananda made his return stop in London to perform at Caxton Hall, then left for America.

Yogananda returned to the United States on 23 October 1936 as a British subject, 'a citizen of India'.[9] Since the time when Yogananda had first entered the US, laws such as the Immigration Act of 1924 had been enacted. Local laws had also been added, which made California a state which 'strictly enforced against relationships between whites and Asians', which made it difficult to establish families. After coming under the surveillance of the British authorities while leaving the US in 1935, the Bureau of Special Inquiry was compelled by California officials to hold a hearing upon his return. Yogananda could not have been surprised as he had already been 'subject to multiple encounters and scrutiny by state and federal officers from 1926 to 1936'.[10]

When he left America the previous year, the US Department of Labor put out a memo which 'requested that a lookout notice be posted for the return of the above-named alien' to determine whether 'he is undesirable' or a 'fit person to re-enter the United States under the garb of a spiritual teacher'.[11] If 'apprehended at a port of entry', then 'his right of admission' was to be 'thoroughly examined'.[12] The California Department was even more aggressive, and looked to 'secure evidence to warrant the institution of deportation proceedings' against Yogananda.[13]

On Ellis Island, across from the New York Harbor, Yogananda encountered the Board of Special Inquiry regarding his residential status, and allegations of financial and moral improprieties. For two days – 26 and 27 October – the Bureau interviewed people who testified on his behalf, as well as those with complaints. The former included Richard Wright and the office manager for Wayside Press, the commercial printer of Yogananda's 'magazine, books and advertising' materials, who wrote, 'I have found him at all times to be a Christian gentleman.'[14] The latter included the Directors of the Los Angeles District of the US Department of Labor, who wrote that he had 'an undue influence on wealthy women' and 'acted with impropriety towards them' and, in general, 'he demanded that his adherents cater to his every need'.[15]

Over two days of hearings, Yogananda vehemently confronted the allegations. The first day was more general.

'What scandal could be brought against you?' they asked. 'Nothing,' replied Yogananda.

Two of the more interesting issues were how Yogananda framed his work. As Christian:

Q: Is your teaching based on Indian religion or on Christian religion?
A: On Christian, and Indian teachings of the Masters of India.

And as physical:

Q: What do you teach in your classes?
A: Just exercises. Just using more will in the movements, that is what I say.
Q: Do you go through a series of physical exercises? A: Yes; simple physical exercises.
Q: Is that all you teach?
A: Concentration and meditation. To sit quietly and concentrate on one thing at a time and to pray to God.

The inspector questioning was unsure of the primary teaching:

Q: Is your church principally physical or is it principally a spiritual church?
A: Both.
Q: Which is predominant? A: Spiritual.

After the first day of hearings, the three inspectors 'received a telegram stating that the file regarding Mr Yogananda was being mailed' to their office. All three inspectors moved 'to defer' the re-entry decision until the "Central Office file" on Yogananda was reviewed. Led by Inspector Magee, the questions Yogananda had to answer got worse on the second day:

Q: I was asking what the forms of initiation were.
A: Signing an information form and after this information form is signed, they get the instructions which are strictly moral and very spiritual.
Q: Do you have any rites or ceremonies to go with?
A: No. None whatsoever. In classes sometimes we have candles and flowers and chants. That is all.
Q: We have information here that one of your rites is sexual intercourse.
A: Oh, good gracious.
Q: And also that there is sexual perversion carried on in that institution.
A: That is an abject lie. It is told by someone who wants to get me into trouble. I am a celebrated lecturer. We don't believe in such things. Good gracious! How can people say such things?
Q: Are there any immoral acts of any kind carried on in the institution?
A: Never.

The Bureau of Immigration was particularly perplexed by his lack of understanding about his own finances, and the sexual indiscretions of other swamis.[16] This involved the alleged scandals of two other swamis from India – Dhirananda and Paramananda – and a thorough examination of Yogananda's financial matters, making for nearly thirty pages of questions and answers. Yogananda and Dhirananda had split, acrimoniously and with lawsuits, in 1929.[17] Paramananda was associated with the Vedanta organization of Vivekananda and was also from Calcutta.

Despite the many questions over sex and money, the Bureau of Inquiry focused on the technicality of his lack of having graduated from a traditional theological seminary. Thus, whether Yogananda could represent himself as a 'professor', which was a title with exemption from the contract labour law under the Immigration Act of 20 February 1907 was under question. His self-given title of 'professor of religion' was without affiliation or confirmation of his teaching at a university or seminary for two years prior to his entry into the US.[18] The matter of whether Yogananda would be allowed re-entry in 1936 came down to whether or not his original entry in 1920 as a 'religious teacher', was valid.

At the conclusion of the second day, with Yogananda present for the hearing, three inspectors voted. The first, Inspector Kaba stated, 'I move to admit as a returning resident in possession of a valid reentry permit.' The second, Inspector Hibler, moved 'to exclude the alien as a person not in possession of a valid immigration visa that he is not entitled to the re-entry permit which he presents, having obtained his original admission' under the 'false or misleading statements' that 'he was a professor at the time of his first arrival'. Inspector Magee, with the vote in balance, was up next.

If Magee voted 'to exclude', Yogananda would have been sent back to India in 1936 and not allowed re-entrance into America. Yogananda, or at least his supporters, must have been nervous, as Magee had been the most rigorous in the questioning, such as the above sample shows. However, the inspector simply stated, 'I second the motion to admit.'[19]

In America and near the ocean, a place Yogananda imagined, had materialized into reality. New land for an ashram was being acquired for his spiritual organization along the sunny coast of Encinitas, California. After months of being in the throngs of India, he was ready for serenity.

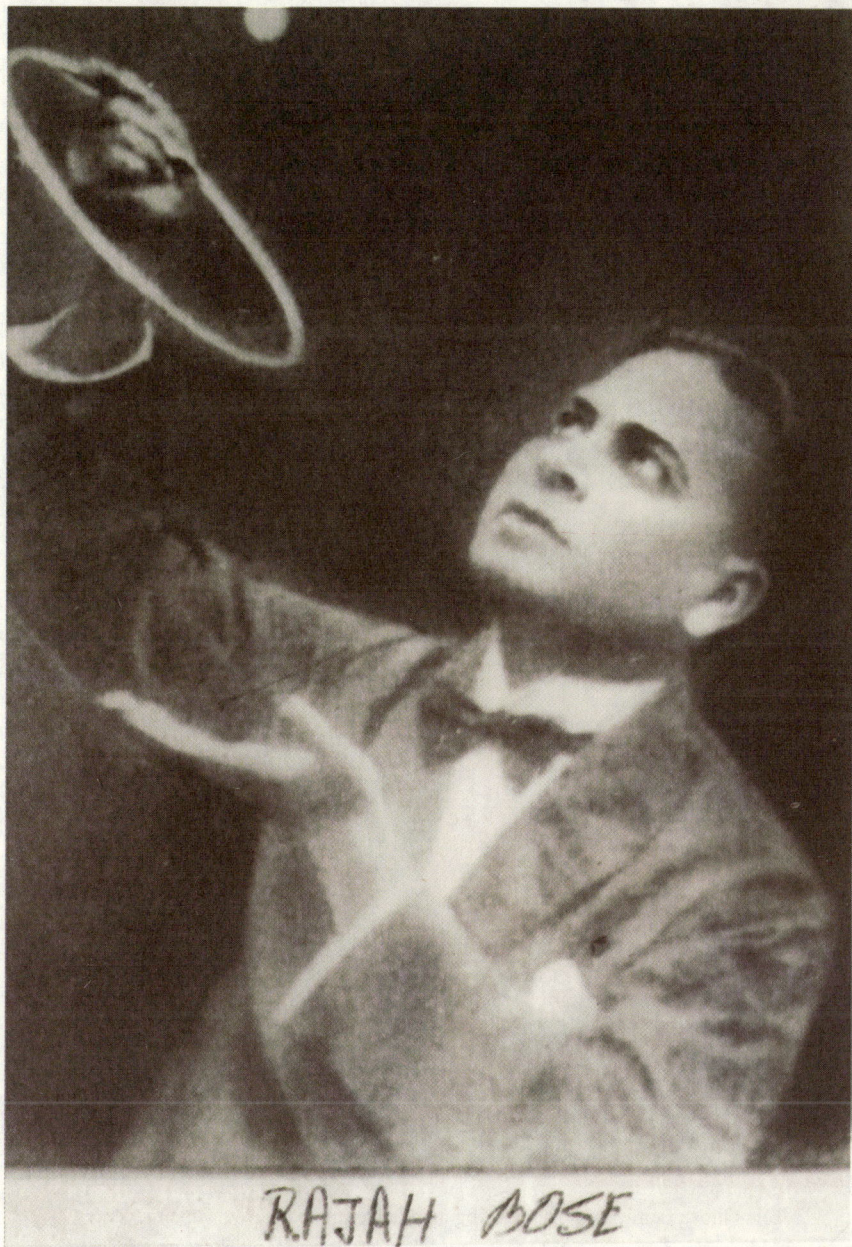

RAJAH BOSE

Magician Rajah Bose, circa 1910.
Source: Magic magazine, 1950 (Magic Circle, London).

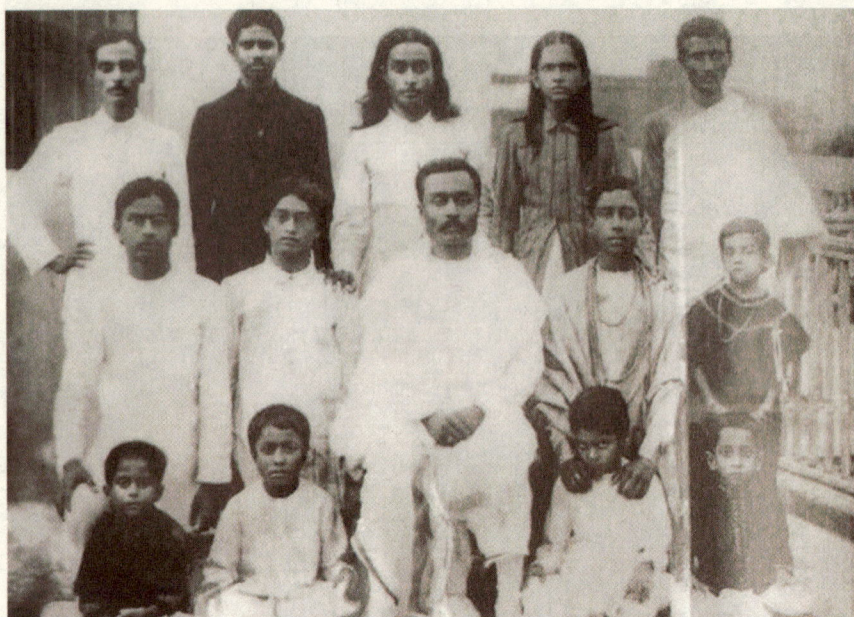

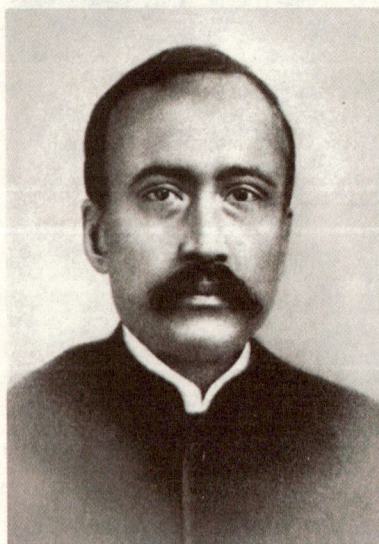

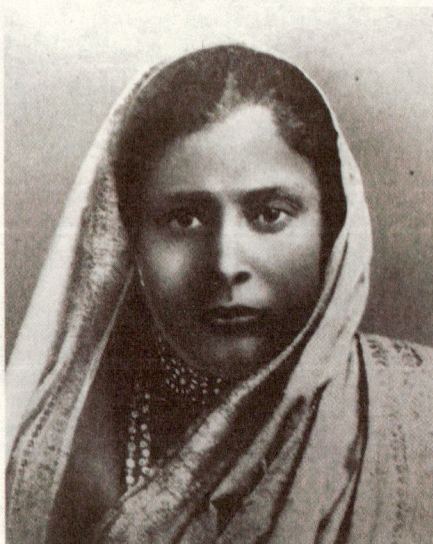

Top: Ghosh family with friends. Yogananda (center, back row), Ananta (center, middle row), Sananda (right center, middle row), Binoy Mullick (seated, far left), Bishnu (left center, seated). 4 Garpar Road, 1914. Bottom: Bhagabati Charan Ghosh, Gyana Prabha Ghosh (Bose), 1900.

Source: Wikimedia Commons.

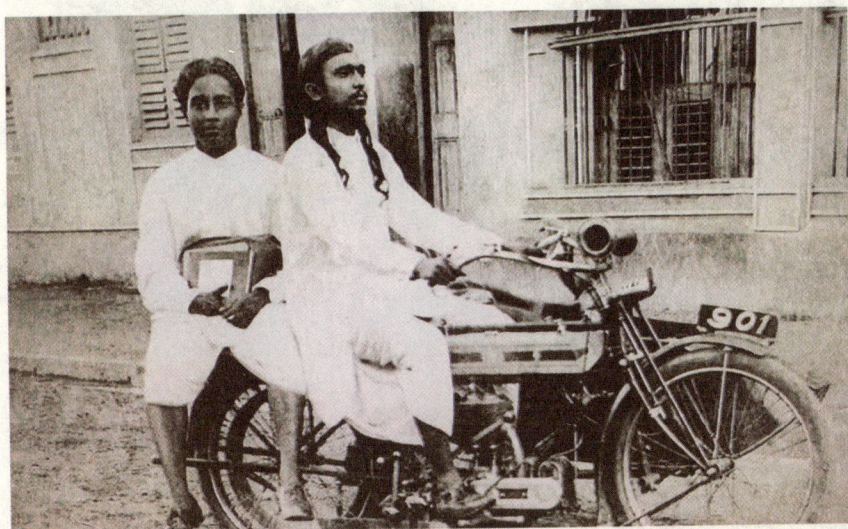
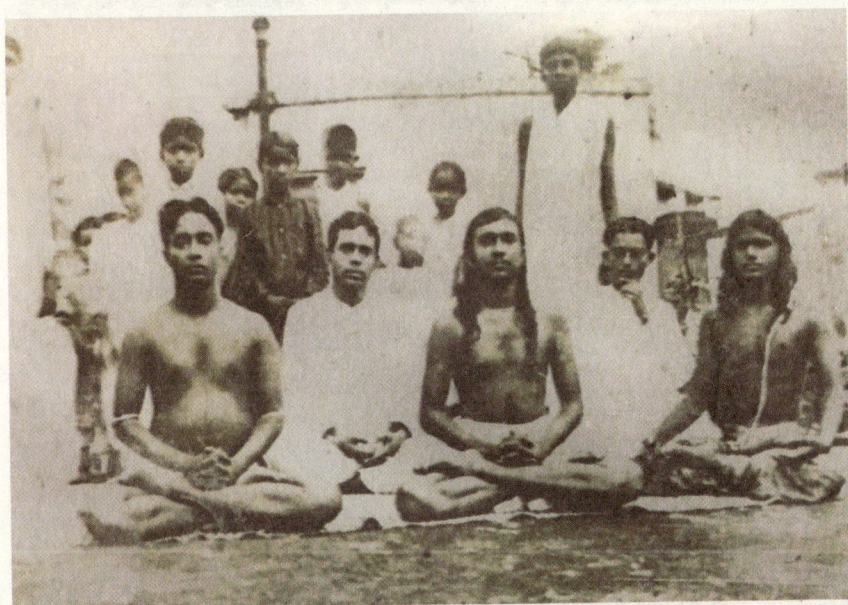

Top: Tulsi Narayan Bose, Yogananda, atop 901 Triumph, 1916.
Bottom: Tulsi Narayan Bose, Yogananda, Dhirananda. 1915.
Source: Wikimedia Commons.

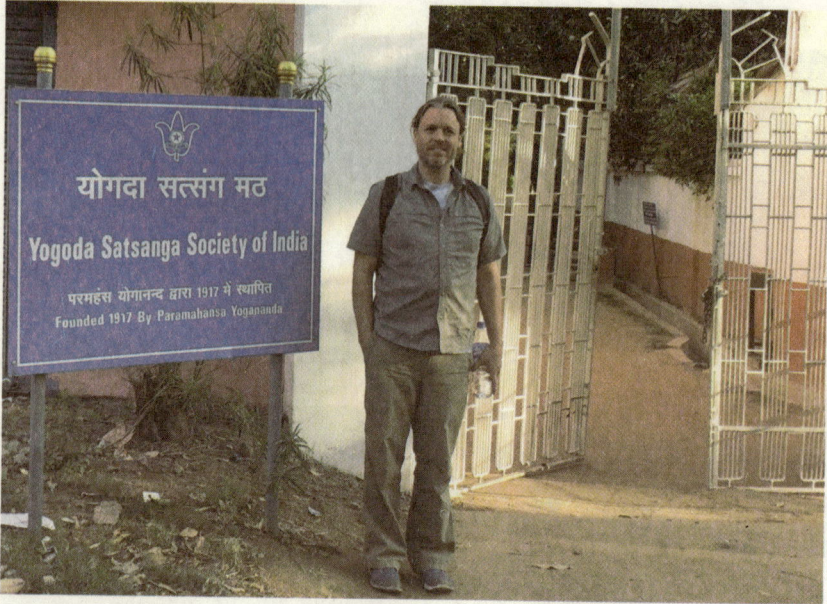

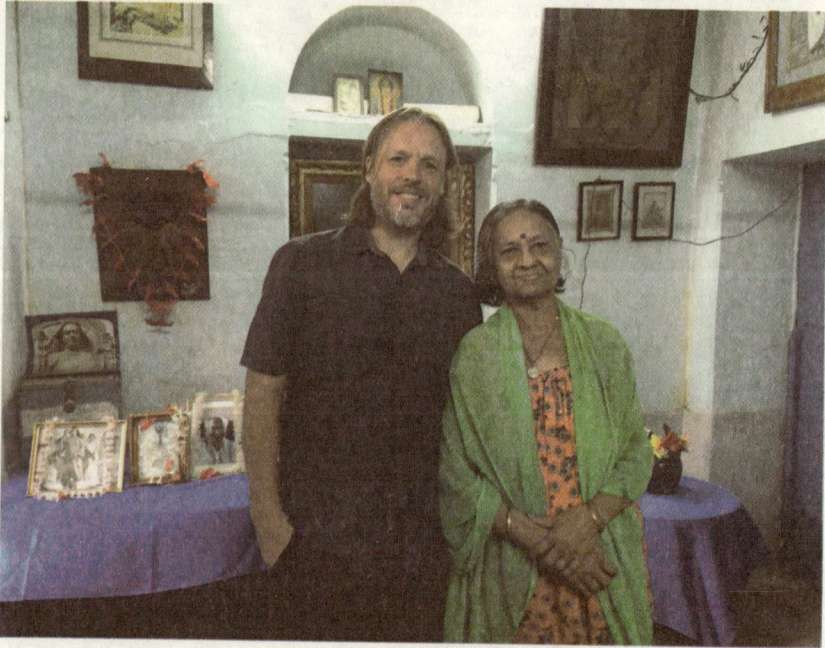

Top: The author in Ranchi, India.
Bottom: The author, with Hassi Mukherjee (Bose). Pitambar Lane, Calcutta.

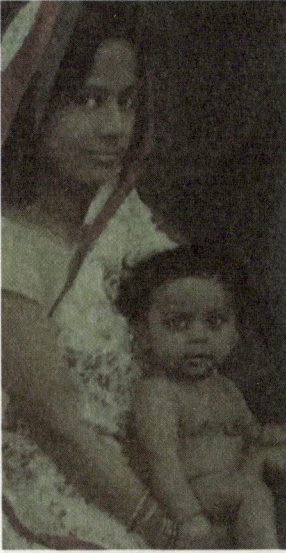

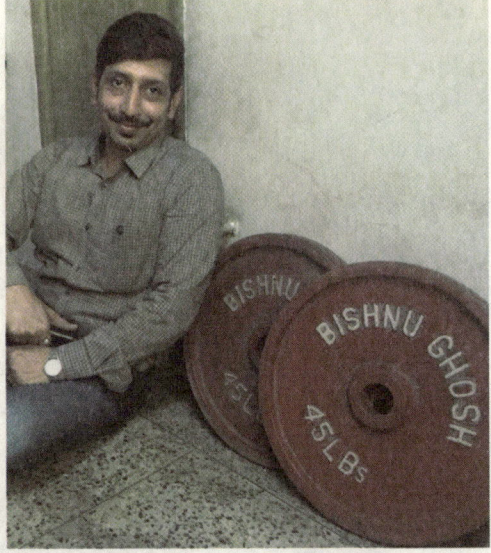

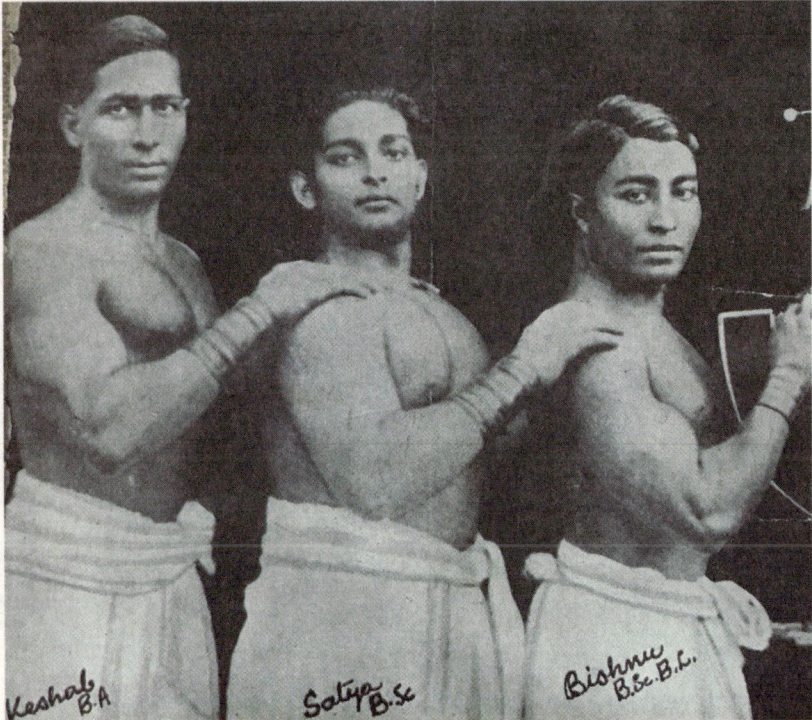

Top left: Ashalata Ghosh with child. Top right: Romit Banerjee at gymnasium nearby Jayanti Mata Mandir in Calcutta, where Bishnu's weights are housed. Bottom (from left to right): Trio of Rajen Guha Thakurta students Chandra Sen Gupta, Bhupen Karmakar, and Bishnu Ghosh, circa 1925. Courtesy of Ghosh's Yoga College; Bayam Charcha.

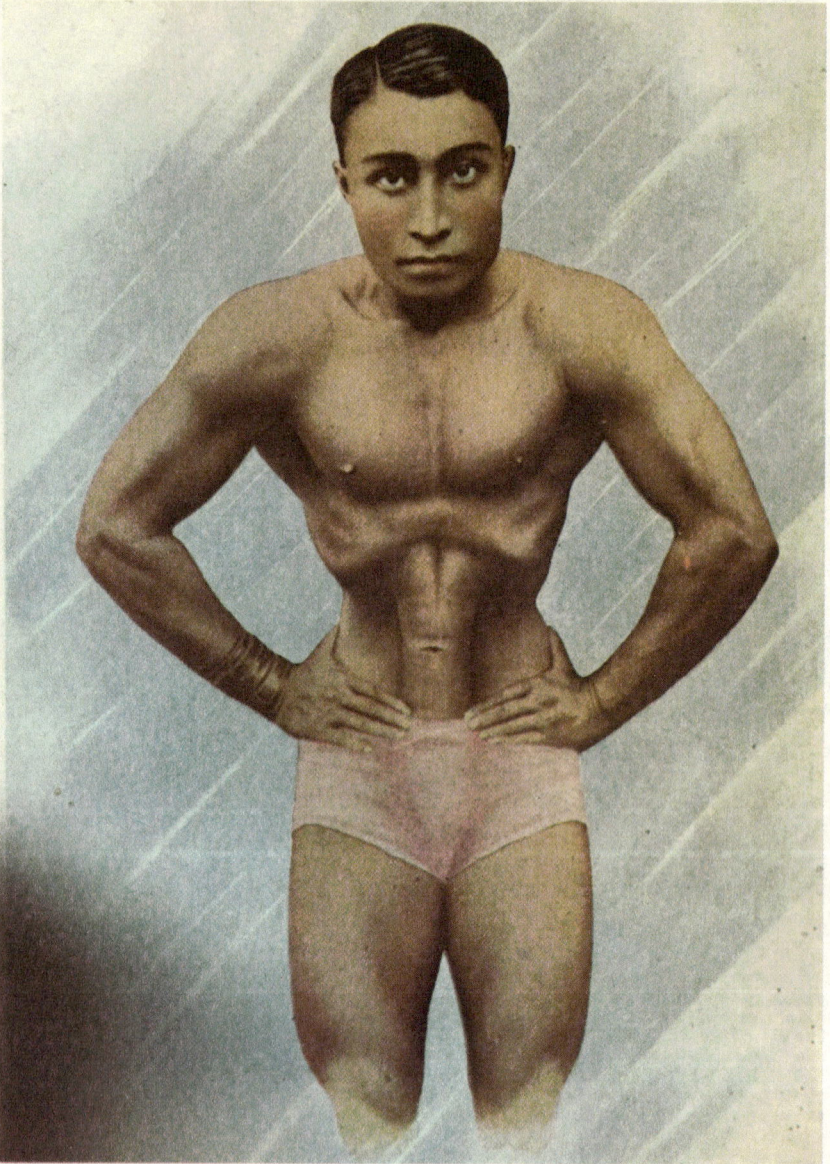

Bishnu Charan Ghosh.

Source: (inside cover) Muscle Control, Calcutta, 1930.

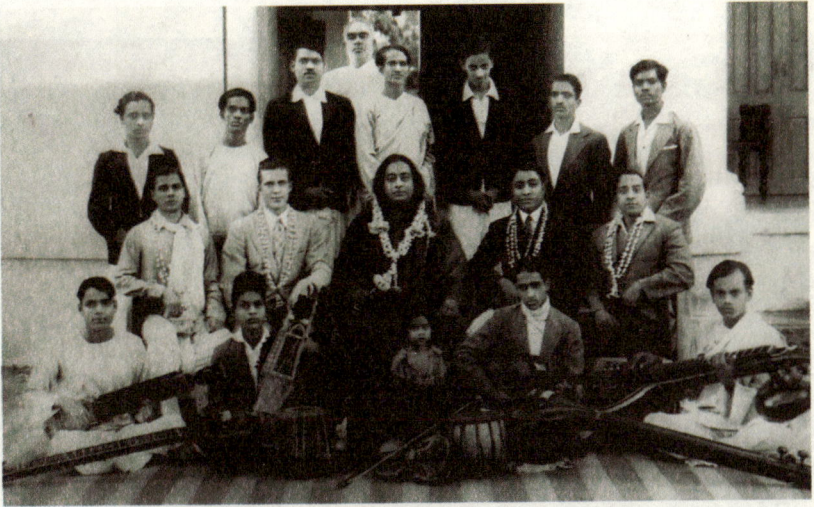
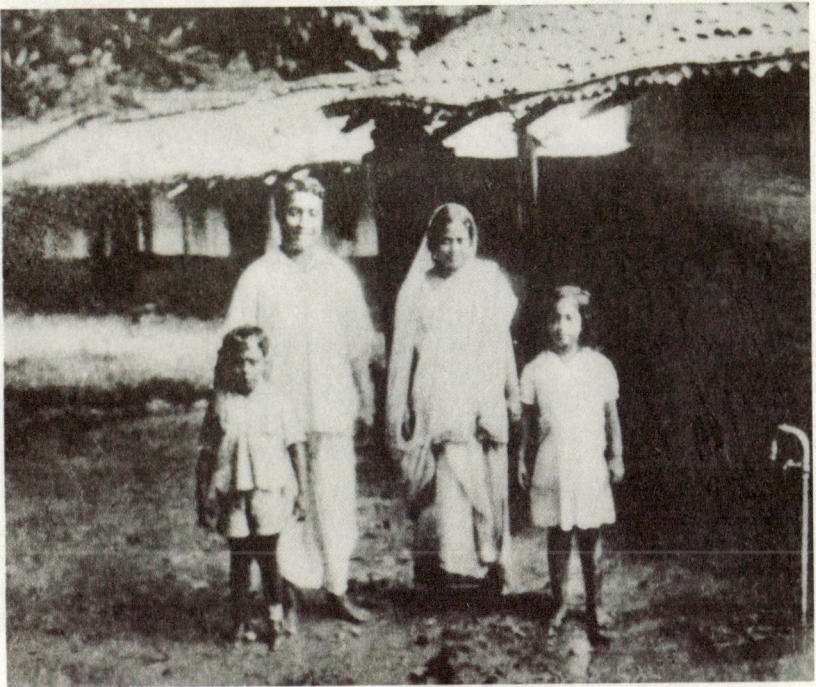

Top: Entourage in Mysore, 1935. Top row, middle: BKS Iyengar. Middle row from left: Buddha Bose, Richard Wright, Yogananda, Bishnu Ghosh, Bijoy Mullick.
Bottom: Bishnu & Ashalata, with children Sri Krishna and Ava Rani, in Ranchi, 1935.
Courtesy of Bijoy Mullick family; Ghosh's Yoga College.

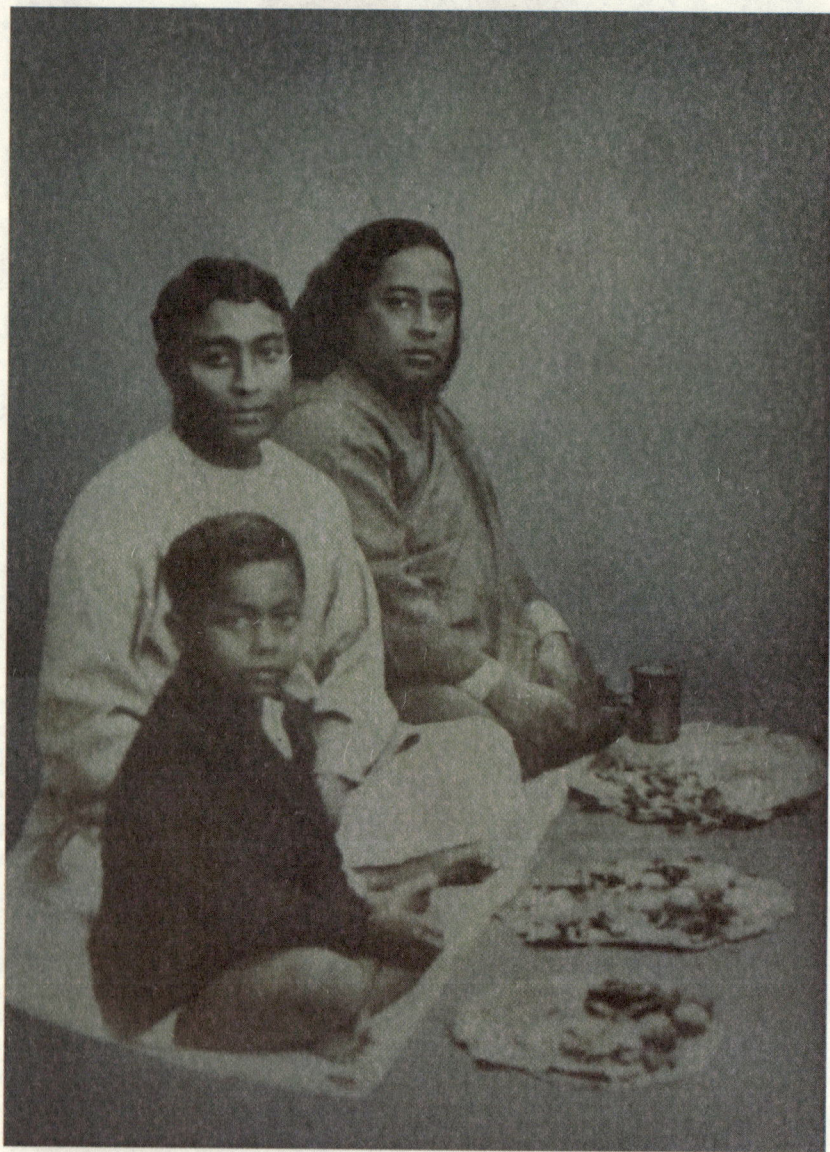

The yoga family of Yogananda, Bishnu, and Srikrishna Ghosh,
Bishnu, and Yogananda. 4/2 Rammohan Road, Calcutta, 1935.
Courtesy of Ghosh's Yoga College.

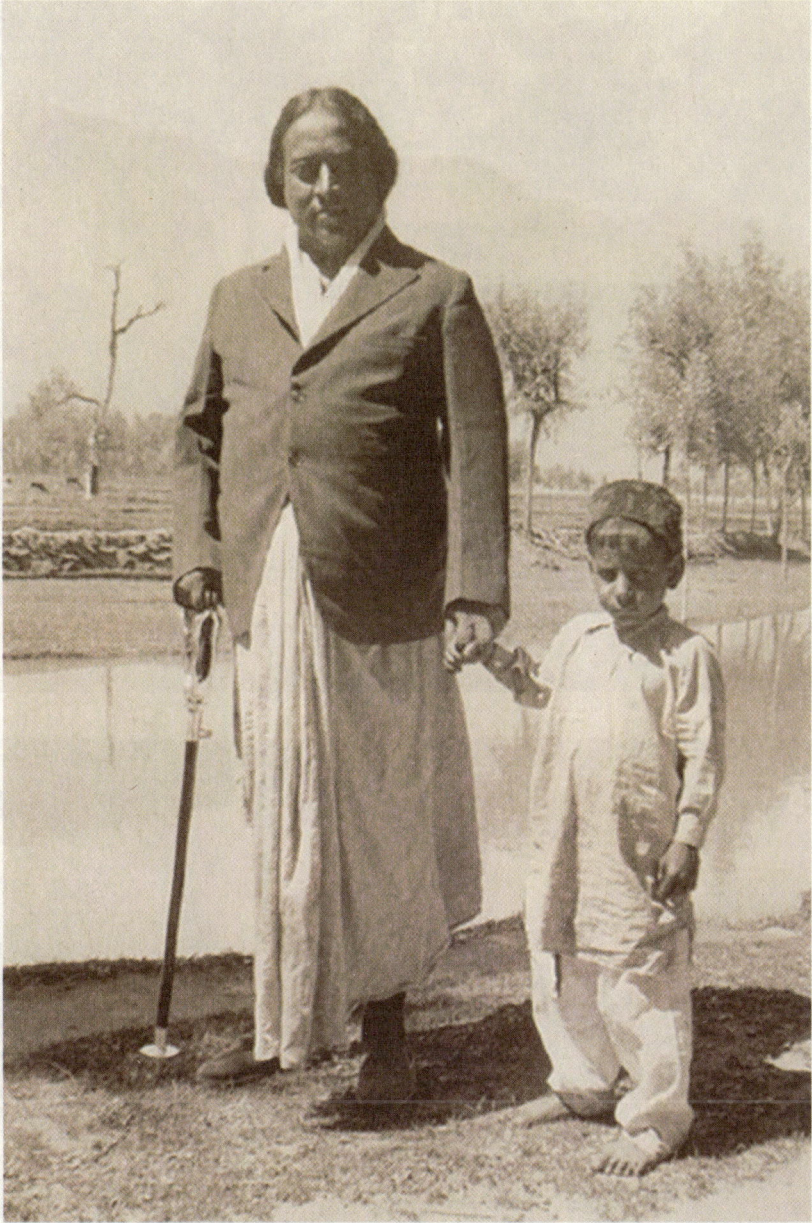

Yogananda with Srikrishna Ghosh, while touring Kashmir, North India, 1936.

Source: Wikimedia Commons.

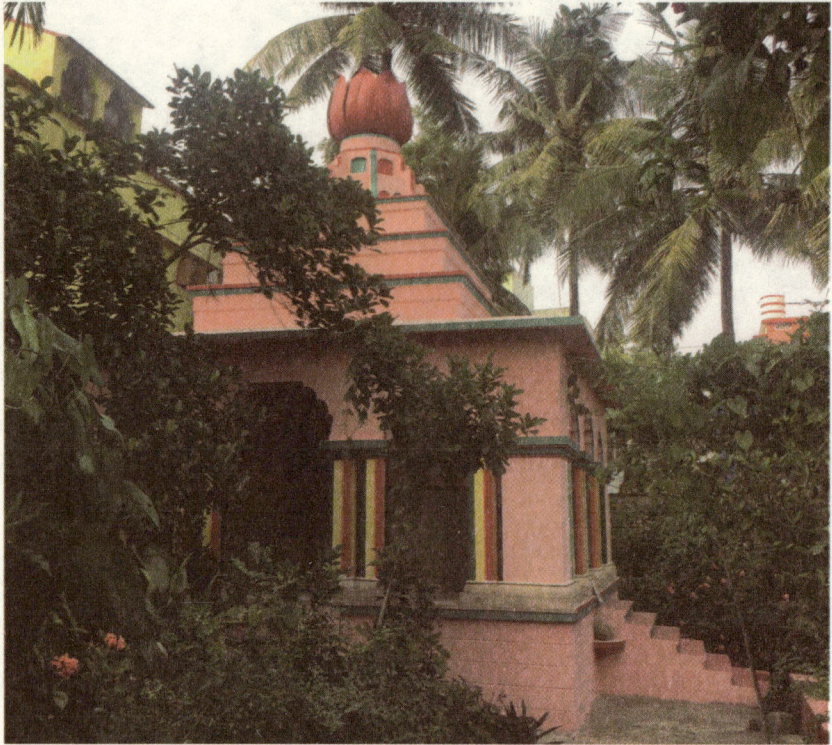

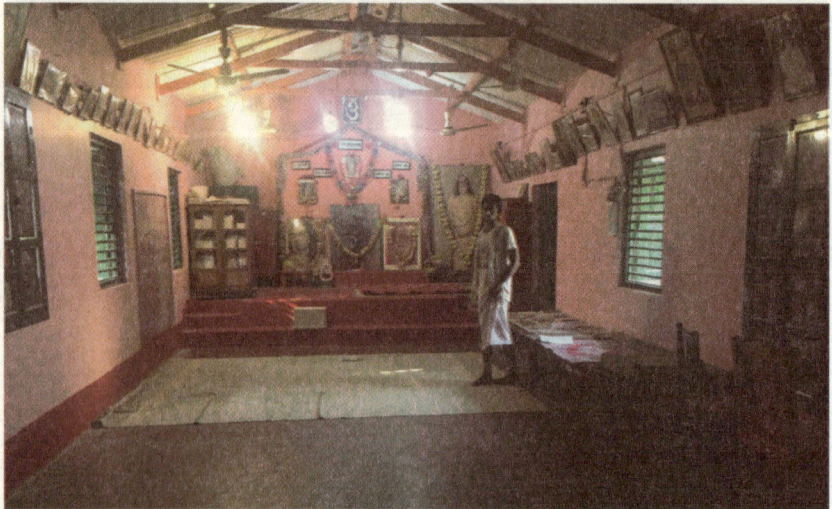

Top: Sri Yukteswar's Samadhi Temple at Karar Ashram.
Bottom: Main Hall of Karar Ashram, Puri.

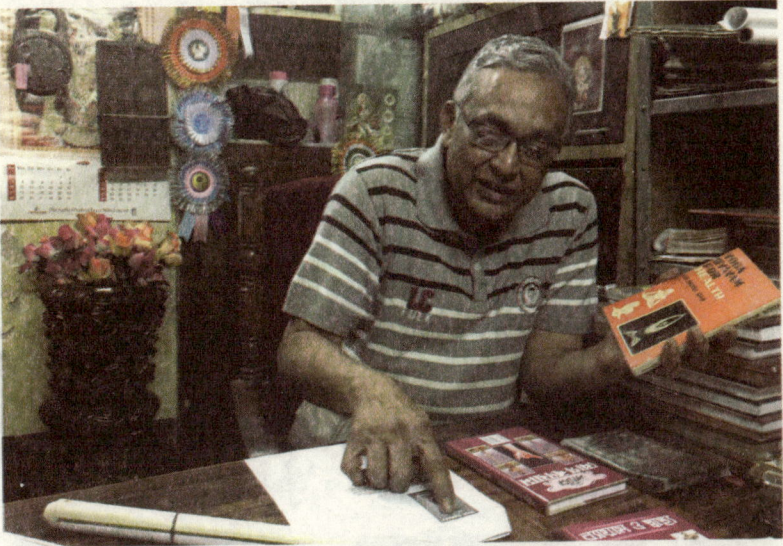
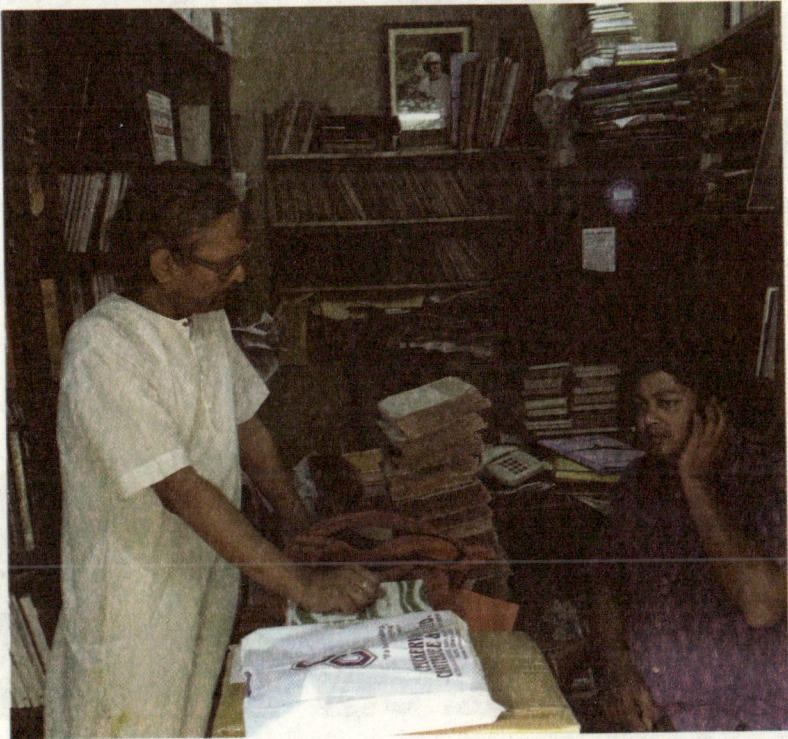

Top: Swapan Das at Ironman Publishing & Yoga, Amherst Row, Calcutta.
Bottom: Arup Sen Gupta with Kamli at Subarnarekha bookstore. College Square, Calcutta.

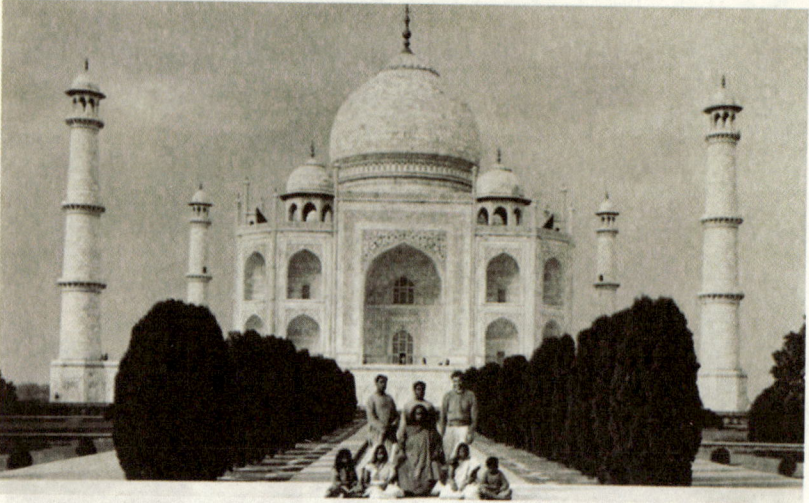

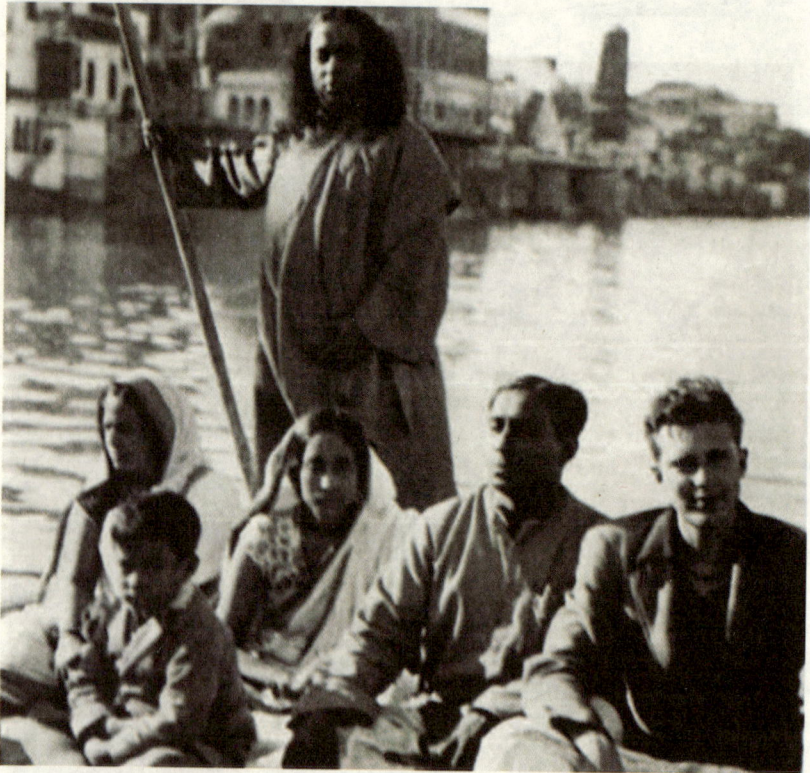

Top: At the Taj Mahal, Agra, 1936. Yogananda (middle seated); Back row (left to right): Sananda, Bishnu, Richard Wright. Front row (left to right): Ava Rani, Ashalata, Parlul, Srikrishna. Bottom: Benares (Varanasi), 1936. Yogananda (standing). Seated (left to right): Ashalata, Srikrishna, Parlul, Sananda, Richard Wright.

Source: Wikimedia Commons.

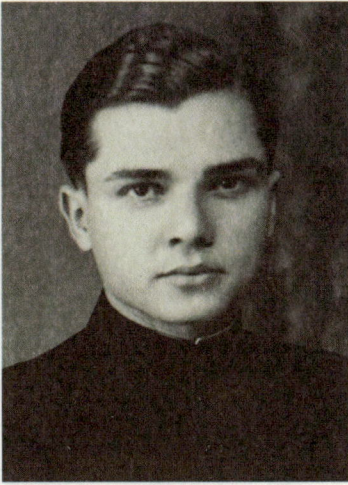

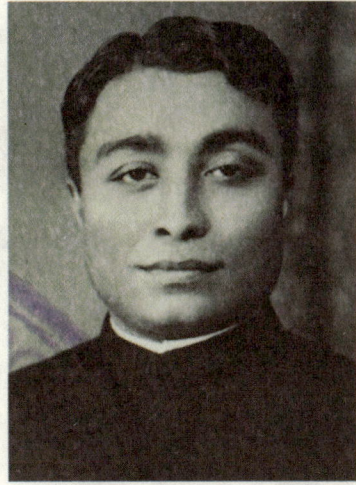

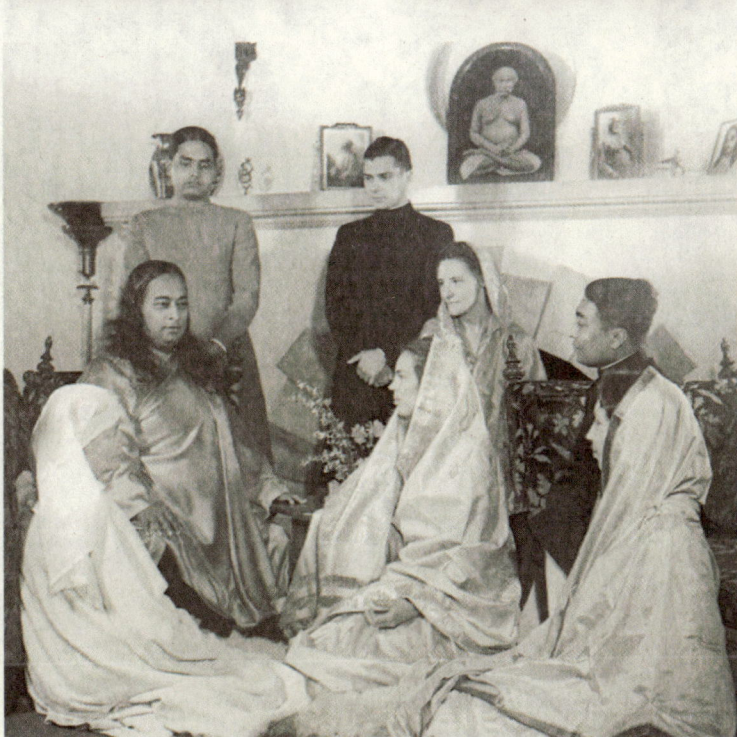

Top: Passport photos of Bishnu (left) and Buddha. Bottom (men from left): Yogananda, Binayananda, Buddha and Bishnu. With (women from left): Gyana Mata, Daya Mata, Ananda Mata, Durga Mata. SRF Mother Center, Los Angeles, 1938.

Source: British Library, London; Wikimedia commons.

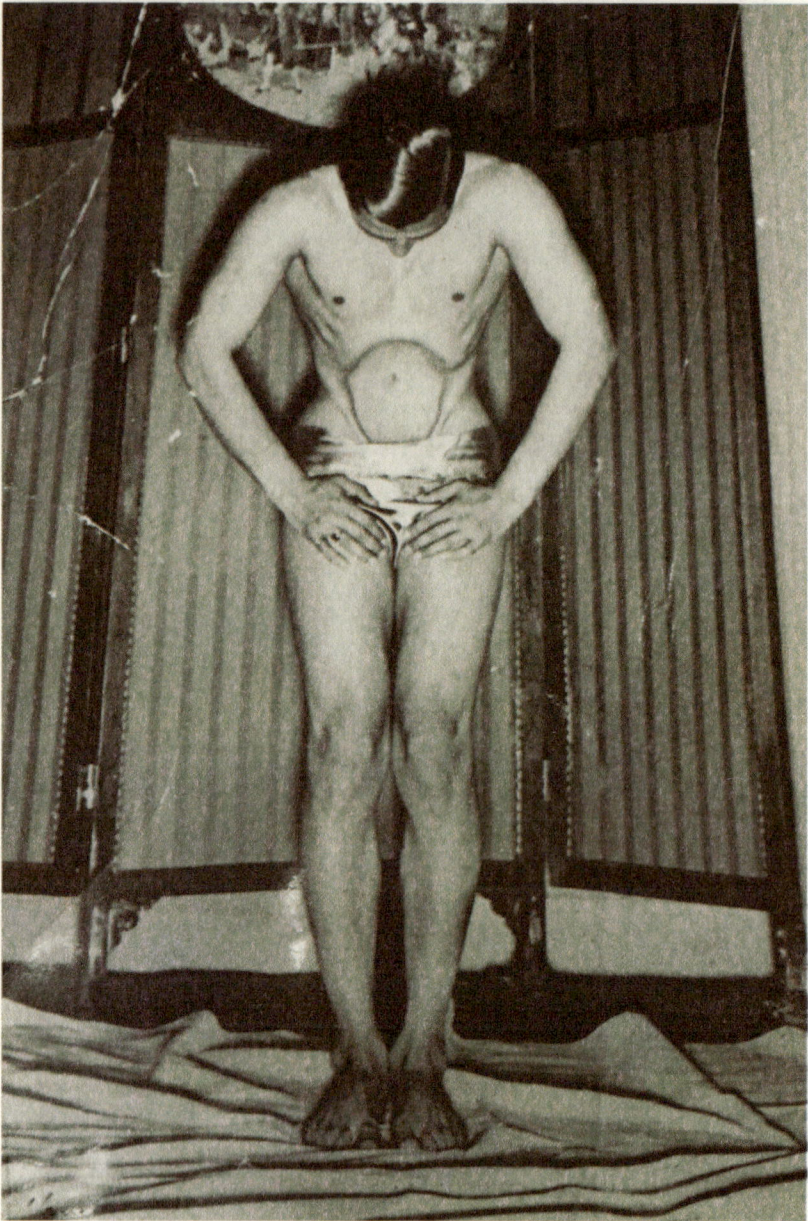

Buddha Bose, performing in Berlin, Germany, 1938.

Courtesy of Soham Heritage & Art Center, Mussoorie, India.

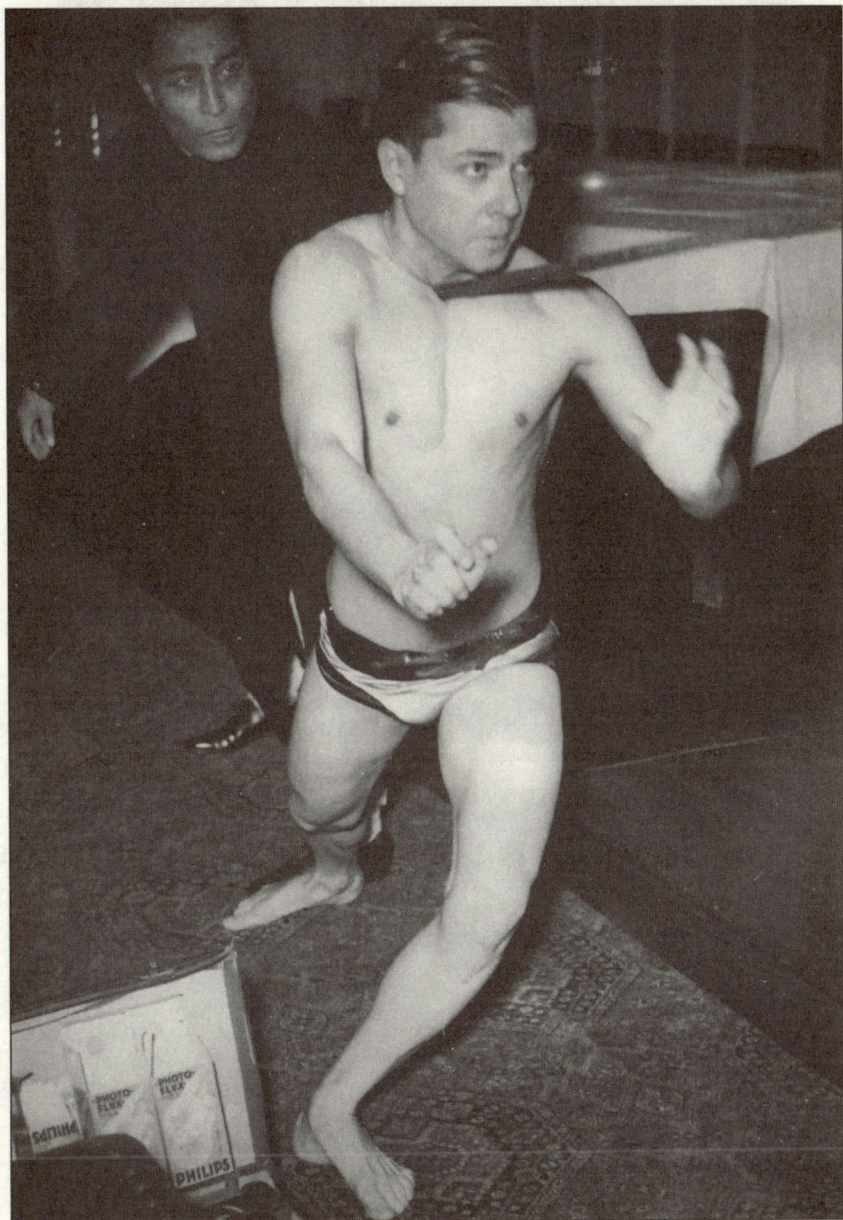

Bishnu Ghosh (left) and Buddha Bose. Caxton Hall, London, 1938.
Courtesy of Austrian Scala Archives.

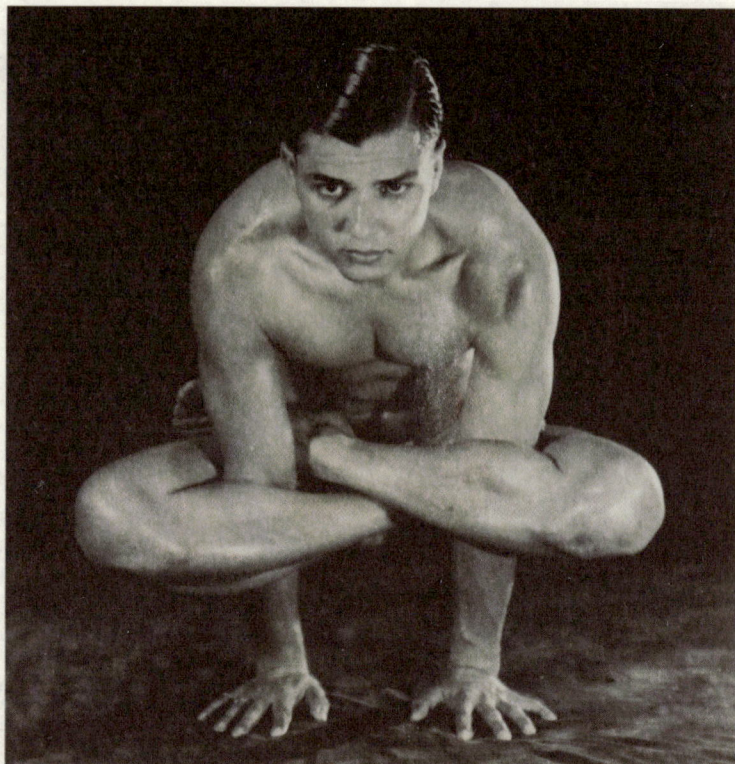

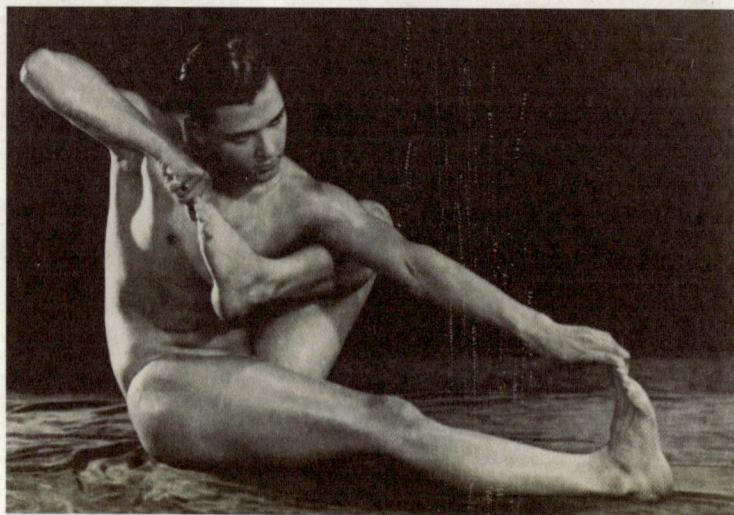

Yoga Asanas images within the previously unpublished 1938
manuscript and album by Buddha Bose.

Courtesy of 84 Yoga Asanas (2015).

PART SIX

ROOTS OF CALCUTTA YOGA

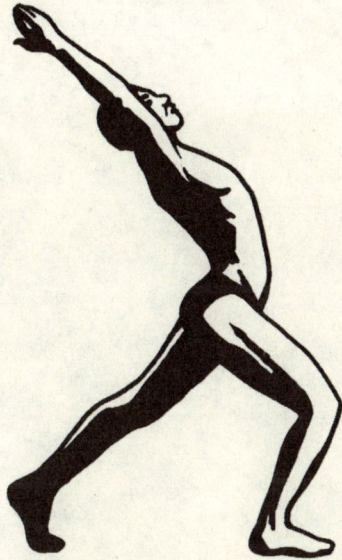

BENGAL HATHA YOGA

I was Eugene Sandow's assistant on the stage for ten long years.
He was superb, extraordinary, but this Bengali boy is more beautiful.[1]
– Captain Knox J.P. of the Calcutta Court, a student of Buddha Bose

Buddha's perception of muscle control practice was transformed when he saw a demonstration of asanas in 1932. He realized yoga asanas were India's indigenous physical culture system, and began learning from Hatha yoga teachers in Calcutta and the publications of Kuvalayananda. As he learned from Bishnu, a primary source of influence was the Hatha yoga Bishnu had been taught at Yogananda's schools in Dihika and Ranchi. This is stated explicitly in the introduction to Buddha's 1939 book on yoga asanas, where Bishnu wrote, 'I myself learned this system of Yoga Exercises at the Ranchi School for boys in India.'[2] Though Bishnu did not reference Dihika, we know from his other writings that the school's first location was instrumental.[3]

At the Dihika ashram school, Swami Alakananda was a Hatha yoga expert who came to train students in the yogic asanas.[4] Bishnu mentioned another person, Swami Kapilananda, who taught him the full array of Hatha yoga methods.[5] Yet another – Swami Kebalananda – was the Sanskrit tutor and *kriyaban* who held 'the position of *Dharmacharya*' at the school. Kebalananda, 'till then a householder' and known as Shastri Mahasaya, 'agreed to don the ochre-robe', in order 'to run the school as per the ideals of the ancient Saints'.

When the school moved to Ranchi, both Swami Kapilananda and Alakananda were left behind (at least from further mentions). Instead, Kebalananda taught Sanskrit, shastras and also Hatha yoga. Kebalananda is not a storied figure, but within the context of the Ghosh family and Yogananda's novice, spiritual-minded, boyhood friends, as well as the Calcutta–Benares *kriyaban* movement, he was an important spiritual influence.[6] Kebalananda was an ardent practitioner and teacher, and well educated.

During his youth in Calcutta, Kebalananda went by the name Ashutosh Chatterjee. His teacher was Vidyasagar, who was famous throughout India for his efforts in social reform and his role in the Bengal Renaissance. Vidyasagar arranged for Kebalananda to attend higher education courses in Benares.[7] Aside from those studies, Kebalananda 'learned Hatha yoga from the Hatha yogis', in Benares (Varanasi). He 'began to practise very seriously and sincerely ... the unique synthesis' of Kriya yoga to obtain self-knowledge.[8]

Beginning in Dihika and continuing in Ranchi, the influence of Kebalananda 'in the newly established school began to expand'. He would 'teach the students' yoga postures, how to chant mantras, and if they were fit, Kriya yoga. In Ranchi, during the early 1920s, Kebalananda became a close confidant of Satyananda, and had a profound influence due to 'the extraordinary power of his spiritual life'. Under his guidance, some people were engaged in learning many different kinds of *sadhana*, or meditation, of *mantra shakti*, or mantra power. 'Some were engaged in learning the Hatha yoga practices.'[9]

How exactly Kebalananda taught the 'procedures of *Karma Kanda*' (Vedic rituals and actions), Hatha yoga and Kriya yoga, with a 'focus on *Dharana*, a glimpse of tranquility, and *Dhyana*, or meditation', is unknown. Each required an immense amount of experience. Even to attempt an explanation under the heading of 'Classical Hatha yoga' would be a bit of a misnomer, as the amount of synthesis of disparate practices he would have done in Benares remains unknown. What we know for sure is that the classical Hatha yoga practices of Bishnu Ghosh, learned from 1917 to 1920, laid the groundwork for his teaching of Buddha Bose.

There were also sources inside the Ghosh gymnasium mentioned as being influential. The 1930 book, *Muscle Control and Barbell Exercises* was co-authored by Keshab Chandra Sen Gupta. In the preface to the 'Barbell Exercises' section, Sen Gupta mentioned his experience learning indigenous physical games, with his elder brother Babu Narendra Nath Sen Gupta, who had a 'well-developed body and phenomenal strength', developed through 'physical exercises' that were 'scientific and systematic'.[10] Bishnu and Buddha would call these same brothers to clarify a particular method or form of the asanas they were learning at Ghosh's gymnasium:

> They would often debate about how a particular posture should be done,
> and when they were confused they approached B.C. Ghosh. The last word

however was always the one of Keshub Sen Gupta, who, according to Professor Bose, was the real brain ... So when B.C. Ghosh was not certain about a particular posture, he went and asked Sen Gupta.[11]

Keshab and Narendra had learned the system of Hatha yoga in their Bengal village, and were the ones around Ghosh's gymnasium with that particular expertise. At that time in Calcutta's development, families would often move from a Bengal village to the urban center. They maintained their cultural connections and even journeyed back and forth. For the Sen Guptas, these connections included the knowledge of Hatha yoga. Whether that knowledge was verbal, passed on through generations or textual, is not known. In Calcutta, first-hand knowledge, originally from remote villages, or those experienced in Hatha yoga, was the primary authority. Bishnu and Buddha also had access to classical yoga texts, specifically the *Hatha Yoga Pradipika* and *Gheranda Samhita*.

39

CLASSICAL HATHA YOGA TEXTS

In Bishnu's *Muscle Control* (1930), yogic exercises, including *nauli* and others, were presented as muscle control. In regard to the benefits, Bishnu commented, 'All these types of abdominal contractions safely heal indigestion and improve the digestive power of a normal man.'[1] This sentence closely resembled a statement in the *Hatha Yoga Pradipika*, a classical fifteenth-century yoga text, which stated, 'Nauli is the crown of Hatha practices. It kindles a weak gastric fire, restores the digestion, always brings happiness, and dries up all defects and diseases.'[2] While the *Hatha Yoga Pradipika* is one of the earliest known references to *nauli*, another Sanskrit yogic text named the *Gheranda Samhita* also referenced the technique. To practise, 'rotate the stomach quickly on both sides. This gets rid of all diseases and the bodily fire increases.'[3]

Bishnu and Buddha's understanding of Hatha yoga practice in general and purification techniques in particular significantly overlapped with these primary texts. The *Gheranda Samhita* is largely about the purification of the body, which leads to the subtler effects of Hatha yoga understood through the progressive meditative techniques of *dhyana* and *samadhi*.

When Bishnu described the teachings of Hatha yoga from the yogi Swami Kapilananda in Dihika, he mentioned 'asana, *dhauti*, pranayam, mudra, *nauli*, *uddiyana*, and *basti*', which are mostly cleansing techniques derived from the *Gheranda Samhita*[4] and *Hatha Yoga Pradipika*.[5]

The prominence of mudras alongside asanas in Buddha's manuscript also stand out as influenced by the classical yogic texts. The *Gheranda Samhita* made the slight distinction that 'asanas bring about strength; mudras bring about steadiness'.[6] Neither Buddha nor Bishnu specifically wrote of the distinction between mudras and asanas.

However, a student of Bishnu, Yogacharya Mukul Dutta of Calcutta, described the distinction he was taught: 'Mudras are the integrated version of asanas and pranayamas. In asanas, postures apart, breathing is not specific. In pranayama, breathing is the focal point. In mudras, however, both the postures and breathing, are equally important. In *uddiyana bandha* mudra the posture and the breathing are inseparable.'[7]

Much of what they mentioned and demonstrated while out on their world tour gave credence to the claim of the *Gheranda Samhita* being a primary source text. They promoted India's 'Sacred Physical Culture Made up of 84 Body Postures', repeating verses 1–2 in the asanas section of the *Gheranda Samhita*: 'Shiva has taught 8,400,000. Of these, eighty-four are pre-eminent.'[8]

A large part of the *Gheranda Samhita* corresponds verbatim to the *Hatha Yoga Pradipika*.[9] However, neither of these texts contain the large number of postures which are not-seated, complex and inverted, which we find in early modern yoga texts and in Buddha's compilation of asanas. The *Gheranda Samhita*, for example, presents just thirty-two asanas. This has led to speculation that many of the more physically demanding postures are modern-day creations. However, with more recent scholarship of lesser-known yogic texts, it has become 'clear that more than eighty-four asanas were practised in some traditions of Hatha yoga before the British arrived in India'. And that these went beyond seated asanas to include asanas 'performed in a standing, supine, prone, twisting, back-bending, forward-bending or arm-balancing position'.[10]

In a 1939 lecture, Bishnu explained that there were 'eight ways to breathe properly'.[11] He gave the example of *bhastrika*, a powerful inhalation and exhalation, as one of the 'eight *kumbhakas*' included in the pranayama section of the *Gheranda Samhita*. The eight types of breathing presented in *Gheranda Samhita* are *sahita, surya bheda, ujjayi, shitali, bhastrika, bhramari, murcha* and *kevali*.

Buddha's assistant for teaching the women at Yoga Cure in the 1970s, Chitralekha Shalom, also the eldest daughter-in-law of his family, detailed seven types of pranayama that were taught, which corresponded to seven of the eight detailed in the *Gheranda Samhita*.[12] Four of the breathing techniques – ujjayi, surya bheda, sitali and bhramari – were nearly identical to the *Gheranda Samhita* and Buddha's teaching circa 1970s. Two techniques from the *Gheranda Samhita*, that of murcha and kevali, differed slightly in the teachings by Bose. Murcha was a form of alternating between less time for inhalation and increased time for exhalation, and was mentioned by Bose under the name *sadharan*. Likewise, kevali, listed in the *Gheranda Samhita*, was a technique that halted the breath, and was similar to what Bose listed as *khechari*.[13]

When Buddha Bose published *Key to the Kingdom of Health through Yoga*, Volume 1 (1939), it contained nearly the same preface that was in his original draft of the unpublished *Yoga Asanas* (1938), except for a few revisions. In the published introduction, Bishnu Ghosh explained that 'we have confined our explanations' to 'the asanas or postures as a foundation stone' and left out the 'higher Yoga training in spiritual development' which 'Buddha Bose and myself have received from Paramhansa Yogananda'.[14] The main item edited out of the original preface written by Buddha Bose was his 'brief mention' about '*Kundalini Shakti*', the 'latent power within every human being' which is accessible through 'the exceptional value of these exercises'. His use of the term came directly from seventeenth-century Hatha yoga texts. As '*Kundalini Shakti* enables the individual to control the mind, the importance of awakening it will be readily understood'. He wrote that 'the practice of certain asanas gradually awakens this power' enabling the ability 'to master' the mind.[15]

Through these references, a connection between the development of modern yoga and the classical medieval-era yoga texts should not be overstated. By and large, 'the yoga connection' for modern yoga's development in the twentieth century, was established through a network of places in India, such as Lonavla and Santa Cruz near Bombay, Mysore in south India and Rishikesh along the Ganges, and the teachers therein. They drew from a multitude of traditions, many of them oral and coming from Hatha yogis who were still around at the time. 'The relationships were personal and as such also subject to preferences. B.C. Ghosh did not like "the Bombay people" and preferred Rishikesh instead.'[16]

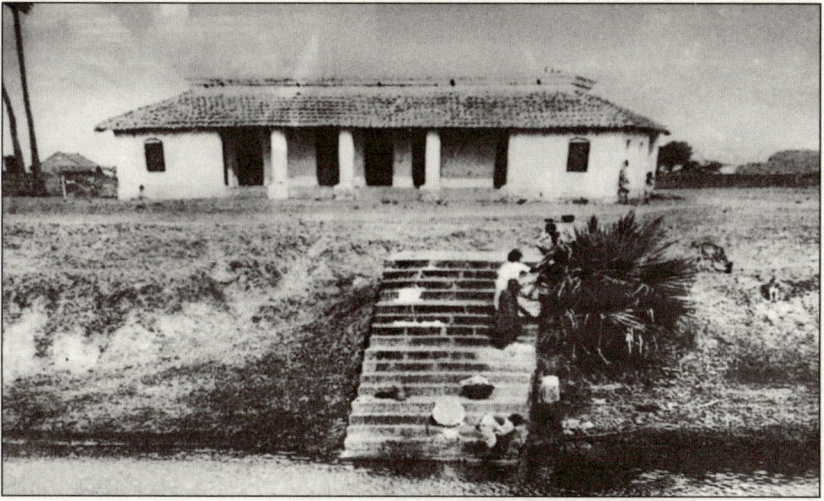

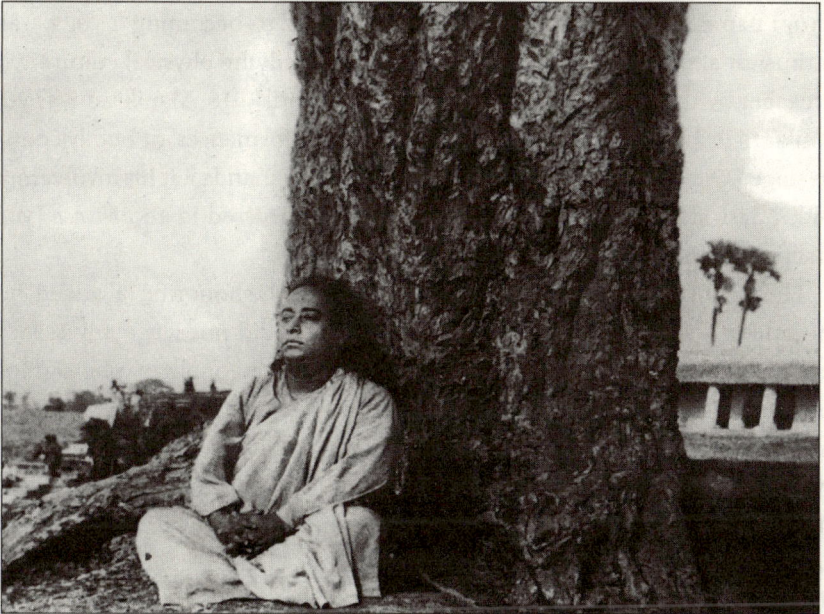

Top: Dihika ashram; Bottom: Yogananda, Dihika, 1935.
Courtesy of Dihika Ashram, India.

40

THE YOGA OF MADHAVADAS

The first modern-era textual influence on Hatha yoga for Bishnu and Buddha came through the writings of Swami Kuvalayananda, who learned from a yogi named Madhavadas. Kuvalayananda, prior to becoming a yoga asana enthusiast and teacher, was deeply involved in studying physical culture with a teacher by the name of Manikrao from 1907 until 1918. Manikrao was very similar to Bishnu, demonstrating 'eye-dazzling performances' of bodily control on stage.[1] Once introduced to Hatha yoga, Kuvalayananda left his involvement with physical culture when he became 'fully engrossed in *Yogabhyasa* [yoga practices]', under Madhavadas.[2]

He became known as Madhavadas, often with the honorific 'ji' added, and the title of Paramhamsa, Maharaj or Yogiraj. He did not write any texts or provide any extensive interviews; he only allowed a couple of photographs to be taken. He was born in 1798 and died in 1921; he lived for 123 years. If one were looking for a proponent of using yoga to live a long and healthy life, then Madhavadas would seem exemplary in this regard. The biographies of Madhavadas, within books on the origins of modern yoga, began with noting that he was the teacher of 'two of the key figures in the formation of modern Hatha yoga' – Yogendra and Kuvalayananda.[3]

Madhavadas was born in Bengal, in a village nearby Shantipur; his family name was Mukhopadhyay.[4] They were devoted to Vaishnavism and followed Chaitanya Mahaprabhu. Beyond Vaishnavism was the influence of the 'school of thought known as Yogis'. Madhavadas excelled in languages, learning Sanskrit, Bengali and English. His mother and father died when he was twenty years old, in 1818. Thereafter, he joined 'Government service in the Judicial Department' in Calcutta, but a few years after having taken the position, and being raised to an officer, he resigned. A particular event in the court 'aroused his indignation' and convinced him to leave the 'worldly way of life', disillusioned and detached. He then secretly left his home to take initiation from a 'guru of a Sri Caitanya sect' in the 'Gaurang Sampradaya by Sri Bhakti Charandas Ji', where he began *sadhana* (practice) and bhakti (devotion) at the age of twenty-three, 'in search of the higher pursuit of life'. This led him beyond bhakti to different paths of yoga. He travelled all over India for thirty-five years, from 1822 to 1857. He was said to have traversed the whole of modern India, and travelled to Tibet, to learn the intricacies of yoga and gain wide knowledge of its practice.

In 1857, Madhavadas was sixty years of age. Having attained a 'great mastery over practical yoga', he retired in solitude in the caves of the Himalayas for the next twelve years, for 'hard Yoga *tapasya*'. When Madhavadas returned from the Himalayas in 1869, 'word about his yogic *vibhutis* spread everywhere'. For the next fifteen years, he lived in various ashrams, and travelled with a very large group 'of nearly 400 to 500 *sadhus* who accepted him as their leader'. In Kanakeswaran, he became 'known as Mirchi Baba', because he would take 'only a lump of powdered chilis and a little quantity of buttermilk' each day, according to the Shiva temple records at the location. In 1885, he settled down along the bank of the Narmada River, near the village of Malsar at the age of eighty-seven.

He was a true renunciant, with his only belonging being a 'cloth on his body'. His ashram started with just 'a pit of fire', but the place soon developed into a hermitage, and he often retired to Ranpur, a nearby place that was more secluded, 'to continue his *sadhana* practices of self-culture'. If not out travelling for a few days at a time, he would guide those who came for his advice. 'It was at these two places that he began to teach the secrets of practical Yoga to a few selected deserving disciples. He also applied many simple Yoga processes for therapeutic purposes.' Multiple stories of his 'miraculous power' and the above account leans towards hagiography, but what is most notable is that when he began to teach others during the latter decades of the nineteenth century, he emphasized 'practical yoga' for therapeutic purposes.

Madhavadas began laying the groundwork for others to become 'modern era' yoga teachers. The reach of two initiates, Yogendra and Kuvalayananda, extended into English print. Yogendra taught yoga as a 'form of physical culture' which functioned as a curative treatment, and promoted the fitness features of asanas, kriyas and pranayamas in a systematic manner.[5] Kuvalayananda had an outsized role in the propagation of the practice of yoga postures, but a clear eye towards maintaining the traditions of yoga and their focus on making 'the channels, the *nadis*, free, so the *pranic* movement can flow everywhere'.[6]

Kuvalayananda, after his initial study with Madhavadas and early publications of *Yoga Mimansa*, put together his book *Popular Yoga Asanas*, 'taken directly from old Yogic textbooks in Sanskrit and ancient Yogic traditions, with only very few minor changes'.[7] From this book, published in 1932, Buddha reviewed the postures, also likely having access to the editions of *Yoga Mimansa*, which had begun in October of 1924. There is a striking resemblance between many of the asanas performed by Buddha in *Yoga Asanas* and photographs within the previous editions of *Yoga Mimansa*. It is particularly noticeable when preparatory stages of asanas are shown.

A secondary appeal for Buddha and Bishnu was the application of scientific rigour to the beneficial claims of yoga asana practice. Through *Yoga Mimansa*, Kuvalayananda published the first scientific experiments, 'using scientific measurements to study the effects of yogic practices'.[8] The pattern of looking to science for validation was also shared by Yogananda as part of the 'new Atomic age' way of thinking. 'The inner science of self-control will be found as necessary as the outer conquest of nature.'[9]

Kuvalayananda ran his yogic studies from a remote ashram in Lonavla, India, and wrote many letters to aspiring yogis around the world. A recent biography of him included a letter, dated 2 April 1934 to the maharajah of Mysore (the benefactor of Krishnamacharya's *yogashala* on the grounds of Jaganmohan Palace), which addressed the maharajah's 'keen interested in Yogic culture'. Krishnamacharya had visited Kuvalayananda's ashram and stayed there for three days, providing 'two demonstrations of "Yogic Asanas" with his pupils'.[10] Palpable tensions emerged in the letters of Kuvalayananda and his students, warning of systems claiming to be yogic that were not part of the Patanjali tradition, specifically, those which were 'very physical'.[11] In a follow-up letter to the maharajah, Kuvalayananda expressed strong reservations about Krishnamacharya and 'his exercises'. Kuvalayananda 'recommended him to keep the Yogic exercises unadulterated'.[12]

This was part of a disagreement Kuvalayananda and his students had with the modifications being made to Hatha yoga to suit the modern era. Kuvalayananda's position was that 'the physical benefits of yoga' were present and provable.[13] However, the more subtle benefits of yoga, such as '*pranic* movement, were not accessible from mere physically oriented exercise. 'As exercise the postures act on a muscular level; they don't go deeper.'[14]

The admonishment of any 'admixture' of the Yogic systems extended beyond the dynamic practice of Krishnamacharya to include 'physical culture'.[15] Kuvalayananda framed the conflict as being between the 'spiritual culturist' and 'physical culturist'. For instance, he discussed the practice of pranayama, and whether it could be practised outside of the 'seat' taken in the 'traditional arrangement' (i.e. a seated, usually in a cross-legged position). The physical culturist 'can practice his pranayama while sitting, or while standing or even while walking' (such as with *ujjayi* breath). However, Kuvalayananda took issue with 'the advice given' by 'particular physical culturists to practice pranayama while taking violent muscular exercises'. That, Kuvalayananda exclaimed 'is impossible'.[16]

Kuvalayananda made the argument that bodybuilders and those practising muscle control were not engaged in true pranayama. 'One may hold his breath for a time during such a work and give it the dignified name of pranayama or *kumbhaka*; but any attempt to claim pranayamic advantages of such a holding of breath, is as unscientific as it is misleading.'[17] This revealed the tension already underway in 1928 between the promoters of traditional Hatha yoga goals like Kuvalayananda (who wanted to add scientific validation to the practices) and those in the public eye that were beginning to utilize yogic techniques for other purposes, such as feats of strength (Bishnu Ghosh and others).

Claims of the 'misappropriation' of yoga had been lodged outside India for decades, but this type of modification was something that was underway in India from the very beginning of modern postural-focused yoga that introduced yogic practices to other physical fields. Bishnu extended yogic practices to feats of strength, done while holding the breath and using *bandhas* (locks) to lock the body in a position where massive weight or force of objects would not crush one's frame. The use of Hatha yoga techniques by the physical culturists brought about backlash among those who thought of yoga, with its asanas and pranayamas, as needing to be pursued from a spiritual vantage point.

Kuvalayananda might be considered a classical yoga purist, since his first general rule was that 'no one will be admitted to the ashram that does not come to it for spiritual evolution'.[18] Bishnu though, did not have this tension, and over time, became much more pragmatic and liberal in his promotion of yogic techniques, both by adding cultural historical validity to the performance of feats of strength and promoting their therapeutic use by the general population as a whole.

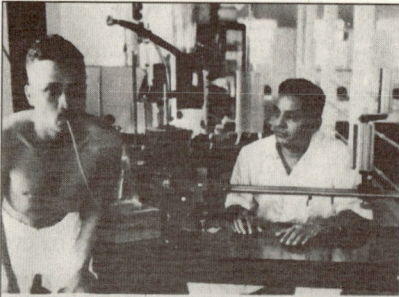

Recording of pressure changes during Madhya Nauli

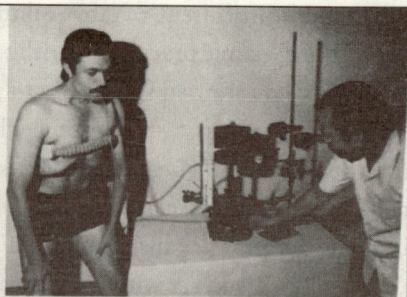

Recording of pressure during Uddiyan

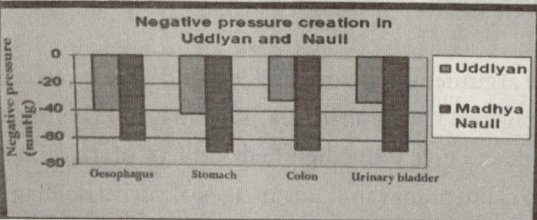

Negative pressure creation in Uddiyan and Nauli

- Uddiyan
- Madhya Nauli

Negative pressure (mmHg): 0, -20, -40, -60, -80

Oesophagus, Stomach, Colon, Urinary bladder

Study on intra-gastric pressure changes in Uddiyan and Nauli

Ref: Kuvalayananda. *Yoga Mimamsa, Vol 1:2, 96-100, 1925.*

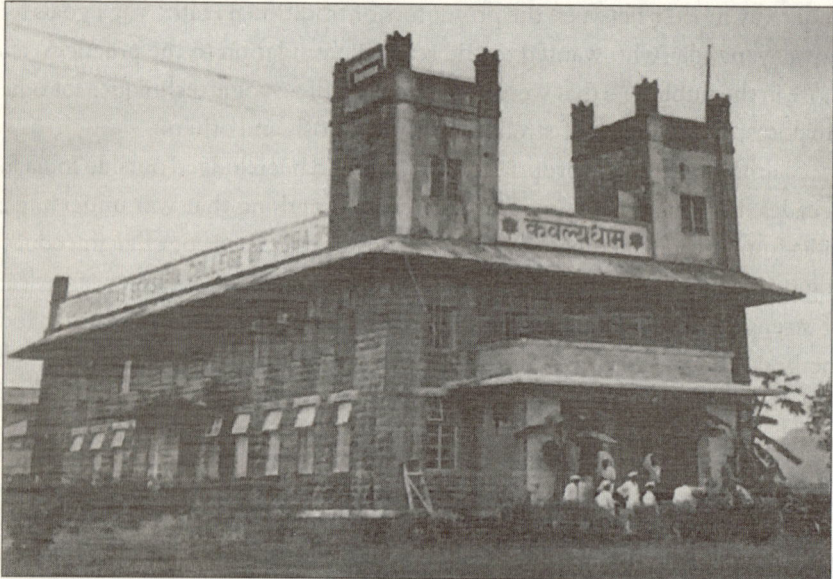

Top: Yogic studies done at Kaivalyadhama Yoga Institute, Lonavala.

Bottom: Kaivalyadhama Yoga Institute, Lonavala, circa 1930.

Courtesy of Kaivalyadhama Yoga Institute.

41

SWAMI SIVANANDA OF RISHIKESH

In Mysore in 1935, Buddha and Bishnu watched Krishnamacharya conduct a performance of purely Hatha yoga asanas with a dynamic flow. The presentation was a bit controversial in the yoga world of India during the thirties; its historical impact would not occur until decades later.[1] Though B. K. S. Iyengar had refused the advance of Yogananda, Buddha and Bishnu were ready to fill the void and planned a visit to America. In the meantime, Bishnu and Buddha readied an asana system.

Starting in 1931, Sivananda of Rishikesh[2] printed his materials through *My Magazine of India*, a small weekly periodical published by P.K. Vinayakam and edited by P.R. Rama Iyengar. It was said to have had a large circulation in India, as well as in Sri Lanka and Burma.[3] The magazine was aimed towards young, study-minded readers, and Sivananda reached many of his key early disciples through it. Each issue provided a page for Sivananda to answer questions in his column 'Precepts for Practice'. The questions broadened the practice of Hatha yoga beyond its previous confines of guru and disciple needing to be in close proximity. For example, one inquirer asked, 'Can I practise Pranayam by consulting books?' Sivananda answered, 'Yes, you must read the instructions several times and understand the technique thoroughly.'[4] These early publications by Sivananda resulted in him gaining a large following through the magazine outlet.

Sivananda's first book that contained asanas was titled *Practice of Yoga* and had two volumes. A first and second edition were published during the period between 1931 and 1933. At this point, influence from the *Hatha Yoga*

Pradipika and other classical yogic texts is not apparent. Instead, in a section titled 'Asanology: A Discourse on Asana', Sivananda reviewed postures taken from *Yoga Mimansa*. He wrote:

> Swami Kuvalayananda is editing a very useful quarterly journal on Hatha Yoga style, *Yoga Mimamsa*, in scientific, modern terms at Lonavla, Bombay … it contains beautiful pictures of asanas. Get the 4 parts of the first volume, wherein all the important asanas are described with fine photos of asanas. It is in English. It will help you a lot.

Yoga Mimansa may very well have been Sivananda's first introduction to written asana practice, as his explanatory text in this first volume closely followed the descriptions given by Kuvalayananda.[5] Sivananda went through multiple pages describing the same postures, using the same names, beginning with 'topsy-turvy pose' or *sirshashana*, the 'pan physical pose' or *sarvangasana*, and all the others which Kuvalayananda covered in his beginning volumes using the same nomenclature. Overall, Sivananda absorbed the volumes of teachings quite readily before turning to traditional Hatha yoga texts, such as the *Hatha Yoga Pradipika*, for his second book.

Yoga Asanas was published by Sivananda in 1934. The first edition 'was exhausted within six months' and a second edition was published in 1935. The original publication was put forth as a 'health-book which was expected to be a real contribution to our national uplift', and published by *My Magazine of India*.[6] The original publisher's preface, discontinued within a few editions, stated:

> As the Editor of *My Magazine of India*, I have had various opportunities of getting to know the taste and the interests of a wide public, all over the Indian empire: and I have noted with a very great pleasure a growing public interest in that ancient form of physical culture known as Yoga Asanas. Letters of appreciation and inquiry received from numerous readers, the encouraging sales of the Yoga Asana Chart, as well as the demand from the public for a complete and comprehensive study of this most important branch of Hatha Yoga have induced me to bring out this publication. The book contains not only the 26 Asanas with illustrations which were regularly published in *My Magazine of India* and also 58 other Asanas with illustrations. You will also find a number of the most important Mudras, *Bandhas* and Pranayams dealt with. Besides the propagation of a good deal of imperfectly known Yogic

literature, the book also offers to everyone practical suggestions for the rooting out of diseases and the building up of healthy bodies.[7]

The number of asanas referred to above, twenty-six plus fifty-eight, made eighty-four. The *Yoga Asanas* introduction presents '90 poses of the body with important *bandhas* and mudras and systems of pranayams, prescribed by the Yoga *Shastras*'.[8] He then repeated, from the classical yogic texts, 'There are 84 lakhs of asanas, described by Lord Shiva. Among them eighty-four are the best and among these eighty-four, thirty-two have been found very useful.'[9]

The list of eighty-four asanas, with its mystical concept of Shiva, the creative force within the Hindu deities, was probably the first such list in the twentieth century of modern yoga. It was very different from classical lists of eighty-four asanas, with its inclusion of more standing postures and considerably less time advised to stay in each posture.

Buddha's 1938 *Yoga Asanas* was remarkable for its photographic display. He looked spectacular, with a well-oiled body, like he was performing for a muscle show. The text was quite ordinary, almost minimal in its instruction. Starting with the preface, the textual similarities between Buddha's *Yoga Asanas* and Sivananda's book of the same name were evident.

Sivananda wrote that there are asanas which can be 'practised while standing', some 'by sitting' and others 'while lying down'.[10] Similarly, Buddha grouped his postures into '*Padmasana*' and 'sitting', then 'lying down', then 'standing', in addition to '*Kurmasana*' and 'Mudras'. The format of listing 'Benefits' and 'Technique' as text columns alongside each asana was used by Sivananda and also by Buddha. And many of the asanas listed without accompanying benefits and techniques in Sivananda's book were done the same way in Buddha's.

Most importantly, the English transliterations of the asanas were exactly the same in nearly all of the postures listed by Buddha. Altogether, seventy-two out of Buddha's eighty-four are identical in name and spelling to those listed by Sivananda. Given the vast discrepancy of spelling from Sanskrit to English, this alone was a preponderance of evidence. Looking at individual asana descriptions, some showed overlapping terminology. For *vatayanasana*, Sivananda gave the direction:

Stand erect. Take hold of the right root and place the heel firmly at the root
of the thigh or at the root of the organ and stand on one leg. Slowly bend
the left leg and let the right knee touch the ground.

Buddha gave the direction:

Stand erect with the heels together, toes pointed outward and forming a
right-angle. Lift the left foot and place it on the upper right thigh. Then
slowly bend the right leg holding the left foot with the right hand until the
left knee touches the floor.

For *yoga nidrasana*, Sivananda gave the direction:

Lie down in *savasana*. Take hold of the legs and fix the feet below the neck
or head. Then slowly raise the buttocks and keep the palm on the ground
below the buttocks or hips.

Buddha gave the direction:

Assume the *savasana* pose. With the help of the hands fix the legs one after
the other behind the shoulders and head. Place the palms on the buttocks.

However, there were many descriptions which were entirely different,
showing the influence of Hatha yoga teachers in Calcutta. A notable difference
was the addition of 'Muscles Exercised' under each asana in Buddha's book.
He did not attribute anything to Sivananda, which is not altogether surprising,
even though it was most assuredly a primary source. Neither did Sivananda
list his sources in later editions.

In the first editions of *Yoga Asanas*, in a section which was dropped in later
editions, Sivananda stated 'at the present moment, there is a great revival of
Yogic system of asanas'. He then went on to recognize individuals 'disseminating
this knowledge of asanas and pranayams, through books, lectures, charts,
magazines, etc.' Two individuals from the Awadh region of Uttar Pradesh
were named, along with a teacher from Bangalore and two individuals near
Bombay: Sri Yogendra of the Yoga Institute and Swami Kuvalayananda with
his 'institute in Lonavla' and 'his magazine *Yoga Mimansa*'.[11]

There was a certain amount of fluidity between yoga schools of different
parts of India in the late 1920s and into the 1930s. Texts written in English were

increasingly common, and there were reported meetings between the schools of yoga asanas. An India-wide circulation of 'how to practise' yoga books had Sivananda's 'Himalayan Yoga Series' at the forefront. English-written newspaper outlets in Lahore (*The Daily Herald*), Madras (*The Hindu*) and Calcutta (*The Forward*), and 'railway station bookstalls' helped propel the emergent 'text-book and field-book for Yoga enthusiasts'.[12]

For Buddha and Bishnu, the goal of publication was to widen the yoga practice to include foreigners and urban dwellers. For Sivananda, the yoga asanas were part of a larger path of a spiritual-minded yoga community.[13] Though there are many similarities between the two texts titled *Yoga Asanas*, by Sivananda and Buddha Bose, there are differences as well. There is a distinct possibility that the two books, instead of being replications, shared an older text of yoga asanas, which has not yet been uncovered.

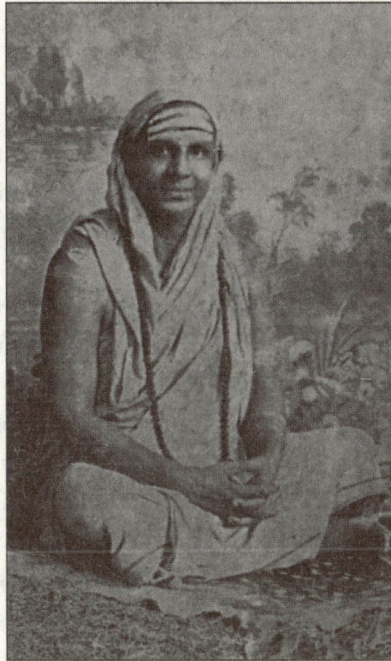

Swami Sivananda, circa 1935.

42

MUSCLE CONTROL TO MODERN YOGA

You can see here the smooth transition from physical exercise to yoga – and vice versa. If you are able to individually activate each muscle of the body and relax it again, then nauli is nothing more than another such exercise – and if this exercise has a certain effect in yoga, then inevitably the same result will follow when performed as muscle control.[1]
– Claudia Guggenbühl

In 1938, Buddha compiled a manuscript, complete with a photo album of himself in yoga asana postures. The full-size black and white photographs, numbering just over ninety, were stunning and strikingly modern, both in their use of light and professional composition.

Buddha never mentioned the photographer of the photos, but he was likely an American named Edward Groth, who became a student of Buddha's in 1937, a year before the photos were compiled, and may be the "Uncle Edward" too (as described in the preface).[2] Groth was an avid photographer, and also snapped yoga-themed photos of S. Muzumdar in Calcutta around this time. Those photos were published in *The Statesman*, for articles on asanas, and later used repeatedly in the seven books authored by Muzumdar, which went through multiple editions and were printed in five different languages. The photos were similar in layout to Buddha's, though likewise uncredited in the newspaper edited by Groth's British friend and fellow student of Buddha, Ian Stephens. Muzumdar did pay tribute to Groth in the preface to one of his books.[3]

Buddha's unpublished manuscript, *Yoga Asanas*, was signed and titled on 15 July 1938. The contents cast all of Bishnu and Buddha's previous accomplishments through the reference of Hatha yoga. The full repertoire of yoga asanas culminated in a complete modern postural yoga system. This resulted in not just Buddha's unpublished manuscript and photo album, but his beginners' book *Key to the Kingdom of Health through Yoga*, Volume 1, published in 1939, which covered twenty-four of the asanas. The period of six years, from 1932 until 1938, then followed by the world tour showcasing India's physical culture system of Hatha yoga, was one of learning, perfection, instruction and changes of lexicon.

In 1938, Buddha wrote that his guru, Bishnu 'always encouraged me to improve my own body and urged me to take up Hatha yoga'. With the desire 'to possess a well-developed body' and the promise of 'a better body than his own', Buddha began 'the practice of Yogic physical culture' in 1929 when he was just 'the age of sixteen'.[4] Up to 1938, when Buddha wrote those statements, however, there hadn't been any mention of his performing Hatha yoga, and neither was the attendant phrase of 'yogic physical culture' mentioned.

As noted previously, Buddha wrote that he was not oriented towards the idea of muscle control exercises as having their origin within Hatha yoga until 1932. Then, while watching a young boy do a demonstration of many asanas and mudras, he realized the techniques, such as the manipulation of his abdominal muscles that he'd performed, were entirely a part of the native Indian tradition. After study of the classical Hatha yoga texts, he further realized the yoga techniques mentioned in the classical texts were the same he'd performed as muscle control.[5]

The progression culminated with the 1938 manuscript and a full adoption of Hatha yoga terminology. What started out as being called 'physical culture' and 'muscle control' in Bishnu's 1930 book, then called 'Yogoda' in 1935 while on tour with Yogananda, had by 1938, changed to 'Hatha yoga' and 'Yogic physical culture'.

The use of a full system of asanas became part of their stage performance, which turned classical yoga on its head. While learning the asanas, Buddha paid an immense amount of attention to the form of the posture, seeking physical perfection. The asanas were traditionally taught with an inward focus, but Buddha's outward perfection, to be displayed in book format with glossy photos, was unprecedented. This new direction, influenced by the stage performance in his family, the strongman feats of Bishnu and the spellbinding lectures of Yogananda, was geared towards the audience. This was also a reflection of the period. Transnational modernism blended yoga's long transhistorical essence with a contemporary system of exercise and performance.

The synthesis replicated the era's utopian beginnings.[6] 'The early twentieth century saw a decisive change in the ways in which the body was thought about, described and represented', with a 'preoccupation, alteration, transformation and even reinvention', as a sign of therapeutic modernity.[7] With this, the quest for hygiene and physical health became a civilized priority.[8]

The notion of perfecting and altering the body was prevalent even before the thirties, but a slimmer and fitter, more active idea of physical culture now took precedence particularly one that was combined with a spiritual aim. All aspects of the physical alignment, including the limb angles and the angles of feet and hands to fingers, were placed in their most perfect-looking position, as if attempting to mimic the modern style of architecture, which was so prevalent in the thirties. Rounded sleekness was seen as clean form, without distraction from the essence of shape.

Posture-based exercise and 'published manuals for use in the home became common during this period'.[9] Buddha Bose, 'the finest specimen' in the 1934 'Body Beautiful' competition in Calcutta, differentiated himself from all previous Hatha yoga publicity attempts through sublime physical display.[10] His attention to perfect outward postural form, precise composition of each physical detail, combined with a magnificent stage presence, was something of an invention within the modern world of yoga. The system was, as one biographer put it, 'a synthesis of Eastern and Western physical culture'.[11] The hybrid encapsulated the idea of perfecting the physical body as spiritual preparation. The yoga asanas, 'as the foundation stone of the Yoga system', became the entire focus when teaching the 'beginner'.[12]

To
Uncle Edward

From
" Buddha".

Calcutta
July 15th, 1938

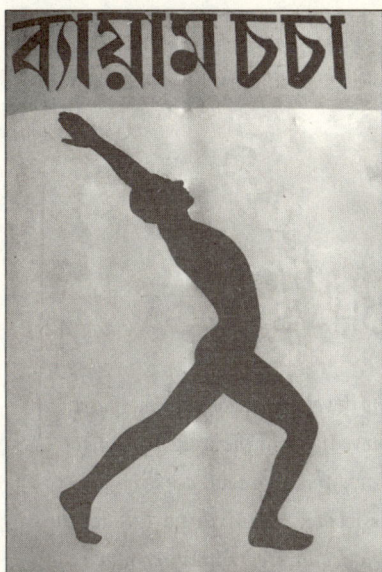

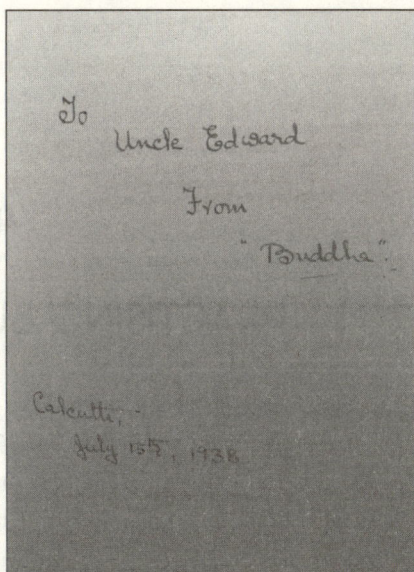

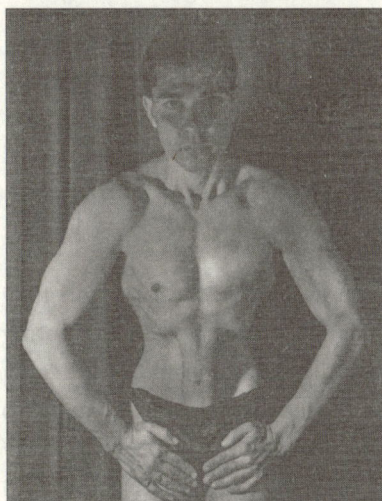

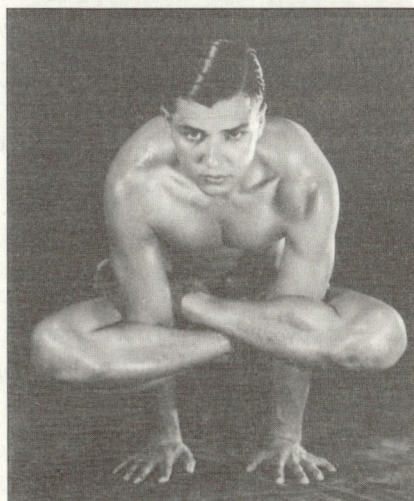

Clockwise from top left: Cover of *Bayam* Charcha; Dedication page
"To Uncle Edward" from manuscript of Yoga Asanas by Buddha Bose;
Buddha Bose in kukkutasana; Buddha Bose in nauli.
Courtesy of Bayam Charcha, Soham Heritage & Art Center, and 84 Yoga Asanas by Buddha Bose.

43

PRACTISING BUDDHA'S YOGA

The student of this ancient art aspires to the development of a slim, smart,
well-proportioned and healthy body. To achieve this end the student requires
perseverance, patience, the ability to concentrate, and above all, a willingness to
adopt healthful and regular habits. If it is possible to practice this art under the
guidance of a competent instructor who is well acquainted with it, so much the
better. There are not now many Westerners who know Hatha Yoga well enough
to teach it. It is for this reason that I decided to publish a book which through its
simple directions and profuse illustrations will enable any interested reader to
immediately begin the practice.[1]
– Buddha Bose, 1938

The underlying system of asana practice presented in the 1938 and 1939
texts by Buddha did not deviate from the significant principle of alternating
contraction with relaxation. Bishnu had applied the technique in *Muscle Control*
(1930), and Yogananda had applied it to the Yogoda exercises first taught to
Americans during the twenties, after having devised it as a personal daily
practice beginning as early as 1916. This principle, of using contraction with
relaxation, found a similar application with the use of asanas for physical culture
contraction, and the use of *savasana*, laying supine, for relaxation. Buddha's
instruction to follow each asana with a period in savasana was a novel concept,
except when viewed in relation to this principle of contraction and relaxation.[c]

In order to follow the contraction–relaxation method previously laid out
by Bishnu and Yogananda, the use of savasana appeared in a prominent role.
Prior to this, savasana as a posture was mentioned in classical yoga texts, such
as the *Gheranda Samhita*, and was presented as one among the many asanas,
not as a special class unto its own.

Kuvalayananda provided primary relaxation instructions to prepare the yogi for the 'pranayamic exercises which come after asanas'.[2] Similarly, Yogendra advised savasana as a 'final exercise'.[3] Buddha explained that the practice of savasana was 'to be practised for a brief period after each contraction, experienced in asana or yoga pose'. And then, going further, 'usually the duration of relaxation in *savasana* posture after each asana is the same as for the asana itself'.[4]

Thus, the underlying connection and continuity in practice was what Buddha delineated in the instructions for his system of yoga asana, in which he took the same principles of contraction and relaxation for the muscles, and applied it to asana and savasana for the body as a whole. The technique followed the same pattern Yogananda described in the Yogoda techniques, which he taught to Americans. A 1925 descriptive outline by Yogananda explained as 'tense with will; relax with feel' and that one should 'remember this motto all through the exercises'.[5] Then in 1930, Bishnu wrote of the 'contraction' and 'relaxation of the body' technique which was employed for bodybuilding exercises.[6]

Used as a practice or technique, this was quite different from the structure of a modern yoga class, which uses savasana more as a means to catch one's breath and as a final relaxation after a series of asanas. Buddha's technique was taught in a one-on-one structure, for a personal practice, where the duration of savasana 'after each asana is the same as for the asana itself'. The practice combined just a handful of asanas – between four and eight –and just one or two breathing exercises, integrated with savasana. Buddha advised to extend the hold time of each posture and to do an increased number of sets, rather than moving quickly from the posture once the basic set-up was achieved. In other words, it was a practice of few asanas, tailored to each individual.

After locating Buddha's yoga teachings, I begin to practise according to the instructions as they are laid out in *Key to the Kingdom of Health through Yoga*, Volume 1. Here is what I wrote about the experience at the time:

I'm hesitant to attribute it too much to the Bose book, but given the changes I've noticed since I started applying his method to my home practice about 3 weeks ago, it seems applicable. There's a quote in Benjamin Lorr's book *Hellbent*, that true balance means exactly 50 percent of the time, less is more. This seems like a total contradiction, but when I started doing the sets and reps as explained by Bose, I got in touch with a softness of the transition, and my expectations of the asana changed. Maybe it's that one goes deeper the 3rd and 4th set (not stretching but mentally relaxed); maybe the longer *savasana* is at work (taking the edge off more); maybe that this way takes up to 10 minutes for each asana; maybe it's a pace one sets up for doing 4 sets rather than 1 or 2 – no need to push it too soon, lots of time here, not striving. It just seems to slow me down enough to really be in the moment with the yoga.[7]

The experience entirely transforms my personal practice of yoga asanas and daily practice in general. It's what begins the journey of unearthing his unpublished 1938 manuscript and photo album, and this historical account.

The yoga asana practice taught by Buddha carries with it a certain adherence to the practice which I encounter while training with Tony Sanchez, the essence of which extends back historically in this lineage, starting with Lahiri Mahasaya in Benares, who would exalt to his students, '*banat, banat, ban jai!*' (doing, doing, one day done)![8]

What started with the nineteenth-century Calcutta gymnasium practices, and continued through the teachings of Bishnu and Yogananda, was put to words by Buddha who stated the 'key to the kingdom of health' is 'patience and practice'. And, 'it is never too late to begin the practice of Hatha yoga', for, 'if one desires a fine mind, a fine body must first be developed'. Through 'the power of concentration', the student 'is perfecting the vehicle through which the spirit can express itself'.[9]

44

YOGA FOR THE WEST

I check into the Calcutta hotel off Russell Street, the colonial-era Kenilworth,
and gaze outside the sixth floor window over the other nearby buildings and then
realize, I'd somehow booked a hotel with a room looking out over the rooftop of
the US Consulate. I know this spot. There, between 1937 and 1942, the American
consulate officer Edward Groth practised his yoga asanas.
Buddha Bose provided the lessons.

Buddha's teaching method laid out a fairly specific process, stating, 'It is
better gradually to increase the duration of practice of each exercise than
to strive to practice a large number of them for a brief period.' He added,
'Those who hope to specialize in this line may learn all of the asanas, but for
average individuals of all ages, a few exercises should be chosen, suitable to
the person's physical condition, age and bodily build.' He grouped the asanas
into six series – *padmasana*, sitting, reclining, standing, advanced (tortoise
sequence) and mudras – and 'arranged the exercises in each series so that the
easiest comes first and the most difficult last', with the exhortation to 'start
practising a few exercises in each group [excluding the advanced series] and
then gradually work up to the more difficult ones'.[1]

Buddha's earliest Hatha yoga students in Calcutta included two Westerners,
Edward Groth from New York and Ian Stephens from London. Groth and
Stephens were not the first Western professionals to travel, work and live in
India, but they were certainly among the first to have a modern postural-based
yoga practice.

In his 1935 biography, Buddha Bose presented himself as a physical instructor, listing his prominent clientele. The biography did not mention that he was teaching Hatha yoga, but a 1939 interview with Bishnu revealed as much. The interview followed one of Buddha's performances of eighty-four asanas. Bishnu told a reporter that Buddha had been 'a teacher himself for the past three years'.[2] In their literary autobiographies, both Groth and Stephens stated that 1937 was the year they began their exploration into yoga asana practice with Buddha, just after he had begun to include them in his teaching. Both Groth and Stephens played a pivotal role in helping Buddha with his professional endeavours a few years later, but their first encounters with Buddha were more practical and instructive for both Buddha's method of teaching and their own motivations for the practice.

Ian Stephens arrived in India in 1937 and was employed by the English daily newspaper *The Statesman*. After a short stint in Delhi as an assistant, he relocated and was promoted as the editor of *The Statesman* in Calcutta.[3] He was from London, having lived and studied in Bloomsbury alongside a crowd of famous writers, but he worked abroad in different parts of Asia throughout his career.

Stephens memoir, *Monsoon Mornings*, detailed his time as the '*sahib* editor' of *The Statesman* in Calcutta, and his encounter with Hatha yoga asana practice. After his arrival, he found European exercises and games, such as squash or tennis, 'exhausting in the Calcutta heat'. And further, 'getting a partner' was not easy with his 'busy writing job not fixed to office-hours'. 'Yoga,' he thought, 'might be the answer' for 'keeping healthy in that hot, humid city'.[4]

Stephens was 'primarily indebted' to an American friend named 'Edward Miller Groth, who was the second-in-command at the American Consulate in Calcutta' for 'his addiction to yoga exercises'. Groth initially took up the practice with more 'enthusiasm' than Stephens, but Stephens was soon persuaded to follow.

In 1937, Groth had been in Calcutta for 'three or four years' and had grown tired of 'tossing the medicine ball on the roof' of the American Consulate office building. 'In a Turkish-bath climate like Calcutta's,' he wrote, a discipline of 'sufficient exercise' was essential for good health. 'After a long, hot day at the office one was tired, but that was just when one needed exercise.' The 'Calcutta's Deputy Police Commissioner' put him 'in touch with Buddha Bose, an excellent Bengali instructor in Hatha yoga'. Groth, like Stephens, 'soon realized' this type of yoga, 'concerned with the perfection of man's physical vehicle', was 'exercise better suited to a tropical climate' than other sports.[5]

When Groth and Stephens began, Stephens wrote that his American friend

Groth was more aggressive, with a condition Stephens labeled as 'transatlantic over-zeal'.[6] Groth 'especially wanted to do the difficult headstand'. However, Buddha 'a qualified teacher … from Bishnu Ghosh's gymnasium in North Calcutta … advised against it and said the shoulderstand was equally beneficial' as an inverted posture.

Despite the warning, Groth wrote, 'my ambition, and probably vanity, had been roused'.[7] In both accounts, Groth started out with an injury, dislocating 'several vertebrae', and wound up 'temporarily in an osteopath's hands for a ricked spine'.[8] He did 'eventually learn to do the headstand', through a more gradual process.

Buddha came to teach Groth 'twice a week', and on the other days, Groth 'would try to master the new technique'. Though he at first 'wanted to learn as many asanas as possible', he eventually took the advice from Buddha, who 'constantly warned' Groth 'that at forty-five it was essential to concentrate on the eight or ten best suited' to his needs.[9] Once adjusted, Groth's routine, aside from his 'two-mile walk home from the office', was to include a daily yoga practice followed 'several times a week' by 'a good massage' from 'an excellent masseur'. Then he would 'sleep soundly' for 'twenty or thirty minutes' in savasana. When he awoke, he would be 'rested and refreshed', ready for 'whatever duties awaited him in the evening'.[10]

In contrast, Stephens took the 'more cautious British approach'. From the first lesson he limited his practice, taking his teacher's advice 'to restrict himself to the 10 or so exercises which seemed right for his physique'. As opposed to Groth's 'comprehensive' goals, Stephens saw himself as more 'limited', without interest in 'a system' for 'exploiting the body as to afford at least glimpses into the Divine'. Instead, 'what [he] wanted … was simply a way for keeping healthy in a bad climate'. He impressed on Buddha his desire for 'an indigenous method' of physical training 'suited to the body's needs when one happened to be living in a tropical swamp'.[11] Stephens, who was described as being 'tall, lanky' and 'often of abstract appearance', took up a daily routine of yoga.[12] Among the ten or so asanas Buddha gave to Stephens for practice, his 'specialties' were *nauli*, with its 'dramatic controls of the abdominal muscles' and the 'knees-ears variant of *halasana* which puts one in a boxed-up posture withdrawn from sight and hearing'.[13]

Stephens kept up his daily practice for decades. His devotion to the practice led one Indian reviewer to note that he was 'probably a believer in yoga' but 'not so ascetic or mystic as to be aloof from the life of the Indian peasants'.[14] Others wrote that he was 'a yoga fiend' who 'lived alone in a local hotel'. And that he seemed a 'real recluse' when not working, 'who neither drank nor smoked'.[15] At times, he 'would startle the staff by appearing in the newsroom in a loincloth'.[16] With regard to his dress, Stephens wrote that for years he 'always wore an Indian *langoti* or loincloth, finding this a convenient garment in the tropics'.

Throughout his 'difficult editorship' at the *Statesman*, Stephens kept up with the practice of yoga asanas taught to him by Buddha. He never adjusted them or changed the routine. Reflecting on it later in life, he wrote that he 'couldn't have got through some of the worst times without them'.[17]

Fluent in English, of mixed origin, and experienced with Western Hatha yoga students, Buddha was able to communicate with a Western audience when compiling *Yoga Asanas*. His goal, stated in the preface of the 1938 manuscript, was ambitious. Buddha wanted to make yoga accessible to a general audience of Westerners, so that they may 'begin the practice' and even learn 'Hatha Yoga well enough to teach it'.[18] Buddha not only wanted to teach but also make teachers of Hatha yoga abroad.

Buddha knew they were going to the West soon enough, and he would attempt to publish the book in London. 'Soon,' he wrote, 'we got an invitation from abroad in the year 1938.'[19]

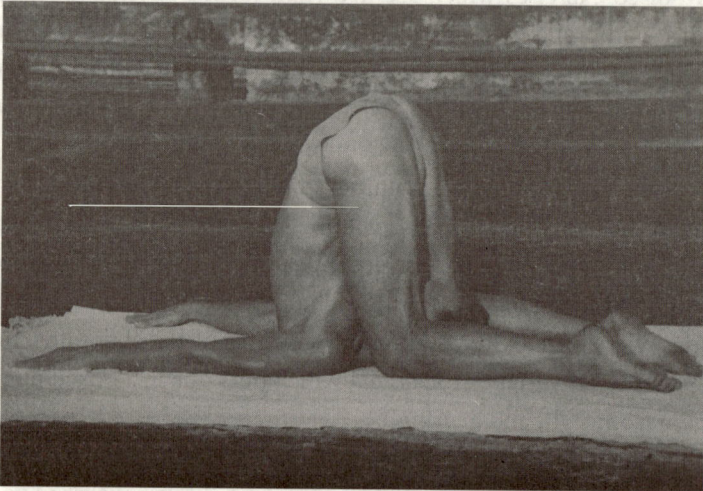

Ian Stephens, British student of Buddha Bose and Editor of The Statesman, practising asanas in Calcutta, circa 1934.
Source: Center of South Asian Studies (Cambridge).

Buddha Bose, 1938 Unpublished Album

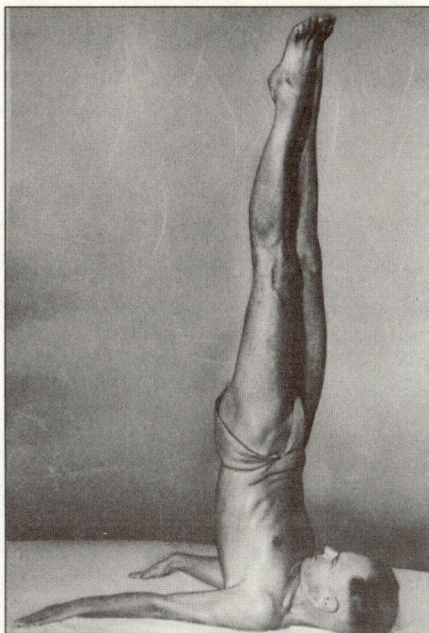

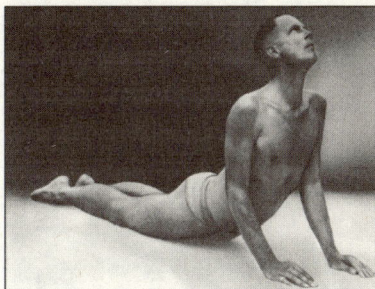

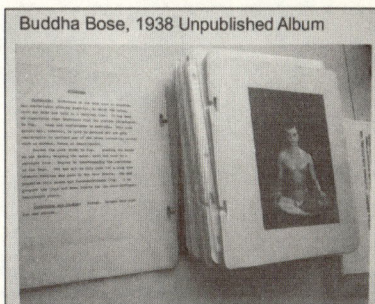

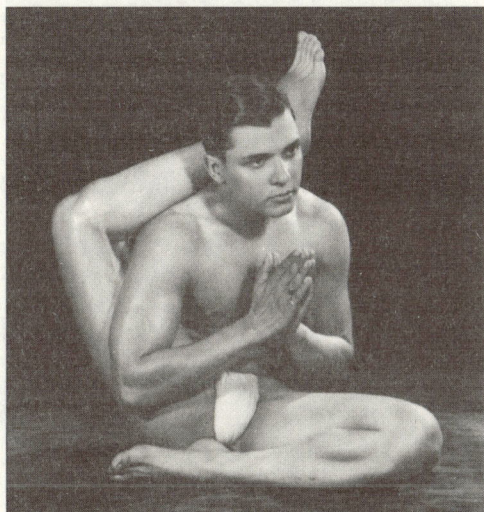

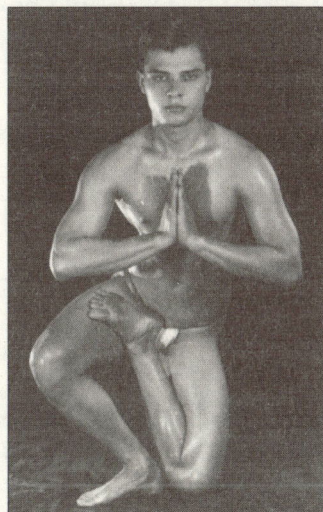

Top left: Ian Stephens; Top right: Ian Stephens;
Middle right: manuscript of Yoga Asanas by Buddha Bose;
Bottom: Buddha Bose.
Courtesy of Center of South Asian Studies (Cambridge),
and 84 Yoga Asanas by Buddha Bose.

PART SEVEN

EIGHTY-FOUR YOGA ASANAS
WORLD TOUR

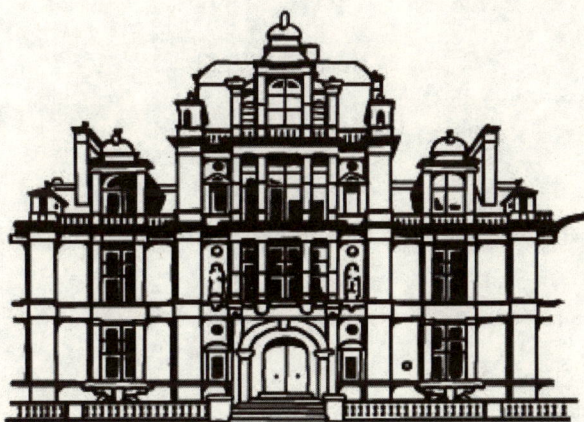

Caxton Hall

The Statesman

Statesman House

Calcutta, July 27th, 1938

A.H.Joyce Esq.,
    Information Officer,
    India Office,
    Whitehall,
    London, S.W.1.

622
1938

Dear Joyce,

I have given an introduction to you to Mr. Buddha Bose, who may call on you some time during the Autumn.

He is an instructor in Hatha-Yoga, and his family has a training institute in Calcutta. He has been teaching me the elements of these exercises this hot weather. He has now left India for a tour in Switzerland, Germany, England and the United States to arrange about the publication of a book. The letter-press, a draft of which I have seen, will not be remarkable, but the book has a good chance of arousing great interest because of its brilliant illustrations. There are few well illustrated books on Hatha-Yoga and Bose, who is exceptionally skilled and has a fine physique, has had taken more than a hundred photographs of himself in the most difficult poses which are in their way works of art.

I have also given him introductions to Sir Frank Brown, to Mr. Richter and to Major F. Yeats-Brown, to whom I am sending copies of this letter.

I am not sure about his financial position but I infer that he has some small private means. He will be travelling with an uncle, also a Hatha-Yoga expert, whom I have not met.

The German and American Consuls here have given Bose good introductions,

-2-

and I understand that the former has arranged to put him in touch with a high Nazi official concerned with physical culture.

Bose is a simple, genuine soul, aged 27, though he looks younger, and somewhat lacking I should say in worldly knowledge. For any help and advice you could give him he would be grateful. Though there is nothing wrong with his intelligence, some risk I think exists of his being taken up by cranky people, since he is good looking and undoubtedly has exceptional physical talent. When you see his proposed illustrations you will, I know, agree with my estimate that his book when published may be of real service in explaining an aspect of Indian culture about which there is ignorance in the West.

He has had a fairly large number of European pupils here including Hodson of the Police and Groth of the American Consular Service.

I hope you and your family are well,

With kind regards,

Yours sincerely,

Letter by Ian Stephens (1938).
Source: British Library (London).

45

BERLIN

People got mesmerized with the art of yoga.
Yoga exercised and benefited the body,
the internal organs and the mind all at the same time.
The West had no idea about this![1]
– Buddha Bose

By the time Ian Stephens mailed an introductory letter to his contacts in London and New York City, Bishnu and Buddha were already at sea, bound for Europe. In the letter, dated 27 July 1938, Stephens introduced Buddha Bose as 'an instructor in Hatha-Yoga', with his family having 'a training institute in Calcutta'. Stephens, then editor at *The Statesman* added, Buddha 'has been teaching me the elements of these exercises in this hot weather' and has 'now left India for a tour in Switzerland, Germany, England and the United States to arrange about the publication of a book'. Stephens declared, 'the German and American Consuls' in Calcutta 'have given Bose good introductions, and I understand that the former has arranged to put him in touch with a high Nazi official concerned with physical education'.[2] By September, Bishnu and Buddha were in Europe and on their way to perform in Berlin at an event organized by the German Oriental Association.[3]

The event in Berlin was just a few months prior to the German incident known as the Night of the Broken Glass (Kristallnacht), where German Nazis attacked thousands of Jews and Jewish-owned properties. This event began the Holocaust, and 30,000 Jews were sent to Nazi concentration camps.[4] Bishnu and Buddha's association with the Nazis in Germany showed their naiveté, as numerous laws had been passed in the first half of 1938 that restricted Jewish persons and their business operations. The world of politics was not their expertise. Stephens noted as much in his 27th July letter, when he remarked that twenty-six-year-old Buddha Bose was 'somewhat lacking in worldly knowledge'.

While the timing of their performance in Berlin corresponded with violent acts of antisemitism, Bishnu and Buddha were there for physical culture at the request of individuals not aligned with Nazi antisemitism. Yogananda had an established Self-Realization Fellowship in Berlin, and the organization provided assistance for Bishnu and Buddha.

A news item by the Berlin correspondent for *Amrita Bazar Patrika* covered their Berlin reception saying, 'We can safely affirm that the performances of Mr. Bose related as they were to the Yoga teachings, left behind a very deep impression on the audience.'[5] Many members of the German government 'whose numbers included representatives from the German Foreign Office, the Propaganda Ministry, the Foreign Organization of the Party and the various Ministries' attended the performance and reception.

Ambassador Werner Otto von Hentig concluded the event by heartily thanking the 'well-known Indian teachers of physical education' for the presentation, stating that 'Germany could learn much from India and the Yoga philosophy'. Hentig was actually a critic of the Nazi regime, but because of his foreign service expertise, he couldn't be ignored or pushed aside by Joseph Goebbels, the Minister of Propaganda. Organizing a demonstration of the Indian system of physical culture was more than mere curiosity for Hentig, given his abundant praise and ideas about how Germany could learn from 'the yoga philosophy'.

Germany had been on the forefront of European choreographed mass drill exercises by students. During the 1920s, Hentig had been involved with leadership efforts for the development of the German Youth Movement. Hentig's movement was started as groups of young people searching for free open space, away from contaminated cities and modern disappointments, where they could develop healthy lifestyles. The movement was based on the longing for a pristine way of being.

At the very time Bishnu and Buddha arrived in Germany, Hentig was intervening at great personal risk, to arrange for thousands of Jews to be transferred from Germany. Hentig had just successfully initiated a favourable decision by Hitler to remove obstacles in the way of Jews emigrating to Israel. He argued there were advantages for Germany in the establishment of a Jewish state, and was negotiating a new programme that would have the first thousand Jewish boys and girls be trained in physical culture in preparation for emigration to Palestine.[6]

Some of the other German government officials who attended the event were more in line with Nazi thinking at the time. The notion that the word 'Aryan' was derived from Sanskrit most likely played a role in the welcoming of yoga and physical cultural practices. Germans had become the first translators and enthusiasts of the Sanskrit heritage of India in the latter part of the eighteenth century. The Nazis felt the shared Indo-European practices needed to be, like the term Aryan, 'resurrected for political purposes in Germany'.[7] After seeing the demonstration by Buddha and Bishnu, 'Von Heinching, President of the Cultural Function at the Principal Reich, Sportsfield College', echoed this sentiment. 'We are fully convinced' from the 'yoga demonstrations that our system of physical culture is incomplete'.[8]

Whatever else was planned for Buddha and Bishnu's trip to Berlin, in coordination with Ambassador Hentig and others, would soon be impacted by events leading to the Second World War.[9] Regardless, by this time it was clear that Bishnu and Buddha felt they had already made an impact. While they were performing 'shows at various universities', Bishnu and Buddha 'realized the country was gearing up for a massive war'. So, 'post haste', they made their way out of Germany, and 'set out on a journey for the other side of the Atlantic'.[10]

Ian Stephens sent his letter of introduction for Buddha out to various contacts in London as well. These included his contacts in the India Office, Frank Brown and the author, Francis Yeats-Brown. The latter had just recently published two books on yoga which emphasized asana and pranayama. They were titled *Lancer at Large* (1936) and *Yoga Explained* (1937). Yeats-Brown had travelled through parts of India receiving teachings and had documented his personal journey. *Lancer at Large* included the path he travelled and detailed his encounter with a 'Paramahamsa Bhagawan Sri', who gave him 'directions' for 'breathings and positions', but left Yeats-Brown seeking more stimulating exercises. He was told by the Bhagawan, 'to meditate' instead.[11] While in Calcutta, and still on his search for the physical component, Yeats-Brown posed the rhetorical question, 'Is there not a Yoga of Action more exciting and more mysterious than the Yogas of contemplation?'[12]

This continued, as Yeats-Brown went to Belur Math, near Calcutta, the same place where Vivekananda had stayed after his return from America. While there he lamented, 'Vivekananda wrote nothing about Hatha Yoga, or practically nothing, and to me the physical basis of mysticism is of great importance.' He went on, 'Why this neglect of Hatha Yoga in both East and West?' He was clearly seeking what Bishnu and Buddha were in the process of systematizing at that very moment. In fact, the next place he went in Calcutta was surprisingly close to 4 Garpar Road, where Bishnu and Buddha lived.

Yeats-Brown visited his 'dear friends', Jagadis Bose and his wife (not related to Buddha) at the Bose Institute, just a block away from where Bishnu and Buddha had practised and taught Hatha yoga by that time. Missing them again in Europe, Yeats-Brown did not follow up on the letter of introduction which Stephens sent him.

Stephens also sent a letter of introduction to Sir Frank Brown, secretary of the East India Association (a collaboration between Indians and retired British officials), in London. Brown followed up on this introduction, which resulted in a high profile yoga demonstration. In a letter that Buddha sent to the India office, dated 21 September, he wrote that he and Bishnu 'were to leave London for New York on the 28th'. However, Buddha wrote, he had changed his plan 'as I am giving a demonstration on Yoga Asanas on the 10th [of October] which has so kindly been arranged by Sir Frank H. Brown'. The yoga performance was held at Caxton Hall in Westminster, sponsored by the East Indian Association.[13]

46

LONDON

Upon arrival in London, Bishnu stated in an interview that he and Buddha Bose had 'been demonstrating in Berlin and are going to America' but were 'interrupting the trip in London, at the request of the Indian Society'.[1] The India Society Association event was one of three events to which Buddha and Bishnu were invited. Prior to it was an 'invitation from the London police force'. 'Many came to learn yoga', and Buddha recounted having 'taught as much as he could in the few days' of the training.[2] The third invitation was for an event at Caxton Hall, located in Victoria. It would be their most acclaimed performance.

Caxton Hall is a storied venue. Located at 10 Caxton Road, close to St. James Park Station, it was originally built for use by parishes, but then was 'used as Westminster City Hall after 1900'.[3] A plaque dated its stone foundation as laid on 29 March 1882. It became the Town Hall for Westminster, and a political venue for groups such as the national Women's Social and Political Union (WSPU). The British Suffragette movement 'held meetings at Caxton Hall at the beginning of each parliamentary session'.

The Hall was the location of prominent concert events, public meetings and famous marriages. Like many of the great halls in London, it was long ago converted for other uses. Since 2008, the red brick and Corsehill stone building, with its pavilion roof and iron crestings, is home to apartments and a few offices.

The original architectural drawing of Caxton Hall, at the Metropolitan Archives in London, showed a dressing room off to the side, which opened onto a stage platform. Buddha and Bishnu's main event was held in what was then known as 'The Great Hall'.

Yogananda had given a lecture in Caxton Hall about both his voyage to India in 1935 and on his return to America in 1936, a few years before Bishnu and Buddha had accompanied him. The events were presided over by Sir Francis Younghusband, the president of the World Federation of Faiths. During his 1935 voyage, Yogananda called it a 'unique response from the people of London who by the hundreds demanded the training of Yoga after my lecture at Caxton Hall'. Yogananda 'promised to teach them on [his] way back to America'.[4]

Yogananda 'was continually interviewed and photographed by newspaper and newsreel representatives'. At one of these events, reporters found Yogananda 'meditating in a dim, heavily-curtained purple suite in a Park-lane hotel'.

He is a short, stocky man with long, lank black hair worn in a bun on the nape of his neck. He appears to be about 25 but he claims to be in the fifties [he was 43 at the time]. He says that he sleeps for only about 2 hours in the 24 and lives on half a dozen oranges and lettuce a day.

The *London Sunday Graphic* columnist, Gordon Webb, went on to further describe his meeting with Yogananda. 'In a quiet room, high above the clamor of London's traffic, a famous Indian mystic, one of the masterminds of Yoga, gave me a remarkable demonstration of his powers.' Yogananda 'can control his sense of touch or eliminate it entirely, and can switch the energy on or off from any part of his body'. Yogananda had told him, 'I control my sense of touch so that I can rest a block of ice on my hand for hours without feeling it. I can stop my heart beating for many hours.' Asked to demonstrate the ability to stop his heart from beating for a brief period, Yogananda acquiesced.

The Daily Mail wrote:

Sitting back in his chair and relaxing, his pulse appeared to stop after about half a minute. Some time later his pulse became normal and stretching himself, he explained: 'I was asleep, and my circulation slackened accordingly.'[5]

It continued:

His condition he attributes to his faith, on which he is to lecture at the Caxton Hall, Westminster, on Tuesday and Wednesday.[6]

Yogananda's two lectures in September 1936 at Caxton Hall were titled 'Removing Fatigue at Will' and 'Highest Technique of God-Contact'. The events were preceded by the singing (in Bengali) of a Rabindranath Tagore song to unfurl the evening.

The audience for 'the classes grew so large' that evening that the organizers 'were obliged to seek larger accommodations' for a second show.[7] Kedarnath Das Gupta, the founder and general secretary of the World Fellowship of Faiths, the same group that had invited Yogananda to speak in Boston seventeen years prior, opened the event at 'the Windsor House to keep the people together', until Yogananda finished speaking next door in Caxton Hall.

A reporter from the *London Star* wrote that he 'managed to squeeze into Caxton Hall before the overflow invaded the Press table'.[8] He went on to write:

The occasion was an address on God by Swami Yogananda, Yoga Master. Hall, floor and balconies were crammed full of people. For an hour-and-a-quarter, attention was held by a remarkable piece of reverent entertainment. I have heard few equals of the Swami as an orator. There was not a syllable of rant or unintelligible metaphysics. His character-acting of a socially distracted lady trying to practice meditation as the Swami ordered, would have brought down any house.

Yogananda illustrated 'his lecture subject with practical demonstrations', and at the end of seventy-five minutes, apparently not the least fatigued, he 'left to address the overflow meetings', inside the Windsor House Hall next door, also filled to capacity. Sir Francis Younghusband closed the event by giving tribute to India 'for producing saints and holy men' such as Yogananda.[9]

After the Caxton Hall event, headlines were made by a statement of Yogananda's: 'I Can Teach Londoners to Live to 100', blared the headline (the *Daily Mail* gave Yogananda the derisive nickname of 'Peter Pan Man').[10] To do that, they would need to practice:

If only English people would spend half an hour each morning and an hour each night in deep concentration, and thus develop their will power and control, there is no reason why they should ever look old or die before the age of a hundred. After six months practice in the art of concentration wrinkles begin to disappear; the eyes get clearer; and strength and vitality increase.[11]

Given Yogananda's success in London, and the connections he made, the doors were opened for his brother Bishnu and Buddha to follow in his footsteps two years later.[12] When Buddha Bose arrived in London in 1938, he was following in his father Rajah's footsteps too. Both were trying to overcome stereotypes, they were each redefining the performance of the magician and the yogi.

Yeats-Brown wrote in 1937 that 'Hatha yogis suffer from a suspicion that their rites include obscenities and black magic'.[13] The word 'yoga' would have been far more likely to have been associated with Indian magic than with the more physical technique of asanas which Buddha performed. When the Hatha yoga teacher, B. K. S. Iyengar, arrived in London sixteen years later, he was to confront this very same perception.

Asked about the inclusion of magic in yoga, Iyengar replied that when he 'got down at the Victoria Station' in London, 'the customs officials asked' what his profession was, and he answered 'yoga'. To that, he was flung spontaneous questions of whether he 'could walk on fire, chew glasses or swallow blades?' Reflecting on the 1954 experience, Iyengar was 'shocked and surprised by these questions', as he only knew of their occurrence 'in India where the street performers' exhibited these sorts of tricks. The forlorn Iyengar replied he did 'various asana similar to calisthenics', which 'they were not aware of' as yoga.[14]

Buddha wrote about the moment they went 'to show the different asanas' and perform an educational display of yoga practice, 'People got mesmerized with the art of yoga; it not only benefited the body but also the internal organs and the mind ... all at the same time. The West had no idea about this!'[15]

Westerners 'often mistook Buddha to be a European' due to his light skin and English complexion. Along with his perfect English, this meant that the 'very high acclaim' he had been given in India 'for his perfect performances of the poses' would continue abroad. People 'gazed at him, fascinated by his handsome and perfect physique and his perfect postures'.[16]

Dear Mr. Joyce,

I duly received your letter of 17th inst. I was to leave London for New York on the 28th of this month, but since I have changed my plan as I am giving a demonstration on 'Yoga Ashanas' on the 10th Oct., which has so kindly been arranged by Sir, Frank H. Brown, so I will be happy to see you on the 5th Oct. at 4 P.M. as fixed by you.

More when we meet.

Yours sincerely,

Buddha Bose

Letter by Buddha Bose (1938).
Source: British Library, London

CAXTON HALL, 10 OCTOBER 1938

*I drop in for a class of Hot Yoga, right around the corner from what was then
Caxton Hall, where Buddha and Bishnu performed the eighty-four physical
asanas for the first time in the West. The yoga studio, called SoHot Victoria,
teaches the tradition of Calcutta Yoga first taught by Bose and Ghosh.*

The Caxton Hall performance by Buddha and Bishnu was presided over by
Sir Francis Younghusband, just as he had for Yogananda's performance.
The event was listed in *Indian Arts and Letters*, the journal of Royal India, as
a talk by 'Mr Bishnu Ghosh on "The Ancient Indian System of Yoga Asanas"
as adapted to modern the requirements with demonstrations, by Mr. Buddha
Bose'.[1] As he recalled being on stage performing the asanas, Buddha wrote, 'I
still remember the enthralled faces of the numerous people in the audience,' and
'the enraptured face of the president of the show, Mr. Younghusband.' Just as in
the other places, 'everyone was enchanted. I saw our victory was riding high.'[2]

One syndicated press column included a photograph of Buddha with
accompanying text: 'An Indian contortionist demonstrates a 3,000 years old Yoga
asana exercise. He is able to tense and relax every single muscle of his body.'[3]

The particular pose in question, *kurmasana* (tortoise), featured Buddha
Bose wrapping both arms under his feet and then extending the feet behind
his head, crossing them and leaning his body all the way forward. With the
head completely under and out of view, the flexion of the spine and significant
shoulder and hip flexibility made it a very advanced display.

Bishnu gave a lecture alongside the performance of the asanas by Buddha.
He claimed that 'the ancient Indian system he expounded is scientific, giving
exercises for all people at all ages and in every station of life, energizing the
body and helping to render it immune to disease'.[4] A London newspaper wrote,

'These feats are not possible to be performed by human strength or by skill but it is possible for the people of India only because it is the land of Yogis.'[5] News of the London event had reached as far away as the United States and Australia when newspapers made mention of it in October 1938. Similar to when Yogananda toured London, the wires had a tendency to over-promote. So alongside factual headlines like 'Physical Culture – An Indian System', they screamed, 'Breath Held for Half-Hour!'[6]

The sensationalized coverage of Buddha holding his breath was elaborated on, stating that 'Buddha Bose, after expelling the breath from his lungs, is able to remain for half an hour' without breathing again. Bishnu explained that because Buddha could 'breathe with his intestines', he could remain buried for that period, 'without inconvenience'. Displays of muscle control with 'weird results' were also described. A London reporter wrote that Buddha could:

Depress his abdomen almost to vanishing point. He can cause the upper and lower muscles of his arm to expand and relax alternately. He moves his ears as easily as a dog. Most remarkable is his power to inflate one side of his stomach while the other remains deflated.

Bishnu was quoted, saying that 'the practice of the exercises put the body so perfectly under the mind's control that diseases like tuberculosis, dyspepsia, rheumatism, and so on can be eliminated even when they have reached a supposedly incurable stage'.[7]

Following the Caxton Hall event came the first mention of eighty-four asanas on the tour. A report wrote, 'Buddha Bose is showing 83 of the exercises in London,' and though it was not demonstrated, one should assume that *savasana* or corpse pose (relaxing on one's back), was the eighty-fourth asana. Savasana, in other historical lists of eighty-four asanas, was either at the end of the list, or listed multiple times and not counted. The demonstration by Buddha Bose, called 'Yoga Asanas', was not yet advertised as eighty-four asanas, but nevertheless was a system that contained the number.

In his speech, Bishnu told the audience that the 'physical Yoga system' they were presenting 'might be called exercise without exercising'. The system of practice was done without 'the usual equipment of physical culture and the paraphernalia of games'. Bishnu stressed that within India, the yoga method always had been 'taught in connection with religion and philosophy'. The demonstration shown in the postures focused on breathing, muscle control and glandular development, which were described as 'the cardinal points' of the system. Bishnu was orienting the yoga asana practice not as a secular exercise, but very much entwined with a spiritual philosophy, without getting into much of what that entailed. Instead, he focused on the rudimentary practice and a description of this Indian physical cultural system.[8]

It was clear that what Bishnu was speaking of was similar how Yogananda described his system of Yogoda. It was the 'energization of muscles by will power, to develop not only the muscular tissues but the nervous and organic tissues of the body as well'. The practice of yoga asanas described by Bishnu, 'teaches perfect control of the body. We can move any muscle at will. The power is attained through deep breathing, concentration, and the practice of exercises which are the result of 3,000 years of experience.'[9] Like Yogananda before them in the 1920s, Buddha and Bishnu quickly transitioned from giving Westerners an incredible show, to laying out a practical format. The Yogoda technique was a means of making Kriya yoga more accessible for the beginner; likewise for the accessibility of the beginner, asana techniques were taught by Buddha and Bishnu to individuals or groups. The term Yogada, as a broad catch-all term, was dropped by the time of this tour.

When '83 of the exercises in London' were performed at Caxton Hall by Buddha, he also posed for a number of photographs of yoga asanas and other oddities.[10] One of them, 'a dangerous and at the same time wonderful feat of strength', was what Bishnu Ghosh wrote about in his 1930 book *Muscle Control*.[11] The caption of the photo mentioned how 'the 25-year-old Indian Buddha Bose pressed an iron rod with his throat, against the wall and bent the rod'. Behind Buddha stood Bishnu, with the side of his foot holding Buddha's during the feat. Another photo was taken of Buddha doing *nauli*, probably just after or before a show, on a stage in front of the curtain.

On 9 October 1938, Bishnu and Bishnu met with political leader, Jawaharlal Nehru, in London. The three of them were photographed while attending an East Indian Association event, the evening prior to Bishnu and Buddha's performance at Caxton Hall. Nehru shared the audience's interest in yoga. About a decade earlier, he'd read *Yoga Mimansa*, and soon after, started to advise others 'to visit Kuvalayanandaji's institution and study this ancient silence'. Previously, in 1929, Nehru had 'taken lessons from that great yogic scientist', and during the 1930s, he had taken up a yoga practice.[12] 'A favourite exercise' of Nehru's, while incarcerated by British officials in India from 1931 to 1935, was *sirsasana*. He would start each day with four to five minutes of standing upside down in a headstand, which he found both 'physically invigorating' and 'a form of psychological stimulus'.[13] Nehru would later comment that the exercise was 'a complete reversal of the normal situation. The body is forced to adapt itself to new conditions.' Without it, one 'sits or walks about all day and forgets about giving the spine a change'.[14]

In later years, Nehru also crossed paths with Buddha's student, Ian Stephens, while he was still editor of The Statesman. Since both were keen devotees of yoga, 'during an interview with Nehru seated on the same settee with India's future Prime Minister, both men were tranquilly doing pranayam, or breathing exercises'. Stephens quipped that 'it was much more fun than politics'.[15]

Nehru had heard about Buddha's success, and had 'prepared a certificate' for him. 'I declined the certificate and the perplexed Panditji asked me why', wrote Buddha. 'I told him I was objecting to this certificate, as it was being given on just hearsay. I would much rather he watched my performance and then give me his honest opinion.' Buddha was unsure of how Nehru would take the argument, but in the end, 'he agreed to see' Buddha perform. After a 'show of many asanas to a charmed Panditji', Nehru 'tore up the earlier letter and wrote a new one'.[16] The handwritten letter, later called by Buddha 'Pandit Nehru's Opinion', included an endorsement of their plans to travel to America:

> Mr. Buddha Bose is a remarkably successful exponent of the ancient Indian system of yoga exercises. It is an education in physical culture and fitness to see him perform. I understand he is going to America. I wish him success.[17]

In the middle of October, Bishnu and Buddha set off for America.

48

NEW YORK

On 15 October 1938, Buddha Bose and Bishnu Ghosh left the British port of Southampton and boarded the SS *Europa*, bound for New York City. They travelled in third class, the lowest available for passengers. Bishnu listed his age as thirty-six, stated he was married and gave his occupation as 'lawyer'. Buddha listed his age as twenty-six, status as single, with the occupation of 'physical instructor'. Both were categorized as being from 'other parts of the British Empire'. Buddha's birthplace was listed as Colombo, Ceylon, and under 'race or people' was 'Ceylonese'. Bishnu's birthplace was listed as 'Lahore, India', and nationality 'Indian'.

They both were listed as being fluent in being able to both 'read' and 'write' in English. Under notable complexion or marks, Bishnu listed the 'scar on the right side of forehead'. Buddha listed himself as 5'6" in height, and Bishnu as 5'5". They both listed Yogananda (Bishnu referencing him as 'brother' and Buddha as 'friend') as the person they were visiting and used his Los Angeles address of '3888 San Rafael Ave'. They also both answered 'No' to the questions of 'whether a polygamist' and 'whether an anarchist'. Unlike Yogananda a few years earlier, they passed through the New York immigration control easily.[1] They didn't have a return ticket for Calcutta, but indicated their 'length of stay' would be six months.

As they arrived in the US, news of their London performances the prior month reached Americans. A *Washington Post* headline declared, 'Deep breathing is a Beauty fad now in London'. Buddha Bose was 'in London teaching it at so much per head to crowds of new practitioners'.[2] Similar articles reached across the Midwest, placed in newspapers out of Lubbock, Texas, Cincinnati, Ohio and Greenville, South Carolina. The headlines read like this one in the *Evening*

Independent of St Petersburg, Florida, which proclaimed: 'Proper Breathing is Way to Beauty'. Recent books and the 'lectures of Francis Yeats-Brown' had 'stimulated' the 'international social set'; 'Yogi exercises are a rising fad in London and arousing increasing interest in New York.'[3]

Among the most prominent press coverage was an article and photographic spread in *Ken*, a New York bi-weekly aimed at intellectual readers. The magazine's content tended to deal with political debates, such as the European situation prior to the Second World War. Its editorial position was 'opposed to left & right dictatorship'. The *Ken* magazine article, and its syndication, gave instructions for alternate nostril breathing as taught by Bishnu and Buddha. The directions stated:

> Close the right nostril, inhale deeply through the left, then close both. When holding the breath becomes a strain, exhale slowly. Take next breath through the right one, with the left closed, then close both, and so on.

Doing this for twenty breaths total was a 'typical exercise anyone could do'.[4]

This exercise was a yoga pranayam technique found in classical Hatha texts such as the twelfth-century, *Yoga Yajnavalkya* and seventeenth-century, *Gheranda Samhita* and *Shiva Samhita*. In the section on 'purification', verse 55, the *Gheranda Samhita* instructed 'inhale through the left nostril and then exhale through the right. Then, after filling yourself up with air by inhaling through the right nostril, exhale through the left.'[5] Nowadays, the Internet makes everything so accessible that simple instructions such as this might seem trivial, but it is remarkable that, on that day in 1939, the average newspaper reader in Lubbock, Greenville and St Petersburg might have learned a classical Hatha yoga breathing technique.

Ken magazine also included large black and white photographs of Buddha Bose performing asanas. This finding revealed the background of the photograph, which appeared in the Smithsonian's compilation, 'Art of Transformation'. While in London, prior to performing on the stage at Caxton Hall, Remie Lohse, a popular freelance photographer in the 1930s who was prominent enough to do fashion covers for *Vogue*, took photographs of Buddha. The four photographs included in the magazine featured Buddha performing a handstand while in lotus, a side-twist and two abdominal mudra postures, *nauli* and *uddiyana*. The caption stated that the 'yoga disciple' who was 'now teaching in London' attributed his 'pulchritude and perfect health to the Yogi regimen', the essentials of which involved a series of 'breathing exercises combined with a form of mental discipline'.[6]

Through Ian Stephens, Buddha had arranged meetings with both the British Library of Information in New York, and the American Consuls who had 'given Bose good introductions'.[7] However, their main point of contact was at Columbia University.

Yogananda, in his 1948 *Autobiography*, only briefly mentioned the voyage by Bishnu and Buddha. In it, he wrote of their world tour, that they 'travelled to Europe and America, giving exhibitions of strength and skill which amazed the university savants, including those at Columbia University in New York'.[8]

Bishnu's role at Columbia University was often mentioned in ensuing years, with his being titled everything from honorary professor, to a faculty member at the university. More realistically, Buddha, in the acknowledgments of his 1954 book *Holy Kailas*, gave him the title 'Yogindra Sree Bishnu Charan Ghosh, Late "Yoga" Lecturer' at Columbia University, New York'.

During the 1930s, Columbia University was at the epicenter of Hatha yoga and its introduction in the United States as a form of therapeutic exercise. Pivotal during that meeting point was a woman named Dr Josephine Rathbone, who was a physical education professor at Columbia University during the thirties and forties. In 1934, she wrote a book titled *Corrective Physical Education*, which focused on 'techniques of progressive relaxation' for, among other things, 'rest and relief from hypertension'.[9] Her 1934 book became a classic text and went through seven editions over some thirty years. A trailblazer in dealing with neuromuscular tension patterns, Rathbone wrote extensively about the medical applications of exercise for rehabilitation and the role of relaxation as part of overall health.

According to the *New York Times*, Rathbone took a year's leave of absence from Columbia University in 1937, and during that period was in India. In her memoirs, Rathbone wrote about her travels to India in the early 1930s, when she met with Kuvalayananda in Lonavla.[10] She was made familiar with yoga through a master's student at Columbia Teachers College, P.G. Krishnayya, a student from Madras. Rathbone, along with other university scholars, was intrigued by the para-medical studies which dealt with yoga.[11]

Kuvalayananda's books and journal writings also reached Koover Thomas

Behanan of Yale, who used a fellowship 'to make a scientific study' of yoga under Swami Kuvalayananda in India in 1932. There, Behanan practised twice daily, 'at dawn and sunset, on an empty stomach'. He began with simple poses such as 'posterior stretching' or *paschimottanasana*, 'sitting with his legs stretched out' and hooking the forefingers over the big toes to touch the knees with the head, thereby bringing 'a rich supply of blood to the pelvic organs and toning up the nerves arising from the lower part of the spine'. The 'plow posture' or *halasana*, was practised next and was 'one of the finest exercises for keeping the spine flexible and the nerves healthy'. 'Standing topsy-turvy' in *sirsasana* 'on one's head for 20 minutes ... clarifies the mind'.

When Behanan returned to Yale, he finished his dissertation on yoga asanas and then published his book in 1937, titled *Yoga: A Scientific Evaluation*, which was hailed as 'the first physiological analysis of yogic exercises' in *Time* magazine. The magazine also gave Behanan the title of 'Yale's Yogin'.[12] A week prior to the *Time* mention, Behanan and his book were profiled by *Life Magazine*, which included nine photos of Behanan and others holding yoga asanas from 'the mystic Hindu practices'.[13]

Rathbone followed Behanan (whose parents were part Indian) to Swami Kuvalayananda, but unlike Behanan's more devotional quest, Rathbone's journey was entirely pragmatic. She did not make the voyage to Calcutta. In fact, while she was out travelling, there was no indication that she met Bishnu Ghosh. Instead, she was introduced to Bishnu and Buddha upon their arrival in New York by Theos Bernard, a fellow Columbia University student of yoga. Theos had been in India in 1935 with his father Glen Bernard, and had connected with Buddha Bose and Bishnu Ghosh while visiting Yogananda in Calcutta. At the same time, while Rathbone was teaching at Columbia, Theos was getting a master's degree, and then a doctorate in religion.

When Rathbone returned from her year-long hiatus, she was part of a fairly small group in the US that intimately knew the physical yoga asanas and part of an even smaller group that had taken a scholarly approach to the practice. She became a leader in presenting the benefits of doing yoga and its 'quieting positions', which rid the body of tension and induced relaxation. She was in an optimal position to bring Buddha's yogic performance and Bishnu's lecture into an academic setting.[14]

In the fall of 1938, Rathbone started a clinic at Columbia University, which treated patients for stress and other ailments, and sponsored 'demonstrations by Yogin at the college'.[15] The 'Yogin' in question was Buddha, who had arrived with Bishnu in New York City just in time for the beginning of the semester.

Having authentic yogis come to Columbia served to legitimize Rathbone's use of the practices and add to the knowledge she'd gained from her time with Kuvalayananda. As an 'early pioneer' in the 'therapeutic stream of physical activity', Rathbone 'was instrumental' in 'pushing open a door to mind-body practices from the East', moving them into a practical approach. Bishnu was very open to this approach, since it was the same synthesizing approach he had taught in Calcutta.[16]

During the fall of 1938, Dr Rathbone taught a class titled 'Art of Relaxation' at Columbia, which was the beginning of integrating her work in yoga with 'her broader goal of alleviating a variety of disorders ... caused ... by the era's pathological level of tension'.[17] The course would be a first of its kind, combining the findings of medical science with yoga – a common sense approach to well being. Following their partnership in the fall of '38, Rathbone arranged for Bishnu and Buddha to return in the spring, for lectures and demonstrations. For the winter months, after their time in New York, Bishnu and Buddha headed to Los Angeles to reunite with Yogananda. They were Yogananda's first family visitors in the United States.

After he returned from his 1935–36 tour of India, Yogananda's monthly (sometimes quarterly) magazine published quite a number of photographs from the visit. His secretary, Richard Wright, also published many of his diary notes in the magazine. This inspired Yogananda's American students to voyage to India themselves, which resulted in headlines like 'American Students Visit Ranchi in India'.[18]

'Free guest-quarters' were provided 'for American Yogoda students and travellers,' the organization stated. And that 'anyone travelling to India may avail himself of this opportunity by writing to the Los Angeles Headquarters for a letter of introduction to the Ranchi headquarters'. Another article 'An American Student in India' presented the interaction between the students of Yogananda in India, especially Ranchi, and the US, where they could take in the relaxing environment. 'The days we spent there were among the happiest of my life,' wrote Lois Patterson Downs.[19] With Buddha and Bishnu visiting Los Angeles, the students of Yogananda would now have India's physical culture system of asanas to view and learn firsthand.

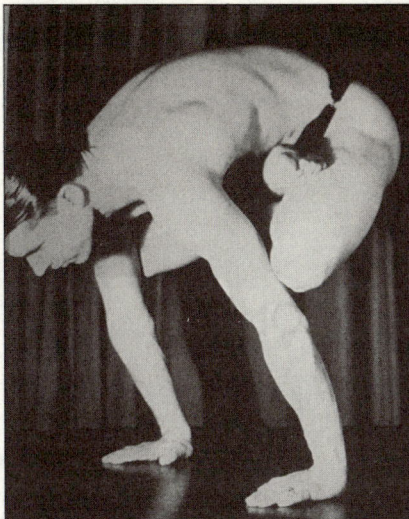

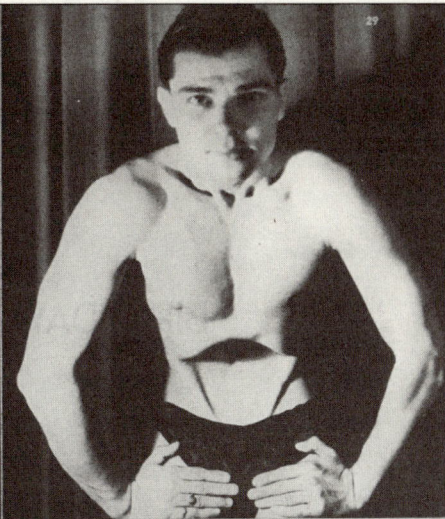

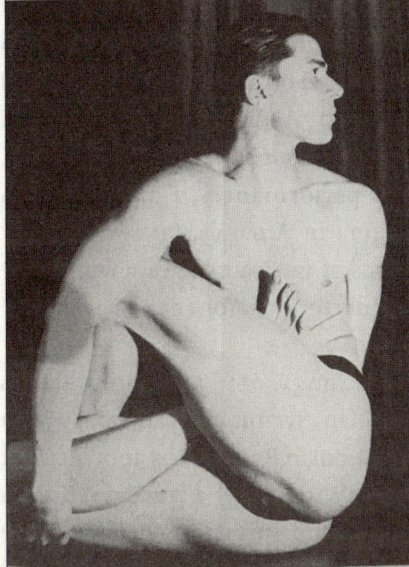

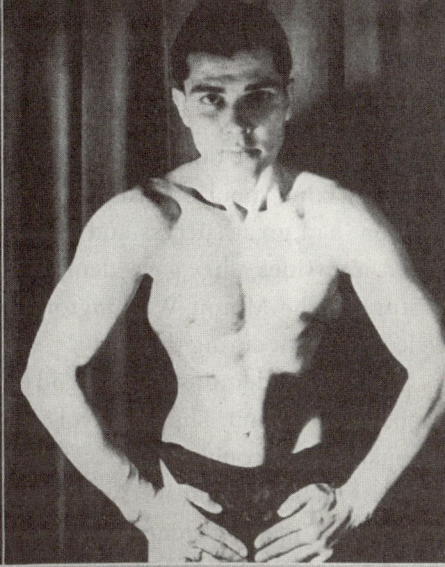

YOGA disciple Buddha Bose, "the most beautiful man in India," attributes his pulchritude and perfect health to the Yogi regimen, the essentials of which—a series of involved breathing exercises combined with a form of mental discipline—he is now teaching in London. (Ken Particles page 9)

Buddha Bose in London (1938).

Source: Photos by Remie Lohse, Ken, Dec 15th, 1938.

49

BIRTHDAY REUNION

Upon arriving at Yogananda's Headquarters in Los Angeles, *Inner Culture*, Yogananda's monthly magazine, proclaimed, 'Yogananda's Brother Now in America'. Bishnu, the 'renowned physical culturist', had arrived 'after an extended tour of Europe where he was acclaimed on all sides as a wonderful exponent of Yoga as applied to the physical body'. And with him was Buddha, 'considered to have one of the most perfectly proportioned bodies in India'. The magazine mentioned their previous performances; Caxton Hall in London 'had great success and appreciation'. In America, 'at several New York Universities', they gave 'demonstrations of intricate life-renewing body postures'. The Mount Washington headquarters of Yogananda 'warmly' welcomed both during their stay.[1]

Besides the demonstrations and the teaching, some interesting things happened to Bishnu. The first involved an Indian, Swami Binayananda, whom Yogananda had brought to the US from his school in Ranchi. His appointment had raised a bit of controversy back in India. 'Within only a few days, Bishnu Charan saw many incidents of unbecoming and suspicious behaviour by Binayananda and made Yogananda aware of these' slights.[2] Yogananda had already gone through other mis-steps with an Indian sannyasi that he had brought over from India and could not take the chance of a troublesome Binayananda causing problems for him in America'. He sent him back to Ranchi, where he became the 'president for the Yogoda Satsanga in India'. The result was that 'the American part of the organization was free of any more complications'; however, the arrangement 'caused noticeable discontent to rise in the Indian part of the organization'.[3] It was to be the last effort made by Yogananda 'to take any more *brahmachari* workers to America from India'.[4]

Yogananda made a huge impact on Buddha's life while in Los Angeles. Buddha's daughter, Rooma, revealed that Yogananda had asked Buddha, 'You have achieved a perfection of the body, but have you given attention to perfecting the inner body?' Yogananda told Buddha, 'Your asanas are perfect,' before prodding him again, 'Have you considered the perfection of the soul?'[5]

The spiritual encounter with Yogananda enriched and transformed Buddha Bose. In Los Angeles, around Christmas 1938, he became an SRF minister, 'ordained by Yogananda to impart Kriya meditation knowledge to desirous persons and train them in Kriya meditation'. Throughout his life, he would consider himself a disciple of Yogananda.[6] This resulted with Buddha making a change in his profession.

Bishnu and Buddha had started their travels in 1932 as a 'lawyer' and a 'physical instructor' respectively. At the time, Bishnu dreamed of 'going to London to be a barrister'. Buddha had listed 'physical instructor' as his occupation on both the 1932 and the 1938 passports. After Los Angeles, they both wrote 'religious minister' as their occupation title.

The spiritual initiation changed Buddha's outlook, as he took to the wholeness of yoga, practising Hatha yoga and Kriya yoga thereafter 'every day without fail'.[7] When 1938 concluded, the SRF magazine noted, 'The Christmas festivities at the Mt Washington headquarters in Los Angeles were made doubly enjoyable by the presence of Bishnu Charan and Buddha Bose.'[8]

A photo with four prominent female disciples of Yogananda showed Binayananda, along with Buddha and Bishnu, dressed in black suits, during Christmas 1938. 'Christmas Day was a never-to-be forgotten celebration', with 'a cross-like table' for dinner; 'Swami Yogananda played the part of Santa Claus.' The day before, on Christmas Eve, an early morning meditation was conducted for 'seven hours without intermission. Those who joined this meditation felt the seven hours pass like seven minutes of unending joy.'[9]

Bishnu's other involvement in LA was more light-hearted, the sort of playful activity that a younger brother would do with an older brother. Though Yogananda had lived in the United States for nearly eighteen years, no one knew his birthday.[10] It was not celebrated, and if anyone asked which day it fell on, he would deflect the question.

In London in any case, he had promoted the notion that anyone who followed his techniques could live to 100 years of age.

By concentration and relaxation I can do with two hours sleep out of the 24. There is no reason why anyone who will give an hour and a half every day to deep concentration cannot do the same. When the heart is quiet consciously, every other part of the body is rested with incomparably more benefit in a deep sleep. It is this rest which prolongs life.

A reporter remarked, 'Yogananda has the appearance of a man in his early 20s.' Yogananda replied, anyone who 'faithfully follows' the teachings 'can attain complete self-mastery and remain young even in old age'.[11] But on occasion, Yogananda would state something that seemed outlandish, especially in hindsight. 'I expect to live forever,' he said as a twenty-nine-year old on 8 January 1924 (three days after his birthday). 'My system brings everlasting youth.'[12] Bishnu though, being the mischievous younger brother, let it be known to Yogananda's disciples over Christmas that his brother's birthday was on 5 January and that there should be a celebration of the event.[13]

For disciples close to Yogananda, learning his birth date was a moment that they welcomed, a chance to gain insight into his personal life. However, Yogananda would still not reveal his birth year, requiring just one candle to be placed on his cake. He joked, 'I still have a little strength of breath. I must take care I don't blow the cake away!'[14]

The pivotal event took place within Yogananda's community of devotees three days after his birthday, on the 'first anniversary of the Golden Lotus Temple'. On 7 January 1939, the *Los Angeles Times* wrote in its listing of 'topics for sermons', that 'a Hindu-American dinner will be served at 3 p.m. tomorrow at the Golden Lotus Temple in Encinitas'. And then, 'following the dinner, demonstrations in yoga will be given by Bishnu Charan and Buddha Bose'.[15]

50

GOLDEN LOTUS TEMPLE OF
ALL RELIGIONS

Settle here for a time. Give all your lecturers and services here.
Let people come to you for a change, instead of forever going out to them.

In 1935, Yogananda travelled the California coast with his disciples, searching for a place to establish a hermitage; one where he could meditate and write. He then left for India, and when he returned to the US, in late 1936, the Encinitas 'Yogoda Dream Hermitage' was presented to Yogananda as a gift from his most advanced disciple, James Lynn. His disciples 'prayed that he wouldn't know about it' beforehand.[1] Yogananda did know of the place, and had sent letters while in India inquiring about whether it had been purchased. Still, upon seeing the location, Yogananda's 'eyes got teary and he was very grateful'.[2]

When Yogananda arrived at the newly acquired property, he wrote, 'I saw a building jutting out like a great white ocean liner towards the blue brine. First speechlessly, then with "Ohs!" and "Ahs!", finally with man's insufficient vocabulary of joy.' He later wrote, 'After my world tour and visiting Switzerland and Kashmir and all beautiful places in the world, I can safely say that this Yogoda Dream Hermitage resting on a cliff overlooking the ocean is the most perfect, most beautiful place I have ever seen in the world.'[3]

The ashram had '16 unusually large rooms, each one charmingly appointed'.[4] It was like a drop of heaven, he thought, and 'Encinitas became his favorite spot'.[5] After fifteen years of travel, he heard an inner instruction which he easily heeded. 'Settle here for a time. Give all your lectures and services here. Let people come to you for a change, instead of forever going out to them.'[6]

Yogananda moved right into seclusion. The Encinitas site, at 215 K Street, sat on seventeen acres of coastline atop a bluff. He wrote extensively and meditated profusely.[7] The land consisted of two buildings, and plans were made for 'a large glass temple' to be 'built on the highest knoll of the estate'.[8] A year later, construction of the Golden Lotus Temple was completed. By 1 November 1937, costs for the construction of the temple, along with other upgrades to the land, and a Yogoda Dream Hermitage, totaled $250,000.[9] Inspired by Yogananda's sense of design, the temple featured four towers, crowned by four large gold-plated copper lotus flowers. The copper absorbed lightning strikes, the ideal material to have placed atop a temple on the edge of a bluff overlooking the Pacific Ocean.

A press release was sent out on 3 November to over one hundred newspapers announcing 'the formal opening of the temple on New Year's Day, 1938'. The PR proclaimed: The 'unique features of the open-roofed temple include its hill-top situation immediately overlooking the ocean, a four-storied glass tower, and a new lotus design, the first in America, with huge lotus buds encrusted with gold leaf, whose glint in the sun is visible for miles around.'

One can detect a note of hubris. It was 'a kind of advertisement, a statement'.[10] The golden spires were 'easily seen by motorists' as they travelled along the Pacific Coast Highway between Los Angeles and San Diego.[11] 'The whole structure', the release stated, was 'mirrored in a large pool by the side of the temple'. Richard Wright was asked whether the design of the Golden Lotus Temple was inspired by the famous Taj Mahal. He replied:

I visited the Taj at Agra last year with Swami Yogananda. However the Taj has no golden lotuses so far as I know. Ours is the only structure in the world with this original lotus design.[12]

The lotus flowers were formed into the shapes of the three stages of unfolding. The largest was placed atop the entrance in the middle and unfolded as a symbol of potential. Two more, one on each side, were bloomed more, a symbol of divine unfolding. The last of the four was on the opposite side of the structure, overlooking the ocean. An octagonal observatory jutted two stories higher, and atop it was the fully opened lotus, like an awakened soul open to infinite potential. Photographs from the time show a wide variety of plants such as cactus, aloe and various succulents, trees including palm, and a Monterey, pine which was given to Yogananda. The greenery lined the paths that wove through the gardens.

The Golden Lotus temple was spectacular, with 'a four-story glass tower and telescope, a rooftop meditation deck' and inside, 'a floor-to-ceiling window that served as a backdrop for its altar'. The altar featured statues of religious figures from many world religions, along with gems in a 'symphony in emerald, opal and sapphire'. After it opened, 'thousands of people flocked to the temple to learn Kriya yoga and seek enlightenment, including celebrities such as Greta Garbo'. Upcoming event announcements and advertisements were regularly placed in the *Los Angeles Times*. 'One hundred miles south of LA on Highway 101', the temple served as a place for Yogananda to showcase his guests of honour, such as Bishnu and Buddha.

On that January day, 'hundreds attended the inspiring Sunday morning services' conducted by Yogananda. The main event was later, during an 'after-dinner program', provided by Bishnu and Buddha as a birthday celebration for Yogananda. More than 200 had gathered for the Hindu-American dinner programme and afterwards, a 'series of yoga demonstrations' by Bishnu and his 'star pupil' Buddha. During the performance, against the backdrop of the endless Pacific Ocean, Bishnu gave a lecture titled 'Yoga-Asanas: The Yoga System of Physical Health and Development', which he explained had, 'evolved in India more than 3,000 years ago as one of the greatest methods of rejuvenation'. Buddha's performance followed Bishnu's talk and was a display of his ability to illustrate 'the power of mind over body'. Buddha 'amazed the audience with his feats of skill and muscular control'.[13] He demonstrated '80 yogic postures', which included the 'difficult' muscle control postures. Other asanas included:

> *Vrikshasana* or Tree Pose, *Halasana* or Plow Pose, *Kukkutasana* or Cock Pose, *Bhujangasana* or Cobra Pose, *Dhanurasana* or Bow Pose, *Beera-Bhadrasana* or Saluting-God-in-Warrior Pose, and *Padmasana* or Meditation Pose, commonly known as the Buddha or Lotus posture.[14]

The Hindu attendees probably had an understanding of yoga asanas from their cultural background, and this display would not have surprised them. For the Americans in attendance, of whom many were in their youth, it was a profound introduction to the world of Hatha yoga. Though they were exposed to Yogoda exercises already, those were less physically demanding than what they saw Buddha perform. The Americans must have been transfixed, amazed and inspired to begin their own practice of the asanas.

Just as he had done in Berlin, and at Caxton Hall in London a few months prior, Buddha stayed in each asana for just a few moments, and while holding the pose, Bishnu would pronounce its name and make a few remarks on its health benefits. Buddha transitioned from one asana to another. From sitting asanas that stretched his body, he would move into variations of asanas in cross-legged *padmasana* or lotus pose. These were followed by lying down positions, and then standing ones. He concluded with postures in handstands, backward-bends and then advanced postures, such as balancing on one leg while wrapping the other behind the head in standing single-leg tortoise pose. Taking only twenty to thirty seconds for each of the asanas, the performance would take around forty-five minutes to complete.

As Bishnu narrated the performance, saying aloud each asana by its Sanskrit name and translating it to English, he would watch with a keen eye, paying attention to Buddha's movements and breath, without interfering. He looked engaged, leaned in towards the student and occasionally lightly touched him, as if he were projecting his own willpower into his student's performance.

After the asanas and muscle control postures were showcased, it was time for feats of strength. A six-foot-long iron bar was taken out, one end of it pressed against the wall to stabilize it, the other end placed against a particular spot on Buddha's larynx. He then 'bent an iron rod with his throat'. This was followed by 'extraordinary demonstrations of strength and mind control' from Bishnu, 'bending an iron rod with his teeth' and 'talking while others held his throat'.[15] Yogananda's magazine reported on the event with an article that included mention of Bishnu 'as one of the first students at Paramhansa Yogananda's School for Boys at Ranchi', in addition to being 'a disciple of his brother and Guru', who 'has trained thousands of youth in health and mind development in Bengal and all over the world'. It was an explicit endorsement for taking up the yoga asana practice that he and Buddha brought to Yogananda's ashram of devotees.

While at Yogananda's ashram, Bishnu and Buddha continued their demonstration and teaching of asanas for a number of months. One of the disciples, Mr James Lynn, had the opportunity to learn 'advanced Hatha Yoga practices'. Lynn, 'if it was clear or sunny' was out on the lawn in Encinitas early, 'doing his tensing and other exercises, such as standing on his head or walking on his hands with his legs upright in the air'. Bishnu, upon seeing the ability of Lynn, 'wanted to teach' him 'all of the asanas'. Lynn thought about it, and asked Yogananda. He was told, 'If you do, you may lose your bliss.'

'At that time', Lynn's 'Hatha Yoga routine was already satisfactory'. Yogananda had advised Lynn 'not to delve in too many physical exercises', which were 'alright for those who do not deeply meditate'. Instead, 'he was advised to concentrate on perfecting his meditation practices'. When Roy Davis wrote of the encounter, he felt Yogananda 'might have responded differently' if it was another person. That was the case for many of the younger disciples, who in the coming years, took up regular practices of Hatha yoga as taught by Bishnu and Buddha. Before they left, Buddha was asked by Yogananda to stay with him in California and to take over his work in America. However, Buddha 'declined, stating that he wanted to serve his Yogasana guru, Bishnu Charan Ghosh, in furthering his physical culture training'. Yogananda said, 'Fine you go with my brother. It is your wish.' Buddha Bose was given permission in writing by Paramhansa Yogananda to initiate *grihis* in the doctrine of Kriya yoga.[16]

Buddha and Bishnu had established the teachings of Hatha yoga with Yogananda's disciples. A few years later, it would flourish in the public through Yogananda's magazine. The February 1939 issue of *Inner Culture* pictured Buddha Bose and Bishnu Ghosh on page two of the issue – Buddha, 'in a very difficult pose known as *dakkhana-nauli* and *uddiyana bandha* together' and 'Bishnu Charan, Yogananda's brother, in *padmasana*', sitting cross-legged atop a Bengal tiger skin. By the time it was published, the duo were back on the East Coast.

GOLDEN LOTUS HOTEL OPEN FOR GUESTS

The Golden Lotus Hotel is the new name given to the Parkview Hotel adjoining the grounds of the Self-Realization Fellowship Hermitage and Golden Lotus Temple at Encinitas, California. This hotel has recently been acquired by the Fellowship. It has been newly painted and renovated and the grounds improved. An attractive palm tree grove has been started.

The climate of Encinitas is, according to Government weather records, the most healthful in the country. Guests at the hotel will also enjoy the glorious ocean stretches and the beach nearby. On Sundays they can attend the services conducted by Paramhansa Yogananda at the Golden Lotus Temple.

Rates for transient and permanent guests are very reasonable. Those interested may write for more information to Manager, Golden Lotus Hotel, Encinitas, California.

NEW CENTERS IN EAST

William J. Stewart, well-known Bishop of the Spiritual Christian Union Churches in Belleville and St. Louis, has converged his churches with the Self-Realization Fellowship. Yogacharya Sri Khagen has recently completed a series of lectures and classes in these cities. A warm welcome is extended to the many new members.

ORDAINED MINISTERS

The following 24 persons are Ordained Ministers of the Self-Realization Fellowship Church, Inc., of America (affiliated with the Yogoda Sat-Sanga Society of India):

Sister Bhakti
Buddha Bose
F. Darling
Frederick F. Downs
Lois Patterson Downs
Sri Ranendra K. Das
Bishnu Charan Ghosh
Sister Gyanamata
Yogacharya Sri Khagen
Brahmachari Jotin
Margaret Lancaster
Yvonne Larson
Sri Nerode
Laurie Pratt
Brahmachari Premeswar
Yogacharya Pretorius
Louise Gunton Royston
Orpha L. Sahly
Bishop W. J. Stewart
C. Richard Wright
Faye Wright
Helen Wright
Virginia Wright
Paramhansa Yogananda,
Founder and President

Buddha Bose and Bishnu Ghosh, ordained SRF ministers.

Source: Inner Culture.

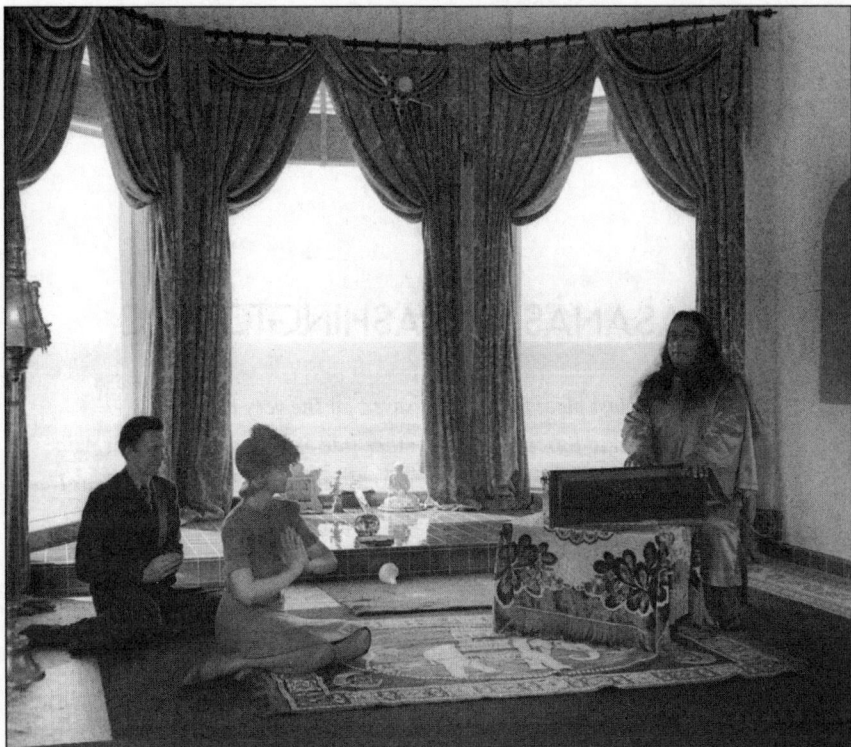

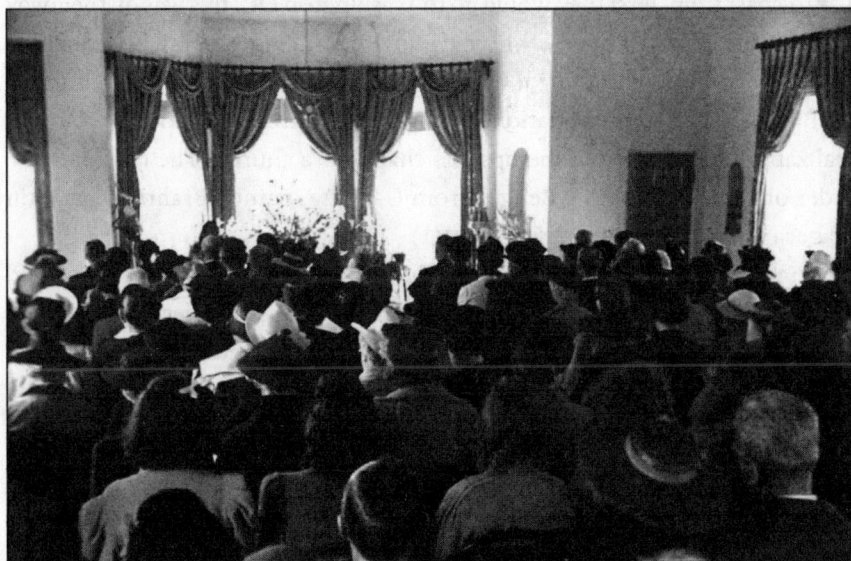

Top: Richard Wright (with his wife) and Yogananda;
Bottom: Service inside Golden Lotus Temple, circa 1940.
Source: Wikimedia Commons.

51

84 ASANAS IN WASHINGTON DC

The last place to visit was saved for the very end.
I didn't need to travel to Europe, or to the other side of the world, India or Asia.
It was nearby, across the Potomac River, near Washington DC. I realized, as I
stepped inside, where Buddha and Bishnu had performed. Not on the ground
floor, but upstairs, in the chapel hall. On the small stage, eighty years earlier,
Buddha performed Eighty-Four Yoga Asanas.

By February, Bishnu and Buddha left Los Angeles for the East via the coast-to-coast train. First they would go to Washington DC; this was on their way back to Columbia University, where they would further work with Josephine Rathbone on therapeutic yoga. On the evening of 20 February 1938, Buddha and Bishnu gathered in the nation's capital, with 'the congregation of the Self-Realization Fellowship', in the upstairs chapel of a church. The reverend and leader of the church was a Bengali from Calcutta, named Brahmachari Jotin (he became Swami Premananda in 1941).

Jotin had been 'educated at the Ranchi school and Calcutta University' and was summoned to America by Yogananda in 1928 to assume leadership of the DC area's SRF centre. Yogananda had deliberately ignored the segregation of African Americans, and Jotin's events had 'started in a basement room in the poor section of Northwest Washington at Columbia Road in the District of Columbia'.[1] It had been difficult, but in 1938, a new Washington DC SRF church had just been dedicated in the section of the city called Friendship Heights.[2] Yogananda told him, 'Jotin, what you have accomplished in Washington, I could not have done.'[3]

What made this DC event special was the newspaper coverage.

The story, by an unnamed author, was placed at the top of page one, in section B, 'Society and General' of *The Evening Star*. It included boldface headlines, three photographs of Buddha and a detailed account of their performance. Similar to events prior, Buddha performed 'physical Yoga demonstrations'. This article of 21 February 1939 is particularly significant because it is the earliest known documentation of eighty-four asanas being performed outside of India. Just below the headline, the bold letters read, 'India's Quasi-Sacred Physical Culture Made Up of 84 Body Postures'. The third paragraph again repeated the description, saying that 'eighty-four different body postures, designed to show the control and development of muscles by the mind were presented', from beginner to advanced. 'He and his teacher are on a world tour', and all together, they performed 'more than 100 postures of the Yoga system of physical culture', the reporter wrote.

Bishnu explained that 'the easier postures make the limbs flexible. When this is achieved, the more intricate postures become easier.' The reporter of the news item quoted Bishnu as saying 'there are eight ways to breathe properly', which included 'breathing by force of the throat which utilizes the full power of the lungs'. And that 'the 3,000 year-old Yoga system of physical culture, developed and handed down in India for countless generations' was being demonstrated by its foremost exponents.[4]

'The Yoga system might be called exercise without exercise,' said Bishnu, who described it as 'energization of muscles by will power' in order 'to develop not only the muscular tissues but the nervous and organic tissues of the body as well,' echoing language from Yogananda. Bishnu pointed out that 'by muscular control' one 'can relax so completely while awake that he requires only six hours of sleep a night and can, if necessary, get by with only a few hours of sleep a week'.

The reporter made an examination of their muscles, which 'showed they were soft, almost flabby, when relaxed, but hard as a rock with contracted'. The 'chest expansion' for Bishnu 'ranges between 7 and 9 inches', and his 'forearm expansion' is 'more than 2 inches when contracted,' he reported.

The article mentioned that Bishnu and Buddha 'speak the Bengalese dialect in their private conversations, although both speak English fluently'. Bishnu, it went on, 'is the head of a system of physical culture colleges that extends through eight provinces of India, including Bengal, holds several college degrees and is a recognized theologian'. The last accomplishment was attributed to his having been 'ordained' by Yogananda to initiate others into Kriya yoga. Bishnu then expanded on his theological accomplishment to explain that in India, 'the Yoga method' through 'breathing, posture, muscle control and glandular development' has 'always been connected with theology and has been taught in connection with religion and philosophy'.

What Bishnu seemed to be pointing out was that only those initiated by a learned guru would be taught these methods. 'The cardinal points' of the '3,000-year-old Yoga system' were only 'developed and handed down in India', as they had been 'for countless generations'. The confluence of Kriya yoga ministry and displays of Hatha yoga 'physical culture' puts the spiritual–physical synthesis on full display. Bishnu and Buddha 'were scheduled to return' to Columbia University in New York City after their DC performance.

Columbia University and Washington DC were likely not the only places Bishnu and Buddha visited during their time on the East coast. A Harvard magazine, *The Crimson*, interviewed a physical yoga student-practitioner, named William Conger, who was from Youngstown, Ohio. Published in February 1939, the student cultivated an ability to withstand sensory changes or other extreme events (such as weather) without reaction.

The article stated that the 'young Yogi has already reached some degree of *pratyahara*, control of the body's nerves. He can be seen around the Yard in the coldest weather without overcoat or sweater.' Conger's Hatha yoga practice of *Kundalini*, he said, was how the 'true Yogi displays his power only to his inner circle of students'. And on that note, Conger told the interviewer, 'I am looking forward to a visit of Buddha Bose and Bishnu Charan who are touring many universities displaying their physical power.'[5]

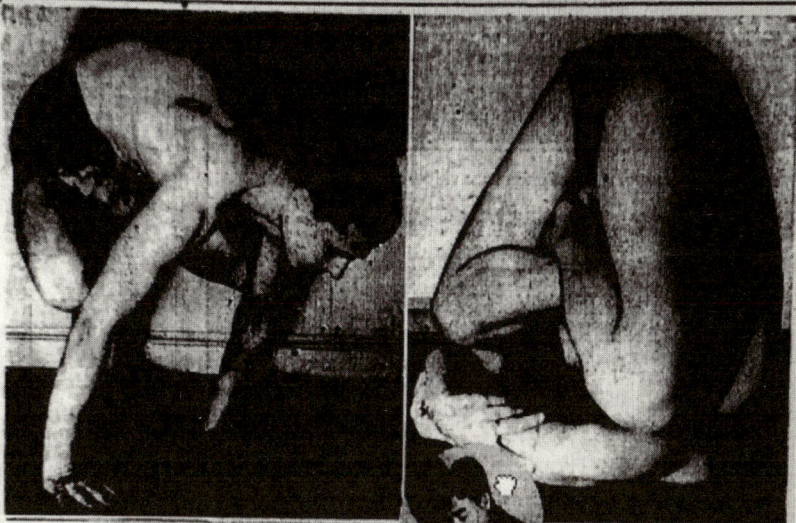
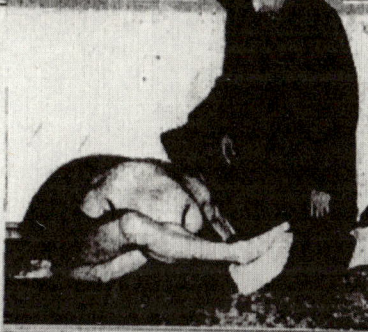

Buddha Bose & Bishnu Ghosh on stage in Washington DC (1938).

Source: The Evening Star, *Library of Congress Archives, DC.*

PART EIGHT

YOGA FAMILY

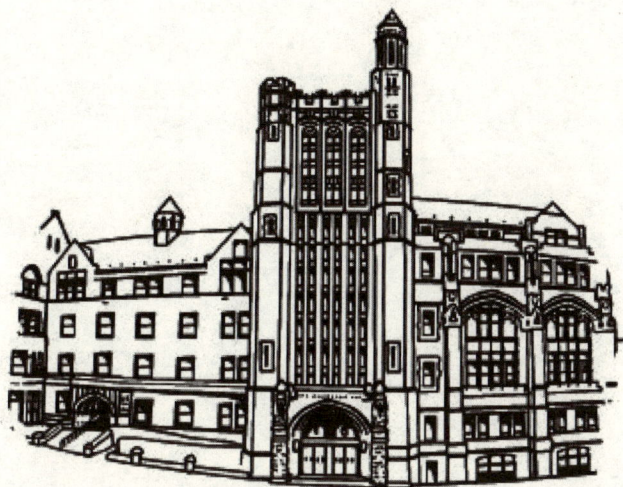

Columbia Teachers College

PART EIGHT

YOGA FAMILY

52

COLUMBIA TEACHERS COLLEGE

Bishnu and Buddha's concept of yoga and it's public presentation transformed while they were at Columbia Teachers College. They were no longer touring. Instead, they were demonstrating, teaching and observing during their four-week residency. Their course had thirty students; all learning to be physical education instructors. The group of American students, used to slouching in chairs and slumping over while reading or writing, learned basic yoga asanas and methods for respiratory control, specifically for the lungs and diaphragm, and relaxation.

Dr Josephine Rathbone said she taught 'individual gymnastic' lessons one-on-one 'for those who wish to build up strength and vitality' and a 'relaxation course'. Her coursework was a clinic for a modern society, one which was 'too keyed up' due to the 'machine tempo in daily life'. 'Bad postural habits and even diet', she wrote, 'impede proper relaxation'.[1]

Her focus on stress and an approach to 'the problem from the psychological as well as the physiological point-of-view' provoked interest, both in the press and at Columbia Teachers College.[2] Members of the community were 'amused as well as puzzled by the intensity of the interest' in her course on methods of relaxation.[3]

The course included instruction of the yoga technique *savasana*, which Rathbone recommended doing in five-minute intervals throughout the day to relieve tension. 'Take more exercise' was a directive to be coupled with 'rest is the great restorative,' she wrote. 'No educational program to offset tension was complete without training in how to relax consciously. Workers needed to be appreciative of the values of relaxation.'[4]

The courses were a success and scheduled to be repeated in the spring of 1939.[5] Titled 'Physical Education 168D: Methods of Relaxation', the course was listed as a means to learn techniques for those 'who desired to improve their posture or to overcome such detriments to health as fallen arches, weak and painful feet, weak abdominal muscles, indigestion, constipation, overweight, underweight, sleeplessness, poor circulation, weak heart ... or for those who desire to learn exercise to do at home'.[6]

Rathbone included yogic techniques, 'physiology' with 'massage and adhesive strapping', 'Methods in Relaxation' and 'Corrective Physical Education'.[7] It was this last course that involved Indian guest lectures and demonstrations.[8]

The class, with Bishnu and Buddha as Rathbone's guest lecturers, was full; with thirty students. The demonstrations were performed by Buddha with lectures by Bishnu in front of a class of future physical education teachers over a four-week period. At the conclusion, their 'friends at Columbia University' provided them with a letter of thanks, dated 4 April 1939.[9]

The coursework over that year proved to be a breakthrough for both the American teacher Rathbone and for Buddha and Bishnu. Rathbone made it a point to supplement 'the therapeutic and educational aspects of yoga' with her background in health and physical education. The two were not just complementary. 'Relaxation therapy and modern yoga emerged in the West at roughly the same moment in history as modern psychology' and helped to deal with the unprecedented nervous exhaustion in a overstressed society.[10]

Rathbone was not interested in promoting yoga as the transcendental theological belief system which Bishnu had talked about in Washington DC, but as a means of 'alleviating a variety of disorders, such as heart disease, neuritis, indigestions and insomnia, which were caused, in her view, by the era's pathological level of tension'.[11]

Rathbone may have been the first to fully appropriate yoga for stretching and relaxation in the West, but she did it with full encouragement from Bishnu. For he had already been on the path of appropriating yoga as exercise, integrating both Eastern and Western systems, since the twenties. The role of lecturer at Columbia Teachers College was validation, and later referenced as a touchstone event, when the institute Yoga Cure was started in 1939 with twenty-nine teachers of Columbia.

Buddha and Bishnu helped make the practice of yoga asana more commonplace, bringing the practices beyond the confines of India. Yoga was catching on.

Soon after they left the United States, *Life* and *Time* magazine coverage and newspaper accounts of yoga became more detailed and beneficial. Indra Devi in Los Angeles opened yoga studios, Theos Bernard lectured and gave lessons and many other authentic first-generation teachers emerged out of their experiences in India in the thirties. For Buddha and Bishnu, the experience in America would be the moment of inspiration to truly begin teaching and promoting yogic exercises suitable for everyone through the setting up of Yoga Cure.

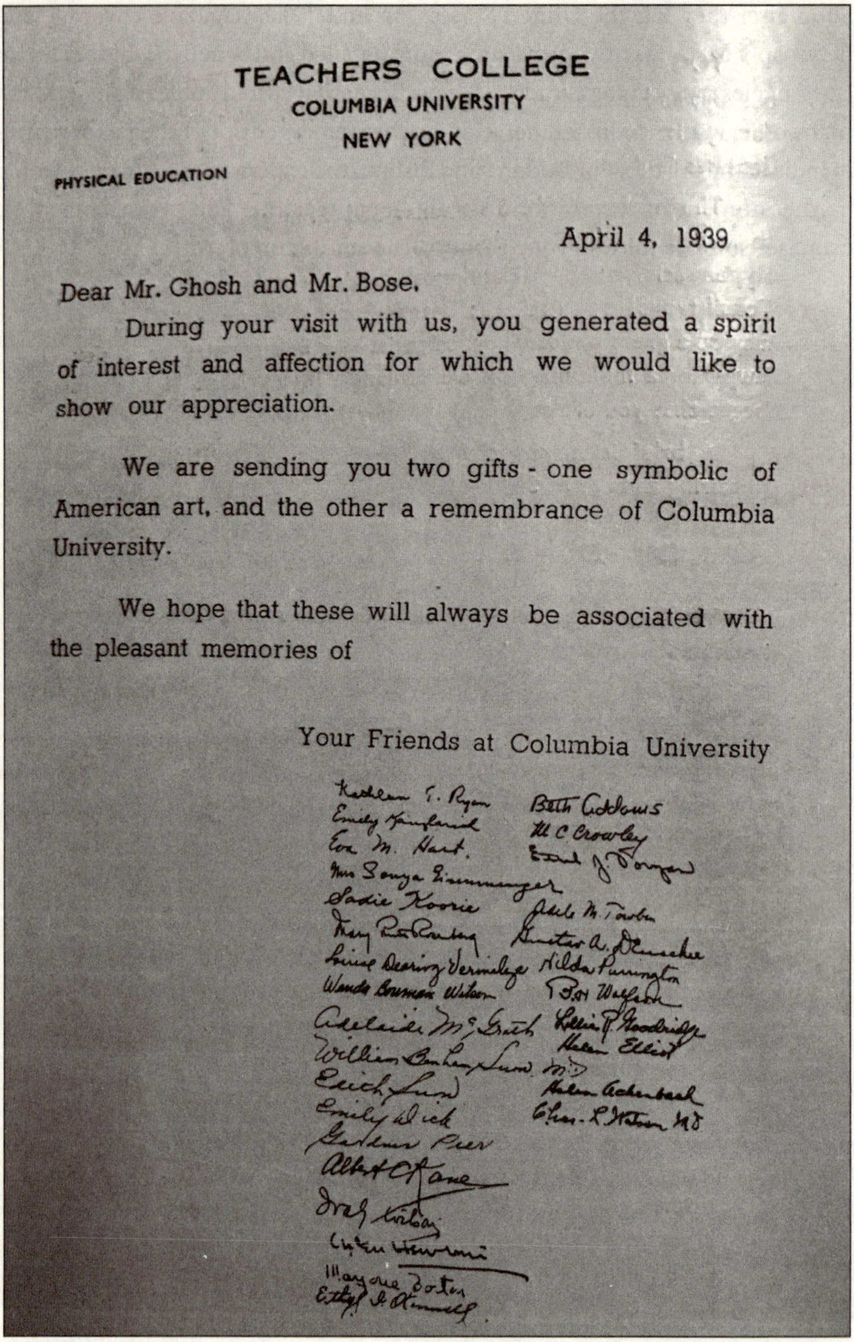

TEACHERS COLLEGE
COLUMBIA UNIVERSITY
NEW YORK

PHYSICAL EDUCATION

April 4, 1939

Dear Mr. Ghosh and Mr. Bose,

During your visit with us, you generated a spirit of interest and affection for which we would like to show our appreciation.

We are sending you two gifts - one symbolic of American art, and the other a remembrance of Columbia University.

We hope that these will always be associated with the pleasant memories of

Your Friends at Columbia University

[handwritten signatures]

Letter from Teachers College,

Columbia NY. Courtesy of Mataji.

53

KEY TO THE KINGDOM

Those who hope to specialize in this line may learn all the Asanas,
but for the average individuals of all ages, a few exercises should be chosen,
suitable to the person's physical condition, age and body build.[1]
– Buddha Bose

Buddha and Bishnu had left Calcutta on 6 July 1938. They returned a year later.[2] By July 1939, their fame had spread. The *Calcutta Municipal Gazette* named Buddha 'the famous Physical Culturist known throughout India'.[3] The *Amrita Bazar Patrika* displayed photos of Buddha performing on the European stage with the caption: 'Three thousand-year old Indian system of physical culture demonstrated in London by 27-year-old Buddha Bose.'[4]

In August 1939, after returning to Calcutta, Buddha had the opportunity to perform the asanas before the poet Rabindranath Tagore, India's intellectual renaissance legend. Tagore wrote of their meeting, 'I have heard so much about the marvels achieved by Hindu Yogis in their yogasana but I have had till today no demonstrable proof of such hearsay. My son, I feel happy and grateful to my creator that I have lived long enough to witness the amazing yogic feats which you have shown me this day.'[5] Tagore confirmed just how rare, private and hidden the practice of Hatha yoga still was in India at the time.

Edward Groth and Ian Stephens continued to help their teacher, Buddha, and to publicize yoga as exercise. Stephens wrote that Buddha wanted to arrange 'the publication of a book'. And further, 'the letter-press, a draft of which I have seen, will not be remarkable, but has a good chance of arousing great interest because of its brilliant illustrations'.[6] The draft which he had seen was the unpublished manuscript dedicated by Buddha to 'Uncle Edward', signed and dated 15 July 1938.

Buddha had hoped to find a publisher for his manuscript while abroad, but it did not happen, and he moved forward to publish it in Calcutta. What Buddha published in 1939, through the bound print organ of Stephens's employer, *The Statesman,* was a book titled *Key to the Kingdom of Health through Yoga,* Volume 1. The book contained twenty-four yoga exercises, with an introduction written by Bishnu. It also contained the note by Tagore, along with a photo of Buddha and Tagore. The slim, sixty-seven-page book was published and 'printed by D.A. Lakin at The Statesman Press Calcutta', a part of 'The Statesman Ltd., Calcutta and New Delhi'.[7]

The draft manuscript, comprising over ninety asanas, with descriptions and photos, was never completed or published in its entirety (until 2015). Why exactly Buddha never published a second volume remains a bit of a mystery. Explanations by Buddha's family on the lack of a second volume seemed speculative. For example, his daughter stated that as Buddha matured, he no longer believed that any further advanced asanas needed to be promoted, as they only served a small population. Another reason voiced was that after the world tour and initiation into Kriya yoga, he became less focused on the physical outward display of asanas and more on the spiritual inner world. Yet another was that some of the photographs, or their descriptions, in the original manuscript were amateur. There was the possibility of truth in all of these statements; however, another reason, the turbulence of the forties, should also be considered. In addition, complicated personal and family events were about to commence that were just as upsetting to the status quo.[8]

There were slight but significant textual differences between the unpublished 1938 *Yoga Asanas* preface written by Buddha and the preface in Volume 1, published in 1939, which, again, highlighted the change of nomenclature described earlier. For example in the latter, 'Yogic physical culture' became 'Yoga system of body culture' and his 'being invited to demonstrate Hatha Yoga' in 1938 became his being 'invited to give exhibitions of these Yoga poses'. In fact, by the time of the 1939 book, the terms 'physical culture' and 'Hatha yoga' were dropped entirely, with neither term being used even once. Given that the contents of the preface were nearly identical otherwise, what was removed or changed was done with a specific purpose in mind. The changes over time were made in order to place the terminology in a specific historical context for a select audience.

Bishnu and Buddha felt the necessity to historically validate both themselves and their stage performance abroad through the lineage of Hatha yoga, 'India's ancient yoga'. Thereafter, they wanted to counter the perception that Western-based physical culture systems were superior to traditional Indian ones, which were closely tied to nationalist efforts underway against colonial rule, hence, a 'Hindu art of physical culture'. And last, there was the desire to break new ground by synthesizing the old with the new, the East with the West, as presented with a unique and thoroughly modern appeal: yoga exercises. The transition only took a few years and seemed to have come about as a direct result of their re-positioning yoga asanas as a 'cure' for common ailments among the masses. This framework had been enhanced by their work alongside Dr Josephine Rathbone the previous year, at Columbia Teachers College.

The exit of the term 'Hatha yoga' in favour of a more neutral 'yoga exercise' was reminiscent of the sentiment expressed by B. K. S. Iyengar, when he mentioned (after meeting Yogananda and seeing a more spiritual side), that modern yoga seemed like a revamped exercise practice which was a replica of 'wrestling and gymnastics' combined with 'physical culture'.[9] For Buddha, whose 'natural love for a symmetrical body' was 'fostered' under the 'encouragement' of his guru Bishnu Ghosh in order 'to improve his own body' by taking up 'the ancient Yoga system of body culture', the physical orientation was natural in his early years.[10] On a more personal note, Buddha changed one other line from the original manuscript, recalling the 1931 correspondence with his brother Dennis. In the letter, Buddha had admonished Dennis for missing the chance to avenge against their father, Rajah, 'on behalf of your brother'. Buddha wrote the curious line afterwards: 'The chance may or may not come again – for opportunity never comes twice.' In the 1938 manuscript, Buddha began the last paragraph with an opportunity for exaltation. 'I offer the reader of this book the key to the kingdom of health and happiness.' The paragraph in both the original 1938 manuscript and the 1939 publication were nearly identical, except for the last line. Left out of the 1939 publication, it now read: 'Can you afford to miss it?'

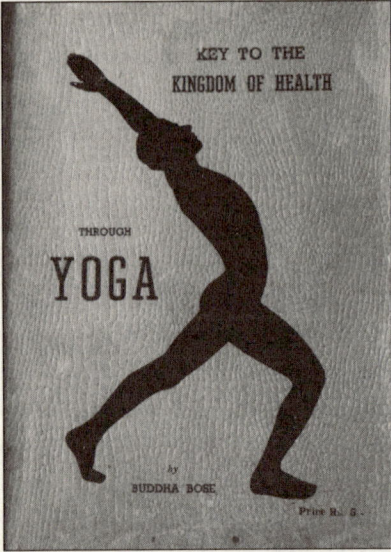

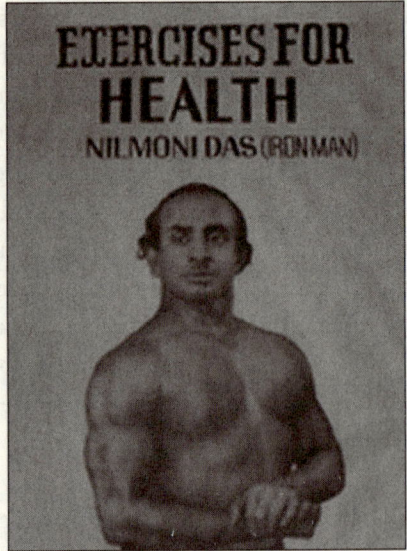

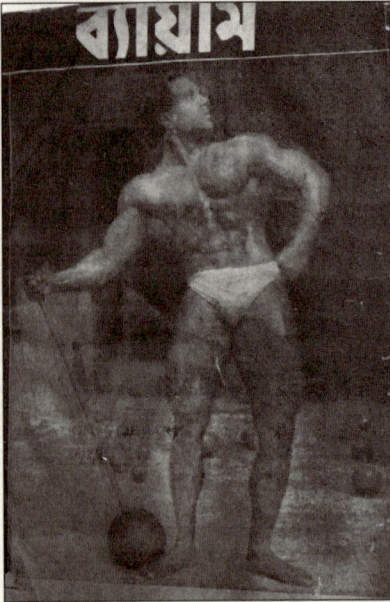

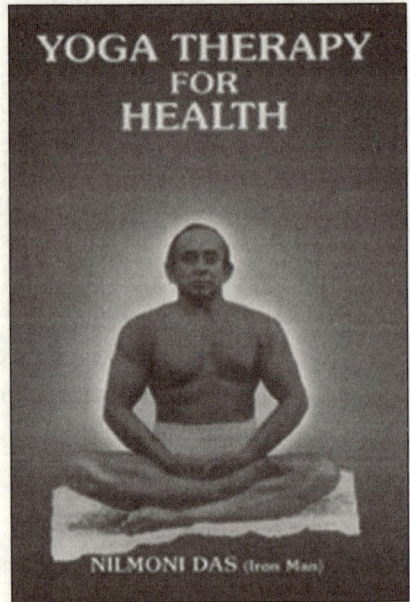

Clockwise from top Left: Cover of Key to the Kingdom of Health Through Yoga, 1939;
Cover of Nilmoni Das's book, circa 1950; Cover of *Bayam*, circa 1950.

Courtesy of Rekha Maharaja-Ivey; Shopan Das; National Library (Calcutta).

54

GRAND PHYSICAL DISPLAY

For Bishnu, the return from a world tour provided fame and celebrity status in Calcutta. He joined the ranks of those who had travelled to America and returned, like Vivekananda, his brother Yogananda and the wrestler Gobar Guho (Jatindra Charan Guha). He had gone to Europe and America, toured, lectured and demonstrated on physical culture. His status became enhanced and the Rammohan Roy Road gymnasium became not only a place for bodybuilding, but also for yoga *bayam* development.

On 8 October 1939, the third annual 'Grand Physical Display' occurred in Calcutta. It would be Buddha and Bishnu's first public event since their journey abroad. The competition was staged and sponsored by the Zionist Institute of Physical Perfection along with the Bengal Amateur Weightlifting Association (BAWLA), whose director was Joe Solomon. At the time, Solomon was the official holder of the title of 'Bengal's Strongest Man' and one of many prominent Jews in Calcutta. At one point, the Jewish community held a presence of 3,000 to 4,000 persons in Calcutta. A lone Jewish bakery, still located in the heart of New Market, and run by Nahoum and Sons, sells fruitcakes and breads. Nowadays, it is one of the only reminders left of the Calcutta Jewish community. In 1939 though, it was still quite strong.

Among Solomon's 'noteworthy performances' was 'the passing of a Buick Limousine car over his abdomen', an accomplishment that was a 'great and unexplained feat which excited the admiration of an audience well over 5,000'.

The first BAWLA competition had been staged in 1936. The annual event was held at the Dalhousie Institute, which was originally in central Calcutta, on the south side of Dalhousie Square. In its third year, there was an 'All India Men's Physical Excellence Competition', but Buddha, with 'the most perfect body' as advertised by newspaper clips around the world, did not enter the competition. Instead, he gave 'a demonstration of the world's oldest physical culture system' titled 'the cream of yoga exercises'. It was not a central component of the programme, being held during one of the intervals between the main events. The mentality of Hatha yoga as not for the common man was something that Buddha and Bishnu encountered when they brought 'the cream of yoga exercises' to the stage in Calcutta. Since it couldn't help but cause a stir among those in attendance, they were careful to bill it as 'a demonstration of the world's oldest physical culture system'.

The programme was extensive, with different displays of physical culture. They ranged from the very unique, such as 'fancy and illuminated club swinging' and acrobatic tightrope feats, to practical advice on how to 'keep fit for women', performed by the ladies section of the Jewish organization. There were also wrestling exhibitions, weightlifting contests, 'spectacular feats of phenomenal strength', as well as Jui-Jitsu and boxing contests. With over twenty names on the programme, each had a story. Bijoy Mullick, 'India's leading exponent in the art of muscle control', like Buddha, gave an interval demonstration. Bishnu was listed as one of the eight judges of the event, alongside Joe Solomon, who opened the show, and Major P.K. Gupta. Gupta was fifty-six years old but still at the top of his game. In the event, he was part of the performance of wooden *gadas* or Indian clubs that were swung around one's body.

P.K. Gupta was also the teacher of strongman Nilmoni Das, still at the beginning of his career at this point. Nilmoni and Bishnu were both contemporaries and competitors, since each had a gymnasium in the same neighbourhood. In the fall during Durga Puja, Bishnu held a similar presentation of yoga asanas, for which Nilmoni Das was in attendance.

Nilmoni was nicknamed 'Ironman' and lived at 2 Amherst Row. For an interview, Arup arranged a meeting with Swapan Das, his son.

On the very narrow Amherst Row, we reach the residence, where a plaque with 'Ironman' Nilmoni Das hangs outside the gym. Next door is a printing shop for Ironman Publications.[1]

Inside, Swapan still regularly conducts classes and trainings in yoga, just as his father and mother did beginning in 1940. In a speech he'd given on 21 June, International Yoga Day, he talked about how his father encountered Bishnu's teaching of yoga asanas. 'To gather material for his books Nilmoni Das always attended any function where physical exercises were performed, sometimes even without being invited. In one of those, in the late 1930s, Bishnu Ghosh and his students performed yoga exercise along with bodybuilding exercises.' The 'common people did not realize the potential of yoga as exercise at the time'. Swapan recalls:

A great number of bodybuilding gymnasiums would crop up everywhere in the city and its surroundings in those days. All were established by renowned bodybuilders. These gymnasiums excelled in training people in bodybuilding, weight lifting, bending of iron rods, tearing iron chains, passing trucks and elephants over the chest, gymnastics and other physical sports. The youth were being trained in these physical activities. These trained and skillful youth would then be invited to various *pujas* and other festival occasions to show off their expertise.[2]

This was exactly the type of event in which Bishnu brought out yoga asana and mudra demonstrations, similar to the previous 'cream of yoga' presentation. The Durga Puja festival performance, held at the Simla *Bayam* Samity in north Calcutta, fascinated Nilmoni and the other bodybuilders:

Other bodybuilders screamed at him and said, 'Bishnuda do we need yoga in our bodybuilding sports?' Bishnu Ghosh made them understand the importance and benefits of yoga. Their support was necessary to promote the practice of yoga among the common people of India. Soon yoga and bodybuilding centers became a common sight in the city of Calcutta. Yoga was being promoted and demonstrated frequently in different places. The surrounding areas of Calcutta, the villages and urban areas soon were flush with yoga pamphlets and letters; all distributed by the great bodybuilders.[3]

Bishnu was about seven years older than Nilmoni, and after having long discussions with him about yoga *bayam*, Nilmoni 'realized its usefulness and without wasting any time started practising'. Swapan recalls:

To know the subject more in depth he went to the yoga ashram in Lonavla and gained a lot of knowledge about Yoga through long discussions with Madhavadas Ji's direct student Kuvalayananda *Maharaj*. Later on and with the same intention, he went to Swami Jagdish Varananda of the Ramakrishna Ashram, and Raghunathpur of 24 *Parganas*. This is how Nilmoni Das prepared himself before writing the books on Yoga.[4]

The Bengali books on yoga that started coming out in 1940 were published by Ironman Publishing. 'Bengali households bought hundreds of thousands of the Ironman books, and the yoga posture charts would hang on the walls in each Bengali home. Many of the youth in this state have learned a few yoga asanas from these charts and practised free-hand exercises reading his books,' Swapan says.

Nilmoni Das's 'Yogic Asana Chart' is remarkable in its similarity to the postures and methods that are now a standard in Hot Yoga classes throughout the world. The chart shows twenty-six asanas, illustrated with photographs, along with these important tips:

- Persons of all ages, male and female, can practise.
- No asanas should be practised with strain and exertion.
- Normal breathing is essential when practising asana.
- Each asana should be practised four times, twenty to thirty seconds at each time with an interval for practising *savasana* for ten to fifteen seconds.
- Practise a few freehand exercises for warming up the body before asana practice.

As I walk along the open-air bookshops in the College Square area, I see multiple copies of the various Ironman publications available for purchase. Swapan has a few remaining of the original English poster. He sells them to me and a few other Americans for five rupees each (the ancient price tag). He could easily ask us for 500 each, instead of what amounts to be a dime.

I find myself a bit sad each time I leave Swapan's Amherst Row yoga place. His son has now left for America, and he's probably not coming back to Calcutta to teach yoga. The place is small, filled with a large office-desk that greets you as you step into the house, bowing low to get through the doorway. An entire wall is filled with books and memorabilia. Swapan sits at his desk, and from the curtains behind him, tea and biscuits emerge, sometimes Indian desserts. Through a side door, I can overhear the classes in the yoga room. It is an intimate space, though large in the impact it has made.

Swapan tells me, 'Ironman yoga and publications is going to shut down within the next few years.' Like so many others, his father's story is long forgotten. As I hang the yoga asana chart on my wall at home and follow his instructions, the teaching and the practice continue on.

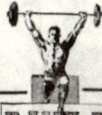

THIRD **BAWLA** ANNUAL

GRAND PHYSICAL DISPLAY

Staged by

THE ZIONIST INSTITUTE OF PHYSICAL PERFECTION

and the

BENGAL AMATEUR WEIGHT LIFTING ASSOCIATION

at the

DALHOUSIE INSTITUTE

CALCUTTA

━ **OCTOBER 8th 1939** ━

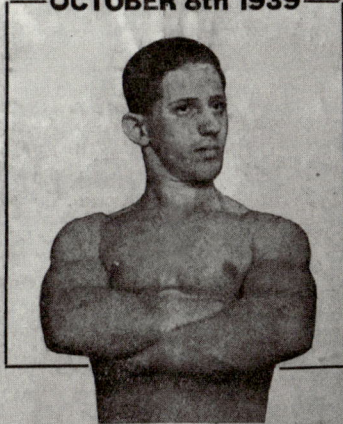

S. G/L. D. O. DR. JOE SOLOMON, (H). M.B., D.P.E., F.I.P.D.

Director of The Institute & Secretary of the B. A. W. L. A.

Official Holder Of The Title "BENGAL'S STRONGEST MAN"

MR. ASOKE SEN, THE EMINENT POET OF BENGAL, has kindly consented
to preside and MRS. SEN to give away the prizes.

OFFICIAL PROGRAMME

This page and next: 1939 promotional pamphlet in Calcutta.

Courtesy of Michael Shapiro.

Programme

1. Dr. JOE SOLOMON, H.M.B., D.P.E., F.I.P.D., the celebrated Health and Physical Culture Authority, will open the Show.
2. NEBLETT KIERNANDER, holder of the Title "India's Most Perfectly Developed Athlete" will exhibit his un-paralleled Physique which enabled him to win this Title.
3. BOXING EXHIBITION—Baby Arratoon, Champion of India and Burma Vs. Leo Thaddeus of All India Fame.
4. KEEP FIT WORK FOR WOMEN—By the Ladies' section of the Zionist Institute of Physical Perfection.
5. INTRODUCING JEHUDA DZBONKOWSKI, Palestine's Strongest Man.
6. PYRAMID PERFECTION IN SPECTACULAR TABLEAUXS,—By Mullick's Health Home.
7. JIU JITSU—a demonstration of Death-Producing Grips and Blows.
8. ALL INDIA BOYS' PHYSICAL EXCELLENCE COMPETITION.
    1. Lgr Charles Abraham.
    2. Lgr. E. Joshua.
    3. Lgr. Dudley Lambourne.
    5. Lgr. Boy Smith.
    4. Lgr. Felix O'Hara.

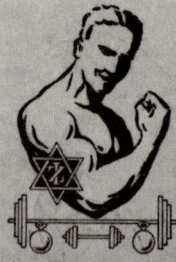

    (In order of appearance)
9. INTERNATIONAL WEIGHT LIFTING MATCH.

    INDIA   **Vs.**   **BURMA**

    S. K. NAIR   E. AIN KYU

    (Champion of India)   (Champion of Burma)

    Referee : Prof. K. Raghavan.

    Staged by the Indian Empire Weight Lifting Federation, under the Laws of the Federation Internationale De Halterophile.

INTERVAL

10. WRESTLING EXHIBITION—Sergt. Pat Burge well known in Wrestling Circles for his Prowess Vs. Battling Mirza. Sochin Bose, Indian Olympic Champion Vs. S. Banerjee.
11. BIJOY MULLICK, India's Leading Exponent in the art of Muscle Control.
12. FANCY & ILLUMINATED CLUB SWINGING—By Mullick's Health Home.
13. THE DEB BROTHERS, India's Premier Equilibrists and Acrobats.
14. A DEMONSTRATION OF THE WORLD'S OLDEST PHYSICAL CULTURE SYSTEM—the cream of YOGA exercises.
15. SPECTACULAR FEATS OF PHENOMENAL STRENGTH—by Renowned Exhibitionists.
16. WEIGHT-LIFTING CONTEST FOR THE MIDDLE-WEIGHT TITLE OF INDIA

    M. P. KRISHNAN.   **Vs.**   **ROLAND LEHANEY & HENRY SMITH.**

    (Holder)   (Challengers)

    Referee : Dr. J. E. Solomon, H.M.B., D.P.E., F.I.P.D. (Certified)

    Staged by the Bengal Amateur Weight Lifting Association, under the Laws of the Federation Internationale De Halterophile.

    Announcer : Mr. S. K. Nair, F. I. P. D.

    Scales by Messrs. W & T Avery Ltd. Official Loaders : Messrs. C. G. Apcar and G. Freiter.

17. ALL INDIA MEN'S PHYSICAL EXCELLENCE COMPETITION—A Parade of the Cream of India's Manhood.
    1. B/Lgr. Himansu Banerjee
    2. Lgr. T. P. Daruwalla
    3. Lgr. Lancelot Joseph
    4. Lgr. Robert Jackson
    5. Lgr. Josh Joshua
    6. Lgr. M. P. Krishnan
    7. Lgr. B. Murtough
    8. A.L. D. O. Joe Mingail
    9. Lgr. Shaik Subrati
    10. Lgr. Henry Smith.

    Judges : Miss Sylvia Abraham, Miss Racheal David, Dr. Joe Solomon, Major P. K. Gupta and and Messrs. N. A. Kiernander, Bishnu Ghosh and David Mordecai.

PRESENTATION OF PRIZES.

GOD SAVE THE KING.

55

GOLDEN LINE

'You never give up, do you?' asks Arup, in a tone suggesting he already knows the answer.

'No.' I reply, 'That doesn't occur to me.' I loosely quote from the Upanishads: 'To get to a destination you just have to start walking and walk on and on and on and you will most certainly then arrive at the destination.' This is without question. It has nothing to do with faith and everything with going forward. The practice is about getting up and moving. The practice is to mentally move beyond where you are now. I have to go, for I am not yet at the destination. The practice is all.

Arup and I are outside the Birla Academy of Art and Culture which houses Buddhist artifacts from Bengal. It's located on Southern Avenue, across from South Lake in Calcutta, which was a favourite outdoor place for students of Bishnu Ghosh to visit. Using the lake water as a backdrop made for good photographs of feats of strength and yoga asanas.

As we stand there, Arup gets a call. Kamli, who is on the other end of the line, owns a College Square bookstore named Subarnarekha. I can tell he has something good.

Each time we go to the bookstore, Arup complains about how lazy Kamli is compared to Kamli's father, who ran the shop when Claudia was in Calcutta a decade ago. He would find everything she asked for in historical publications on yoga. Kamli was supposed to have gone through some boxes in storage, looking for old issues of *Bayam* magazine, which Bishnu had edited. He thinks they are around, somewhere or another. Arup tells me that Kamli's father would know exactly where everything is.

'This one,' he shakes his head, 'he should die; shall we kill him?' I laugh and say no, with the hope he might one day might find the old magazines of

Bayam, of which only 200 copies were printed each month. Kamli tells Arup that he's got a signed copy of the 1930 book by Bishnu Charan Ghosh for us.

I can barely contain my excitement. 'Let's go right now!'

The only problem is the time and Calcutta traffic. It's 4 p.m., and though it's not many miles away, it will likely take well over an hour to get there, and Kamli wants to leave by 5 p.m.

We still try.

Forty-five minutes later, we are barely halfway there, our yellow cab hasn't moved in ten minutes, and everyone is honking. In the midst of the incessant noise and heat, Arup calls the bookstore, shouts aloud into his decade old flip mobile phone and gains another fifteen minutes.

I can't stand it any longer. I tell Arup I'll meet him there, get out of the cab and start walking. I know where the place is by foot and tell Arup it will take me fifteen minutes to walk there. I am going to cut through the alleyways. I feel liberated.

Six months ago, I couldn't have walked alone through the streets and alleyways of Calcutta. There are few signs, street markers or indications. It is overwhelming at first, like an urban jungle, the sun is lost behind a city haze, and a feeling of desperation arises without a guide. Now though, I can feel the direction of the city. There is nothing quite like it.

I make good time, and arrive before Arup. I duck into a small opening and walk up the back stairs into the bookstore overlooking College Street. Below, a cacophony of sounds from horns, autos and buses mixes in with the grind from the steel wheels of the hundred-year-old tram line that hulks along. Arup arrives, and we go in to see what Kamli has found.

I'm pleasantly shocked. He's found an original copy of Bishnu Ghosh's 1930 book *Muscle Control and Barbell Exercise*. The copy is badly damaged on the outside cover, but inside it is in fine condition. Tucked behind the cover is a small coloured-pencil print of Bishnu in the *nauli* pose. And he's signed the book: 'Presented to Rabin Ghosh, by B. C. Ghosh'. Rabin was one of Bishnu's key bodybuilding students in the forties and fifties.

Arup negotiates and brings the price down to 1,200 rupees, about $20. Then we celebrate by manoeuvering through the makeshift stalls along the side streets, the *boi para* (book colony) of second-hand books, over to the Coffee House, where we drink milky coffee.

The next morning we have an interview scheduled, but Arup is a no show. Arup never forgets. I call and get no answer, until I try again later in the day. I remind him of the interview, and he's beside himself for having forgotten.

It's painful. He's a professional and knows he can no longer trust his mind the way he used to. I tell him it's no biggie, and we can reschedule, but he's quite amiss over the development. Hoping Arup would continue, I blow it off. He doesn't. I have felt this coming with Arup. The ending.

It is Lakshmi Puja day, a quiet and serene puja done inside Bengali homes. I choose to go to the coffee shop, taking my laptop with me so I can write out details. I recall when Arup would ask me to say 'Lo-na-va-la'. I would hesitate, trip my tongue, and repeat it incorrectly, every time. Arup would add, 'You are not a true yogi until you can say Lonavala.' We would laugh.

So many days he would tell me that he had been making calls all morning long and that it was nearly time for his rum. As I sit at the coffee shop, Arup calls. I ask him if there is anything he wants to send to his daughter in Switzerland, perhaps a package or something. I can tell by his harshness he has something to say.

He says there is nothing to send and then, 'I want to finish this with you now.'

'What about …', I ask about so many things but he isn't listening.

I barely make out 'You can hear my sorrows' and wonder if that's really what he said. But then it hits me with a pause, when he says, 'Do you understand what I am saying?'

'I understand.' 'Keep well.' 'Goodbye.' 'Goodbye.'

It's over. I let him have that closure. After the conversation, I feel remorse, suddenly longing to call home but knowing it's the middle of the night in the States. I feel like I failed somehow. Whatever light I had, whatever got Arup out of bed, to be near, has left me, or not shone brightly enough for him to pull it together for another day. But I know it's not me, it's his challenge to overcome.

Arup's physical degeneration has led to his wearing the steel belt, and his alcohol dependency has led to organ illness, affecting his mind. He knows what he faces and tells me there is no reason to feel sorry. He's right, of course. To come out purified on the other side, he will have to travel through that tunnel alone. But I can't help feeling a part of me leave too. An innocence perhaps, a knowing that everything is ending a little too quickly for us. Perhaps some things are meant to be left undone, or passed on to another to do on our behalf.

As I walk back to Ghosh's Yoga College along Raja Dinendra Street, I stop across the street from a water spigot. It always flows, straight from the Ganges River. Throughout the morning and all day long, men squat on the sidewalk to take their outdoor bath. It doesn't matter what time they choose; the water is always on.

I realize what I've gained. I've learned to stop striving, a lesson learned while practising yoga according to how Buddha Bose had originally taught. I've replaced the American workout style with a daily practice according to the system originated here in Calcutta. In turn, I've become more receptive, developed subtler senses. I just mingle with everything. The entire process, I realize, is one of letting go of control, letting things come to me on their own. All I have to do is set it in motion, to practise and the rest follows.

56

HIMALAYAS

The easiest route to Holy Kailas and Lake Manasarovar is from Almora.[1]
– Buddha Bose

Even 'the average Hindu believes that these Himalayas are sacred'. Goddess Parvati and her husband, Lord Shiva 'live there with many other gods' and deities. 'At the foot of these Himalayas are the sacred places', Rishikesh and Haridwar. 'Swamis, yogis, *sadhus* and *babas* come here and sit in *samadhi*, some wearing no clothes.' Alongside generations of pilgrims, they hike to temples in the Himalayas 'along the banks of the Ganges and Yamuna', and along other rivers, 'such as Badrinath and Kedarnath'.[2]

When Buddha wrote of going to the Himalayas for the first time, he did not include the motivation for his voyage. He only said, 'In the year 1940 I was there and had the opportunity to see the spiritual power of those Holy Places.' According to a retelling of the story by Mataji, a disciple, Buddha's inspiration to visit the place came from his Bengali mother.

'At that time his stepmother was sick. She had tuberculosis.' Buddha was told that his Bengali mother 'could survive only if she went to the mountains. She needed fresh air, and Almora was the preferred spot. But there was no money to take her there, which worried him.'[3]

Edward Groth, the American Hatha yoga student who studied with Buddha beginning from 1937, was in Calcutta from 1934 until 1941.[4] Even though the difficult postures proved to be too ambitious at first, he did 'eventually learn to do the headstand', and it was while he was holding this asana one day that a fortuitous event occurred. It was 1940, and Buddha was at the American Consulate office to teach him. He was in *sirsasana* and Buddha forgot the timing. When Buddha did not continue counting, the American came down from the pose on his own. Having realized that his teacher was worried about something, Groth asked, 'Mr Bose what is the problem? You do not seem to be in a normal state today?'

Buddha replied, 'I am sorry I forgot the timings of the *sirsasana*.' Groth said, 'Never mind, but what is the reason?'

Buddha then told him he was worried about how he would take his mother to Almora as he did not have the money. Groth offered to pay for the journey and told Buddha, 'Do not worry. You have given me a lot of training, now just take your mother to the hill station.'

Buddha left with his Bengali mother. While at Almora, as they 'were sitting in the sun alongside a road', his stepmother asked, 'Do you know where this road goes?' He did not, and she went on, 'This is the way to go to Kailas and Manasarovar.' Buddha 'realized that if his stepmother said this, then he must go'.[5]

The idea of going to the Himalayan Mountains had been growing inside Buddha, who had begun to realize 'the profound effect yoga-*bayam* had on the mind'.[6] It was only natural that he became interested in following the spiritual pull of the Himalayas. Others around him, both in Calcutta and on his recent world tour with Bishnu, kindled the notion. Compared with Yogananda, whose desire to trek into the Himalayas presented obstacles and never fully materialized, Buddha's quest was supported and encouraged.

Groth himself knew quite a bit about the place too. He had completed an '8-page report by the American Consul to India on September 13, 1939', which detailed the story of the 1939 K2 American expedition. The report provided a gripping account of the mountain adventure, with the goal to scale the second-highest mountain in the world. It had 'all the hallmarks of a great novel, with intrigue, drama, personality clashes and gripping mountain adventure'.[7]

Upon his return to Calcutta, Groth 'showed a very beautiful film of a journey from Srinagar to Gilgit and Hunza, and then through Chitral to Peshawar'.[8] This film likely inspired Buddha to document his own 1940 voyage with a camera and film equipment, probably borrowed from Groth.

Yogananda never entirely grew out of his desire to visit the Himalayas, and influenced Buddha's notion of this spiritual adventure. While Buddha was at Yogananda's Los Angeles ashram a year earlier, he saw a series of headline articles in *Inner Culture*, Yogananda's magazine.[9] They were written by Nicholas Roerich, an American disciple of Yogananda. Consecutive issues featured titles such as 'Hermitages in the Himalayas' in August and 'Ascending the Heights' in the October 1939 edition. 'The sacred hermitages at Manasarovar, Kailas, Badrinath, Kedarnath, Triloknath, Rewalsar, these glorious gems of India, always fill the heart with special blissful tremor.'[10] Roerich had voyaged to these places with a caravan of travellers and passed on the legends of the rishis. The articles comprised the 'miracle men' and 'strange tales' he encountered on the Himalayan mountain paths.

In 1938, while Buddha was in London, it was Francis Younghusband who arranged for Bishnu and Buddha to perform in Caxton Hall. Called 'The Last Great Imperial Adventurer', Younghusband was a former British Army official who had gone to Tibet in 1904 and had become the president of the Royal Geographical Society. Younghusband was one of the first colonialists to conceive of the 'idea of climbing Everest' as he 'was marching to Chitral in 1893'.[11]

Younghusband was renowned for his encouragement regarding voyages to the Himalayas, since he himself was said to have had a spiritual experience there. He considered the Himalayas the source of India's religious feeling, a place for pilgrimage, 'where the glaciers would shine like gold as catching the first rays of the rising sun and the last rays of the setting sun'.[12]

Bishnu would go on a later pilgrimage with Buddha, but not this first one. Though Buddha may have travelled there alone, there are records of who he met while there. Swami Pranavananda, in his historic 1949 book titled *Kailash Manasarovar*, made mention of the voyage Buddha took by writing, 'Sri Buddha Bose of Calcutta, the well-known Yoga-Asanist, visited Kailas and Manasarovar by Niti-Hoti pass in 1940 and returned by Lipu Lekh pass.'[13]

The books by Pranavananda were written as pilgrim guidebooks, and the contents had both scientific and spiritual observations. Though many travelled there, the spiritual vibrations were not easy to find. He wrote, 'It is no wonder that a person devoid of any spiritual tendencies cannot perceive or feel the effect of the spiritual vibrations, existing in a particular place.'[14] 'Nowadays', he went on in the 1949 book, people 'pay a flying visit and go back in a day or two, without taking proper and full advantage of the spiritual vibrations existing in those places by staying there calmly and quietly for some time and taking to spiritual practices.' Explaining the beauty of Kailash and Manasarovar in his books, he relayed how he would hear the sound of bells, cymbals, and other musical instruments on the top of Kailash.[15]

For the 'benefit derived from the spiritual vibrations existing there ... there is an injunction in the *shastras* that pilgrims to the *tirthas* should stay there for at least three nights' he wrote, adding, 'Kailas and Manasarovar are the holiest of the several *tirthas* in the Himalayas.'[16] Buddha's writings revealed, in much a similar way, that he was able 'to see' the mountain's 'spiritual power'.

In 1940, Buddha went to Kailash and Lake Manasarovar. He brought the camera and the film equipment borrowed from Groth with him on the trip. At one point, a *sadhu* came towards him unannounced. As Buddha saw the saint nearing, he told his porters to give the sadhu some alms. The sadhu replied, 'I am not a beggar. I have come to talk to you.' He then told Buddha, 'I've noticed you are taking films of these places for quite some days now. You are doing good work but you must be present at the time of showing the film to all the devotees.' Then the *sadhu* left, without saying anything more, though he granted Buddha a photo of the two of them together.[17]

When Buddha returned to Calcutta, he was twenty-nine years old and lived on the first floor at 4/2 Rammohan Roy Road. He returned from his journey to a life of occasional performances, but mostly of taught his students. His daily routine included rising early in the morning, drinking some water prior to attending to the bathroom, and then beginning his practice.[18] He'd travelled the world, and had now published a book on yoga in Calcutta; his future seemed wide open.

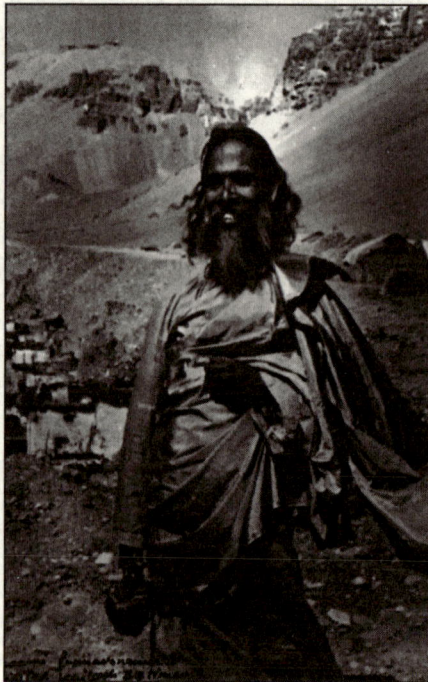

Swami Pranavananda, circa 1950.
Courtesy of Mataji and Soham Heritage & Art Center, Mussoorie, India.

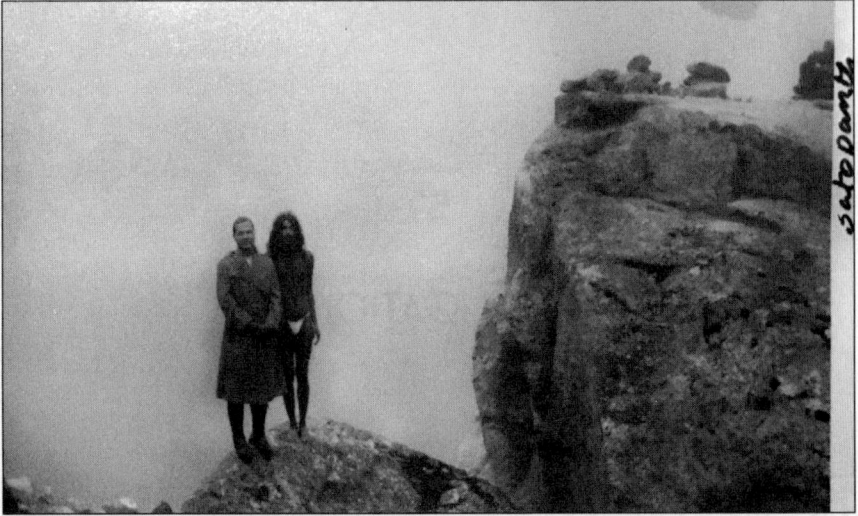

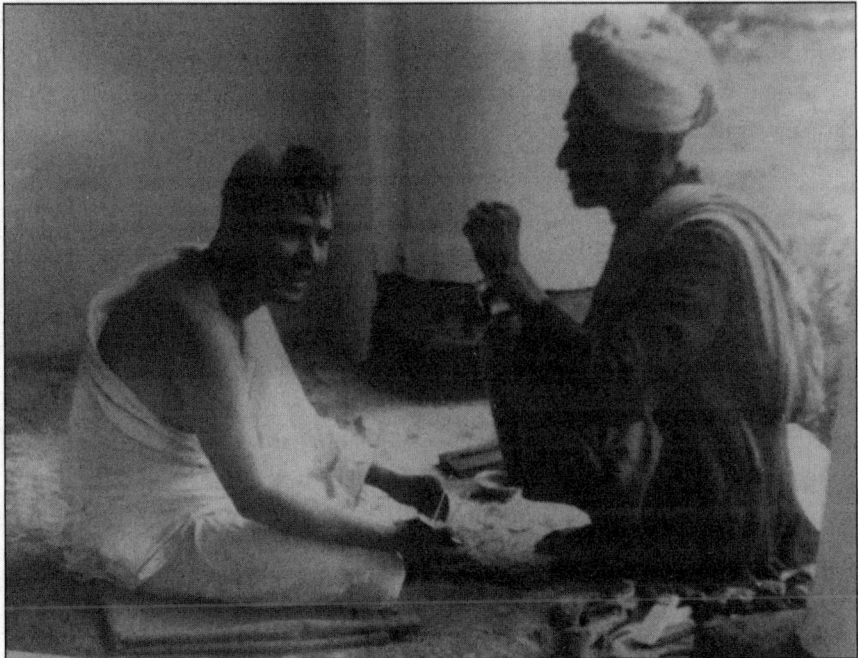

Top: Buddha Bose with yogi in the Himalayas.
Bottom: Buddha Bose being given darshan in Himalayas.
Courtesy of Mataji and Soham Heritage & Art Center, Mussoorie, India.

57

OBLIGATION

Bishnu's wife Ashalata looked all over Calcutta to find a match for their daughter, Ava Rani, but to no avail. The patriarch of the Ghosh family, Bhagabati, was now eighty-eight years old and had a suggestion. There's a saying, *'bagal me baccha gav bhar dhandora'*, which means 'the child is right under the armpit while the village is beating drums looking for the child'. The right choice was under their nose while they were out looking for a match all over town.[1] Bhagabati was suggesting Buddha.

A flabbergasted Bishnu asked, 'Really? Would Buddha accept Ava Rani, a girl half his age, as his wife?' He knew how easily Buddha was able to converse with and teach Europeans and Americans; he had seen Yogananda offer him organizational responsibility; he knew the boundless opportunity awaiting Buddha.

Buddha later pointed out to his children that when Bhagabati asked him whether he was willing to marry Ava Rani, Bhagabati told him to not feel obligated to marry, that he could refuse.[2] Given the circumstances though, it would have been difficult for Buddha to have felt anything but obligation. He accepted the proposal and married Ava Rani.

When Buddha, at the age of sixteen, had moved into the Ghosh home, he said, 'I owe everything to that old man,' referring to Bhagabati. With the marriage, a second refrain was added, 'I sacrificed everything to this old man.'[3] (Buddha Bose's grandson, Pavitra Shekhar Bose, flat out told me, 'He married out of obligation.') A sense of obligation was a family trait, passed on from Rajah, and now Buddha's to relive. As his eldest daughter-in-law Chitralekha said, 'He owed this to his guru.'

For Bishnu, it fulfilled the love he held for Buddha, which rivaled that for Srikrishna (Gublu), his own son:

I respect him and I would do anything he asks. He is God's light, he is God-given gift and grace in my life; he is incomparable in physique, looks and qualities – he is Sri Buddha Bose. Buddha was my student once upon a time and now he is my dearest – he is my son-in-law now.[4]

Buddha became even more a part of the family, moving to the second floor of the family's house. The family consulted astrologers, and the marriage was consummated at a time that meant they would give birth to a son on a particular date, the idea being that he would be a great yogi. While it was very common for an astrological chart to be drawn up at the birth of a child, the attempt to construct both fate and destiny was more difficult.

It was a fun time at the 4/2 Rammohan Roy Road house for Bishnu. His favourite pupil had become his son-in-law, and his own son, Srikrishna, turned thirteen. Bishnu was careful with 'Gublu', as the boy was called.

'If he was bit by a mosquito I would not let him go to school. I would take care of him the whole day and let him stand only when the swelling went down,' wrote Bishnu.

The grandfather, Bhagabati, responded, 'What is this madness? Why are you not letting him attend school?'

Bishnu replied, 'Baba you do not know, what if he scratches the spot unmindfully?' Bishnu 'checked his stool every day', and often neglected his work to spend time with the boy. He would 'playfully practise wrestling with him for one hour every day'.

Initially we would wrestle on the bed, but the mattress got destroyed. When the new mattress was made, Gublu's mother would not allow us to play on the bed anymore.

I told Gublu, 'So what if she will not allow us? God has given our bodies enough spring and mattress we can wrestle on the ground.' So the bed was pushed to one side and we wrestled on the ground. My father would dedicatedly be a spectator and laugh joyfully at Gublu's antics.

My daughter, Ava, who is two years older than Gublu also wrestled every day. She had enormous strength but she always lost to him in the twists. Ava defeated many young men at the *akhara* even a few months before her marriage. Gublu and I wrestled any time of the day, maybe 3–4 times in a day. My *chhotda's* youngest son, Putu, was also an expert in wrestling and Gublu would catch him at 9 a.m. to go to the *akhara* to wrestle and learn from him. Gublu was very punctual and disciplined.[5]

The duo engaged in 'marble games and kite flying' as well. The son was Bishnu's pride and joy.[6]

Buddha, who Bhagabati welcomed into the house as a son over a decade prior, had married his granddaughter. Bhagabati had not only kept the Ghosh family together after his wife, Gyana, had died with the children still young, but also made the family grow and prosper. Even though Bishnu once felt himself 'a problem', with which his father had to deal as a single parent, the two developed a very close relationship. Bishnu told of an incident which happened later in his father's life:

My father had crossed seventy-two years of age and yet I saw him practising his *bayam* every morning – his ten times *dand* and *baithak* and then swinging two cudgels ten times. I used to do 300 *dand* and 400 *baithak*, wrestle and do weight lifting with barbells.

So my father's *bayam* practice seemed laughable and one day I asked him jokingly, 'What is the point in doing this little *bayam*?'

My father said softly, 'What happens? Actually nothing and this is not suitable for my age. I have been practising this for years to hold up an ideal for you. See you have followed and that is why you used to wake up at 4 a.m. and go for your *bayam* to City College; and then be back to sit down for your studies at 6 a.m. I had decided I would continue till such time you asked me this question. Now that you have asked I shall not do this from tomorrow. Hope you have learned a lesson from me today and will teach your own child so that he or she grows up to be an ideal child. My pranayama and *mahamudra* that I do for an hour every evening is quite enough for me and very suitable.'

Bishnu wrote, '[It was] a great lesson for me … if parents of today follow this ideal they will surely bring up their children in the most ideal way.'[7]

PART NINE

THROUGH FALL,
FIRE AND FLIGHT

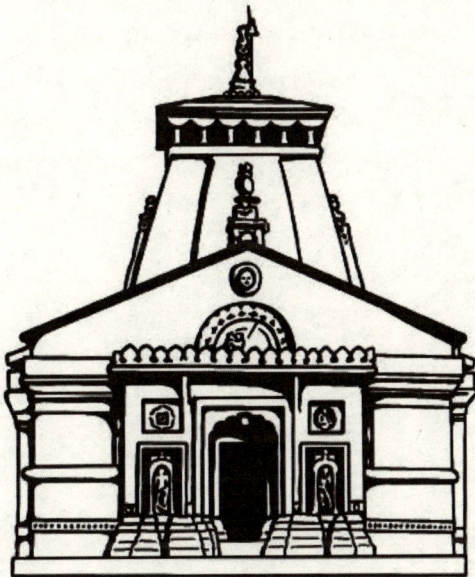

Kedarnath Temple

58

SWAMI'S POINT

The Golden Lotus Temple was built in 1938, on Southern California's West Coast, alongside Pacific Coast Highway 101. Situated atop the highest point along the coast in the Encinitas stretch, it was a landmark. The octagonal observatory with its white frame, rose up three stories and stood out against the background of the blue sky. The four gold-plated lotuses atop the structure glistened in the sunlight.

After Yogananda returned to the US from India, the hermitage in Encinitas became his favourite spot. The local surfers often spotted Yogananda 'with his long, flowing hair and orange robe', atop the bluff at 215 K Street in Encinitas and started calling the overlook 'Swami's Point'.[1] The main Self-Realization Fellowship (SRF) operation was further north, near Los Angeles at Mount Washington, and had become an active organizational beehive. In Encinitas, Yogananda could benefit from the quieter location and spend his days finishing his autobiography, meditating in the caves built into the bluff and walking on the grounds.

Richard Wright, his devotee, had been with Yogananda in India from 1935 to 1936 before serving as his secretary and treasurer in the US for four more years. Eventually though, he 'fell in love' and 'went to work for a living wage at the Lockheed Corporation' in Burbank. A photograph showed the young couple inside the Golden Lotus Temple, sitting in front of the eight-foot windows that opened to the Pacific Ocean, enraptured, as they listened to Yogananda play his harmonium and chant.[2]

Yogananda loved to be at the Golden Lotus Temple to meditate. A void of deep friendship had left his 'life after Dhirananda's departure'. It was with James Lynn that he rekindled a close relationship. Lynn (or Saint Lynn, as Yogananda referred to him) changed the atmosphere of the ashram 'with his deep devotion 'to the practice of Kriya yoga'.[3] The two would go to the edge of the property cliff, then take a few stairs down to where 'two man-made caves with a partition' were carved into the hillside.[4] There, placed straight westwards overlooking the Pacific Ocean, with the waves thundering hundreds of feet below, the Swami and Saint would enter *samadhi* and meditate for hours on end.

Disciples made pilgrimages to the temple in order to be initiated into Kriya yoga by Yogananda. Brahmachari Jotin, the leader of the 'Eastern Headquarters' of SRF in Washington DC, visited Encinitas in 1941 and called it Yogananda's 'dream temple of golden lotus and blue marble'.[5] On 6 July 1941, Jotin was 'ordained and consecrated' in the 'ancient Swami Order', being given the new name of Swami Premananda during 'an inspiring service' at the Golden Lotus Temple.[6]

Those who became initiated or even just attended services on each Sunday, left with a tangible sense of the mystical. It was 'just like seeing paradise without dying,' a visitor once remarked.[7] Ramananda, a disciple of Yogananda, reflected on the place years later by saying, 'People could see the ocean through the huge window ... They could see the stars and the moon, and Yogananda would be talking there. They would just be swept up into this beautiful vibration. They got intoxicated, really.' In hindsight, it was a risky spot to build such a temple, right on the edge of a 300-foot bluff that overlooked the sea. It was a bit 'too perfect and beautiful to stay in an imperfect earth for long,' lamented Yogananda.[8]

Stories surround the temple's fall. On 19 March 1942, during an Easter Sunrise and Morning Service in the Golden Lotus Temple, Yogananda and his devotees were sitting still, deep in meditation. Yogananda abruptly yelled, 'Get out of here at this very moment!' Nothing had happened, but a few months later, a slight movement of the temple occurred and cracked the concrete. In the May of 1942, just four years after it was built, the temple began to slip off of its foundation.

Accounts vary of why the temple started to move. The Fellowship placed the blame on the city of Encinitas; for waste-water runoff. Environmental groups blamed the SRF organization for its constant irrigation of the garden grounds near the temple, where they also placed pools of water. From above, the grounds looked immaculate, but underneath, things were slipping. Whatever the cause, the soil, which was in a very dry climate, became soft, and 'once the 2-foot layer of clay beneath the temple was moistened by water' the weight of the temple sank towards the setting sun.

It was just a few inches at first, and Yogananda made an attempt to rectify the situation. In the month of May, workers were called in, and they readied an attempt to move the building from its foundation, away from the bluff. But, preoccupied with other matters, they did not respond immediately. In June, before Yogananda left Encinitas for Los Angeles, he wanted to hold one more worship in the temple. Later on, he called it 'a temptation', which he avoided when he 'realized it was the purpose of Satan to cause him and his congregation all to go down with the temple with the added weight'. He instructed that services inside the building be postponed for a month, and instead, Sunday worship services at the Encinitas hermitage were held outside on the lawn.[9]

On the afternoon of Sunday, 22 June, students in Encinitas heard 'the stucco and frame building creaking'. They called Yogananda and were instructed to 'speedily' remove the remaining oriental rugs and ornaments from inside the building. A large brass bell which hung atop the building was removed. The weighted four golden lotuses atop the building had already been removed in the hope that the workers would arrive on time.

It was too late. By the time the building movers arrived on 23 June, one day later, they could only watch the inevitable happen. That evening, Yogananda called from Los Angeles. Bernard Cole answered the phone and heard, 'All is finished.' He replied, 'Yes.' The temple had slid and a few hours later, *Associated Press* reported an ominous headline over the wires: 'Temple of Religions Sliding into Ocean'.[10] Over the next two days, a photo of the leaning temple appeared and was syndicated to newspapers across the country, reaching other countries too. In the photograph, the building was still together, with the stairs leading up to its pinnacle, but the entire structure was 'tilted over at a 45-degree angle'. The *AP* syndication reported that the 'magnificent domed temple' had shifted on the unstable foundation of clay and dirt, 'moistened by seepage' and 'slowly slipped over the bluff's edge'.[11]

Having already salvaged the furnishings, rugs and emblems, there was nothing to do but watch as the structure 'plunged ungracefully part way down the cliff, its walls cracking and immense windows shattering'.[12] By the time the photograph reached many of the readers on 24 June, the Golden Lotus Temple had fallen over the bluff onto the beach below.

In Calcutta, the Ghosh family was awaiting the birth of a child. It was the first born for Bishnu's eldest daughter, Ava Rani and his star pupil, Buddha. In the days leading up to the birth, Ava Rani, who played the harmonium and often sang songs, had stopped singing. Her mother Ashalata told her that singing, with the force of exhalation, might produce a baby before the due date.

On 24 July, a month after Yogananda's temple crashed to the sea, Buddha's wife, Ava Rani, gave birth as astrologically planned. The boy was named Ashok Kumar Bose. After birth, he suffered from severe convulsions and needed to be sedated with Gardenal to keep epileptic episodes at bay. This had its own severe side effects later on, but the immediate concern was alleviated. Ashok was not the only boy in the family, as Ava Rani's younger brother Srikrishna was thirteen years old at the time, two years younger than Ava Rani.

Bhagabati Ghosh passed away on 1 August 1942, at eighty-nine years of age. He had outlived his wife by nearly forty years, and his passing was not totally unexpected. The Bengal–Nagpur Railway executive had long ago left his career, and as his children grew, he turned more and more towards meditative detachment as his preoccupation. Seven years earlier, when he was eighty-two, Bhagabati had 'strangulation of a hernia' and needed an operation. With 'no anesthesia at that time' Bhagabati replied, 'Arrange for the operation. I will do my pranayam and I won't feel any pain.'[13]

When news of his father's death reached Yogananda, he wrote a three-page tribute in his magazine. He recounted his fatherly interactions and the beatific simplicity with which Bhagabati lived his life. In that same issue, Yogananda published a commentary on the *Bhagavad Gita*, titled 'How to Live in the World But Not of It', which he surely saw as a reflection of his 'earthly father'.[14]

At Bhagabati's *Shraddha* ceremony, Bishnu read aloud a poem of last rites which stated, in part:

This home was lit up with your deeds.
Looking after everybody's needs ...
You were like the great oak tree ...
Giving shelter to all for free.[15]

59

HALSIBAGAN FIRE

'On 8th November, 1942,' Bishnu recalled, 'my whole life turned upside down.
So long I was envied and now suddenly I became the object of their pity and
sympathy. That day my crown fell off my head.'[1]

By 1942, Bishnu's son Srikrishna was quite a joy for the entire family. Bishnu would take him out on his daredevil motorbike stunts and 'would playfully practice wrestling with him for one hour every day'.[2] Bishnu wrote, he 'was very punctual and disciplined. He studied at the time of study, played during playing hours, wrestled at the right time, flew kites at the right time. There was no loophole to scold or reprimand him at all.'[3]

When Yogananda had visited his family in Calcutta seven years earlier, he had taken a liking to Bishnu's son. The boy, then six years old, would pose for Yogananda, showing 'muscles and postures and extraordinary feats'. His small eyes sparkled 'with joy' when Yogananda expressed appreciation.[4] At meal time, Srikrishna would sit with his father and uncle, just the three of them together. He was the heir to the world they were building.

Srikrishna excelled in sports and was athletic and charming. He shared Bishnu's love for performing before audiences. Bishnu and his students would perform feats of strength to paying crowds, through a circus named Gemini, especially during the puja events in Calcutta. He could not keep his son from following him to the events, and Srikrishna himself would occasionally perform feats and asanas on the stage with his father.

That fall, Bishnu had arranged a performance in north Calcutta at the Halsibagan pandal during Kali Puja. The circus was held inside a tent, and of course there were always some looking to get in for free, so the lone entrance was tightly secured to hold them off. Once the owner of the tent had admitted all of the paying guests, the entrance was tied off. He went to dinner, planning to return towards the end of the show to open the doors again.

The place was made entirely of dried bamboo and canvas, with thatches from palm trees to help cover the roof, like tinder. During the performance, a short-circuit in the electrical wires started a fire.[5] Flames quickly engulfed the inside of the tent, choking off the air. People scrambled for the exit, only to find the main exit tightly locked. They would have to crawl out from under the tent or rip through its strong canvas. As they did so, the air was sucked in, oxygenating the fire and increasing the heat. The structure was about to collapse.

Amidst the chaos, Bishnu was frantically looking for his son, and Srikrishna was screaming for his father. Bishnu was helped out of the tent. Initially, Srikrishna had been able to exit, but he ran back into the tent yelling for his father, not realizing Bishnu had already escaped. The tent collapsed, and the screams of those trapped and burning alive could be heard all around the building. Adults forged into the fire, putting their own safety aside, picking up and throwing aside the burning bamboo poles. By the time they reached Srikrishna, his skin was burnt and blackened.

Even though the fire happened over seventy-five years ago, it is still recalled today in Calcutta.

'It was a terrible tragedy. People never returned home,' said Mukul Dutta.

Hundreds of people died on that night. The roof of the tent fell on the people and there were hardly any survivors. All those North Calcutta families with their wives and daughters in gold jewellery – all burnt to ashes. And in all this, there were people who snatched off what they could lay their hands on from the dead bodies. Truckloads of dead bodies were being fished out from the site and taken to the crematorium for mass burning, without any rituals. After that incident the government passed an order that if any public functions would be organized after this they must provide multiple exits. The Halsibagan function had only one gate.[6]

The thirteen-year-old Srikrishna was not burned to death that day. It was a death that lingered on for a few days. Maybe there were moments of hope, but those were lost as he slipped away. His body charred, after a few days, unable to eat or drink, his mother attempted to have him sip a drink of milk. Others in the room watched as the white fluid visibly leaked out of the boy's throat. There was not enough flesh left intact even to ingest a fluid. There was no rush to the hospital for skin grafting and intravenous tubes because, sadly, that was not in the realm of possibility. Everything possible was attempted, but it was not enough.

Trying to find meaning in the senseless death, Bishnu wrote in a poem meant for his lost son, 'People call you unlucky but I know how lucky you are. Fire charred you, scourged your eyes, your flesh hanging out burnt – and yet, my dear son, I could not stop you from chanting God's name!'[7]

Srikrishna endured the pain for days, 'in full consciousness and bore the unbearable pain with elan'. He 'was fond of flying kites' and 'was lying there burned and blind when he suddenly cried out, *bhomara!*' In Bengali, the word *bhukatta* means one is successful in cutting off someone's kite string as a cry of joy or victory; *bhomara* on the other hand, means death has come with its whistle and another journey awaits.[8]

Bishnu asked, 'What? You did *bhomara*?'

Srikrishna, with his eyes closed and blinded due to the burns, replied from far away, '*Nischoi* (of course), 'and his life passed away as he finished this world'.[9]

'I had to witness this in horror and awesome wonder,' Bishnu wrote, as 'you ignored your burning pain, and advised me again and again to remember God, not in vain.'

After the 'horrific death' of his only son, he wrote, 'I restrained myself from committing suicide when I thought of Buddha and how his life would be destroyed if I died.'[10]

Of course there had been deaths before. The mother of Yogananda and Bishnu, Gyana, had died; even children of the Ghosh family had been lost. Two of their brothers, including Ananta Lal, who was the eldest, also died in their youth. Bhagabati had not reacted with a show of grief; he was so enshrined in the impermanence of life that he was neither uplifted by his wealth nor drowned by moments of loss. Srikrishna was likely influenced by his grandfather, Bhagabati, in his display of detachment.

Bishnu though, was not like his father in that way, and was much more attached to the moment. He was passionate, eager to engage, competitive and loved a big moment with his huge heart. This moment though, the death of his eldest and only son, was devastating for Bishnu.

In a poem titled 'To a *Sannyasi*' he reflected on the experiences 'a householder goes through' which the sannyasi will never know. 'How do I describe the loss of a son? The pain, the heart-wrenching pain sensation? Heart broken, despairing loss?'

He also reflected on the condition of his wife, Ashalata, who was just as forlorn. 'How do I describe a wife's estranged behaviour? A mother who has just lost a child? Or, depict a grieving wife's slavish, dutiful, cold, submission in the most intimate moment?'[11] The death of Srikrishna tore open the family with as significant a loss as that of Gyana in 1904, and came just months after the household patriarch, Bhagabati, had died.[12]

Yogananda, whom Srikrishna called 'Uncle', transcribed 'a broadcast to Gublu in the Astral World'. For his young nephew he wrote:

I felt your loss here, along with the loss felt by your father Bishnu and all who loved you. Of all my earthly brothers, Bishnu has been dearest to me. And you were very dear to me, you lay an example of a perfect model youth of Bengal. As your father Bishnu trained thousands in India to possess Sandow-like bodies, so you, his star student son, though gone from earth, will ever shine in the memory of all who knew you. You demonstrated your feats of strength in public gathering, even though you were only thirteen, just before death was hovering over you. And when the tent caught fire and so many perished and you were badly burned, you were telling your father not to grieve and that you were praying to God.[13]

'Plucked,' Yogananda continued, in 'the rosebud of your life.' And then, 'you will come back … to decorate the garden of human life, you will come as a special rose to make others rosy with health and a champion of freedom from weakness and disease'.[14]

Decades later, Bishnu described the lingering pain from that moment. 'I still remember that day – it plays like a picture in front of my eyes. I still go through that pain.' The way he died 'is still etched in my mind, comes in my dreams and dances in front of my eyes when awake'.[15] Immediately after the death of Srikrishna, Bishnu 'abandoned his law practice at the Alipore court'.[16] He could 'not go to the *bayamagar*' (his gymnasium) either, and instead 'just sat around thinking for two and a half years'.

Bishnu poured himself into writing Bengali poems to process the calamity of what he had seen transpire in those few days. He worked through the loss, and 'sought peace through rhymes and rhythms as his pain translated rhythmically'.[17]

His poems numbered well over hundred, and were compiled years later.[18] Drenched in raw emotion, the first lines of a few included: 'No death in the poet's voice; People call you ill-fated; The day my eyes stayed awake; The day when our eyes met in curiosity; You are my dearest, so; and, Dear ones do not die.'

At Ghosh's Yoga College, photos of Srikrishna still hang on the walls. In them he seems fully in the moment, content and without a care. On one wall, a framed tribute hangs. The letterhead is from the Atheneum Institute at 100A Garpar Road, where Srikrishna had attended school, dated 21 November 1942.

While I stayed in the house and studied therapeutic yoga, I would see the small frame above the bedroom door when I entered. I wonder how long it has been there, perhaps seventy-five years. The enclosed print, with the title, 'In Memory of late Srikrishna Ghosh', has a round, black and white school photo of Srikrishna. Then below, a tribute to his life reads:

Death's blazing finger touched you, and you slept; Sudden and irreparable our loss; How deeply we regret! A dense gloom has spread over the school and all – Boys go about with sad and noiseless football.

Your urbanity, kindliness, refinement and sweet temper. Good breeding, serenity, truthfulness and your culture – All these had endeared you to everyone you met; Your sweet memory! Ah! one will never forget; As a student in the school, you were second to none; A boy of your caliber is a pride of an institution.

Well-built frame and herculean strength you possessed – Marvelous were the feats, a boy of thirteen displayed. Worthy son of Bishnu Ghosh! Flower of Bengal! How soon you left us in response to Heaven's call!

Yogananda losing his temple paled in comparison to the loss Bishnu suffered, but both would have to find a new way forward in their lives after the losses of 1942. The death of Srikrishna was the end of Bishnu's future as he saw it, and with what was happening all around him in Calcutta during the forties, it was difficult for him to imagine a new beginning.

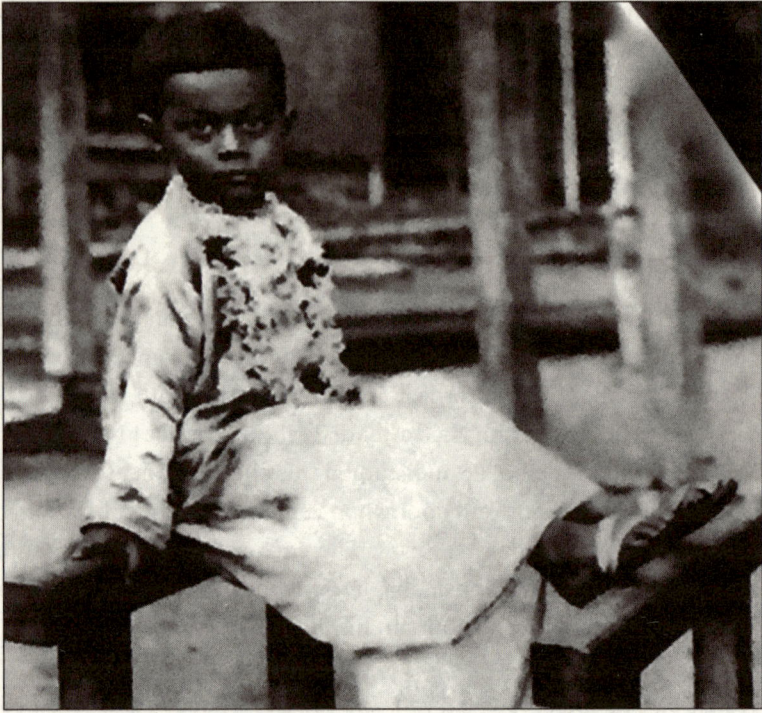

Srikrishna Ghosh, circa 1942.
Courtesy of Ghosh's Yoga College.

60

CALCUTTA'S CLOUD OF WAR

During the hot summer months, monsoons come barrelling into Calcutta
from the Bay of Bengal. 'Clouds heap upon clouds, and it darkens,' wrote
Rabindranath Tagore. Heavy rain, followed by a period of sunshine, and then, it
rains, seemingly non-stop, and everywhere becomes flooded.

No part of life in Calcutta was left untouched by the forties – everything changed. The Bengali film director Ritwik Ghatak, who came of age at that time, captured the sentiment of the changing turmoil that shocked the city. 'Life was placid in 1940 and '41,' he recalled, then 'suddenly, during '44 and '45, a series of events took place … things changed so fast.'[1]

First, war approached.

Back in Encinitas, CA, prior to the collapse of Yogananda's ashram, naval authorities persuaded his organization to 'cover the glinting, gold domes with white cloth after the U.S. entered World War II'. Visible from the Pacific, 'the domes were thought to be a potential enemy target'.[2]

Yogananda began to publish political statements in his magazine that were decidedly pacifist. In one, titled 'Right Patriotism', he warned against 'politicians being blinded by their patriotism' and that the true use of patriotism was only 'to protect your country'. Instead, he wished that 'people follow the laws laid down by Christ: "Love thy neighbour."' To do otherwise, he wrote, would bring 'an avalanche of miseries upon the nations of the earth'.[3] In the 'Book Reviews', Yogananda promoted books by Pearl Buck (*American Unity* and *Asia*) and Wendell Willkie (*One World*), advocating for 'spiritual statesman'.[4]

In the spring of 1940, as Buddha left Calcutta for the Himalayas, the signs of a world war were becoming imminent. When Paris fell to the German invasion, Rabindranath Tagore wrote a letter from Bengal which was published in the

New York Times on 16 June 1940. It both summed up India's minor role, and the plea for America to stem 'the tide of evil' that had arisen to menace 'the permanence of civilization'.[5]

Then, in September of 1940, the British seized the German Consulate in Calcutta, ensuring that India would play a role against the axis. By the time Buddha returned from the Himalayas, the war had officially reached Calcutta. Imagine the shock of coming down from Kailash and Lake Manasarovar, the heights of the earth pulsing with divine spiritual vibration, to the depths of fear in the eyes of the people, and the ignorant froth of international warmongering drifting through the air of Calcutta. He must have thought about turning back and leaving Calcutta for good ... that thought would be saved for later.

The death of Tagore, an icon of Indian and Bengali culture, in August 1941 was the end of an era, the end of the Bengal Renaissance. At first, the European war seemed a long way off. However, once Japan shocked the world by bombing Pearl Harbor in December 1941, matters quickly changed. In short succession, the Japanese overtook the European possessions of Malaysia and the colonial fortress city of Singapore. Then, after less than a month of bombing Rangoon, Burma was also taken by the Japanese.

By the early months of 1942, the world war crept closer to Calcutta, and it seemed nearly inevitable that it would come into the city. Panic took over. The Japanese had their sights on securing the Bay of Bengal and cutting off Calcutta's port from use by British forces. It was estimated that if Calcutta was taken, 70 per cent of India's war capability would be gone.

Suddenly, the second city of the colonial era found itself on the front line, facing a seemingly unstoppable force.[6]

The war with Japan in the early forties exposed deep fissures in Calcutta too. 'It will be to India's lasting shame and disgrace if she stabs England in the back when she is so sorely pressed,' said Gandhi.[7] Subhash Chandra Bose was part of the movement that believed that with the war, the ideal time had come to snatch Indian independence away from colonial Great Britain.[8] Yogananda backed the non-violent campaigns that Gandhi led but, overall, was not public about his political leanings within India.[9]

In the spring of 1942, many believed the Japanese would attack India when the monsoon ended – that when the hot, humid, water-clogged delta lands began to dry, the Japanese would invade India with warships and planes heading into the Bay of Bengal. But before the monsoon ended, the US had arrived in defence, swamping Calcutta with British and American troops.

Americans brought a different lifestyle with them to Calcutta, especially compared to the traditional European aristocrats that Bengalis were used to seeing. The Americans had a different attitude towards Indians and their culture. 'Many Calcuttans were surprised and even shocked and offended by their disregard for age-old colonial and Indian traditions. Others found them refreshingly efficient and modern, and lapped up everything they brought with them, from their money and materials which swamped the city, to their Magazines, Movies, Swing & Jazz.'[10] The April arrival of thousands of US troops brought military operations to the outskirts of Calcutta, places such as Dum Dum to the north, and Barrackpore and Alipore to the south.

The Americans were given strict guidelines of travel in Calcutta, with all of north Calcutta in the 'out-of-bounds area'.[11] Bishnu sought out interaction with Americans. Prior to the death of Srikrishna, he 'trained the American air-force men in jiu-jitsu at the Dumdum airport'.[12]

After initial successes, the Japanese were pushed back by Allied forces.[13] Calcutta was just within the range of Japanese bomber planes, who targeted the operations of the port, but the threat of invasion receded. The war, as far as India, Bengal and especially Calcutta were concerned, would not become a center of the conflict, as it was winding down to completion.

The first couple of years in the decade belied the storm. Calcutta was spared from the battlefield of the world war, but the tumultuous decade was just beginning.

61

HUNGRY BENGAL

The tragic Bengal famine of 1943 played out on the streets of Calcutta. With Bhagabati passing away in 1942, all of his savings, which were considerable, were handed down to his sons and their households. While there was no indication that the famine affected the Ghosh family directly, it was a pivotal moment for Calcutta. Specifically, it impacted Buddha's student Ian Stephens,

In the May of 1942, four years after he had begun training under Buddha, Ian Stephens saw the results of his daily yoga asana practice. Stephens, while undergoing a routine medical test, was asked to blow 'to one's full lung-power' to raise a mercury-column in a tube. 'Do that again!' the doctor exclaimed. Stephens had 'exceptional lung-expansion'. He had developed this through his daily practice of *nauli* and 'breath-holding'. Topping the 'mercury-column height' mimicked the 'exhale totally before you start' nauli. He found the 'breathholding feats' enjoyable, and since 'the better you get at it the longer your breath-holdings last', they had a lasting impact on him physically and mentally.

Stephens would write years later that it was only through his daily practice of yoga that the strain of covering the 1940s events in Calcutta was manageable. 'Throughout these stressful times, due perhaps in the main to Hatha yoga, I kept consistently almost disgustingly fit. So life remained a continuous rush and reflective pauses didn't come in,' he wrote.[1] From 1941 to 1946, 'in strenuous times' it was 'my addiction to yoga exercises' which preserved the 'editor from the loony-bin'.[2]

The strain of the war had increased demand and reduced the supply of food. Then a cyclone occurred in 1942, which forced prices of rice out of reach for many of the poor. Further drought made the situation even more untenable, causing much hoarding until the lack of food peaked and a famine ensued throughout Bengal. There had also been deliberate decisions made by British authorities to route food destined for Bengal to other places. In 'Famine in India', Yogananda's publication faulted the government, writing that the 'cessation of imports of rice from Burma' and the exportation of 'Indian wheat to the armies' fighting the Second World War left 'landless peasants' and millions of Bengali's without food.[3]

Most Bengalis then and even many today, live with little savings and subsist on a seasonal, or even day-to-day, basis. They were disproportionately affected by the food shortage. Eugenie Fraser, wife of a jute mill owner, reflected about Calcutta in 1943, writing, 'The whole of Bengal was in the grip of a devastating famine.' People from the villages rushed to Calcutta only to find the same shortage prevailing there as well. In Calcutta, the pavements and stations became crowded with masses of dejected people, sitting, lying, begging for food, but hopelessly resigned to their fate of starving to death.[4]

Stephens focused on leading an international awareness campaign and was later acclaimed for his efforts. On 20 June 1943, his paper's editorial warned that Calcutta was lacking an arrangement for food rationing. Calcutta, at the time, was 'full of troops from all the nations' as it was geographically strategic. Yet, its 'food-shortage and rocketing prices for essentials' required that 'drastic action' had become imperative and should happen without delay.[5] And yet, even with awareness growing, the famine continued. Yogananda began calling for members to send funds, arranging 'to send proceeds' to the famine-stricken in Calcutta.

Amidst the backdrop of the World War, the Bengal famine struggled to capture the attention of the world powers. Over two million people died a slow death of hunger in Bengal. In Calcutta, without resorting to violence, the poor and hungry 'died without ransacking a single grocery, restaurant or sweetmeat shop,' recalled Ashis Nandy, then a Calcutta schoolboy. Harry Tweedale of the BBC provided context:

Famine on such a scale is not common. When something comparable happens today, money, relief foods and drugs are poured in – not always very efficiently or effectively. I am afraid that not much help came to Calcutta and the rest of Bengal. The world was fighting a war and killing was more important than saving life.[6]

In August 1943, still with no supplies incoming, further 'famine was caused by speculators buying up all the rice and hoarding it'.[7] A month later the *Statesman* illustrated 'the plight of a Province once regarded as India's foremost' by publishing 'terrible photographs' to force the famine into the discussion. Hopefully this would 'alter opinion' among 'readers in Northern India', who were still 'largely ignorant of Bengal's state'.[8] The famine continued into the next month, with the city's daily death rate doubling and the famine spreading throughout Bengal.[9]

Yogananda wrote again about the shortages, through *East-West* magazine, in 'The American Famine Mission to India'. The column mentioned that 'thousands are migrating. They are moving towards the areas which have more food.' This usually meant Calcutta.[10] A previous issue of the magazine echoed the remarks of Eleanor Roosevelt, who 'stressed the need for funds in her column', and wrote of the American men 'fighting in India today' who 'will come home and tell us of the people there and their difficulties'.[11]

By the November of 1943, outside help reached Bengal and food rationing had finally begun in Calcutta, but the famine continued into 1944. After countless avoidable deaths, stored food began to reach the hungry and the famine lessened, but even the living were psychologically impacted. The famine left a deep and hardened face on humanity in Bengal.

62

MANDIR RENEWAL

The season of failure is the best time for sowing the seeds of success.
– Yogananda

When the Golden Lotus Temple was constructed, the December 1937 issue of Yogananda's magazine compared it to the Taj Mahal and the Golden Temple of the Sikhs in India. During the dedication of the temple at 11 a.m. on 2 January 1938, Yogananda explained that the Lotus was 'one of the most important symbols of spirituality in India, as its unfolding petals signify the expansion of the soul, and the growth of its pure beauty from the mud of its origin is a beautiful spiritual promise'.[1] Mud had become the undoing of the Golden Lotus Temple, four years later.

When the 'first church of all religions' slid off the 'hilltop by-the-sea' and into the ocean in June 1942, there was only a discreet note on the calamity in the next issue of Yogananda's magazine. On the inside cover, an article written by Yogananda was titled 'The Cosmic Motion Pictures'. It portrayed a firsthand account of being 'chosen to play both tragic and comic parts' in 'the talking pictures' to 'keep all of our senses and thoughts deluded and entertained'. The 'Magic Operator' played 'the cosmic pictures' on 'the screen of our consciousness' through the senses, resulting in a 'daily-changing drama' of a 'vast dream-vitaphone presentation'.

Yogananda appealed to the divine and magic operator, 'give me a few days of respite from my task now and then' to retire to introspection 'and behold with a laughing heart' the tragedies or comedies being enacted. Yogananda ended with one more request:

Teach me to look upon the tragedy-pictures of my own life with a thrilling, interested attitude, so that, at the end of each terribly sad picture, I may exclaim: 'Ah, that was a good picture, full of thrills and life. I am pleased to have seen it, for I have learned much from it.'[2]

That the tragedy was viewed through the metaphor of a cinematic experience, complete with a Great Oz like operator behind the scenes, was a symbolic feature from the period. On the back cover of the same issue was an announcement of the 'second church of all religions', located in Hollywood, CA – home to where the stars played their roles in the movies and society. This was his way forward.

Swami Kriyananda, an American who became a disciple of Yogananda in the late forties, called the collapse of the Golden Lotus Temple 'a major tragedy' in Yogananda's life.[3] Its slide into the ocean was broadcast throughout the newswires in such a publicized way that many who learned of the temple came to the conclusion that Yogananda and his organization were finished. The popular perception took Yogananda and his organization by surprise and 'forced him once more to become outwardly active'.[4] In response, he took to publicizing their resilience. In August, Yogananda made an announcement that a new edifice would be rebuilt at the Encinitas location, right next to Highway 101.[5]

It wasn't that easy; for a time, the Encinitas ashram was plagued with conflict. In the days following its collapse to the sea, mementos of lumber, concrete, plaster and tiles were taken away by those who made the surfside beach excursion. Plans were made to rebuild the temple in the same location, further back from the cliff, but the hermitage found itself embroiled in other matters.

Surfers in the area started to carve paths across the property, along the fragile bluff, as 'they took shortcuts down to the surf'. The Self-Realization Fellowship (SRF) attempted to cordon off the property and bulldozed the slopes 'in an effort to stabilize them with landscaping'. The non-approved action put them in hot water with the city of Encinitas. Things came to a head that following summer in 1943, when a forty-five-year-old man who was climbing down the cliff fell fifty feet to his death on the rocks below, the site where the Golden Lotus Temple had 'toppled and crashed'.[6]

Soon after, government regulators charged SRF with 'gross violations of state laws' in 'causing a major bluff collapse and blocking access to the beach'.[7] A compromise was finally reached when 'the fellowship gave a public easement along its bluffs to improve access to the popular surf spot' and abandoned immediate plans to rebuild the temple on the bluff.[8]

Yogananda claimed that Satan had played a role in the catastrophe and perceived it as a royal battle playing out. If Satan took away a one-of-a-kind prized temple, then God, through him, would build more. He had removed the Golden Lotus figurines from the temple and would reuse them. Yogananda took the event for a sign that he should expand his worldwide hermitages.[9]

Two locations were focused on immediately. The SRF temple in Hollywood was opened on 30 August 1942.[10] The San Diego site was acquired in January 1943, with the announcement:

SRF intends to make this place the future site for a centrally located Golden Lotus Temple to be created after the war, to take the place of the one in Encinitas.[11]

In June 1943, on the first anniversary of the temple's collapse, Yogananda wrote a column titled 'One Year Later', which announced that the two new temples had been built. One in San Diego, another in Hollywood.[12] But it was still just the beginning, with new temples, ashrams and centres being announced in each successive issue in the years to come.

One year after the Golden Lotus Temple fell into the ocean, Yogananda was told in an interview, 'What a pity you lost your Golden Lotus Temple in Encinitas!'

Yogananda replied firmly, 'It was the best thing that ever happened to me!'[13]

63

YOGA FAMILY RENEWAL

Do not get attached to the happening surface,
you will only stay afloat, flapping around;
the deep, silent and peaceful depth will never come near unless
you seek and go deep down.[1]

– Bishnu Ghosh

The Bengali poems of Bishnu Ghosh, most of which were composed during the mid-forties, were not published until many years after Bishnu's death, by his son Bishwanath. The above poem was written with an orientation towards *sadhana*, the means of accomplishing something in life. Most of the poems, though, dealt with the death of his son Srikrishna and his attempt to find a way through that tragedy, to go on living with purpose.

In the first poem, titled 'Offering', Bishnu wrote that though his child was 'gone forever', he would collect 'your [Srikrishna's] pearls of wisdom' and 'put them in verse content for all to read and benefit'. This offering was so Bishnu could be a vehicle for his son's wisdom, with the intent that it carry on. In another poem, titled 'Promise', Bishnu wrote, 'I weave a web of longing that is a lie, to heal my silly yearning.' He could not stop Srikrishna who 'paid heed to the call from above' but 'now I promise to persevere the path of strength severe'. This, ultimately, was the path forward for Bishnu.

A similar message from Bishnu's poems in Bengali is inscribed in marble, under the statue of Bishnu placed on Upper Circular Road. Translated to English, it reads:

Man is not born for leisure
He has tremendous responsibility on his head
I have no complaints if I get only grief
I shall go wherever duty takes me

Bishnu turned his efforts towards his gymnasium and students with renewed commitment as a tribute to his lost son. It was around this time that Bishnu joined the Bratachari movement, which emphasized physical development for both boys and girls.[2] Within the next few years, a trio of young students arrived, around whom Bishnu would shape his life for the next fifteen years. The first two were Gouri Shankar Mukerji and Monotosh Roy.

In 1944, a nineteen-year-old Bengali named Gouri Shankar Mukerji entered Bishnu's life. Gouri 'was like a son to Bishnu'.[3] He had first met Bishnu prior to the calamity and death of Srikrishna in 1942. Gouri had bought a ticket to a Gemini circus show, which Bishnu conducted in north Calcutta. Bishnu noticed Gouri because of his keen sense for finding youth who were ready to bloom, and also because 'he looked similar to his own son'. Gouri wasn't interested in taking up physical culture training at that moment, but the invitation stuck in his mind.[4]

While studying for his exam at Scottish Church College, he became ill with asthma and decided to visit Bishnu. Gouri found the gymnasium was closed, learned the story of Srikrishna's death and sought out Bishnu to pay his regards. Bishnu initially declined but listened, and could not resist Gouri, whose resemblance to his lost son opened his heart. Shortly thereafter, Bishnu took Gouri under his wing. When Bishnu reopened the gymnasium, he accepted Gouri Shankar Mukerji as his first student. Many others followed, and returned, but none would have greater impact and fame than Monotosh Roy.

Monotosh Roy was born in 1926, and started under Bishnu's tutelage in 1945, several years after Bishnu saw him working out.[5] 'There was no looking back' for Monotosh. He was 'interested in bodybuilding from his childhood' and 'had a natural body for the purpose. And though he practised on his own, his systematic way of doing bodybuilding started with Bishnu Ghosh. There he learned the proper way of building his body and bringing it to shape.'[6] Monotosh, like a lot of Bishnu's students, was poor, and survived on whatever food his family could find. At that time, the gymnasium was 'open and free'. It was 'a very simple gym' and 'the instruments were all manual'. It was 'in the open and everyone could see inside the gym'. Afterwards, Bishnu fed his students. He brought in a few cows to live under a nearby shed on the property, 'so his students could drink milk' after they worked out.[7]

Years later, Monotosh recalled what his teacher had told him: 'Monotosh, believe in your work and yourself – then you will never make a mistake – you will never lose. Do something new every day. Never stop. The day you stop, the devil will make home in your heart.' From the beginning, Monotosh had the 'desire to know the fundamentals of muscle movements' and wondered whether Bishnu would become his teacher, but he could 'not gather the courage to ask him the question' aloud. Bishnu explained 'the fundamental creation of our muscle movements and gestures' in a rhythmic manner. Monotosh recalled:

It was 1945 and 10th or 11th of August when I realized my heart's desire had somehow tuned in with Bishtuda's heart. It was past 10 in the night. On the way back home I again stopped by at Bishtuda's place, it was close by and I had been there in the evening doing my regular exercise. He just kept looking at me for some time and then just said, 'Sit, we have work to do.'

There was no one else in the room, only Bishnu and Monotosh, who understood he was being 'initiated into the secrets of muscle movement fundamentals!' He wrote, 'I sat there mute, listening without batting my eyelids. Shivers ran down my spine and I got lost in his powerful lecture on the subject.' Bishnu's talk with Monotosh, which made him realize his potential, was highly motivational.

You are a hard nut to crack, you are the ripple in the beautiful melody, you are the statue made by the great sculptor, you revolve, turn, overturn mental freedom. You are the silent leader of yesteryears. You are the deathless warrior on the great battlefield ... You are a thinker, you are an artist. You are the prisoner, you break rules and become free. You are Rahu, devour the sun with your arms ... you are the traveller in life's battlefield blowing the conch-shell, you are the pilot, you are the worshiper of every changing new discovery of all ages.[8]

After just one year of training under Bishnu and his top assistant, Tapas Bhattacharya, Monotosh 'won the title of Mr India for best physique' during a competition in Nagpur in 1946.[9] The accomplishment brought a wave of excitement to Ghosh's gymnasium, as fellow bodybuilders sought out Bishnu's teaching.

Also in 1945, a second son was born to Ashalata and Bishnu. He was named Bishwanath. In the same year Ava Rani gave birth to a second son, Arun. Following the death of Srikrishna, the three boys, especially Ashok, were heavily doted on and pampered by the women.

Buddha's children were also great looking. Ashok and Arun, with clear blue eyes 'and the fair skin' were 'too handsome'! 'If and when Ashok sat on the floor, someone would immediately make him sit on a silk mat.'[10] Following the trio of boys, two girls were born: Karuna Ghosh and, a year later, Rooma Bose.

Nearly a decade earlier, in 1938, Buddha had left Calcutta for the world tour, still naive and immature in some ways. On tour, he had gained confidence and self-worth by demonstrating before hundreds of people; he gained a more worldly outlook. He had found a deeper family connection in London, a meaningful spiritual connection with Yogananda, and now, a family in Calcutta. He never showed any resentment for being obliged in marriage to Ava Rani. Later on, Buddha would tell the story of how when he was in America, being hosted by Yogananda, people 'started telling him to get married'.

Buddha replied, 'If I get married, I wish the girl to come from a yogi family.'

They responded, 'What? How can a *sannyasi* have a daughter? They can have no family.'

Buddha said, 'I didn't mean it that way; I meant she must come from a *sannyasi* family.' In marrying Ava Rani, a niece of Yogananda, he felt he had fulfilled those remarks.[11] Ava Rani too, despite the difference in age, 'was a woman who stood by her man. She was the firm and steady backbone that Buddha leaned on without even being aware of it.'[12]

Buddha also gained employment during this time. He signed on with the Calcutta Corporation, which held a variety of subsidiaries. One of them was named American Indian Co., which soon involved Buddha in the international trade of porcelain products. After the war, Buddha's position as a 'merchant' provided him the opportunity to travel abroad. He flew to London, and while there, visited his mother in Brighton along the coast, before returning to Calcutta. The business planned to expand, with its eyes set on America. This held the promise that Buddha would soon be able to travel abroad again, teach Americans yoga and visit Yogananda; the future was bright.

A large field connected the backyards of the Ghosh residences at 4/2 Rammohan Roy Road and 4 Garpar Road, which sat on opposite sides of the same block. Children's voices were heard while they played; new students came in and out of Bishnu's gym; and soon, Independence arrived for India. But alongside the hopeful future, the communal division of Calcutta loomed over the city. The Ghosh family, Bishnu's students and the Garpar area neighbourhood, were in the middle of the conflict.

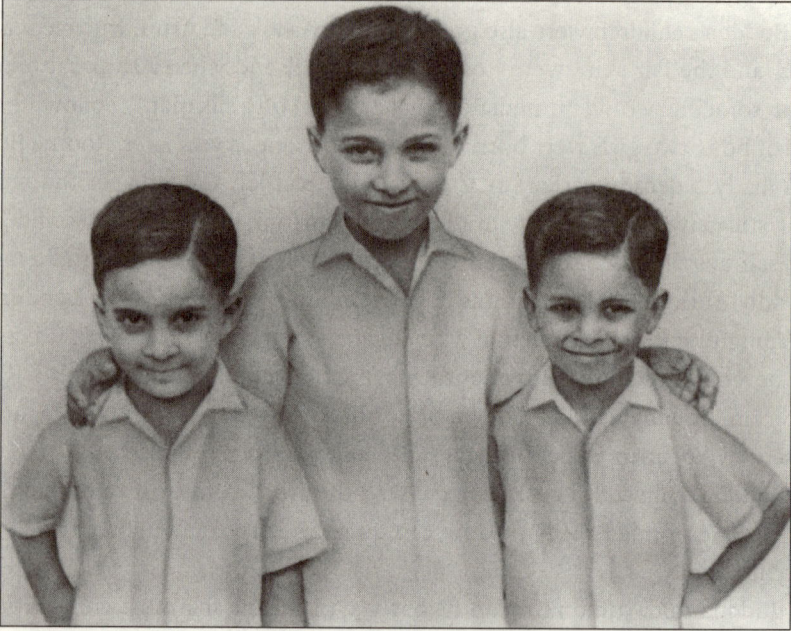

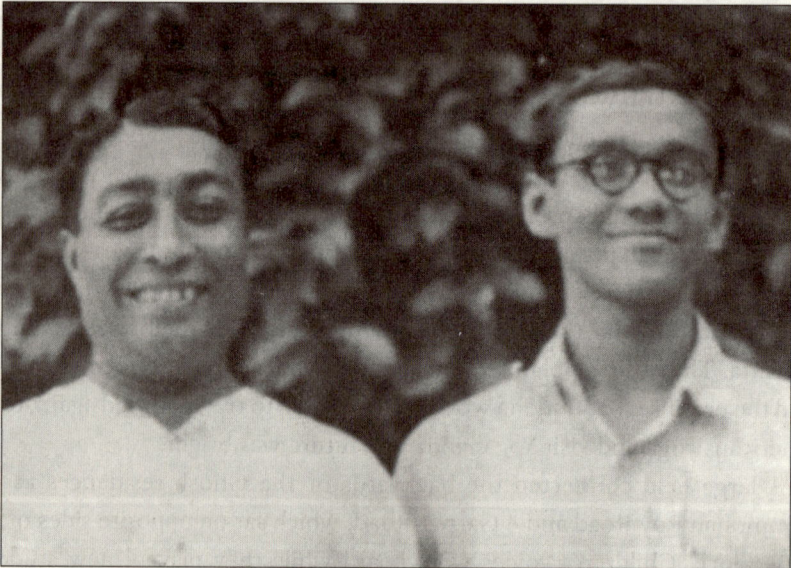

Top: (left to right) Arun Bose, Ashok Bose, Bishwanath Ghosh (Circa 1948).
Bottom: Bishnu Ghosh (left) and Gouri Shankar Mukerji (Circa 1950).
Courtesy of Ghosh's Yoga College.

64

GARPAR PARA

We were born in a deceived age. The days of our childhood
and adolescence saw the full flowering of Bengal. Tagore,
with his overpowering genius, at the peak of his literary career;
the renewed vigour of Bengali literature in the works of the 'Kallol'
group of young writers; the widespread national movement in schools and
colleges, among the youth of Bengal; the villages of Bengal, with their folktales,
folk songs and festivals, brimming over with the hope of a new life.
Just then came the war; came famine.[1]
– Ritwik Ghatak

The threat of the Second World War did not materialize, even though it
struck fear into the city. Calcuttans were evacuated, but the bombing,
mostly in north Calcutta near the river port of Baghbazar, was sporadic and
not severe. Then the Bengal famines arrived, and it brought about a hard streak
among the masses. Millions of hungry farmers deserted their villages and left for
Calcutta. Instead of finding food they found *bustis*, with slum-dwelling masses.
Then came fighting, neighbour against neighbour – 'The Calcutta Killings'.

The communal riots of Calcutta are a controversial and difficult topic to
traverse.[2] And unlike the previous city-wide calamities, the Ghosh and Bose
families were directly affected and involved in the communal riots. Long before
the riots in the 1940s, the Hindus and Muslims were not without their tensions
and previous clashes.

Bishnu remarked about an incident in 1926. While he was a student in Hindu
School, his friend 'Jatin was killed in Mechua Bazar in a firing by the *gurkha*
police'. Bishnu and Jatin 'had studied together' at the Boys School in Ranchi
and shared a passion for neighbourhood akhara practice. After his friend was

killed in the Muslim-dominated streets through which he passed for school, Bishnu wrote of taking 'a sword in a scabbard and a *bhojali* tucked inside my *dhoti* under my *kurta*' for his own protection. Once, school officials thought Bishnu had hidden a stolen book. When confronted, Bishnu stripped to show his armament and said:

> 'I hope now you believe it is not a book.' The head guard was stupefied and then uttered, 'My God you are a dangerous boy.' I said, 'This is nothing, now see this,' and took out the sword from the scabbard and flashed it around, then swiftly put it back inside. Then I told him, 'I am not a dangerous boy, these are for my self protection. I am a member of the seven hundred strong Voluntary Servicemen.'[3]

In 1947, Muslims were a slight majority in Bengal (which included what is now Bangladesh), but a minority in Calcutta. The 1941 Calcutta census records 73 per cent of the population as Hindu and 23 per cent Muslim. There were some who stressed unity.[4] The slogan of '*Ek Ho!*' (We Are One) could be heard during street marches in Calcutta.[5] However, in the lead-up to Independence, Hindu public opinion was also being mobilized and 'revisionary history' tended to reconstruct 'nationalism' from what had always been a 'scrambled' situation.[6] Calcutta Hindu elites, since the 1860s, had been cultivating a nationalist consciousness.[7] Jugal Kishore Birla, an active funding source for Bishnu Ghosh, financed 'training and physical culture for the Hindus'.[8] The gymnasiums would be a focal point for the communal riots.

As 1947 and Independence neared, the formative stages of an Indian government began. Muslim political leaders resisted being a minority, which led to a breakdown in negotiations.[9] An event called Direct Action Day was mobilized by Muslims throughout India on 16 August 1946.[10] It was promoted publicly to as a peaceful demonstration but quickly turned violent. The Muslims wanted to retain Calcutta within a new partitioned state, while Hindus felt that if Bengal was not to remain whole, Calcutta should stay within India. Events spiraled out of control and there was little effort to quell the killings.[11]

> The 'suddenness' that day was the beginning of what afterward was called 'the week of long knives' and the 'great Calcutta killings'. It was a long week of mass murders and civilian on civilian attacks. India was on the verge of Independence, and this was a fight 'over who was to be master

over Calcutta'. Would Calcutta become 'the capital of a Muslim Bengal' and a part of Bangladesh, or remain within the Hindu-dominated India?[12]

The outbreak of communal violence between Hindus and Muslims plunged the city into despair and horror. 'Weapons of gunnery were short to come by', and fighting with *lathis* (sticks), spears and knives, even hand to hand combat, ensued. 'The iron rods used in reinforced concrete building works were all stolen and sharpened at both ends ... there were brick bat fights all over North Calcutta ... there were fights in every street and alley from Sealdah to Shyambazar. There were corpses all over North Calcutta, they were in the river, canals, side lanes, in fact, everywhere.' [13]

Margaret Bourke-White, journalist and travel writer, covered the August 1946 incident in Calcutta.[14] On the first day, Muslims rioted, looting shops, stoning and setting fire to Calcutta's British district. They then went after Hindus with knives and clubs in north Calcutta. 'Before the disastrous "Direct Action Day" was over, blood soaked the melting asphalt of sweltering Calcutta's streets.' Some three to five thousand people were dead.[15] After the initial day of Muslim attacks, Hindus organized and began to counter-attack, retaliating by setting mosques afire and burning Muslim slums.[16]

It was a battle for territory, and the murders of innocent people described most of the casualties.[17] Mother Teresa, then a teacher in a city school, remembered, 'We were not supposed to go out into the streets, but I went anyway. Then I saw the bodies on the streets, stabbed, beaten, lying there in strange positions in their dried blood.'[18]

Ten days after the killings began, the toll of the dead was between six and ten thousand, and 'the streets were full of bodies'. Corpses lay rotting in the streets or were 'crammed down the manholes to block the drains'.[19] Police were unable to stop the fighting. One weary police officer said at the time, 'all we can do is move the bodies to one side of the street'.[20]

At first, the outbreaks were reported as 'spontaneous and inexplicable', but as the *Statesman* explained, 'both sides in the confrontation came well-prepared for it'. Four days after the killing began, the *Statesman* further reported:

This is not a riot. It needs a word from medieval history, a fury. Yet 'fury' sounds spontaneous and there must have been some deliberation and organization to set this fury on its way. The horde who ran about battering and killing with 8 ft *lathis* may have found them lying about or bought them out of their own pockets, but that is hard to believe.[21]

The riots were well-organized from the start on both sides.[22] During the previous generation, Indian clubs in north Calcutta had been formed for various purposes, ranging from health, typified by Ghosh's gymnasium, to nationalist positioning against the British. Ghosh's College of Physical Education, with its gymnasium being a focal point in the neighbourhood for young men, was sandwiched between Muslim communities.

'The riots turned the club into a new kind of formation.' Strongmen were the protectors.[23] Bishnu 'and another famous person called Pulin Behari Das, a famous legend with the *lathi*, in the same area fought back the attackers and protected everybody'. Bishnu, 'along with Nilmoni Das, Keshub Sengupta, Bhupesh Karmakar – they all resisted the Muslim attack'.[24]

The Ghosh family *para* (neighbourhood locality) was also stricken by the communal conflict. Sananda, the middle brother between Yogananda and Bishnu, had three sons. The first died in infancy; the second, Harekrishna, lived a long life into the 2000s at 4 Garpar Road, meeting many pilgrimage travellers to Yogananda's home. Sananda's third son, Shyamsundar, 'at the age of twenty-four, was fatally wounded by a stray bullet during an uprising in Calcutta in December 1946'.[25] One can only imagine the state of Bishnu's mind, after losing his own son, to then see his brother also lose a son.

Aside from the usual remarks about Bishnu, the writer of a short Bengali biography added something quite different. 'Bishnu was behind bars for a brief period during the reign of Bidhan Chandra Roy as the Chief Minister of West Bengal.' The police station of Calcutta had no record of this in their database. The only thing indicated was that Bishnu was arrested, for 'joining campaigns of disruption'.[26] Interviewees were not shy to defend him: 'Bishnu would stand up to fight when needed,' a student of his recalled. 'This was his courage.'[27] Multiple accounts described his participation in glowing terms.[28]

A police officer, Shakur Al Hosain, admitted that if they had the forces, the police 'would have placed a picket at the crossing of the Garpar Road and Bipradas Street', to divide the Hindus from the Muslims living in Raja Bazar.[29] It was at this spot, one interview revealed, where Bishnu, his weapon in hand, 'stood at the crossroad and shouted, "If you come over here, I'll kill you all." Nobody came against him.'[30]

The reprisals 'were savage'. The members of the Hindu neighbourhoods 'became the protectors of their community and some of them openly and proudly turned into killers'. Whether 'savages' or 'heroes' depended on the perspective.[31] In the aftermath of the riots, Hindus solidified 'physical control of the city', ensuring that Calcutta, upon Independence, would be the capital of 'a separate Hindu state in West Bengal'.[32]

Until the late thirties, Calcutta enjoyed the status of the 'Second City', after London. The yogic writer, Francis Yeats-Brown, visited Calcutta again in 1937 and remarked that, as a whole, the 'great city, with its solid, comfortable air, is reminiscent of those eighteenth-century days' of Englishmen. Then he added, 'Those times have ended, never to return, but it is still the richest and most European city in the East.'[33]

A decade later, Bengal was torn apart by communal fighting, upended by a shortage of food, unemployment and a large flow of refugees in the wake of the creation of East Pakistan. The 'Twilight of Bengal' had arrived.[34] Calcutta stayed with India as part of West Bengal, but the state lost a large part of its cultural and rural economic bases with the division of Bengal. What had happened to Calcutta and Bengal during the forties shocked its inhabitants.

After Independence, with the British leaving, a Bengali 'Boom-town' developed in central Calcutta, and then a new decade began. The future looked brighter, certainly for Bishnu.

FORGOTTEN YOGI, 18 JUNE 1947

Tragedy was all around Buddha Bose in the 1940s,
but it was as if he skimmed through it all.
He was on the periphery, not at the centre, until this point.

When Buddha and Bishnu brought their style of Hatha yoga asana practice to the US in the late thirties, Buddha, being half-British, was embraced entirely by Yogananda and his disciples. Buddha's ability to relate to the Western audience, and as an accomplished physical culturist and a master in yogasana, pranayama and Kriya meditation, he found an immense number of opportunities. He was poised to become the iconic yogi to bridge the East and West, through a modern therapeutic-based asana yoga practice.

On 18 June 1947, Buddha Bose boarded the *Clipper Eclipse* in Calcutta, on Pan Am Flight 121, bound for New York. In the passenger manifest, his occupation was listed as 'businessman'. The previous year, Buddha had 'stopped taking part in any shows', as the 'concentrated practice of yoga-*bayam* helped to change his mind'.[1] He had become more spiritually focused and was orienting his teaching towards those he would encounter abroad. The plane stopped in Karachi to refuel; the next leg of the flight was to Istanbul, then London, before the scheduled arrival in New York.

Flying in the forties was somewhat precarious, but Pan American boasted its 'perfect safety record in 1946' as 'proof that flying is safe'. The same year, Pan Am completed a '13-day circumnavigation of the globe', another 'first' for 'the pioneer of trans-ocean air travel'.[2] However, the *Constellation*, their newly built four-engine fleet of 'gigantic air liners' for commercial flights, had 'a series of conflagrations in the air' in 1947.

That March, President Truman had initiated a board of inquiry on air safety. The safety bureau was quoted, 'Should any of these planes burn up and kill its occupants, our only alternative will be to ask for a Congressional investigation.' On the very same day that Flight 121 left Karachi with Buddha aboard, a separate Pan Am Pennsylvania-bound flight in America was forced to land when 'one of its four engines caught fire'.[3]

Buddha's flight from Karachi to Istanbul was overnight. Five hours after take-off, trouble developed in the number one engine due to failure of its cylinders, forcing a shut-down. Company radio in Karachi advised the pilots to land in Habbaniya, Iraq. Flight 121, however, affirmed its intention to continue, and added that if it were unable to reach Istanbul, a landing would be made at Damascus, Syria.[4]

The decision to continue on after the first engine issue was not outside of normal operations. An emergency landing in Iraq would mean days lost, waiting for new cylinder-replacement parts. Most of the pilots had been aviators during the Second World War, and were not shaken by a single engine's loss. Thirty minutes later, the 'fasten seat belt–no smoking' sign came on in the passenger cabin.

Suddenly, 'the entire cabin became illuminated'. The crew had 'no warning at all' of the impending engine trouble; engine number two had also overheated and caught fire. The fire spread to the wing and shortly afterwards, the number one engine separated from the plane. This ruptured the gasoline line and fed the fire. Passengers were 'awakened by flames whipping past the port windows'.

The plane, 170 miles from Iraq, with still 290 miles to Damascus was unable to maintain altitude. The pilot would attempt a forced landing in the Syrian desert. 'Everybody sat still, waited, each thinking his own thoughts.'[5]

There was no one in the seat next to Buddha. Across the aisle were two fellow Calcuttans, with whom he conversed softly as the plane descended. In the night sky, he watched the fire through the window and assumed his life was about to end. As he looked out the window he 'had a vision of his wife in a widow's garb'.

Then he noticed the seat beside him was no longer empty. 'When the plane was about to crash I saw a saintly person next to me. It was the same person I had seen at Kailas Manasarovar.' Kathia Baba, 'who wore little except for the wool garment across his waist', was there sitting next to him. He 'could see this person sitting next to him and felt his cold touch. Very cold. As if coming straight from Kailas.' He could feel the touch. He heard the words of Babaji, 'You are thinking of wife?'[6]

Rapidly descending from 18,500 feet, the plane was on fire. A crash was coming. A stewardess, Jane Bray, recalled, 'We hit hard on the belly with an awful jar which would not stop. We slid across the sand. The plane swung hard around to the left and split in two. Flames poured in and the heat became terrific.'[7]

The Pan Am plane 'plowed into the flat Syrian soil along the Euphrates river' just after midnight.[8] The impact killed the crew in the cockpit and ripped the sides of the fuselage away from the plane. The airplane split in two. A survivor from Calcutta, Dr Rafiden Ahmed, told a reporter in Lebanon that when the plane first hit the ground, 'both sides of the plane blew off'.[9]

Buddha was seated just behind the plane's fissure. In landing, the airplane's left wing hit first, then ground-looped sharply, 'the cabin breaking open'. Buddha was ejected from the plane. To his front, the cabin rows and cockpit continued forward about 100 feet, then burst into flames as the fuel was dislodged. No one from that part of the plane survived. The passengers to the rear, behind Buddha, survived.

'The horror was still evident in his eyes while he related the accident,' wrote Chitralekha. Buddha told her, 'when he regained consciousness he realized he was immobilized and quite sunken into the hot desert sand. Fire was raging, people were screaming, he could hear the painful cries of small kids who were also travelling in the plane.'[10] His clothes aflame, Buddha used sand to put out the fire. He then thought, 'I am saved. My life is saved.'[11] 'Again, he saw the Himalayan yogi who said, "Foolish person you have forgotten who has saved you. Is this your work?"[12] Buddha realized a saint was speaking to him.'

The passengers who survived moved quickly away from the burning, hot wreckage to a hillside overlooking the crash site. They huddled together and watched the blaze through the night, wondering how they had survived. Fourteen persons died and twenty-one lived. One flight officer, named Gene Roddenberry, also survived the crash. For Roddenberry, like Buddha, that fateful night would change his life forever. Roddenberry decided 'he didn't want to be a pilot anymore, he wanted to do something different with his life. He resigned from Pan Am to pursue a career in writing, and ultimately, television.' Most of Roddenberry's fans know him as the creator of Star Trek, a TV and movie series spanning decades. 'A symbol of humanity's unlimited potential and the countless adventures that await us in the cosmos', Star Trek became 'a cornerstone of popular culture' for future generations.[13]

Roddenberry, having been assigned to sit to the rear, remained alive, and became the officer-in-charge of the chaotic crash scene.

The horrific events that transpired next were described by Buddha and Roddenberry. Shortly after the plane crashed, Roddenberry interacted with the 'desert tribesmen', to influence them to rob the dead only and to spare the survivors. After they left, other looters from a nearby town arrived, leaving the survivors with only their clothing.[14] Buddha's remembrance of it was vivid:

All of a sudden he saw the notorious Bedouin bandits emerge from no-where on horses and start looting the completely helpless passengers. He still remembered how the bandits snatched the earrings off a woman's ears while she was burning and crying out for help. He remembered with horror how a pregnant woman's stomach burst and threw out the unborn baby.[15]

When asked why he never attempted to take this experience to the screen, Roddenberry responded, 'I don't think it's possible to capture the feeling of the survivors as they experienced the sunrise on that morning so many years ago. There was a small group of us who were alive and thankful that we had survived what was an unsurvivable crash.' Despite all of his skills, he admitted he 'could not capture that moment, nor display the impact surviving had on me and others'.[16]

When daylight arrived, two surviving English passengers swam across the Euphrates, locating a Syrian military outpost, which sent a small airplane to investigate. By noon, the desert temperature climbed to 125 degrees. Life rafts were inflated and used for covering before 'aid began to arrive from several sources'. Roddenberry radioed a report to Pan Am, 'who sent out a stretcher plane to rescue the survivors of the crash'.[17]

Twelve of the survivors required medical treatment. 'The most seriously injured of them were transported by plane to Beirut.' This included Buddha.[18] At the American Hospital in Beirut, he was treated for his facial and burn wounds, then flown to Brussels for more procedures. His mother Emily, 'heard about the accident' and left London to see her son. 'She turned away when she saw him.' Unrecognizable, she said, 'He cannot be my son.' She asked to see a birthmark, and only 'then she was assured this was her son'. Buddha 'thought there was no reason to live anymore. He looked at himself in the mirror and then threw it.'[19]

'An air crash, a fractured spine, a mangled face. Months in a hospital, in plaster cast', was how a reporter described Buddha's experience.[20] Years later,

Buddha wrote that his exposed skin had been burnt, he later wrote, 'Medical science did a wonder cure to my face and hands.' However, a much more serious issue was that 'the spine was fractured'.[21] Since he already had a visa to go to the United States, he was flown to New York to consult doctors there about his damaged spine.

Buddha Bose was not in Calcutta for India's day of Independence, 15 August 1947. Instead, he was laid out in a New York City Hospital. His visa was time-stamped on 26 July and was good for one year, but Buddha stayed in the US for only three months and visited different doctors. At the end of September, he left the US via San Francisco, returning to Calcutta in October 1947.[22] Broken and disabled from the crash, after 'months of hospitalization abroad', his spine had not healed.[23]

Buddha would need to wear a 'belt to support his spine', the American doctors told him. Only thirty-five years of age, having been born at sea, atop the German 'Iron Dogs' ship deck, the alloy marked his fate again. A 'steel jacket' was placed around his waist. 'The belt,' he was told, 'had to be worn for the rest of his life.'[24]

66

KEDARNATH

One day, early in the research, while looking through one of Yogananda's magazines
from the 1940s, I find a photo of the Himalayan mountain temple Kedarnath.
The deep sense of beauty strikes me just by looking at it.
Little do I realize its significance at the time.

Bishnu and Buddha's wife and children heard news of the plane crash right away. For days, they did not know whether Buddha had survived, and feared the worst. Upon his return months later, India was independent, but Bengal had been split in two – partitioned. Like Buddha, who was broken, alive but not whole.

'After my return to India,' Buddha wrote, 'I suffered a lot with my spine which was gradually becoming worse. I consulted many doctors but to no effect. I was getting fevers.'[1] He was told he had 'tuberculosis in the spinal cord' and 'paralysis in the legs'.[2] After six months, amidst the conflict of communal fighting of 1948, his health, specifically his spine, remained uncured. He was in severe pain and bedridden.[3]

Buddha's father, Rajah, died in the spring of 1948.[4] Rajah had made his withdrawal from magic a few years earlier, and his fame quickly faded after 1945, even in Calcutta. His business as a 'dealer in is in glass in Giridih, in the state of Bihar', where Buddha had worked as a child, which had likely been sold or given to his Bengali son, Ambar.

Buddha thought to tell his mother of Rajah's death, but before he did, Emily revealed that 'she already knew' Rajah's 'soul had departed'. 'Your father came to see me', meaning 'his spirit had come to see for the last time before his soul passed away'.[5]

Buddha likely never reconciled with Rajah. Nevertheless, the death of his father must have further sapped his will at this moment in his life. 'What is the use in living like this, totally dependent on others?' thought Buddha. 'After realizing that I was beyond human cure,' he wrote, 'I decided to go to Sri Kedar and Badrinath.'[6] He had 'decided to give up on his life and go to the Himalayas'.[7]

Buddha had been to the Himalayan mountains during his 1940 pilgrimage. At the time of crisis, he wrote, a 'divine influence made me think to go there', having already experienced 'the spiritual power of those Holy places'. His planned pilgrimage was desperate. He plotted out 'the 21st of May, 1948' as his 'scheduled date to leave Calcutta'.[8]

Just two days before the departure, Ashok, his eldest son, 'dropped from a swing and broke his arm'. It was not that traumatic of an event, but nevertheless, his family asked him 'not to go to Kailas'.[9] Buddha broke down. 'I was broken-hearted and cried out, "Oh God why are you doing this to me? Just when I am about to leave for Kedarnath and Badrinath why am I having to go through this test?"'[10]

'The condition of my mind at that time may well be imagined', he wrote, as he 'gave up all hopes of getting cured at the Holy places of the Himalayan Ranges by Divine Power'. At that moment, though, he wrote, '*Bivak* (conscience) gave strength to my mind and said, have faith.'[11] Surrendering completely, Buddha left Calcutta on 21 May, the scheduled date, having decided 'to go to Kedar-Badri and have God's shelter'.[12]

Sitting at the head of a valley, the temple has a stunning backdrop of the Himalayan peaks. Kedarnath is the end of the road, accessible only by walking or riding a mule or a pony. Only little-used remote passes continue from there, with the ice peaks and snow-covered Himalayan mountains above. Kedarnath, one of the twelve Jyotirlingas named in ancient Sanskrit texts, is said to be where Lord Shiva lived and passed on yoga.

According to popular belief, the Kedarnath temple was built in the eighth century. It was hidden under ice for 600 years during the Little Ice Age, between 1300 and 1900 AD. During that period, the temple was interred within the glacier. Buried and forgotten, it then re-appeared. The earliest photographs show the isolated temple amidst a few sheep-herding huts lower below.

To get to Kedarnath nowadays, a road takes one to Gaurikund, about nine miles away, and to the trail kept up by the government. Though steep, it takes only a day or two to hike it. The road to Gaurikund did not exist in 1948, only forty-eight miles of trail.

For Buddha, unable to walk the mountains easily, only two or three miles of laborious progress was possible each day. Following the riverside leading to the temple, 'for 21 days he walked – or tried to – the 48 miles to Kedarnath from Rudraprayag.'[13]

With 'only a few miles journey left to reach Sri Kedarnath', Buddha suffered 'an attack of high fever and was running a temperature of 103 degrees'. Forced to 'give up all hopes to reach' that day, he rested. 'With no recovery in sight he had decided his life would end in Kedarnath.'[14] Buddha had reached his nadir.

The next day, his condition still the same, he 'got strength of mind' and 'decided to go ahead', even at the risk of his life. Somehow, he managed to reach Kedarnath 'in spite of high fever'. Buddha described his moment of arrival: 'The sight of the snow peaks of the Kedarnath Range and the age-old Temple which was built by the Pandavas to mark the place where they met Sadasiva on their way to Mahaprasthan thrilled my mind with Spiritual Vibration.'

Yet, as he stood before Kedarnath Temple, awe-inspired against the backdrop of snowy peaks, he did not at first 'have the fortitude to enter'.[15] Instead, he 'stayed at a *dharmashala* (rest-house) near the temple' for the night. 'My condition was such that I could not move and I was very sad.'[16]

The following morning, 'after washing my face, hands and feet in the holy river Mandakini I sat down inside the *dharmasala* to do my regular prayers', wrote Buddha.[17] Then, 'as usual', Buddha 'sat to do pranayam'.

After I had done pranayam 4 or 5 times I saw a vision of Lord Shiva, it was an auspicious day for me and I hadn't the least idea of it. When I was about to get up I heard a voice tell me, 'Wait. Stop. Sit and repeat this mantra one *lakh* [hundred thousand] times and your ailment will be gone.' I sat down to do the mantra *japa* as told.

Buddha committed: 'I threw off the steel jacket I was wearing and obeyed the Divine Voice. When his chanting of the special mantra was over, the vision was also gone.'[18]

When I got up after doing it for one *lakh* times, I realized more than 26 hours had elapsed. I got up, had a bath in the Mandakini river and went inside the Kedarnath temple. I did my *stotra* (verses) recitation inside the temple and came out. I realized that I had no pain in my back now![19]

'Since then,' he wrote, 'I am without the steel jacket.'[20] No longer needing it, 'he threw it into the Mandakini river'.[21]

Was this a miracle? It obviously cannot be verified, but Yogananda had an interesting take on these sorts of instances:

What seems to be a miracle is explained by a law whose secrets man has not yet discovered. Besides, he remarks, is there not a tendency for the word 'impossible' to lose its sense with the progress of atomic science? He explains, for example, that the power of dematerialization of the body is a result of a yogi's ability to combine and disintegrate atoms at will.[22]

There was no scientific explanation for what happened to Buddha at Kedarnath, but there was a yogic one. Writings on classical yoga state that 'when one engages oneself seriously in ascetic *tapas*', such physical changes could happen.[23] Only 'complete surrender to the Divine' enabled overcoming the 'resistance'. *Tap* means 'to heat' and *tapas* means 'straightening by fire' or a 'voluntary self-challenge'.

In an interview with Buddha, about a decade after the crash and his healing from it, the interviewee surmised that for most individuals, it was generally 'not until the boat was about to sink that one remembers Nearer My God To Me'. For Buddha, 'always religious', he 'found himself struggling against scepticism after the tragedy'.[24]

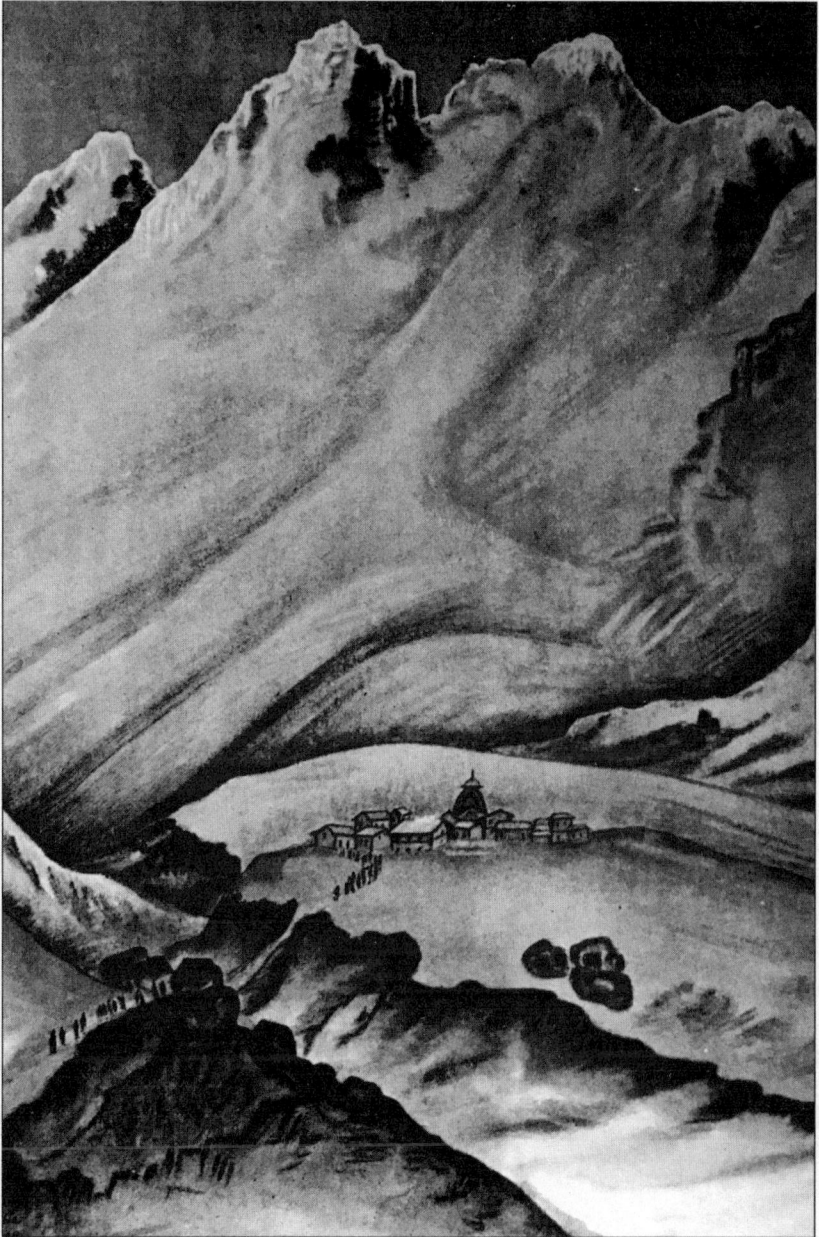

"Pilgrims Last Climb to Kedarnath."

Source: Theos Bernard Papers. Courtesy of the Bancroft Library (Berkeley, CA).

PART TEN

STUDENTS OF SAMADHI

67

GHOSH'S COLLEGE OF PHYSICAL EDUCATION

When I email Professor Narasingha Sil about going to Calcutta, he replies, 'Bishnu (aka Bistu) Ghosh was the pioneering founder of a gymnasium (not in the Greek sense nor style) at his home in Garpar in North Calcutta. You need to visit the area and ask any young man there to direct you to Ghosh's *akhara*.'

At the corner of Rammohan Roy Road, a statue sits next to the main roadway. Once called Upper Circular Road, the busy road is now known as AJC Bose Road. Sitting in *padmasana* (seated lotus), Bishnu is iron-cast and magnificent in size and shape.[1] Just a few steps beyond the statue is 4/2 Rammohan Roy Road. The house is set back from the road by about twenty yards, and at the end of the alleyway, an archway announces the school's name in blue lettering: 'Ghosh's College of Physical Education'. Below that, in red lettering: 'Ghosh's Yoga College' and 'Estd 1923'.[2]

On each side of the archway, *nagas* (snakes) have been carved and painted in the cement near the top of each of the side columns, as symbolic protectors. A large jasmine vine climbs up one of the columns, with white flowers and their pleasant smell wafting through the air, especially after the rains in the evenings and mornings. Just beyond the entrance to the left, sits another, more recent, bronze statue of Bishnu Ghosh, again in *padmasana*. To the right, next to a jasmine vine, is a statue of Hanuman, the Hindu monkey deity that called upon as a source of strength.

To my dismay, after following the professor's directions, I find that the gymnasium part of the college was shuttered fifteen years ago and the property sold to the neighbours. The entrance has been closed with bricks and painted over, but with a bit of focus I can make out the outline of where it used to be. The only remaining evidence of the gym's existence is in Hanuman's encasement, where the word *Bayam* is engraved on a piece of marble. The neighbours are generous enough to grant me access through a side door. I step into Bishnu's old gym and it feels like stepping into a temple. It is the September of 2015 – eighty years after Yogananda held his first group initiation in India in this very spot.

Unlike so many other rooms in the main Ghosh house, the old gym is a vast open space. At ground level with a concrete surface, it is naturally cool. Beyond the bricked-up doorway is a staircase, which leads up to the first floor of the main house, where many of Bishnu's students stayed, including Buddha Bose, Monotosh Roy, Gouri Shankar Mukerji and later, Bikram Choudhury, who would become famous in America.

The new owners left the space open, inserting a marble-tiled temple in place of the gymnasium. It is sparse, not gaudy, and much of the original concrete flooring is still visible. The room has a sense of solace and solitude.

The Ghosh family is happy that the space is now a temple. How better to enshrine the place as a tribute to Bishnu? His former presence, so determined, is left to the silent and shoe-less, with reverence and an attitude of respect.

One of the few students of Bishnu still alive is Hiten Roy. More than eighty years old, he remembers the gym well and shares his stories with me over multiple interviews.

Hiten and his best friend, Kamal Bhandari, started going to Ghosh's gymnasium at the same time, in 1949, when they were both sergeants with the Calcutta Police. They were non-vegetarian, eating fish, eggs and milk, but they did not consume alcohol, tobacco or coffee. Every day, six times a week, they would come to the gym after work, doing *bayam* to warm up, then weightlifting with barbells and other contraptions to build strength. Every other day, their workout would be for three hours, and included 'a series of deep-knee bend exercises, bench presses and triceps and biceps curls'.[3] They did this up until the day Ghosh's gymnasium closed.

I also locate Bishnu's second Calcutta gymnasium in the southern part of the city, in Ballygunge.

A very wealthy philanthropist of India, Sri Jugal Kishore Birla, was so highly pleased with [Bishnu's] work with India's youth that he purchased land in Ballygunge and constructed ... a large gymnasium. It was called Bajrang Gymnasium.[4]

In 1935, Bishnu 'convinced Jugal Kishore Birla that the Indian youth needed to do exercise to keep fit mentally and physically. Birla then gifted this property for the *bayamagar*, a place to do exercise. The property was placed under a trust committee.'

At first, no one I asked knew anything about it, but when I shared the information with Chitralekha, she recognized it, just a few blocks from her home off of Southern Avenue. It's a large structure, three stories high, with a large courtyard. The name, Bajranga Vyayamagar, is written in red atop the archway. Hanuman is known as *bajrang*, the god of might. 'Hanuman's Exercise Gymnasium' is an apt translation.

After a few visits to the gymnasium, a man named Balaram, who has been working out in this space for 'more than forty years', agrees to an interview. Another student chimes in on behalf of Balaram's credibility. 'These people here love this place and have been coming for more than 40 or 50 years. I have seen this guy not miss a single day of workout'.

Balaram 'used to work with a the tea company, Lipton' but has retired and is 'busy as a physiotherapist from morning till nine at night'. His afternoon workout consists of *bayam* – free-hand stretching, followed by barbells and weightlifting. He mentions two characteristics I've heard often about Bishnu. First, his ability to find and train students:

Bishnu Charan Ghosh made many young men famous with his body building techniques. He would spot the right boy – whether in the village or town – and then bring him over to his house. He would train him, feed him, put him through all the training required and then place them in competitions. Many of these young men became world famous.

Second, within the wider society:

Later Bishnu Charan would help them get government jobs in high profile places. The police and the ministries – all of them respected and honored Bishnu Charan and when he would send a candidate, they would gladly employ him because of his guarantee. You don't find such people any more.

I ask Balaram what the place was like in the old days.

'Wrestling was a huge affair back then. *Kushti*', as it's called in Bengali. 'It was all here,' Balaram tells me, pointing out a place, now covered with a concrete floor, where the mud-pit once was. In the 1990s though, 'It all disappeared. Memberships have come down. Attitudes have changed, people go for other types of workouts.'

I ask whether yoga was practised.

'Yes, upstairs, the first floor was totally dedicated to yoga. In one room we had yoga, one was for workouts, one for meditation and so on.' Dibya Sundar Das, one of Bishnu's yoga students from the 1960s, was among the last to teach yoga here. Before him, Balaram saw Bishnu's students, who 'would come here and practise. Like Kamal Bhandari, Hiten Roy and Monotosh Roy', all the 'big stalwarts' from before. Kamal and Hiten only focused on weightlifting until they got involved with organizing yoga asana competitions in the seventies. From the beginning, in the forties, Monotosh Roy combined yoga with weightlifting, even in the bodybuilding contests.

The original weights from Bishnu's gymnasium are still used today in north Calcutta.[5] The place is next to the Jayanti Mata Mandir, once owned by Gouri Shankar Mukerji, a prominent student of Bishnu. Gouri opened a gym there in 1998, but it did not have weights. Half a year later, after Gouri's death, his nephew, Romit Banerjee, inherited the gym.

Not long afterward, Romit learned that Bishwanath (Bishnu's youngest son) was 'closing down the gym' at 4 Rammohan Roy Road. 'Spontaneously', Romit 'took all of the antique stuff – Bishnu Charan Ghosh's dumbbells and barbells' to the gym in north Calcutta. When he took the weights, he asked if he should also take the Hanuman statue. It was 'the original Hanumanji of Bishnu'. Bishwanath 'was sad at seeing him take all of his father's weights and said, "Let the Hanumanji stay with me."'

'All these dumbbells and barbells had been used by stalwarts of bodybuilding', Romit said, 'if I had not taken them I don't know where they would have landed.'[6]

I walk into Romit's gymnasium for the first time and see many men using Bishnu's weights, so I do too. Interestingly, weightlifting here is done with no shoes.

68

MR UNIVERSE

Bishnu would recall that when Monotosh Roy returned from London, people were stunned at his win, and a reception was arranged at Albert Hall. At the same place, in a different time, 'people applauded when Swami Vivekananda' spoke, but here, with Monotosh Roy, Mr Universe, 'the Albert Hall crowd was exploding with a roar of approval'.[1]

The post-Independence generation of Calcutta youth were brought up with the belief that a healthy mind could only exist in a healthy body. This reached its height in the fifties, a period known as the Golden Age of Physical Culture.[2] Kamal Bhandari, one of Bishnu's students at the time, said, 'Bodybuilding was fun. We practised for four hours from Monday to Saturday and Bistuda [Bishnu] would be there to inspire us. Braving the summer heat we practised for hours together and felt a deep sense of satisfaction when people praised us for our well-defined muscles'.[3] Bishnu's student, Monotosh Roy, became a legend in this era, performing yoga asanas and feats of strength on the stage, becoming Mr Universe.

The highly competitive Mr Universe contest started in 1950 and garnered global publicity, which reached the physical culture proponents in Calcutta.[4] Heading into the 1951 competition, everyone expected the contest to be between London's, Reg Park and the Americans.[5] Park, having just missed winning the '50 contest, was heavily favoured to win the '51 Mr Universe competition.[6] No one expected anyone from India to contest for the title. Bodybuilding was in the pre-anabolic era. Physique was 'combined with muscular density and shear strength' and a focus on 'grace and beauty' to produce results achieved through training and determination. The best exercises and movements from the West with the traditions of India were integrated; Monotosh, training under Bishnu, had integrated weightlifting with yoga asanas.

The 1951 Mr Universe contest was held in London on 1 September in a hall near Russell Square. It was organized by the National Amateur Bodybuilding Association (NABBA), under the auspices of the World Federation of Bodybuilding. The NABBA in London accepted Monotosh for the Mr Universe contest and also invited Bishnu Ghosh to be one of the seven judges.

When Monotosh Roy began his performance, the lights shone to reveal him in a pose 'as Jesus Christ'. This had the potential to be controversial with the London crowd, but instead it 'created an unprecedented response among them' as it was seen as 'a religious theme' used imaginatively, and was instead 'cheered by the people of London'.[7] It might be questionable as to what the Mr Universe contest had to do with yoga asanas, but only until what Monotosh did next. Rather than traditional body poses of muscle alone, he combined them with yoga asanas.

Monotosh 'performed the *sirsasana* (headstand) in the body agility category, then he did *urdha padmasana* (shoulderstand in lotus), then *urdva kukkutasana* (hand balance between the legs in lotus)'. The latter two were advanced postures, requiring a level of flexibility and agility one would not expect to see on the stage of a bodybuilding contest; 'the European audience had never witnessed such a performance before'.[8]

Overall, reports stated that he 'gave wonderful performances of muscle control and feats of suppleness associated with their country'; his 'symmetrical build was art'.[9] He then added the feat that Buddha Bose had done before. A dagger was 'tied to a rod and the pointed part was placed' on his throat as he 'applied full pressure of his body to bend the iron rod'.[10] The performance by Monotosh, whose nickname was 'Tarzan of Bengal', blew the crowd and judges away.

Monotosh scored 384 points and Juan Ferraro came in second with 383 ¾ points. Reg Park came in third, with 381 ½ points. Monotosh had won the highest score and was slated to be named Mr Universe. It was unprecedented. In a remarkable upset, 'the impossible had happened and Monotosh Roy had been selected as Mr. Universe, 1951'.[11] 'Everyone expected a walkover victory for Park', and the upset was unacceptable to the 'backroom' observers of the decision. The seven judges, two from England, and five from abroad, including Bishnu Ghosh, were thrown into chaos, 'a row blew up amongst them' with 'many sharp exchanges'.[12] Those in favour of overturning the result argued that the judges had mistakenly made it a 'test of athletic ability' and had 'based their judgement on performance rather than physique'.[13]

In a second vote, 'the judges were each asked to write on a sheet of paper their first and second placings for the overall winner. Six out of the seven judges had Reg Park down for the supreme title'.[14] This resulted in them 'taking the title' away from Monotosh.[15]

The NABBA President, D. G. Johnson, took the microphone and announced, 'Ladies and Gentlemen, I give you Mr. Universe 1951 – Reg Park of England!'[16] The 1951 contest did not come down to English vs American; instead, it was Englishman vs Indian, and there was no way the sponsors of the event were going to disappoint the English crowd.

Monotosh Roy won the most points for the Mr Universe contest. Then the rules were altered, in spite of the scores, to award the Mr Universe contest to Reg Park instead. A couple of years later, another such instance occurred, with the contestant in class two ending the contest with more points than anyone in class one, two or three, and he was awarded the overall title of Mr Universe.

There were only hints of 'certain dirty work behind the scenes' related to the tainted results of the competition.[17] A photo from the event had the caption, 'B. Ghosh of India, and Monotosh Roy, winner in the Small Man class' discuss 'the contest at the dinner to officials and competitors'. Bishnu, of course, was right in the middle of the exchange, but no mention was made of the controversy in print until 'more than ten years later', when *Health & Strength* recounted the incident.[18]

Indians agreed that 'all in all, the '51 Universe was a great and memorable occasion'. An English reporter 'heard several people say that they wouldn't forget it as long as they lived'.[19] Neither would Bishnu. Monotosh went home a Mr Universe in Class Three, even though he did not win the overall title for the year. However, the 'full results' remained, which showed him leading in points for the contest. Even in the late sixties, Bishnu still felt the sting and would talk about the chaos of judging Mr Universe 1951, telling Monotosh Choudhury that 'Monotosh Roy beat Reg Park'.[20]

Afterwards, Monotosh Roy continued to perform with Bishnu. In 1951, at the Anatomical Society of India, the *Calcutta Medical Journal* reported that 'Bishnu Ghosh and his pupils' gave a presentation on the 'external anatomy of the human body as influenced by the Yogasana system of physical culture'. While Bishnu lectured, Monotosh 'gave a demonstration of different muscles of the body' to the session attendees.[21]

After returning from London, Monotosh branched out, opening his own gymnasium. The 1951 performance of Monotosh broadened the reach of yoga, as he was the first to showcase yoga asanas with his bodybuilding performances. The combination reached the mainstream in 1964, in two magazines which were at the centre of the bodybuilding universe at the time. In the January issue of *Strength and Health*, the cover article was titled 'The Secrets of Combining Yoga and Weights'. The very same month, its competitor, *Health & Strength*, published its January issue with the cover article titled 'Common Sense Yoga'.

A couple of decades later, in 1972, Monotosh was 'selected as the lone judge from India for the ensuing Mr Universe competition' in Baghdad. He also produced a promotional magazine for the Indian Bodybuilding Federation.[22] In the magazine, 'The Mother' Aurobindo, endorsed the effort of making 'our body strong and supple so that it may become in the material world a fit instrument for the truth force which wills to manifest through us'.

Sitting at the Coffee House, I flip through the pages of the 1972 magazine. I have no idea where Monotosh's gymnasium might be; then inside the magazine, I find an ad listing the place. Not surprisingly, the address of 1 Naya Ratna Lane is in north Calcutta, just on the other side of Vivekananda's family house. I head out to find it the next day.

Crisscrossing streets and alleyways, following Google maps, I find the location of Roy *Bayam* Yoga, but no one is there. I call the number and arrange for a meeting that evening.

I get back to the Roy *Bayam* Yoga studio at 6 p.m., go inside and take some photos of the place. I'd called again during the afternoon and arranged to meet Monotosh's daughter and one of his students, Salil Burman, at the house. Inside, photos line the walls, quite aged, probably how Monotosh left it a decade ago when he died at the age of eighty-nine. He had an immensely successful bodybuilding career, but I am interested in his yoga.[23] The family brings out the memoirs, and I read through the articles and look at the photographs.

A set of photos show Monotosh with telemetry electrodes placed on his body. There are individuals who look like doctors measuring him. I ask, 'When were these photos taken?'

'He went to visit Japan for the demonstration of yoga and pranayam, to promote India's physical culture activity,' responds Salil. 'The scientists and doctors examined Monotosh Roy thoroughly and observed he was "dead" and then he once again came back to normal life.' Salil talks this over with Monotosh's daughter in Bengali, and they agree it happened around 1970 to 1972 in Tokyo. Of course, it cannot end there. He adds, 'Japan offered Mr Roy to stay in Japan permanently to lead a high-class stylish life but, as a great Indian nationalist, he refused that offer'.[24]

Monotosh's book, *Yoga-O-Jiban*, was translated in 1970 from Bengali into English. Titled *Cream of Yoga*, the book taught yogasana postures, from beginner to advanced. Bodybuilding and yoga, 'both are indispensable,' he wrote, 'the secret of building super human bodies.'[25]

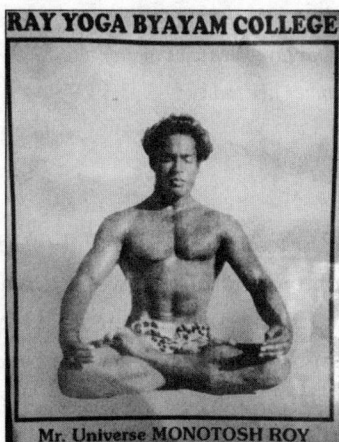

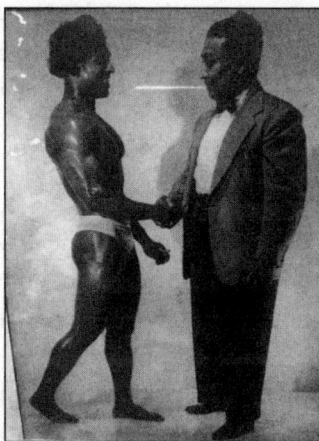

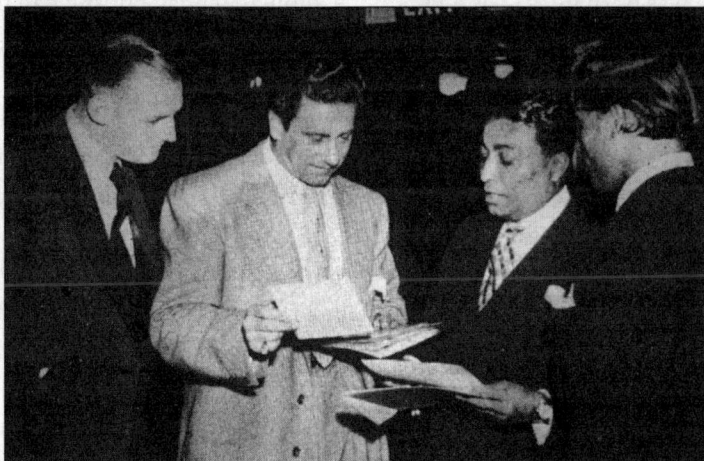

Top left: Monotosh Roy. Top right: Mr Universe contest (1951).
Courtesy of Ghosh's Yoga College; Monotosh Roy family.
Bottom: Joe Weider (middle left) with Bishnu Ghosh (middle right).
Source: Your Physique, Dec, 1951.

69

DEVI CHAUDHURANI

Reba Rakshit, that Bengali star of the big top,
could bear the weight of elephants and large vehicles on her chest.
But few seem to remember her today.[1]

It was not just strong*men*; there were also women. To date, all of Bishnu's top students had been male, but soon he would meet a woman who 'was tall, graceful and quite feminine. Yet she had amazing strength'.[2] Her name was Reba Rakshit; Bishnu would call her 'my favourite student'.[3] And like other students, Bishnu had first seen her from afar, while she was up on the stage, performing in the circus as a teenager.

Reba was born in 1933 as a Hindu in Comilla, Bengal, but she had fled her homeland after the 1947 partition, when Bengal was split into Bangladesh and West Bengal. She was said to have come 'from a very ordinary background', and she 'worked at the Kishore Bangla Press while pursuing her studies with earnestness'.[4] In her youth, 'she excelled in yoga, *bayam* and bodybuilding'. She was compared with another 'shining star in the female category from the glorious past', Sushila Sundari, who had 'broken the social barriers'.[5]

Halfway through the twentieth century in Bengal, women involved in physical culture were unique. Sushila Sundari was one such woman. Another, from the twenties, was named Aruna Bandopadhyay. As a young girl, she had suffered 'from typhoid and pneumonia' and recovered as 'she practised *bayam* regularly'. At the age of fifteen, 'she stopped a speeding car at the Rammohan Roy Centenary Celebration' held in Calcutta, and she was 'an expert in jiu-jitsu, *lathi khela* (a traditional Bangladeshi martial art), and fighting with swords and knives'. Such women were 'not to be found easily'.[6]

In Bengal, 'women who were initiated to the world of sports formed a tiny percentage of the elite section of society'.[7] Bishnu was part of the forefront of "improving"; or "widening the gap" that effort to include both genders:

> Yes, Reba had to face the same societal prejudices and obstructions as did Sushila in the past, but nothing deterred this young woman from achieving her goal. No amount of snags, objections, slanders and acute poverty could make Reba drop out from her chosen path – her guru giving her all the encouragement she needed.[8]

Reba was well known for her feats of strength, and in her prime, the Nizam of Hyderabad bestowed upon her the title of Devi Chaudhurani, a title used in her *bayam* articles.[9] 'The college of physical education ... would receive invitations from several *puja* committees to see Reba Rakshit, a favorite pupil of Ghosh'; she left them 'spellbound' with her ability to withstand heavy weights upon her body, such as fully loaded cars.[10] At circus events, a reporter proclaimed, 'Miss Reba Rakshit can put an elephant on her breast!'[11] She was also profoundly influential in spreading yoga *bayam* among women.

Bishnu had many students before her (even women), but Reba – along with Labanya Palit – was the first woman he taught to teach others. Less is known about Labanya, who wrote *Shariram Adyam* in 1956, a Bengali book whose title was based on the Sanskrit saying attributed to Shiva: '*sariram adyam khalu dharma sadhanam*' (the body is the primary cause of *sadhana*). Labanya and Reba were contemporaries, and during the fifties they became the first women from Bengal to broadcast the practice of yoga asana under Bishnu Ghosh, proclaiming 'to take care of your physical health; that is your primary duty'.[12]

Bishnu was the editor-in-chief of *Bayam*, the leading monthly magazine in Bengali on physical culture, which was published prior to and around 1950. Later he edited *Bayam Charcha Patrika*, which began publication in 1964 and lasted into the nineties. A couple of choice articles, written by Reba for these publications highlight her role during the fifties in the dissemination of yoga in Bengal.[13]

'The difference between normal exercise and yoga-*bayam*,' Reba wrote, was that 'asana revives the sick and ailing organs' and other 'parts of the body. Things start working normally again. Then the *savasana* evens out all odds and makes the whole constitution work the way it should. Resulting in every part of the body working according to its normal and natural process.'[14]

People flocked to the city for its industries and the availability of working in places other than in the rural fields. As a result, ailments and all sorts of diseases or recurrent injuries, became commonplace. Pollution and filth were rampant. Here was a system of India's past to address these issues. 'Now let me talk about curing through yoga and destroying the attack of ailments,' wrote Reba. Though 'cholera, tuberculosis, typhoid, etc. cannot be cured or healed by yoga', it can 'heal ailments' such as 'blood pressure, asthma, and digestive problems'. If one becomes aware of tuberculosis entering their system, 'pranayam and asana will stop the bacteria doing further damage, because it will revive the lungs rapidly'. 'Rest assured,' she wrote, 'if you have been practising yoga from before,' then 'germs and bacteria can go no further than the entrance, because you are well protected beforehand!'[15]

> The truth about yoga is that anyone can do it – a small child, a young person or an elderly person. There are asanas for every category giving the same results ... one just needs to do a few asanas in addition to their regular regime of exercises to revive their youth and vigour. A person does not need to do more than 5 or 6 asanas every day to keep himself or herself healthy and fit.

Reba went on to point out how yoga would be especially beneficial to women, who did not have a gym to take care of the needs of their health. 'I recommend yoga-*bayam* for them ... yoga-*bayam* is for all ages and genders,' she wrote, advocating practising 'for about 20–25 minutes' daily.[16]

Reba's advocacy of yoga practice spurred on, in the fifties, the practice of yoga among even those who could not afford to go to the gym, writing, 'the best part is that asana practice does not need contraptions or machines, and you don't need to go anywhere, just practise at home!'[117] (Women and girls were unable to attend the clubs and gymnasiums. This would change with the first yoga centre for women opening in 1967.)

> Now I shall talk about females, who do not have the privilege of going to a gym for the needs of their health. I recommend yoga-*bayam* for them – they do not need to go anywhere, and instead, can practise at home in privacy. I hope now it is clear that yoga-*bayam* is for all ages and gender.

And to younger girls on the benefits of *bayam* (exercise):

> *Bayam* removes all diseases and brings comfort and rest to mind and body. This is known to everybody – even little children are aware of this. Young people should not avoid *bayam*. Girls have time to spend on dressing and

grooming but just cannot find time to practise a little *bayam* every day for about 20–25 minutes. When they avoid exercise, it becomes a sad state of being for the child.

On the topic of what to practice:

It is advisable to check with the yoga advisor every 15 days or a month. You can correct if you have done anything wrong or alter the yoga asanas to suit your present condition. The best part is that asanas do not need any contraptions or machines, neither does it need you to spend money unnecessarily. And you do not need to go anywhere to practise your asanas, just practise at home!

Bishnu's 'protégé', as he called her, 'achieved a high level of success and fame'. Under Bishnu's guidance, Reba became 'an expert on motor bikes' and 'won a prize in racing' in 1953 in tandem with Bishnu.[18]

When he was fifty years old, Bishnu went to attend a motorbike race in Behala, south of Calcutta. Participation in the two-person race involved the condition of a potato held between the two riders, between 'the pillion rider forehead and the front rider's back of the head over an uneven racetrack'.

The race started and plenty of the racers sped in high speed; many fell off and many lost their potatoes. I started on the second gear to get a feel of the road and after experiencing a couple of bumps I told Reba to grip my neck hard. Now I took speed and reached the winning post much before anyone else. In fact, Jack Willis, who has been a winner of the past few races, had not even crossed the half line mark. I was the only Bengali participant and even though I won they gave the prize to Reba. According to them if it was not for Reba's encouragement I would not have won the race.[19]

Reba excelled not only in those feats but also 'in yoga, *bayam*, and bodybuilding'.[20] In the circus and at puja events, she 'combined hair-raising endurance feats with yoga'.[21]

Wanting to get my hands on the *Bayam* magazines which Bishnu edited, I think 'Well, this will be easy.' Just locate the copies, have them translated from Bengali to English, and it's done.

Arup scours the old libraries. He looks everywhere. 'There is not a trace of this in Rammohan Roy Library, Sahitya Parishad, Bagbazar Reading Library, or Chaitanya Library, not even with the families. I even went to Uttarpara to look for it in the Jai Krishna Library. Not even in the Federation Hall,' he writes after finding nothing. There were only 200 copies of the magazines printed per month. Even the family of the co-editor, Moti Mondal, is not able to produce more than a few later copies.

Eventually, issues from about ten years of *Bayam Charcha* (1964–74), with some gaps, and a few of the original *Bayam* from decades earlier, turn up. Once copies of *Bayam Charcha* magazine are found, examples of Reba's influence and cultural impact on the adoption of regular yoga practice are readily apparent.

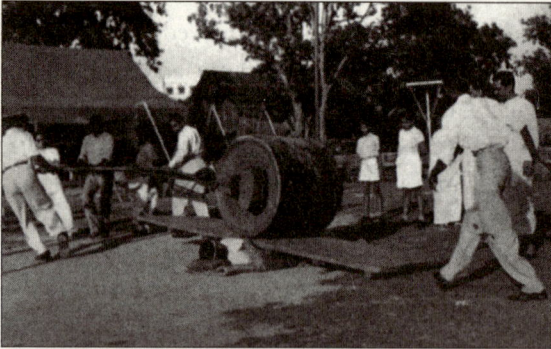

Gouri Shankar Mukerji.
Courtesy of Yoga and our Medicine : 84 Yoga Asanas, Romit Banerjee.

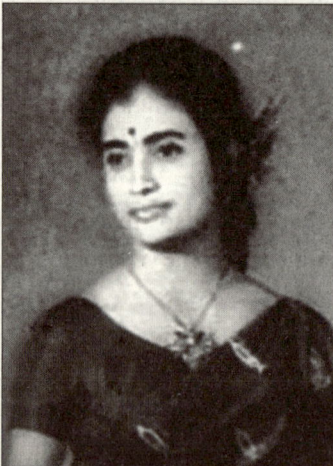

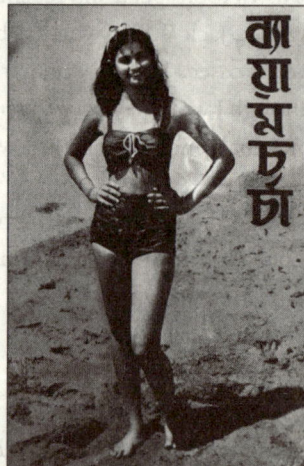

Reba Rakshit, circa 1955.
Courtesy of Bayam Charcha; Romit Banerjee.

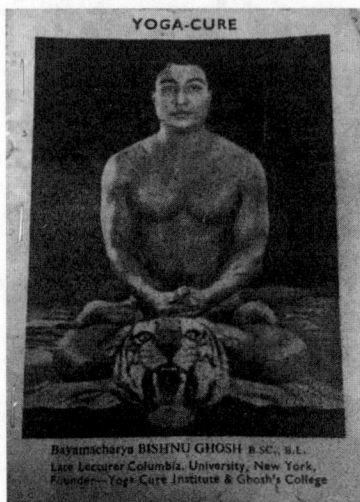

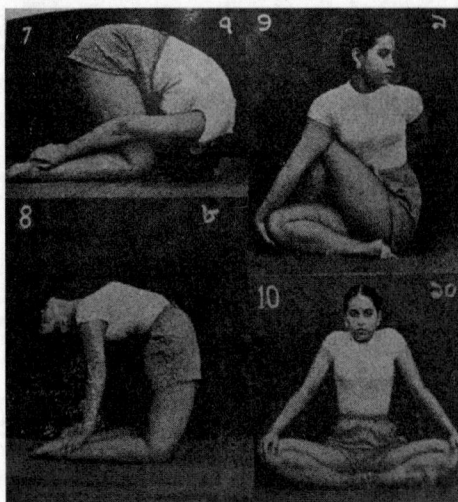

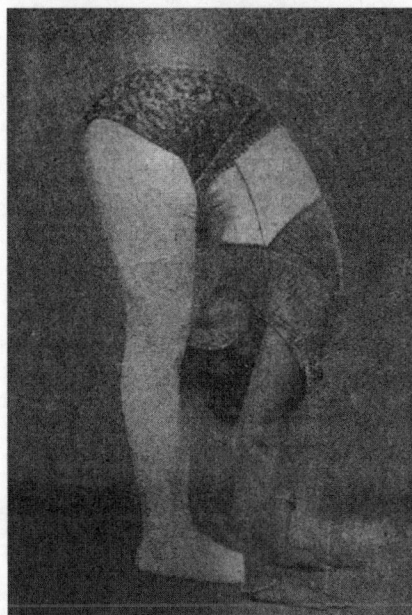

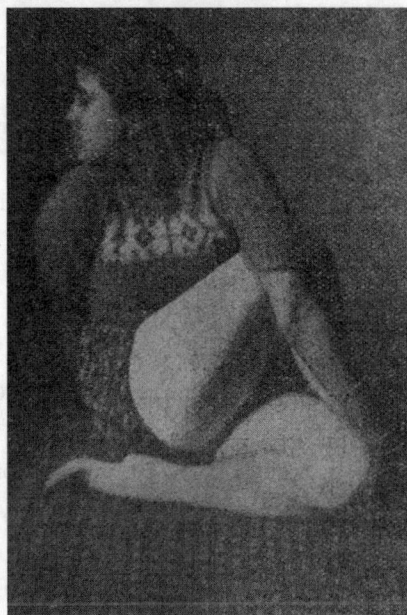

Top left: The cover of Yoga-Cure. Top right: Photos of Karuna Ghosh in Yoga-Cure (1960).
Courtesy of Ghosh's Yoga College, Yogacharya Mukul Dutta.
Bottom: Labanya Palit, Shariram Adyam (1956).
Source: National Library, Calcutta.

70

YOGI RAJ

Gouri told Bishnu, 'I have done something,'
to which Bishnu asked, 'What have you done?'
Gouri replied, 'I have mastered all the 84 asanas.' Bishnu could not believe it,
'It takes years of practice to learn these asanas, show me what you have done.'

Gouri Shankar Mukerji began training under Bishnu Charan Ghosh in 1943 at the age of seventeen, and in 1950, he went to Germany to become a Western-educated medical doctor. His specialty was in yoga and its medical application for curing ailments.

In the March of 2015, when I arrive in Calcutta for the first time, I know nothing of Gouri Shankar Mukerji, not even his name. The first I hear his name is while interviewing Rooma Bose, daughter of Buddha Bose. She asks, 'Have you heard of Gouri Shankar?' After I display my ignorance, Rooma goes on, 'Gouri was another star pupil of Bishnu Ghosh. After Buddha, and before Bikram, there was Gouri.' That seems impressive. Rooma ends her comments about Gouri by saying, 'He has written a book in German; you should find it.'[1]

I add his name to the list of people and books I am looking to find. When I return home, I can't find the book, only a reference from Dibya Das who wrote that after learning the fundamentals of yoga asana from Bishnu Ghosh, he 'took lessons on Therapeutic Yoga from a great teacher, Dr Gouri Mukherjee who was an MBBS doctor by profession and completed M. D. from Germany'. Dibya Das, along with his brother Prem and sister Kushala, learned yoga from Bishnu Ghosh in the sixties.

I return to Calcutta a few months later and seek out the Das brothers for interviews, and also to track down this elusive book. With my research assistant and translator, Arup, I arrive to interview Dibya Sundar Das at his World Yoga Society clinic in Golpark. Dibya and his brother Prem have what amounts to a yoga empire in Calcutta, with branches all across the city.

Arup and I wait behind a line of thirty or so 'patients' waiting to meet Dibya Das at his head branch, for one-on-one yoga consultations. When we finally speak with him, he does not have a copy of the book. However, he gives Arup the location of an ashram in north Calcutta near Dakshineswar that had been associated with Gouri.

The next morning, we head to the north Calcutta ashram named Sri Jayanti Mata. Gouri wound up at this ashram, living a celibate life, with a tantric guru and a personal practice of yoga asana. Members of society came to him for medical and prescriptive yoga advice. One of the ashram's caretakers takes a framed photo of Gouri off the wall, and we move into a side room to place it in the sun. It seems, from the colour and type of photographic print, to have been taken in the seventies. In it, Gouri has gray hair and is about fifty years of age. He was born in 1927, I am told. He lived until 1998, to about seventy-one. He is extremely fit in the photo. He was unique in his practice of yoga asanas at this ashram. He continued practising and giving medical advice well into the nineties.

That same afternoon, Arup and I interview the elder Das brother, Prem Sundar, in the main office at Ghosh's Yoga College. On the bright pink door, a small bronze nameplate reads 'Prem Das, Vice President'. Above it, the title 'President' reads 'Biswanath Ghosh', who was Bishnu's son, now deceased. The office is in the same place where Buddha had his office in the seventies, and before him, Bishnu Ghosh.

When I ask Prem about Gouri he replies, 'Gouri Mukerji was like a son to Bishnu Ghosh.' Prem Das does not have a copy of the book either, but when I ask him what's in it, he replies, 'eighty-four asanas' and something about the medical benefits of the individual postures. When he replies 'eighty-four asanas', I become quite taken with locating the book, though it doesn't seem like I will find it in Calcutta.

That evening, Arup and I have a meeting scheduled at the West Bengal Yoga Association in Wellington Square to talk with an elderly man who was a student of Bishnu Ghosh. While there, we meet a student of Gouri who, in the nineties, had sought out treatment for a debilitating physical ailment. He happened upon Sri Jayanti Mata Ashram, where he found Gouri running a 'Yogic Culture Institute'. Gouri prescribed him a set of exercises to perform daily, which he did, and soon found recovery. The man is able to show me a copy of his yogic prescription. Despite not finding a copy of Gouri's book, I now have the title, know the contents, and have learned much about his life and impact.

Eventually, I find a reference to the book in a German catalog. When I finally hold *Yoga and Our Medicine* by Dr Gouri Shankar Mukerji, I find that it lists four pranayama techniques, followed by eighty-four asanas and then four mudras, each with photos and descriptive explanations. I feel like I've finally found what I have been looking for all this time: a vital connection to the yoga taught by Bishnu Ghosh within two previously unavailable books. First, from the yoga's beginnings with Buddha Bose in the thirties, to this – its culmination with Gouri Shankar Mukerji in the sixties. It is like finding the bookends of transmission for Bishnu's yoga asana teachings over his lifetime.

On a subsequent visit to Calcutta, I meet Romit Banerjee, a descendant of Gouri. Romit provides the inspiration to make the English translation of *Yoga and Our Medicine* available and fills in many more details about the life of Gouri Shankar Mukerji.[2]

Yoga asanas were not Gouri's primary area of practice under Bishnu, at least not at first. He began with a focus on weight-lifting, muscle control and jiu-jitsu. These were the primary strength-building and martial arts practices with which Bishnu trained students. Buddha Bose, when he first trained under Bishnu at the age of sixteen, began in the same manner. The training of asanas was more exclusive and spiritually focused, and it would come later.

On 25 September 1946, at the All-Bengal Birastami Competition sponsored by Calcutta's Ward 23 Durga Puja Committee, Gouri competed and 'secured first place in jiu-jitsu'. A year later he 'secured first place in Best Physique Competition in Group B', competing with the mid-weight/height contestants.

At the end of the forties, Gouri was ready for something new. After a few years of other physical pursuits, he discovered yoga asanas.[3] At Bishnu's house, 'he came across some yoga posture pictures sent by Yogananda'. Though 'the pictures were sent by Yogananda, he was not doing the asanas'. What the book was, or who the photos were of, wasn't clear; but when Gouri asked Bishnu about the photos, the latter replied, 'This is yoga, and only meant for sadhus and saints, not the common man.'[4] Gouri was intrigued and took them home. He was a natural, and having already gained the strength and flexibility from other physical pursuits, he was quickly able to do all the eighty-four asanas.

Once he had mastered them, he showed Bishnu what he had done. After the performance, Bishnu felt he needed to contact his brother, Yogananda, to see how to proceed. At this point in time, still in the forties, the practice of yoga asanas was not widespread. It was still, as Bishnu had said, a practice of the sannyasin and few others. The only way to learn them was to take vows and learn from a guru, or to be in a family-line that had a tradition of yoga asana practice passed down through the generations. Buddha Bose was a rarity, and though he had performed abroad, within Calcutta, he restricted his teaching to foreigners and dignitaries.

Bishnu asked Yogananda, 'Can I teach?' He was referring to teaching the asanas to Gouri.

The reply from Yogananda was brief, 'You can teach.'

Bishnu took this as an opportunity to teach Hatha yoga asanas and pranayam, not just to Gouri, but the populace in general. Bishnu said, 'Bengalis only eat rice, fish, dal and sleep; from now on every Bengali will also do yoga.'[5]

Thereafter, the performance of yoga asanas became a significant part of Gouri's practice and performance. Romit explained that from then on:

Gouri travelled with Bishnu on trucks and lorries to remote villages and towns showing yoga asana. He would demonstrate yoga on top of the trucks to draw crowds, while Bishnu would describe the asanas over the speaker. Thus the promotion of yoga was started and soon became popular among the masses. People would come up with their ailments and illnesses to be cured through yoga. Gouri Shankar and Bishnu would make a chart there and then and teach the patients. It was like a small revolution.[6]

This work culminated in an auspicious event in August 1950. Gouri travelled with Bishnu Ghosh to Rishikesh and while there, Sivananda of Rishikesh, founder of the Divine Life Society, presented the title of 'Yogi Raj' to Gouri Mukerji 'for the mastery of the intricate technique and processes of yogic sciences'.

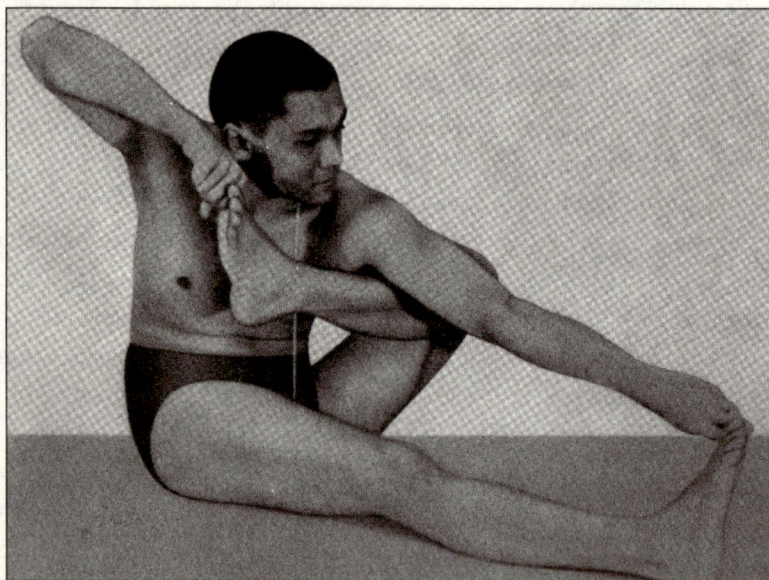

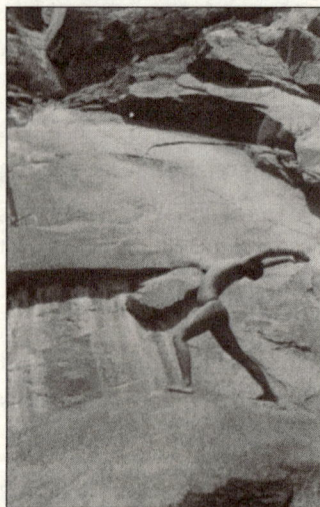

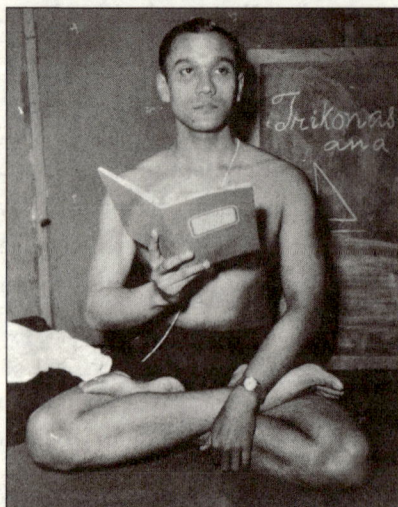

Gouri Shankar Mukerji.
Courtesy of Yoga and our Medicine : 84 Yoga Asanas, Romit Banerjee.

71

REV BERNARD

'Each of the eighty-four basic body-positions is intended to facilitate the attainment of a definite and characteristic result,' wrote Bernard Cole. In this and 'subsequent issues', they will be explained 'in full'.[1]

There is little recognition of the role Yogananda's organization played in the growth of modern yoga outside India during the second half of the twentieth century. After the publication of *Autobiography of a Yogi* in 1946, his organization grew noticeably, and with that growth came changes to meet the broadening appeal. Curiously, beginning in 1949, a substantial part of that change was the frequent inclusion of Hatha yoga in Yogananda's magazine. The writing was done under the guidance of Bernard Cole.

Cole was born in 1922 and arrived in Los Angeles as a student of Yogananda in 1938. It was a few months after Buddha and Bishnu had performed and taught yoga asanas in Los Angeles, but Cole readily picked up the practice from the others.[2] Cole was mentioned in *Autobiography* as one of 'a number of American students' who 'mastered various asanas or postures', and recognized as an 'instructor in Los Angeles of the Self-Realization Fellowship teachings of the asanas'.[3] Yogananda wrote about Cole in the context of Yogoda at the Ranchi School in 1918. He most likely viewed the practice of Yogoda as more beneficial, with its 'extraordinary ability to shift the life energy from one part of the body to another part, and to sit in perfect poise in difficult body postures'. This reference showed he viewed asanas and Yogoda as being similar too.[4]

Overall, *Autobiography of a Yogi* did not present Hatha yoga in a favourable light. Yogananda downplayed its physical focus, as seen in his follow-up comment to the psychologist Carl Jung, who said: 'purely bodily procedures of yoga also mean a physiological hygiene which is superior to ordinary gymnastics and breathing exercises'.[5] It was not merely mechanical, Jung stated, the practice was 'also philosophical'.[6] By 'training of the parts of the body, it unites them with the whole of the spirit'. Jung gave an example, whereby '*prana* is both the breath and the universal dynamics of the cosmos'.[7]

Yogananda responded that the 'bodily procedures of yoga' referred to 'Hatha yoga, a specialized branch of bodily postures and techniques for health and longevity. Hatha is useful, and produces spectacular physical results, but this brand of yoga is little used by yogis bent on spiritual liberation.' 'Forms of yoga proper' begin after the preparatory phases, such as the asanas of Hatha yoga. Clarifying what he meant by 'Yoga proper', Yogananda explained that it was the practice of momentary concentration, sustained focus and absorbed perception, which has a 'final goal' of 'realization of the Truth beyond all intellectual apprehension'.[8]

Yogananda made a similar comment (which revealed his preference for asanas that enhance meditation) while in India during the mid-thirties when asked about numbness of the legs 'during a long period of meditation', and 'what can the yogi do to prevent this?' Yogananda answered by recommending *mahamudra,* a 'spine stretching asana that is done before the practice of Kriya proper', both 'during and/or after a long meditation'.[9] *Mahamudra* helps the body to adapt 'to long periods of meditation', he stated.[10] 'It is considered the best of asanas, and is called *mahamudra* (the great posture).'[11]

However, Yogananda knew of all the asanas from the Hatha yogis who brought them to his schools in Dihika and Ranchi. A 1932 American newspaper report described him performing *kukkutasana* (crow posture) on the stage for example.[12] But the tradition of Kriya yoga, as taught by his teacher Sriyukteswar and, before him, Lahiri Mahasaya, did not lay much emphasis on the physical practices beyond pranayama.

When Yogananda taught the boys in Dihika and Ranchi, he included Hatha yoga practices in an already durative physical component of exercise, which was oriented towards the exercise of youth. In America, with an older audience, he was a proponent of physical exercises such as the energization exercises (what Yogoda came to be called) which were less demanding.[13] After Buddha and Bishnu visited Los Angeles in 1938, they taught additional yoga asanas, thereafter practised by American diciples in Yogananda's organization , where the practice was encouraged. During the forties, modern yoga, with its emphasis on the broader Hatha yoga asanas, took root among the organization members.

Bernard Cole arrived at Yogananda's ashram at the exact moment. He picked up the practice alongside other students who had learned from Bishnu and Buddha. This did not gain much attraction immediately. In 1941, Yogananda offered a 'Yoga University' diploma from Mount Washington. Coursework included his class 'on Patanjali's immortal aphorisms on Yoga'.[14] The second semester, in 1942, was held in Encinitas 'at the Golden Lotus Temple', and 'yoga' and 'physical culture' were among the courses.[15] In the next issue, it was announced that 'Bernard Cole would conduct a Yoga Physical Culture class' in Encinitas and Los Angeles, which, in July 1942, was the first mention of Bernard teaching yoga asanas within SRF.[16] The university was short-lived, but the practice continued.

Two Americans who visited Yogananda were new Vedanta Society members. They interviewed him 'over a long lunch', upstairs in his Mount Washington room. After the 'egg curry and vegetarian' lunch, the guests readied to leave when Yogananda told them: 'Oh, no. You've only heard about my work, now you will see some of it.' Swami Vidyatmananda recalled that space was made 'and a scene ensued that made me think of life in the court of some oriental potentate'. About twenty boys 'barefooted and wearing gym outfits proceeded to do a series of yoga postures' that neither of the two had ever seen before. Yogananda commented on the exercises, explaining their value. After the asana exposition, they even performed feats:

At one point some of the advanced students thrust needles through cheeks and tongue and removed them without drawing blood.

This struck the stoic-minded guests as unpleasant:

'Was this something I should have to accept in becoming an adept of Indian religion?' I asked myself. I hoped not. What we had witnessed struck me as intensely unaesthetic and moreover carrying with it an unmistakable odor of eroticism.[17]

An SRF pamphlet from 1949 advertised the ashram at Mount Washington as 'an opportunity for quiet meditation and the practice of bodybuilding exercises – an ideal atmosphere to encourage all-around development'.[18] The former tennis courts in front of the main structure at Mount Washington were filled each morning with students performing the Yogoda sequence and other yogic exercises. Photos from Encinitas at the time showed students performing yoga asanas on the mound of lawn towards the end of the bluff, under Yogananda's guidance.

Led by Bernard Cole, SRF magazine issues began featuring lengthy in-depth articles about individual postures. In each issue, Bernard Cole, using the name

'Rev. Bernard', wrote four to six pages on a single asana. The first article was titled 'Padmasana: The Lotus Posture'. He began with, 'This is the first in the series of articles dealing with the art and science of the various asanas or body-postures of yoga,' and then stated he would eventually cover 'each of the eighty-four basic body-positions'.[19]

Cole compared yoga asanas to other 'systems of physical exercises' and concluded with the assertion that the Yogoda exercises and asanas of yoga (grouping them together) were more efficient at developing 'body control' than the others.

The asana practice was not linked with either Hatha yoga or Patanjali's system, but rather within the already existing context of Yogoda practice. To be complimentary he stated, 'While it is true that not all can practise these asanas,' the more 'simple, refreshing energization exercises' of SRF 'will accomplish for everyone virtually the same result'.[20]

It is remarkable that the focus was not on beginning asanas but advanced postures. In the very first issue, Cole proceeded to explain the benefits of padmasana, how the 'locked' position was able to 'preclude the possibility of the body's sprawling on the floor or swaying sideways, or to and fro, during certain ecstasies when the body becomes rigid'.[21] The article came with the recommendation to ease into it and only 'if it does not produce discomfort'. Regardless of the instruction, padmasana in its difficulty was quite the introduction to his column. The instructions stated that one should draw 'the right foot towards the body and place it, with the sole of the right foot turned upward, upon the left thigh. The left foot is then drawn towards the body and placed in a similar position upon the right thigh.' Most Americans, used to sitting in chairs and automobiles, would not have such flexibility. The SRF issues released sporadically, sometimes monthly, bi-monthly or quarterly, and had a circulation of about 20,000 copies per issue. Photographs were included, and the first issue pictured a young Norman Paulson, an American disciple of Yogananda, seated in the posture. Cole ended the four-page article stating the next issue would contain 'the special benefits which accrue from the practice of sarvangasana, or the shoulder stand'. Cole concluded, 'Each of the eighty-four basic body-positions is intended to facilitate the attainment of a definite and characteristic result.'[22]

Bernard Cole had a cadre of students perfecting advanced asanas, both for personal practice and for demonstration. Mostly in southern California, his monthly articles reached across the nation and into other parts of the world. These were serious American yogis practising asana, way ahead of their time.

72

MESSAGE OF UNITY

One of Yogananda's main reasons for returning to India was to fulfill the task of writing a book about India's saints. When Bishnu and Buddha stayed with Yogananda in California in 1938, Yogananda was immersed in the effort. Buddha remarked, 'Yogananda used to dictate it to his disciples at times when he was not writing it down, and whenever he was dictating he was in an extempore mood.'[1] The process of writing, dictation, multiple edits and drafts went on for nearly a decade.

When *Autobiography of a Yogi* came out in 1946, its popularity greatly expanded the reach of Yogananda. The book was marketed as one about India's 'gurus and masters' and very quickly became a success, but the book had a deeper message than just stories of Indian saints.

As *Autobiography* began being translated into other languages; the preface for the October 1950 German version contained a post-war unification message. Yogananda wrote, 'I travelled by car through Germany. What a marvelous country! And how friendly its people! To my German readers I send this message: Let us walk forward together – Germans, Indians, the whole human race!'

This was a call for 'spiritual growth' through transnational unity, global peace, even with a recent foe of America (Germany) that was the seed of thought throughout the book. 'The yogic message will encircle the globe,' he wrote. It will 'aid in harmonizing the nations' into a 'nameless league of human hearts'.[2] He aligned the political unity with a spiritual foundation. This unity, according to Yogananda, had its basis in the 'Science of Kriya Yoga', an ancient, global lineage which spanned the world's mystical traditions.[3] It was a commendable effort to combine the story of India's spiritual masters with the role of yoga as a global unifier. It was not a new angle but one that newly progressed from a pragmatic position.

When Yogananda had met with President Coolidge in 1927, he said that even if 'the machine guns' were destroyed, 'people would still fight, if their weapons were but stones'. 'Lasting peace' needed a 'spiritual understanding'.[4] By the forties, after the war, the world was coming to hear his message, and he found an increased adoption of the lifestyle he advocated.[5] Within his own circle of influence, Yogananda fostered the ideal of a worldwide colony of spiritual disciples, and he had been working towards that goal for over three decades in America. After the publication of *Autobiography*, it began to come to fruition.

In India, Yogoda Satsanga Society (YSS), like the Self-Realization Fellowship (SRF), was growing. Many of the dozens of new centers and temples being built during the forties were in India. When Yogananda had left in 1920, his interaction with his home country had been minimal but that changed after his return in 1935.

He wrote to his followers that he had been 'working incessantly for creating a permanent center in Calcutta, the crown city of Bengal, and I think I am almost successful'.[6] It would not happen while he was there; instead the YSS 'Students Home' opened and then moved to a location on Vivekananda Road next to Maniktala market. Just a few years after Yogananda left India, Tulsi Bose purchased property along the Howrah River, just a short walk away from the famous Kali temple in Dakshineswar. In *Autobiography*, Yogananda wrote of the place:

> A stately Yogoda Math in Dakshineswar, fronting the Ganges, was dedicated in 1939. Only a few miles north of Calcutta, the hermitage affords a haven of peace for city dwellers. The Dakshineswar Math is the headquarters in India of the Yogoda Satsanga Society and its schools, centers, and ashrams in various parts of India.

He wrote to tell Prakash Das, who was a director of YSS, that the name of the Calcutta ashram should be 'Tulsi-Yogoda Ashram'.[7]

Yogananda continued to interact with his family in Calcutta as well, in particular with Sananda. A number of the letters between the two were published in Sanada's memoir. More than any of the other members in the Ghosh family, Sananda was a 'close companion' of Yogananda and the one who met the various yogis that influenced their upbringing. When they were both young, he had gone with Yogananda to meet Mahendranath at 50 Amherst. The two of them, along with Tulsi Bose and Satyananda, had 'learned the sacred meditation technique of Kriya yoga' from their Sanskrit tutor, Shastri Mahasaya (Kebalananda). Sananda had also gone with Yogananda to Serampore, where he was 'initiated into Kriya by Sriyukteswar'.[8] After the death of his son during the communal fighting in 1946, Sananda had a spiritual crisis, which brought him closer to his brother.

Their letters, from 1946 to 1952, are affectionate. Yogananda implored his brother, 'Please come out of your sorrow. This is a drama of God ... play your part of sorrow or joy in the best way you can ... in spreading YSS in India.' Sananda listened, and with a renewed focus took up Kriya meditation. He went to Puri to 'take initiation in the higher Kriyas from Sri Bhupendra Nath Sanyal, the last living disciple of Lahiri'. He then started a YSS centre at 4 Garpar Road in 1947.

'Aren't you happy to see that from the very place which you are occupying now a worldwide movement has started which is continuously developing?' wrote Yogananda. A 'center in 4 Garpar Road' and construction of organizational facilities in Puri became a frequent topic in their letters over the years. 'Every place on earth is a place of tragedy', and 'the thought of past tragedies must be wiped away by clinging more and more to God and by doing some religious work ... erase all memories of tragedy by establishing the altar of meditation for God'.[9]

Sananda spearheaded multiple developments at the Karar Ashram in Puri during this period, including the building of its main meditation hall. Then, in 1950, Yogananda wrote to his brother:

> I would like you to undertake construction of a temple over the burial site
> of my beloved Gurudeva, to whom I owe everything. If God wills, I wish
> to bring many devotees from America to spiritual India; but before we visit,
> I want a beautiful *samadhi mandir* constructed in his memory.[10]

Yogananda was said to have resisted flying in airplanes, but he may have contemplated the trip by plane. A 1949 letter from Yogananda told Sananda to please 'keep it confidential that if God wills, by the end of the year I propose to visit India'.[11]

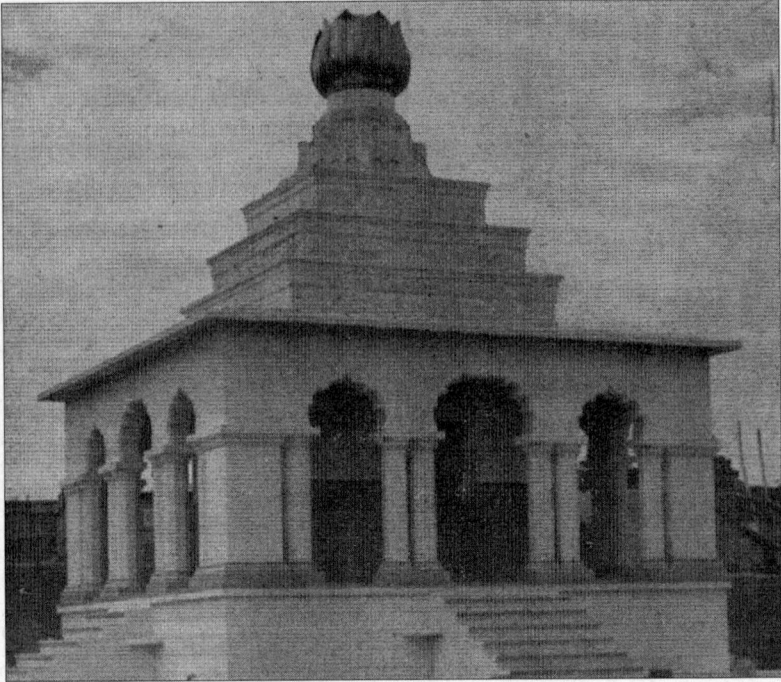

Samadhi Temple at Karar Ashram, Puri. Just after completion, 1952.
Source: Self-Realization Fellowship Magazine.

73

THE LAST SMILE

Today the eighty-four centers of the Self-Realization Fellowship and its affiliates
(in India) represent Paramhansa Yogananda in action.[1]
– Tribute from Swami Sivananda, Rishikesh, March 1952

The 7th of March 1952 marked the death of Yogananda. The day is commonly referred to as *mahasamadhi* or great *samadhi*. At the end of a public speech, Yogananda collapsed on stage. The death was unexpected, as he was just sixty-one years old and his practice of Yogoda claimed to bring longevity.[2]

When B. K. S. Iyengar came to America for the first time a few years later in 1956, 'still nobody knew' of yoga asanas. He recalled that in some places demonstrations were 'banned after Swami Yogananda collapsed' for fear that another yogi from India might also perform and die while on the stage.[3]

Yogananda's autopsy showed his death to be the result of congestive heart failure. Heart problems were passed along within the Ghosh family, as were problems with weight-gain in their later years. Growing up in Calcutta, Yogananda had a sweet tooth and would visit Nandalal's Sweets, across from his home, next to Sukia Street. Abroad, he adapted to the American habit of eating cheese as a vegetarian. By and large though, he seemed well, even putting an emphasis on a healthy lifestyle. He advocated for and ate a vegetarian diet, even having a vegetarian cookbook sold alongside regular SRF publications, but his inclusion of dairy products made the recipes quite rich in fat. A recipe for nutmeg loaf combined a cup of walnuts alongside a potato, onion, carrot, with rice, milk, tomato juice, butter and spices, all in a 'well-buttered baking dish'.[4]

'Fresh fruits and raw or barely cooked vegetables are your best friends,' was the advice Yogananda gave. 'You can eat whatever you want, actually, if you do it in moderation.'⁵ Hilda Charlton happened to share a car with him from Encinitas to Los Angeles and was surprised by his demeanour. She thought, 'Holy people should talk holy, they should talk God, you know, heaven.' But instead, Yogananda talked about how she 'should drink carrot juice and eat carrots and raw foods. He was really holistic.'⁶

Yogananda loved narrating how he had invented the mushroom burger and the 'history of how this meat substitute item had been conceived and popularized'.⁷ There were food advertisements in the magazine (the burgers were advertised in the magazine as having been 'prepared with pure butter') for the Lotus Cafe, which was run nearby his Encinitas hermitage. The cafe had a huge sign on the front, saying 'Mushroom Burgers' right next to the Lotus Gateway. Anyone driving along the Pacific Coast Highway would see it.⁸

There are many stories about the aftermath of Yogananda's death and the miracles which were believed to have occurred. The one most quoted dealt with his body showing no signs of decay. There were even ideas 'to enshrine it on SRF grounds for future viewing', a 'plan rejected by the Los Angeles Health Department'.⁹ It was later revealed though that 'Yogananda's body was embalmed twenty hours after death' and 'the uniqueness of the phenomenon had been greatly overstated'.¹⁰ Three weeks after the death, his casket was sealed by fire and placed inside the Great Mausoleum at Forest Lawn Memorial Park. There were many other fascinating accounts of supernatural events which his disciples claimed to have happened. For these, there were no easy answers.

Bernard Cole, the SRF Reverend and Hatha yoga teacher, reported an experience during the three-week period when his disciples watched the body, prior to his burial, 'Bernard started to realize that his guru had really left his body' and was gone for good, a hard thought for him to accept. Bernard reported that as he was watching Yogananda in his casket for a shift, he looked out the window at sunrise and had a vision:

While he was looking out over that beautiful scene, his spiritual eye opened and he found that he was seeing the physical reality and its astral counterpart at the same time... as the sun rose, Bernard saw another light moving through the mountains. It was, he said, an astral highway of light that was winding its way through the mountains, coming ever closer to Mt. Washington. And on that highway of light, Bernard saw figures moving.¹¹

The saints were coming for Yogananda. Of course, this was Bernard's own story, his own vision.

Another event, witnessed by multiple persons, was a vivid account of the aftermath of Yogananda's death as told by the Swami Premananda, the Bengali who led the Washington DC SRF organization. Premananda wrote, 'upon my arrival at Mount Washington six disciples of yours, my sister disciples, took me to your quarters upstairs'.[12] The seven of them stood in a semi-circle around the upstairs bedroom, where Yogananda lay:

> I was near to your heart on the left side. We all remained quiet in silence. I gazed upon your mortal form, and the thought of your immortal soul rose in my mind. I longed to commune with you once again. My soul prayed that you, your soul would come to us. You appeared before me, and I knew you were with us in the room. I placed my right hand upon your heart and motioned to my fellow sister disciples to do the same. Our hands jointly rested upon your heart and we all took a sacred vow. I uttered the words and all followed me. I felt your presence. To assure us of your presence among us, and the joyousness of your soul, you shed tears. Tears of love and joy trickled down the corners of both of your closed eyes. The disciples stood transfixed observing this unbelievable occurrence.[13]

The next day, Premananda was informed that Yogananda's brother Sananda 'had sent a cable from India', with a simple request that Premananda send the body home to be cremated at Nimtala Ghat in north Calcutta. Sananda had been in Puri, having just finished the construction of the *samadhi mandir* at Karar Ashram, and was 'beginning work on the floors of the veranda surrounding the temple' when the telegram arrived.

In the last letter from Yogananda to Sananda, which arrived 1 March, Yogananda had seen 'pictures of the temple, its interior, and the lotus made of copper', which were placed at the top. When Yogananda saw the pictures, he wrote back, 'I am ever grateful to you. I have had lotuses made here in America, but they are not equal to the one you made. What I couldn't do in America, you have done there.' His last written words to Sananda were, 'Life is ever ebbing away.'[14]

The burial decision was left to Premananda, since he was the 'Guru's countryman'. He recalled how Yogananda had 'made the final disposition' of the body of Sriyukteswar at Puri, so he decided that Yogananda's 'body should not be cremated – that it should be kept in the USA.'[15]

Yogananda's 'last smile' was one of four photographs taken of Yogananda 'just before being called to the dais' to take a seat prior to his last speech.[16] In the untouched photograph, he did not have even a wrinkle on his forehead, his eyes looked both bright and benefic. His smile was soft, yet vibrant. Seated next to the ambassador's wife, in front of him on the banquet table, were iced water, cookies and a dessert dish he had not touched.

His last speech, at the Biltmore Hotel in Los Angeles, welcomed the ambassador of India. Yogananda recited a poem of his titled 'My India' for the ambassador and the other guests assembled. It was a heart-filled poem about his personal love of India and what he felt he had received by being raised there. In it, he spoke of his hope for rebirth. 'If I must put on mortal garb once more,' then, 'would I there, in India, love to reappear!'

The poem concluded with two often quoted lines, which hearkened back to the days of his youth in Calcutta and the years when all he could think about was an escape to the Himalayas to live out his spiritual quest. 'Where Ganges, woods, Himalayan caves, and men dream God – I am hallowed; my body touched that sod.' One can easily imagine that as he spoke these last words, then lifted his eyes and fell to the stage floor, his life flew from the body to that place.[17]

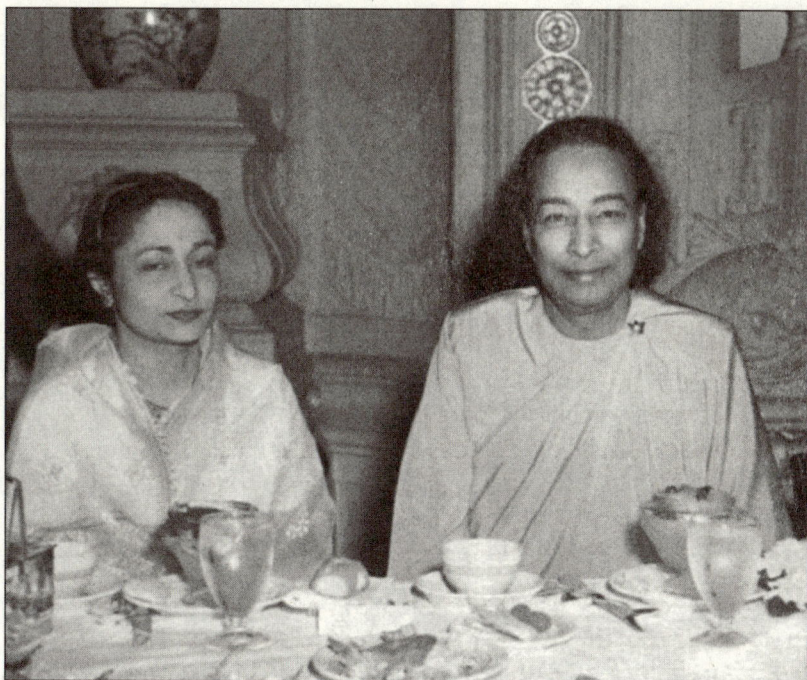
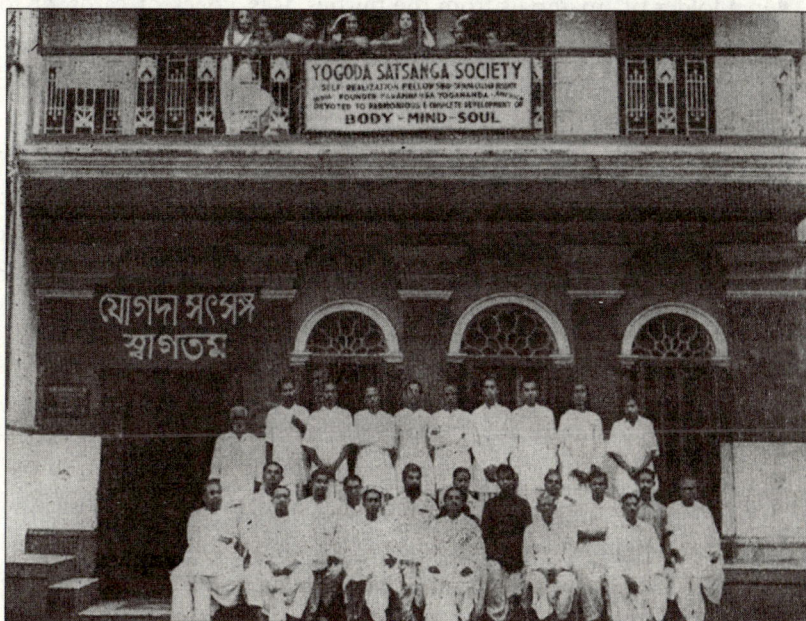

Top: Yogananda, March 7th, 1952. *Source: Wikimedia Commons.*
Bottom: 4 Garpar Road, Calcutta, circa 1950. *Source: Bayam Charcha.*

74

MAIDAN VIEW

If you get out into the center of the Maidan you will understand
why Calcutta is called the City of Palaces. The travelled American
said so at the Great Eastern.[1]
– Rudyard Kipling

Near the end of my library research, I find some lessons from Yogananda in a folder of materials from the thirties. It is a deck of cards, or so it seems to me, called 'Par=a=Gram'. After a quick look at a few of them, one titled 'Devotion' and two others, 'Balance' and 'Purity', I suddenly have the thought, 'Choose one'.

I pick up the entire set of cards, perhaps about thirty of them in total, all different colours. I slowly shuffle the deck a few times, trying not to be noticed by the librarians. I need to mix it up a bit, I think to myself, add some magic and loosen or tighten the fate to whichever one I choose. I split the deck; a few are left in the middle. I choose one from underneath, and see it is yellow. The Par=a=Gram is 'from Paramhansa Yogananda' and reads:

Whatever your position in life, it is you who put yourself there. The human will, when led by ignorance, causes nothing but confusion and trouble, but if it is tuned in with wisdom, it will be guided by Divine Will. Constantly carrying a thought with dynamic will-power means enforcing that thought until it becomes an outward form. When your will-power develops to that extent, you can control your destiny. Always be sure that what you want is right for you to have, then use all the forces of your will power to attain your objects, all the time keeping your mind on God. You will then find that your efforts will be crowned with success.[2]

Everything in it makes practical sense to me. I've seen it at work while collecting the materials for this book, over and over again. However, to me, the talk of 'God' has little practical value. What does 'God' have to do with it? I wouldn't describe myself as an atheist, but having grown up in a Christian theistic environment, I went through a detachment of such concepts after a heavy dose of Buddhist thought and practice. I can't relate to the language, at least how it comes across in my mind.

'What do you think about all this talk of God?' I ask Scott Lamps. We'd been walking around central Calcutta, having taken off the Sunday from training, and were discussing Bengali spiritual teachings. After getting online access at Oxford Books for emails and catching up, and a late afternoon British-style breakfast at Flury's, we walk along Park Street, then decide to escape the noise and walk to the Maidan of Calcutta.

It's been said that 'noise is life, and an excess of noise is a sign that life is good. There will be time for us all to be quiet when we are safely dead.' Well then, that makes the streets of Calcutta very much alive![3] After a few hours of walking around Calcutta, with its incessant honking of horns everywhere, a wonderful recourse is to escape to the massive empty acreage of the Maidan, about 1,000 acres in sum. It dates back to the mid-eighteenth century, when it was cleared by the British occupiers.

We come to rest in the shade, under a large banyan tree near a wide, open field. I sit atop some open roots about a foot above the dirt. To the left, across the grassy plain, the Victoria Memorial looks majestic, like it was held up in space – massive white marble against the backdrop of a rare blue sky. An old man comes by with his contraption; he's a chaiwala. I don't care for one, but buy it anyway, just to watch him pull out the different containers, mix the chai by hand, making it fresh with heat generated from a few coals underneath. He hands me the small earthen *kulhad* (terracotta cup), and afterwards, I place it near me on the ground between the roots, where water and time will melt the clay back into the soil for the tree.

The conversation with Scott moves from Yogananda to Sriyukteswar, then Ramakrishna, whose followers founded the Vedanta movement in Calcutta, which then spread around the world. Ramakrishna constantly spoke of God and Love of God, and went into states of *samadhi* in public, complete with spontaneous, yet obscure, bodily mudra formations as he stood transfixed in time.

'When they speak of spending every moment focused on God,' Scott explains, 'I think of it as realizing the fundamental connectedness of everything to every moment, without judgment or even reflection, just pure awareness and ultimately, the feeling of love.' The thought reminds me of something I've heard from Erich Schiffman, a yoga and meditation teacher based out of Los Angeles.

The very first research trip I undertake for this project is to Los Angeles in October 2014. It's for one week, from Tuesday until Sunday. My plan is to meet someone named Sando Pande, who is apparently, as far as I can make out from the website, a student of Buddha Bose. It is also clear that Sando has some sort of relationship with Bikram Choudhury (of Bikram Yoga), but since he is the only person I've found in America with any sort of tangible relation to Buddha, I fly to Los Angeles to meet him and show him a copy of the *Yoga Asanas* manuscript and photo album of Buddha Bose. Sando, I think, may be the one to help me bring forth the unpublished manuscript, but I don't know what to expect, since he hasn't replied to my email.

On Tuesday night in Westwood at 7:30 p.m., I wait at the local recreation centre on Sepulveda Blvd, where he unceremoniously teaches a weekly Hatha yoga class. He is teaching yoga at Recreation Centers this week, all close to central Los Angeles, in Westwood and Pasadena. I have great plans in mind, a schedule that has me attending all three of his classes in four days. In addition, I hope to have a private interview to record his responses to my long list of excited questions. This plan is short-lived.

At first, Sando is overbearing, angry, and threatening to sue if I publish. 'It's a fake!' he shouts to my face. He is built with a strong physical presence from weightlifting. (Probably why he's been given the nickname 'Sandow' in Calcutta.) I calmly persist, with explanation and details of how I've come across Buddha's work.

Though he has not replied to my emails, he does tell me that he's seen what I've written. Not wanting to put him on the defensive, I explain to him, repeating what I said in the email. 'I've come across the Buddha Bose album of 84 *Yoga Asanas* and want you to take a look.'

He just shakes his head, 'It's not true.'

The experience feels like I am showing a relative a treasured heirloom that they don't even know exists. 'Yes, it is true, I have a copy, please take a look.' I pull two chairs out from the table, hoping that he will take a seat. He declines, so I proceed to show him the album, flipping through its photocopied pages as we stand.

'Is this the only copy?' he asks.

'Well, yes, that I have. These are not the originals, if that's what you mean.'

He looks at me sternly, 'You cannot share these. They are stolen. You cannot publish these.' I haven't even brought up the notion yet of publishing the book. 'He's my uncle, family, these are not yours.' He makes some remark about my being an American and that this does not belong to me. I don't want a confrontation, and he is getting pretty hot.

Just then, a student, having showed up to take his class, informs Sando that the classroom door is locked. He goes to grab the key, and this gives me a moment to collect my thoughts before proceeding.

When Sando comes back, I show him the inscription at the front of the album, Buddha's dedication to an 'Uncle Edward'.

'Do you know who this is?' I ask, 'Uncle Edward?' He shakes his head no. I go on a bit more with details and mention something about Bishnu Ghosh's yoga alongside Buddha Bose.

'Those are different, not the same yoga.' I sense that there is quite a bit of family drama, that this isn't just about the yoga and maybe Sando himself has left some sort of conflict behind in Calcutta. 'You need to meet with Rooma; she is Buddha Bose's daughter. Have you talked with her?'

I had emailed Rooma and gotten no response from her either. 'I will, I will talk with her. I have no intention of publishing this without the family of Buddha Bose being involved,' I tell him.

He becomes a bit more inquisitive at this point, and we start to go through the copy of the album, with me sharing how I came about it, and eventually, he lets down some of his barriers and starts sharing information. Perhaps, I think, he can sense that I am not bringing this forth for greed, fame or any other distraction. I am just genuinely excited about it and want to share it with others that love doing this asana practice.

I ask him a personal question, 'Why don't you teach more people?' He replies curtly, 'That's for Bikram. I just teach in places like this, Hatha yoga, that's all.'

I can't understand it. 'But you have so much knowledge, having studied under Buddha Bose, and you learned the yoga from him.'

He shakes his head, 'No, that's not for me.'

We come upon the page of Buddha in the posture of *virabhadrasana* (warrior). Sando smiles and replies, 'That is the logo of the school.' I get the sense that he knows this is authentic now and feels connected to it all. I offer him the photos and scanned copies I've made, knowing I can get better ones. He's grateful and once again mentions that I should go to India. 'There is also a granddaughter of Bishnu Ghosh, she teaches yoga there too.' He's lessened his agitation towards me, and I tell him I will reach out further to him, if he wants to talk more.

I'm in two minds coming out of this meeting. On the one hand, I really don't want to do something in putting this out that is going to make anyone angry at me, or, who knows, get Bikram with his lawsuits involved, or his daughter in India to start claims about it being stolen. I want no part in a drama; just want to see it shared, but I can also feel how detached I am from everything.

I leave the meeting with Sando and say to myself, 'The whole thing is over, finished.' I have no idea what to do with the remaining time though, so instead I just take to roaming around southern California for the next five days. I relay the conflict and outcome to Scott and Ida Jo. I'd previously invited the two of them to help with the potential publication. 'What do we do with the album project now?'

75

AWAKE

The next morning, I go to visit Erich Schiffmann in Venice for a yoga and meditation class. Erich learned yoga under Iyengar and Krishnamurti, but he credits Yogananda with putting him on the path of spirituality. As a young surf-teen growing up in Los Angeles in the seventies, he came across a copy of *Autobiography* and couldn't take his eyes off the cover photo of Yogananda. He realized, 'What this guy's got ... I want some of that too!'

Now he teaches a style called Freedom Yoga, which integrates asana series with free movement, mudras and meditation. The postures, he explains, naturally came about from yogis in India, who would spontaneously move into them after sitting for long periods. I know, from my own practice of attending long meditation courses where I would be alone in a cell for hours just with breath and awareness, that at times the body begins moving without any thought to initiate it. Freedom Yoga is a way to begin the process of getting past a routine and into the present moment. I connect with it because it combines the static with the dynamic in a way that moves beyond viewing something as stillness or movement.[1] But, there is something else I am coming to terms with too.

'God...' Erich starts to explain. Then, as he must sense the resistance to this word, he gives a prologue:

OK, let me put it this way. First – the word, God. Try to wash your mind clean of what you think the word 'God' means. It's hard. Essentially, though, the word 'God' means Being with a capital 'B'. Being. It means Supreme BEING, the Supreme I AM, Existence – that which is being, everything that's being.

He goes on, posing the question:

Therefore, when you ask the question, 'What is the truth here, really?' and you put the pause in there, then that which is really Real is going to start becoming obvious.

The answer to 'What is the truth here really is God Is. OK?' I'm not there yet, so Erich changes the words:

Now, if the words, 'God Is' trip you up, then the answer is, 'Life, live.' What is the truth here, really? 'Life, live' – and then pay new attention to the experience you are having. Something is happening. Something Real is happening. 'Life, live' is happening. And the deal is to be in the middle of 'Life, live' with less ignorance, less of your usual mindset.[2]

Words and concepts get in the way of how to do yoga, and really, how yoga works. 'It's a way of listening', and of 'being guided from within'.[3] Afterwards, I think about going to Yogananda's Mother Temple at Mt Washington, which I had marked on the map as being close to where Sando teaches. A month ago, I listened to *Autobiography of a Yogi* for the first time, but honestly, I couldn't find the thread, skipped through places; it seems archaic in its language. As I leave Venice, I skip the freeway turn to Mt Washington. 'Why bother,' I think, feeling drawn to continue east. I drive out of Los Angeles on the freeway, towards Joshua Tree.

I will head for the desert, I decide, and a few hours later, I am in Twentynine Palms, at a resort hotel I find discounted on Priceline. I mull it over – what to do next. The answer doesn't take long. After a soak in the outdoor natural hot spring, back in the hotel room, an impulse overcomes any thoughts I had of abandoning the project. I log on and email Scott and Ida, 'I am going to Calcutta, India in March. Tickets are under $900 right now, which is a terrific deal.' I am surprised to hear back from them quickly. They agree to come along, so we all buy tickets for Calcutta, leaving in five months. That night, I feel a shift, with dreams of a distant land and a long voyage.

The next morning, I wake up and think, 'What have I done?' I am mildly excited but unsure of what is happening. It feels like I am guessing. I drive south, towards the Salton Sea to a place called Salvation Mountain, where artists have dumped buckets and buckets of donated paint on the hillside, making a sort of 'Beatles meets Jesus' collage of saintly portraits and spiritual slogans painted atop dirt. The scene is strangely discombobulated against the background of stark desert plains and scattered trailers where people live in seclusion. It is a good place to let go of my thoughts and recollect myself for the next move. Again, through my moments of uncertainty, a thought comes which I feel certain to follow: I will go back to the ocean before the evening is over.

I glance at the document that I prepared before travel, where I typed, 'Yogananda Places – Encinitas', along the Pacific coast, and this becomes my destination. The traffic is smooth through the outskirts of San Diego. I reach Highway 101 and look out over the ocean, the sun low on the horizon. Sooner than I thought possible, I am in Encinitas. Pulling up to the small hotel, I check in. A few minutes later, at 4:59 p.m. exactly, I am amazed to find myself walking into the Yogananda ashram one minute before the gates are shut to visitors for the day.

I walk around the 'Yogoda Dream Hermitage', with its 'entrancing Encinitas Elysium shore', as Yogananda called it, and watch the sunset. I find a plaque commemorating where the Lotus Temple had stood, before its fateful slide into the ocean; its concrete entrance steps all that remain.

The ashram is a pleasant and calm place, with a rich feeling of history. The next morning, I practise asanas on the beach, then return again to the high cliffs and sit facing the ocean. Meditation is followed by a stop at the bookstore and cafe, but all along, it seems like I am in a daze. I am just moving through the motions, not able to fully shake the experience with Sando or fully comprehend how spontaneously I've decided to go to Calcutta. It feels like I am being pulled along, with a sense of willing detachment, to go with the flow.

I didn't know it at the time, but when I decided not to visit Mt. Washington, and instead to drive to the desert, I was getting closer to, not further away from, Yogananda. From 1950 to 1952, after he reached a stage of deeper meditation, Yogananda spent a lot of time in seclusion at his desert retreat in Twentynine Palms, writing his commentaries on the *Bhagavad Gita*. And now, here I was in Encinitas for three days at Yogananda's Golden Lotus ashram, also something I'd not previously planned.

I wander into a tourist shop next to a Whole Foods, and stare whimsically at the art on the walls. A particular one catches my eye, showing a photo of a beach alongside a ridge, titled 'Cardiff by the Sea'. A nice name, a stunning photo and just for a moment I think about whether I should purchase it. The next moment, it feels like I have awakened from a dream, as if a light bulb turns on. Something inside me says, 'Hey, why buy this? Go to this exact place in the photo right now.' The photo was taken just a walk away from where I stand. I move … no, I take off, like a spark has shocked me. I head south, jaywalking across Highway 101, then speed down a long flight of wooden stairs all the way to the sand, I remove my shoes and go to a spot near the southward cliffs, from the photo. The place is called Swami's beach by the locals who surf its waves, and up to the north was Yogananda's Encinitas ashram.[4] It is early afternoon, and I stay well past sunset, just breathing and then meditating on the beach. Afterwards, in the dark, I stride slowly in a sublime state by the water's edge along the shore beneath the hermitage cliff, back to the hotel in Encinitas.

That next day, I call a cousin of mine that lives nearby, and we arrange to go and view the movie *Awake* in Encinitas. The biopic just came out a few weeks ago and is showing nightly in the town's La Paloma Theatre, built in 1928. The movie tells much of the life of Yogananda, in a way that I have not seen before.

I thought I was arriving in Los Angeles for a week of yoga asana practice with Sando. Instead, the short California trip has led to the places most significant to Yogananda. I decide that when I return to DC, I will go over to the Library of Congress and read the volumes of his organization's newsletter, which dates all the way back to 1925, with up to a dozen copies a year. I know I'll find some sort of interaction with Calcutta yoga through those writings, and so the research begins.

PART ELEVEN

PILGRIMAGE AND YOGI SCHOOL

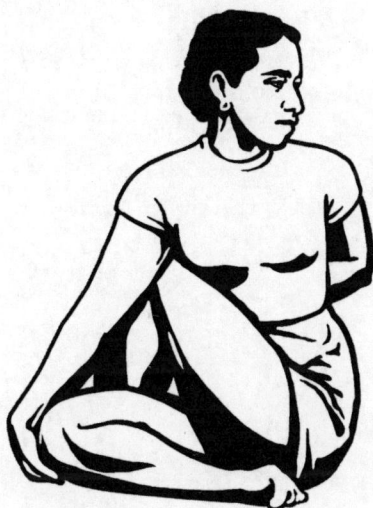

PART ELEVEN

PILGRIMAGE AND YOGI SCHOOL

76

HOLY KAILAS

*As I looked for the next phase in Buddha's life, I realized that to follow his path,
I would be led outside Calcutta, to the Himalayas.*

Near the beginning of the research I find a reference to a book titled *Holy Kailas*, authored by Buddha Bose. I have no idea about the contents and can only locate a single copy in the entire world, which is in the Indian National Library of Calcutta. I ask my research guide, Arup, to arrange for us to go there the first day in Calcutta. I also ask a grandson of Buddha Bose, Pavitra Shekhar, to come along.

Pavitra's father was Ashok, the eldest son of Buddha. Buddha died when Pavitra was seven years old, but he can recall a few memories from their time together: 'The disciplined manner in which all of us would practise yoga, each to his or her own prescription, sharp at 7:30 every evening. Sundays off!'[1]

At the National Library, we encounter a labourious process, our first taste into the bureaucratic protocols of Calcutta. First, we must locate the wooden pull-out card catalogs, find the book number and fill out a long form. We place the form onto a desk and wait for several hours as they search for the book in the vast underground archives. Once the book is located, we sit down to look at the contents. It is apparent from the time-stamp with the day's date that the book has not been checked-out recently, if ever.

What follows is deeply moving, as Pavitra reads through the introduction by his grandfather. He whispers, 'I didn't know this ... it is my first time knowing this, reading it here.' It reinforces in me the feeling of sorrow; how much of Buddha's life is unknown. What happened, I wonder, which all but made this part of Buddha's life forgotten, even among parts of his family?

When I locate the lone public copy of *Holy Kailas*, it feels like I've found the holy grail, with its second-hand access into what Buddha had experienced. After I read about Buddha's film, inspired by *Holy Kailas*, and having exhausted the search in Calcutta, I realize that there isn't anyone in Calcutta who knows a whole lot about this period of Buddha's life. To know Buddha after Kedarnath, I needed to go into the Himalayan Mountains, to find someone who can tell the rest of the story.

Just when this becomes evident, a curious news article crosses my path about a Himalayan museum that just opened. The article mentions photographs on display at the museum in Mussoorie.[2] The display, it says, includes 'a rare photograph of the Viceroy of Tibet', revealing much about the holy shrines during the pre-Independence era, including 'the other three temples with Kedarnath, the Yamunotri, Gangotri and Badrinath'. The museum's curator, Sameer Shukla, said, 'the rare pictures of Garhwal and Tibet were passed on to me by Swamini Guru Priyananda, who had received these from Buddha Bose, an adventurer and disciple of Paramhansa Yogananda'. The curator went on to explain that the photos captured Buddha's extensive travel in the Garhwal Himalayas and Tibet, 'capturing the culture and tradition of Himalayas in his camera'. They 'reveal that the earlier route to the Manasarovar Lake in China went through Badrinath', along with many photos of the famous Kailash Mountain peak.[3]

Obviously intrigued, I make the voyage to the museum in Mussoorie to see the photographs first hand. While there, Sameer explains to me, as I look over each of the hundred photographs, that he had been given the photographs by a Swamini named Guru Priyananda, affectionately known as Mataji.[4]

The year after Buddha was healed at Kedarnath, he returned to the Himalayas in the summer of 1949. Buddha covered treks throughout the Himalayan range, visiting 'Himalayan religious shrines' and mountain peaks '13 times on foot', making annual treks that took much time and planning. He went to 'Kedarnath, Badrinath, Nandan Kanon, Amarnath, Gangotri, Rakshastal, Manasarovar and Holy Kailas'.[5] Nearly every year, from 1947 until the early sixties, Buddha would trek in the Himalayas.

Sometimes, with up to half a dozen porters, he brought along relatives from Calcutta for the pilgrimages spanning months. For one of the treks, Bishnu joined him. A photo showed them standing in front of Kedarnath Temple, most likely in the early fifties. In the snapshot, Buddha and Bishnu stood near the front of the temple where Buddha was healed. At the entrance, beside the large stone-carved Ram Bull, Nandi, the gatekeeper, faced the temple. The Kedarnath Temple priest, Pandit Bahuguna, stood between them. Buddha has a large smile, and Bishnu has his palms pressed together in *pranam*, perhaps giving thanks for the healing of his son-in-law.

Buddha's elder sister, Haydee, also travelled with him to the Himalayas. Haydee had married an Indian military official and moved to Ranchi in the early fifties. In the photo, they were hiking up from Gangotri to Gaumukh, the glacial origin of the Ganges River.

'After knowing the power of Kedarnath,' Buddha thought, 'there must be thousands of people who would love to come to Kedarnath but cannot do so for some reason or the other.' He wondered, 'Many have become old and weak. How can they come here?'[6] He began to bring photography equipment to share the captured moments. At first, he made a slideshow of black and white photographs, accompanied by his own narration. Inspired by his family and others who heard the story, he 'decided to make a movie' but 'not an ordinary film'. He embarked on making a 'holy picture'.[7]

Buddha 'took more cine-film to supplement the first consignment'. More and more people wanted to hear the narration and see the film. 'I took a colour movie picture of those holy places so that I might give a little glimpse of these places to those who might not be able to undertake the travel in spite of their wishes,' Buddha later wrote. By viewing the film and listening to the narration, the moviegoers could experience a pilgrimage to these holy places, one they may never have the opportunity to make themselves. 'It was a silent movie. Buddha would give live commentary with a microphone from behind the stage.'[8]

Swami Pranavananda wrote that the 'very interesting Technicolor cine-film' ran 'for about two hours'. Many watched the film.[9]

Sunanda Bose, recounting the experience of her childhood, recalled that 'his slide show was very popular in those days. It was like a documentary, not exactly a professional film.' She remembered, 'His first slide show was black and white, pictures in the Himalayas.' When Buddha got hold of a movie camera and 'took the photographs in Technicolor', which 'was a new discovery in those days', it made for a 'very beautiful', captivating experience, as 'at that age we were not exposed to such films but found this nice and new'.[10]

After Buddha showed the film for a few years, to friends and family, he started showing it at larger venues. He wrote that 'everywhere my patrons requested me to write a book giving a detailed description of the route to the Holy Shrines'. This is what prompted him 'to bring out a publication', making it as 'illustrative as possible'.[11]

Holy Kailas was published in 1954, and a copy of it was placed in the National Library of Calcutta in 1956. It laid out the route taken to the different pilgrimage destinations, as if it were a descriptive guidebook for those about to take up the pilgrimage themselves. It included thirty black and white photographs, a detailed 'route map' drawn 'to include railways, bus routes, paths, passes and rivers' and descriptions of each place.

The book proceeds from east to west across the Himalayas. It began with the 'western Himalayan shrines' of Yamunotri, Gangotri, Kedarnath, Badrinath and then Nandan Kanan. Afterwards, the reader was told of Rakshas Tal, Lake Manasarovar and Holy Kailas Mountain. The proceeds of the film revenue went to the Yoga Cure Institute.

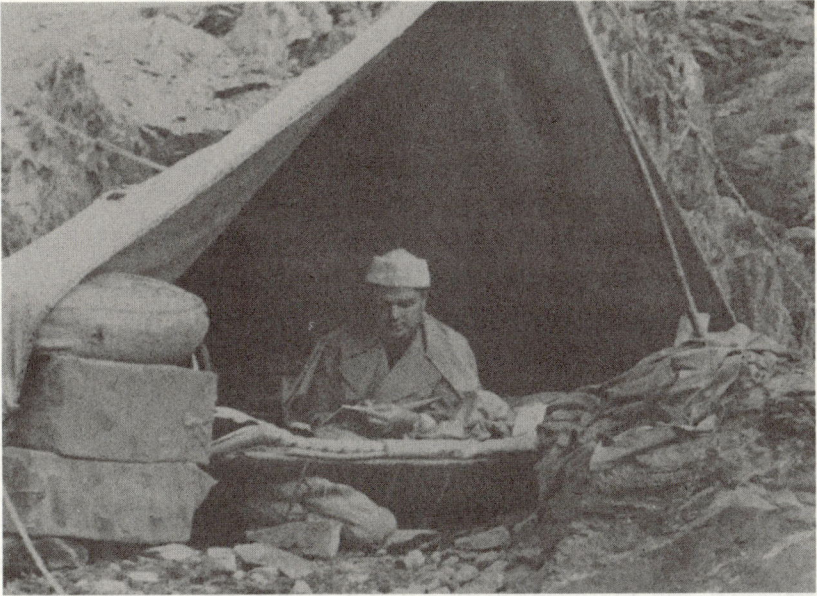

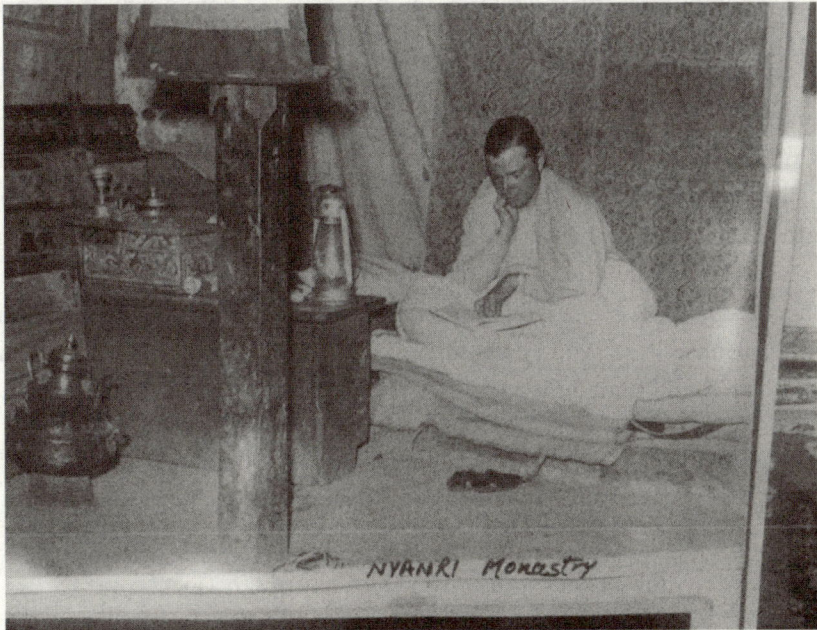

Top: Buddha Bose at Himalayan Monastery. Bottom: Buddha Bose at campsite.
Courtesy of Mataji, Soham Heritage & Art Center, Mussoorie, India.

YOGA CURE, 1 FEBRUARY 1953

We have named our institution Yoga Cure Institute because we cure diseases.[1]

The children of Bishnu (with his wife Ashalata) and Buddha (with his wife Ava Rani) grew up together in the house at 4/2 Rammohan Roy Road. Somewhat surprisingly, both of Buddha's siblings returned to India during the fifties. His younger brother, Dennis, because he was born in Calcutta, was required to join the Indian Armed Forces. His elder sister Haydee, married an Indian, Jagjit Singh, in London and, in 1948, had a son she named Ranjit.[2] Their move to Ranchi brought Haydee and Buddha closer together, and their mother, Emily, joined them in India, boarding a steamer from Sussex to Bombay in March 1956. Ranjit, Haydee's son, stayed in India for a few years, until his father died in 1958. He had fond memories of the time in Ranchi, interacting with his Uncle Buddha and even staying with his cousins at 4/2 Rammohan Roy Road. Ranjit remembered:

I used to visit for stay-overs as a child during school holidays on a few occasions. My uncle had a film projector and would show children's cartoon movies sometime during my stay. This was before the days of television. He used to show movies with no sound, of his trips to Tibet.[3]

Ranjit, later known as Ray, recalled that at night he and the other children would be lined up 'like sausages', laid next to each other to sleep. During the monsoon season, Ranjit watched from the second storey as the palm trees swayed so far over he thought they would snap. He fit in well with his cousins. He would play with Ashok and Arun, 'who both seemed the same age', and

Bishwanath, along with Karuna and Rooma, the youngest of the Ghosh and Bose children.

What is now called Ghosh's Yoga College was once called Yoga Cure Institute, which was founded by Bishnu and Buddha, and their wives, Ashalata and Ava Rani.

The Yoga Cure Institute was formed in 1953 according to the official documents retrieved.[4] While this might be looked at as an extension of what was already ongoing, the registration codified how yoga could work as a commercial family-run business – a yoga family. The registration outlined that the 'object' of Yoga Cure was 'to improve the mental and physical health of the people by Eastern Yoga System, to cure diseases and mental deficiency by said system, to carry on research in the Yoga system, to promote charitable dispensaries and charitable institutions, to help poor students, to construct *dharmashalas*, to repair temples, *Devsaba*, and to help *sadhus*.'[5]

Yoga Cure was a relatively simple formation – a family-run business which provided exercise routines for Calcutta's urban residents, with this message: 'If you can control your mind, you can control the results of the physical karma. Yoga-*bayam* gives one the control.' A marriage of religion and exercise was completed with therapeutic yoga that offered a 'cure' to the suffering people living in the city of Calcutta.[6] The cure was through a 'prescription' for each patient, similar to the Western techniques of physical therapy.[7] Most likely, this was instituted by Gouri Shankar Mukerji after he returned from Germany as a doctor of medicine.[8]

The system of Yoga Cure was, broadly speaking, designed to be an alternative to any other medical treatment and claimed to be a cure for disease. In the beginning pages of the publication *Yoga-Cure*, written by Bishnu, forty 'different diseases that could be treated and cured through Yoga' are listed.[9] As if there were any doubt, Bishnu added a note at the end of the list: 'If you are suffering – contact me personally or by correspondence – and let me prove the truth in my statement made above.' Above all, what Bishnu taught was about the 'little things' or habits of our 'daily life'. The 'stress and strain both nervous and muscular and even of your brain' could be kept at bay. Yoga provided the daily 'good habits for health' in order 'to live a long life'.[10]

From the beginning, the intention was to expand. In general, the organization was a means for money to come into the family via the institute, through propagation of the yoga system. Any person was eligible for membership with an annual subscription of six rupees, 'which shall be paid in 12 monthly installments'. Patients would come 'for cure of diseases and mental deficiency', through 'advice and guidance' and sign up for 'donations and subscriptions'. The proposed 'income and properties' of Yoga Cure went far beyond individuals to include research and 'print and purchase' of 'journals, periodicals, books, leaflets, etc.' This is how the formation of Yoga Cure intersected with the Holy Kailas Pilgrimage Tour done by Buddha Bose. Admission fees and purchases of the book would be managed through this new family organization.

After India's Independence in 1947, integrating the practice of India's physical culture system – Hatha yoga – took on national importance. Shortly afterwards, Ironman Publishing put out two books. *Exercises for Health* and *Yoga Bayam for Health*, previously only available in Bengali, were printed in English, which, alongside their popular charts, reached many throughout Bengal. Within the issues of *Bayam Charcha*, not a month went by without multiple articles on the subject of developing 'healthy citizens' of India:

> It is a fact no nation can survive without healthy citizens. Therefore, the health of its citizens should be of paramount concern to the society. That is why religious preachers like Swami Vivekananda as well as the great heroes of our great freedom struggle laid stress on physical culture, sports, etc. Any effort by any association towards this end is a welcomed step. Towards the goal, *Bayam Charcha Patrika*, a leading magazine on physical culture, sports, *yogasana*, etc. has been doing commendable work by publishing its edition in Bengali for the last three years.[11]

The emphasis was on healthful living and daily exercise, with the intention of integrating this into the schools:

> When Bishnu began recommending that children begin doing yoga, his approach was to limit the number of asanas to those being suitable for their age and bodily needs, such as *bhujangasana*, *sasangasana* and *matsyasana*. He was quoted that the practice of these and others that he recommended be used to give 'proper proportion to the limbs' to facilitate 'the steady growth in children without making the body muscle bound'.[12]

Bishnu's role as integrator, organizer and promoter of yoga as exercise within Indian society was immense, particularly in Calcutta. He even had a radio show. Monotosh Roy assisted Bishnu with his lessons on yoga, broadcast from the Calcutta radio station All India Radio. Another student told of how Bishnu 'was so passionate' to 'awaken the spirit of doing yoga and other easy exercises that he couldn't resist himself to take the microphone on public demands'. Bishnu 'used to deliver talks on "Early Morning Exercises" every morning at 6 a.m. from All India Radio, with lots of humour.'

I find Yogacharya Mukul Dutta online. He is described in a customer review as 'a disciple of the great yoga guru Bishnu Charan Ghosh ... a pleasure to interact with and knowledgeable' and that 'his classes are held at Pearl Clinic at Hindustan Road in the mornings and at his residence at Moulali in the evenings'. After I am able to locate him, I send a message asking him about his background.

Born in 1953, Mukul 'received training directly from Bishnu Ghosh'. He finished training in 1970. I ask what he did next.

'My master recommended me to teach yoga to the school of Paramhansa Yogananda's Ranchi centre', Mukul replies. Bishnu also directed Mukul to a formal education in physiology, which he has taught for the past forty-six years in Calcutta. Mukul describes Bishnu as extremely witty, quick to bring laughter to a situation, with a jovial and friendly demeanour, and down to earth. It feels to me as if, the more I interact with Mukul, the more he embodies his guru's characteristics.

After we meet in Calcutta for a first interview, Mukul's engine of devotion to his teacher Bishnu Ghosh is reignited, and he begins sharing information, helping me set up interviews and posting further information online. Eventually, he posts that he found Bishnu's book, titled *Yoga-Cure*.[13] The preface of the hand-sized pamphlet announced yoga's preventive and rehabilitative effects:

Yoga teaches you to shake off stress & strain both nervous and muscular and even of the brain, quickly before damage is done to your system and before your immunity to disease is destroyed.

The booklet, first published in 1961, contains thirty-two asanas, mudras and pranayama techniques. Very much a 'Yoga Family' booklet, the postures were the work of Bishnu's children. Karuna, '14 years, my daughter', posed for the photos, which were taken by Bishwanath, '16 years, my son'.

GHOSH'S COLLEGE OF PHYSICAL EDUCATION

Sends

Experienced Instructors & Lady Instructresses

POSSESSING PERSONALITY

Trained by **Shri Bishnu Ghosh,** *Presonally*

IN

YOGIC ASANAS, AGILITY AND
FAT REDUCING EXERCISES
AND

To Take Care of

**Polio Cases, Rickets, Corpulent Boys and
Girls of All Ages**

And Also of people Suffering from

**Gastric Troubles, Chronic Dysentery,
Constipation, Flatulence, Hyper-
Acidity, Hysteria & Nervousness**

KALIKA PRESS (P.) LTD.

Advertisement, *Bayam* Charcha.
Source: Yoga Cure. Courtesy of Ghosh's Yoga College.

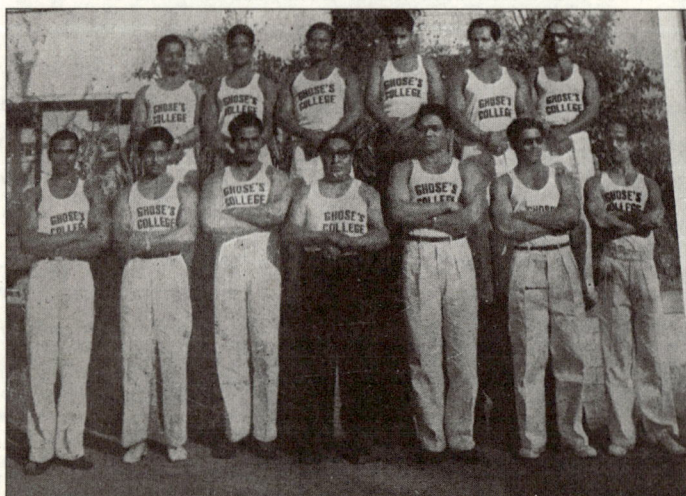

Bishnu Ghosh with his bodybuilding students, circa 1962.
Courtesy of Ghosh's Yoga College.

78

MAGIC AND SCIENCE OF YOGA

There is a strong link between magic and yoga, which extends deep into the past. The central theme of the *Ramayana*, an Indian epic poem from thousands of years ago, 'hinges on the magical performances' of its characters in its teachings.[1] In the first millennium texts, we find magic, trick or deceit being synonymous in meaning with the usage of the word yoga – the 'attainment' of 'supernatural powers by means of psychophysical methods'.[2]

> The medieval practitioners of asana and pranayama were interested in the acquisition of supernatural power in the context of material, worldly existence. It was not until the early nineteenth century that a discourse of spirituality was employed to replace magic and esoteric sexuality in the practice of asana and pranayama.[3]

During the medieval Hatha yoga period, an array of seemingly bizarre metaphysical alchemical practices among yogis would enable the *siddhi*, a type of elemental magician, to provide 'the power of performing miracles, of commanding the elements'.[4] The meditative yogi could choose to adapt 'to a super-sensible reality and to affect this adjustment by an increasingly aloofness from the world of fleeting shows'.[5] The yogi, 'by becoming a master of his inner forces', could also become a 'master of the forces of nature'.[6] Their intersection with the wider society had always been subtle, part strange, part alluring and part sinister. When the world opened up, the representation in the early eighteenth century became a syndicated promotion of magical yoga-related interactions.[7] The mysteries of the East, first espoused to the West through the magical and supernatural feats of yoga, were debased to conjecture and trickery.[8]

The bodily practice was lesser known until its revival in the twentieth century, and by the thirties, scientific study began to encourage the healing uses of yoga.[9] Asanas were 'reconfigured as ancient forms of movement cure, with individual postures prescribed for specific diseases'.[10] The science of a cure became the magic.

The ancient yogis and rishis are said to have presented asanas as cures for villagers who sought them out, and medieval era texts tell of their cure for disease. There were therapeutic notations in the classical yoga texts that we can take at face value. This was something that occurred experientially, as generational knowledge was passed down from guru to disciple, or among the yogis themselves during conversations or teachings, without a written record.

With modern yoga, the fusion and use of medical terminology served to validate the claims of Hatha yoga as India's physical culture system and its ability to cure. The validation of science was seen throughout the early development of modern yoga, from the disciples of Madhavadas to the monthly columns in Yogananda's magazine on scientific developments, which complemented the spiritual understanding of Kriya yoga. As Buddha Bose and other Indian yoga teachers sought to explain the practice to the West, they used science.

The anatomy section of Buddha Bose's book from 1938, Sivananda's from 1933 and earlier books from Kuvalayananda and Yogendra utilized Western anatomical sources to add scientific heft to their claims. Yogacharya Mukul Dutta, a trained physiologist, remarked that the medical descriptive text found in Buddha's 1938 yoga asana book reminded him of Cunningham's *Manual of Practical Anatomy*. First published in 1896, the manual went through a dozen editions and was the prime British text for Bengalis in Calcutta who were pursuing study within the anatomical sciences.[11] Before Cunningham's *Practical Anatomy*, it and other forms of science had been 'part of the curriculum for medical students' in Calcutta, but Cunningham seems to have been Buddha's source for the anatomical discussion in his 1938 *Yoga Asanas* book.[12]

The claims of an anatomical-based 'yoga cure' became standard promotion in the early to mid-twentieth century yoga texts and at the Yoga Cure Institute. For example, around 1950, an article titled '*Paschimottanasana*', by *Bayamacharya* Bishnu Charan Ghosh in *Kishor Bangla*, provided detailed instructions on the seated posture. It ended with the claim, 'All of you who have problems in the morning with bowel movement will find this asana extremely beneficial and the problem will disappear after a few days of practice. This asana is also beneficial in the initial stage of dysentery; liver and spleen problems can also be solved by this asana.'

For a broad number of ailments, case studies were supplied, and the Yoga Cure Institute added yearly statistics. In one year, out of thirty cases of asthma, seventeen were cured.[13] In-depth articles on individual asanas were written in *Bayam Charcha*, and pamphlets were produced:

> The practice of Yoga Asanas and Pranayama cures so many so-called incurable diseases, such as chronic dysentery; hyperacidity; flatulence gastric troubles; constipation; tonsil troubles; asthma; nervousness; allergies; colds, etc. You may be a great philosopher, scientist or educationalist, or a clever lawyer, or a millionaire, or a successful industrialist. But do not forget that you are still prey to physical ills.[14]

This style became more rigorous when Gouri Shankar Mukerji returned from Germany in the mid-fifties as a medical doctor. Gouri brought with him a new physiological understanding for the treatment of disease through yoga. During his time at the German Sports University in Cologne, Gouri, together with his colleagues, W. Spiegelhoff and W. Hollmann, researched the physiological effects of yoga asana practice to determine its best use, safety and possible contraindications. The results were preliminary and not statistically evaluable, since the experimental test group was small, consisting only of Gouri and two other test subjects (athletic individuals without yoga experience). The effort showed that the collaborators were the scientific vanguard in the study of yoga.

Gouri, with his European colleagues, was part of the initial movement of publishing research results in scientific journals on the benefits of practising yoga. Scientific research into yoga asanas had begun before this with *Yoga Mimansa* in the twenties, but had stalled significantly around 1930. By 1940, at Columbia University, Western references to 'relaxation techniques' were prevalent within physical education curricula and literature. However, they did not have a quantitative experimental focus. Instead they were more on the cutting edge of physical exercise and its therapeutic benefits.

In 1960, *Sports Illustrated* kicked off the American medical discussion of the 'scientific analysis' of yoga practice, with a couple of 'Yoga Comes West' articles. They examined the practice in the light of science and asked certain relevant questions. In a subsequent issue, a reader-response explained how Dr Gouri Shankar Mukerji had already addressed many of the questions in a 1956 German article, which 'took electrocardiograms from a yogi who had perfected the respiratory control of his heart to such an extent that he could accelerate, decelerate and even stop his cardiac beat. In this case there was incontrovertible evidence of alteration of impulse formation.'[15] The German article done collaboratively by Gouri in 1956 was among the very first articles to explore the field of yogic asana research.[16]

The studies formed the basis for the 1963 book describing eighty-four asanas, which Gouri co-authored with Dr W. Spiegelhoff. It was titled *Yoga and Our Health* and subtitled 'Medical Instructions for Yoga Exercises'. Gouri gave instruction for eighty-four asanas, along with four breathing techniques and four mudras. The book details scientific experiments they performed in twelve of the different postures, complete with graphs and analyses. The 1963 publication was the first Western book on yoga with an emphasis on scientific and medical research.[17]

79

INDIA'S SCHOOL OF YOGA

The paramedical validation of yoga through science in places such as the Yoga Cure Institute of Calcutta did not happen in a cultural vacuum. It was right alongside India's political popularization of yoga as exercise. The chief proponent of this effort was India's Prime Minister Jawaharlal Nehru. Along with his daughter, Indira Gandhi, he went to visit Swami Kuvalayananda at his Kaivalyadhama Ashram in 1958. 'On the occasion of this visit the prime minister applauded the Swami', because 'Yoga would not progress unless it was examined in light of the advances in modern science'.[1] Nehru played an important role in the modern therapeutic-based yoga as exercise movement, especially within cities and schools.

'Yoga became popular in the 1950s ... because Nehru practised it', though his relationship with yoga asana practice started much earlier.[2] Nehru first met with Kuvalayananda in 1929, which formed the basis for his personal practice. Nehru had begun practising yoga asanas seriously while in and out of the Almora Jail – seven times – from 1931 to 1935.[3] After he was released from prison, he came into acquaintance with Indra Devi, the yoga teacher who learned asana practice from Krishnamacharya and popularized it in the West. The two began a letter correspondence that would last several years.[4]

In 1939, when Nehru met with Buddha and Bishnu in London, he recognized that 'the ancient Indian system of yoga exercises' was 'going to America'. He didn't keep his practice entirely private. Nehru once shared a moment of pranayama with Ian Stephens, then still the editor of *The Statesman*.[5]

When Nehru was imprisoned again from 1942 to 1945, he wrote *Discovery of India*. First published in 1946, the book delves deep 'into the sources of India's personality'. Nehru was very practical in his approach to yoga, and described it as 'an experimental system of probing into the psychical background of the individual and thus developing certain perceptions and control of the mind'.[6]

Nehru interpreted yoga through the historical theory of Patanjali's yoga system. The 'latter stages of Yoga are supposed to lead to some kind of intuitive insight,' wrote Nehru. But Nehru was more focused on the prior stages, where 'the discipline of the body and mind' were to be practised. Here, Nehru mentioned that calling these 'exercises' would be 'the wrong word' to describe the practice, as it was not about 'strenuous movement'. The postures instead 'relax and tone up the body and do not tire it at all'.[7] This 'old asana method' and the 'breathing exercises' formed the basis of 'the discipline of the body' which Nehru practised whenever he had the chance. With Nehru as a leading example, India began to integrate yoga practice in areas of society.[8]

When Sir Paul Dukes collected research for his *Treatise on Hatha Yoga Adapted to the West*, he was invited for a private interview with Nehru to discuss the topic of yoga. Nehru praised the 'essentially scientific' training in Hatha yoga, which promotes 'a sound and healthy body' with 'poise and equilibrium' for the mind. Nehru told Dukes:

> I am glad you are carrying the message of Yoga to other countries. I have been invited to attend an All-India conference on the teaching of physical Yoga in India, the object of which, as the invitation states, is to collect knowledge and experience from various Yoga physical culturists and formulate a national program of Yoga suitable for the masses.[9]

The well-known *Encyclopedia of Indian Physical Culture*, published in India in 1950, included yoga asanas alongside other various exercises. Research done by Claudia Guggenbühl revealed a 'National Plan of Physical Education and Recreation prepared by the Central Advisory Board of Physical Education and research under the Ministry of Education, Govt of India'. The plan, which included 'yogic exercise' was 'created in 1953 and implemented in 1955' but ended when funds ran short. Then, between 1961 and 1964, the Government of India created another program, called "Physical Fitness", but this also disappeared after a short while.'[10]

In the researched materials I encountered, there were no references to *surya namaskar* (sun salutations) being practised in Calcutta-based texts or traditions prior to about 1950. Instead, the *bayam* technique of *dand-baithak* was often mentioned, as well as a four-directional yoga asana series (half-moon stretching to both sides with backward and forward bending), as an initial warm-up.

More notable were the enterprising methods in the forties and fifties, such as the yogic chart and free-hand *bayam* exercises by Nilmoni Das, which became so popular that the younger generation in Calcutta today still refers to these exercises as a part of the identity or lifestyle of the older generation. More recently, within a global context, Prime Minister Modi has led a national push towards popularizing yoga practice within India. However, before this, the role which Nehru played in the fifties was pivotal for the widespread adoption of modern yoga practice within India.

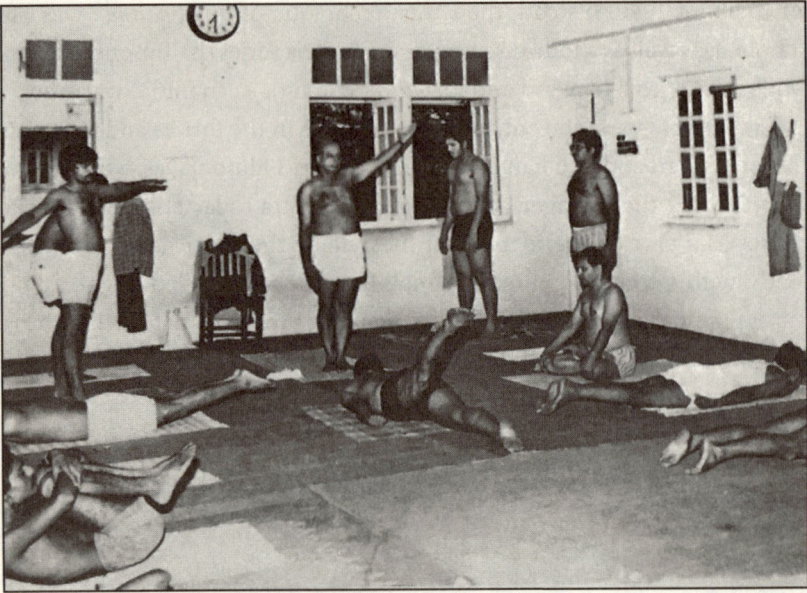

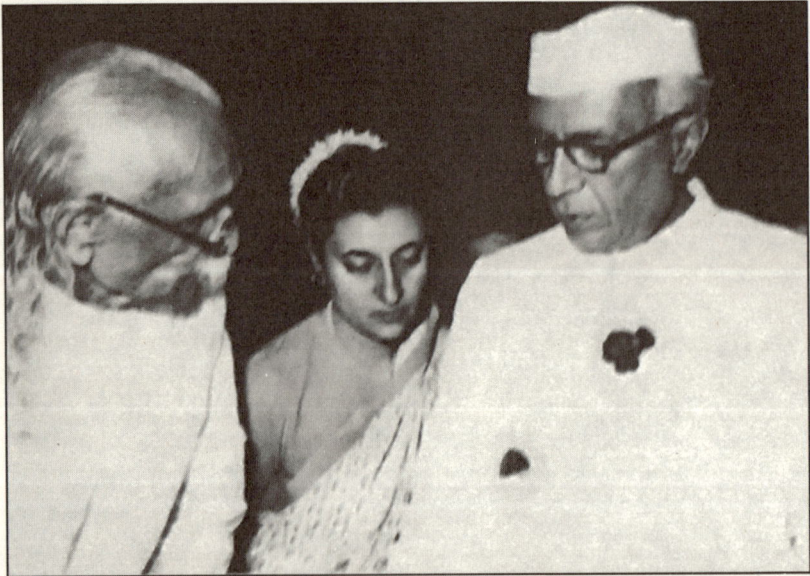

Top: Hatha yoga class, with students doing their own practice, Kaivalyadhama Ashram, circa 1955.
Bottom (from left to right): Kuvalayananda, Indira Nehru, Jawaharlal Nehru, circa 1955.
Courtesy of Kaivalyadhama Yoga Institute.

80

AMERICAN KRIYA HATHA YOGIS

Some of the women renunciates practice the asana of Hatha Yoga and become
proficient in them. Occasionally, at Convocation the men resident disciples
demonstrate their skill in these Yoga postures. They are not a part of Master's
Praecepta studies, but detailed instructions for
the various asanas appear in the SRF Magazine.[1]
– Kamala Silva

Following the death of Yogananda in March 1952, Yogacharya Bernard Cole took a break from publishing further Hatha yoga articles in the *SRF* magazine. Then, in the November 1952 issue, Bernard restarted the effort by discussing an asana in each publication. In July 1953, Cole covered *sarvangasana* (shoulder stand), calling it 'the one asana that would reward him the most for his effort'.[2]

After five years of articles, Bernard had 'many inquiries' about a 'practise list of asanas' that was 'not haphazard' but instead 'systematic and functional'. Finally in November 1954, Bernard introduced 'a practice routine for learning postures' for his American readers.[3]

Bernard followed the method that Buddha used to teach asanas when he'd visited California with Bishnu. Like Buddha, Bernard ordered the postures into three groups: sitting, lying down and standing. He explained that students should 'not practise all the asanas listed in this article at any one time!' Instead, only use the list 'as a sensible guide from the simple to the more difficult asanas'. Bernard gave the advice to 'practise only a few at any one time' until 'you perfect them' and to thenmove on to 'attempt another group'.[4]

Savasana was covered in the January 1955 issue. Again repeating what Buddha had suggested, Cole wrote that the beginner should allow 'ample time between each one for the practice of *savasana*'. He explained that the beginner makes the mistake of practising 'one pose after another'. The 'efficacy of asana practice is dependent on the sequence of muscular stretching or contraction alternating with relaxation'. Bernard then promised 'in the next issue of *Self-Realization Magazine*' he would 'explain in detail' how to accomplish the enigma of 'learning how to not tense the muscles' while in savasana. Sadly, the article was never written.[5] Shortly after the January 1955 issue, on 20 February, the successor to Yogananda, James Lynn, died. Cole again stopped writing articles, this time for good, and left the SRF organization.[6] From 1949 to 1955, twenty asanas and mudras were covered in detailed articles by the pioneering yoga teacher, Bernard Cole.[7]

For a short time, this put an end to the 'Yoga Postures for Health' articles in the magazine. However, students kept practising Hatha yoga within the organization. In addition to the teachers with the title of Yogacharya – Oliver Black and Bernard Cole – other well-known practitioners were Norman Paulsen, Daniel Boone and Donald Walters. They and others were pictured performing asanas on the stage at the annual convocation and featured within pages of the magazine throughout the fifties and sixties.

Walters, also known as Kriyananda, shared his unique way of learning the advanced postures through Yogananda's spiritual assistance. One time, while demonstrating the yoga postures, Yogananda energetically conveyed 'to Kriyananda the ability to do the Hatha yoga postures with ease'. Before that point, some of the postures had been difficult for Kriyananda to execute, but from then on, he 'became recognized as SRF's Hatha yoga expert'.[8]

Kriyananda shared a common sentiment within SRF, that Hatha yoga was 'not spiritual but physical' in application.

The writer, Rev. Bernard, one of SRF's ministers, emphasized how this posture helped by pressing on a certain gland, and how that one stretched the vertebrae and increased circulation – that sort of thing. I'd never voiced any objection, but I couldn't help feeling that, inasmuch as Hatha yoga is the physical branch of the meditative yoga science, Bernard was missing the real point.[9]

The 'real point,' Kriyananda wrote, was a more 'spiritual slant'.

With the September 1955 issue, articles on yoga asanas began again. The style was different from that used by Bernard Cole. The articles were written by Leland Standing and Bernard Tesnière, both newer disciples who joined SRF after the death of Yogananda, presenting 'the medical aspect' of the postures. They also included 'to some extent the spiritual influence of each posture'. Kriyananda 'wasn't wholly satisfied with the way' in which the two 'handled the subject either, but at least it was a step' in what he 'considered the right direction'.[10]

The yoga asanas were presented as one of 'the steps of Patanjali's Eightfold Path'. The third limb, 'Right posture (*asana*)', was explained as 'holding the body in a comfortable, stable position with spine erect for meditation for as long as the yogi wills'. By practising the right posture, 'together with scientific methods of meditation, the yogi is able to accomplish the first two' steps: self-control (*yama*) and moral observances (*niyama*). Readers were informed that a brief outline is 'available free upon request to SRF headquarters' for the 'General Directions for Asana Practice'.[11]

The November 1955 issue featured 'the basic meditation posture recommended by Paramhansa Yogananda'.[12] The text and the directions were decidedly oriented towards meditation and included variations to make them more accessible (such as using a chair instead of *padmasana* for meditation). They were also more rigorous with scientific claims (Tesnière was a medical doctor from France).[13] Similar to its precedent, the articles by Standing and Tesnière were usually around four pages (although they got much longer later on when it was just Tesnière), with detailed information of each pose, photos, directions and modifications. The practice of asanas was also relegated as less effective than the energization exercises:

> Self-Realization Fellowship Church teaches to students a system of SRF Energization Exercises that can be practised more easily than asanas, and that have many superior characteristics. However, the asanas offer certain unique benefits.[14]

The editorial notes continued this dichotomy (Yogoda versus Hatha), which continued throughout the lifespan of the articles on yoga asanas in the SRF magazine.[15]

In 1960, Standing stopped contributing, and Tesnière began authouring the articles solo. The monthly issues on yoga postures continued until 1965. By this time, Tesnière had reached a level of technicality that included a list of references from different scientific journals and anatomical details to support his conclusions. He was writing articles which, in all likelihood, were met by glossy-eyed laymen.

The article on 'Technique of *Savasana*' was particularly illuminating, as it both seemed the sort of follow-up Cole had mentioned he'd write and was reminiscent of the guidelines for practice presented by Buddha Bose.[16]

There were three issues in a row on *padmasana* (lotus pose) in 1963, which covered a combined thirty pages of 'theory and technique' and 'routine of practice'. In the October of the same year, a 'History of the Yoga Postures' was written. Increasingly, Tesnière began referencing archeological artifacts, which showed certain postures in rock carvings.[17] He also referenced Gouri Shankar Mukerji and Spiegelhoff, with their German edition of *Yoga and Our Medicine*, showing a continued collaboration between Calcutta and SRF. The earlier offering was done by mail, of 'general directions for practising yoga asanas', was placed inside the magazine.[18]

The January 1965 issue was on *siddhasana* (adept or success pose). Tesnière concluded with a simple statement, 'Anyone may experience the general benefits of this ancient pose simply by practising it.'[19] At first glance, there was no recognition of this being the final issue to cover yoga asanas. However, among the contents of the combined eleven pages on this seated asana, it included the advanced stages of *samadhi* and how they related to the seated asanas, a natural ending point.[20]

Asanas became an integral part of the SRF organization for a time during the fifties into the sixties. Youth groups 'demonstrating asanas' often appeared in the magazine, even featuring children in the issues. An article in January 1955 titled 'Yogis, Junior Style' described how 'many earnest SRF students who have children train them to follow a daily routine of exercise and meditation'.

One young boy became trained in this daily routine and then was brought to another church's Sunday school by his parents. When the class at the new church began, the boy, Rickie, rose and staunchly declared his loyalty to SRF: 'I am a yogi and I want to go to my own church!' His parents acquiesced and told the interviewee that 'Rickie is now an expert in some of the yoga postures, and meditates faithfully every morning and night'. Another child, Eileen, did 'all the SRF exercises with her parents'. Eileen, the article notes, saw to it that her parents joined her in the daily 'practice of eight yoga postures'. 'A conscientious vegetarian', she once 'refused her favorite soup – vegetable – because it had not been made completely with vegetables'.[21]

In 1965 (alongside immigration changes), Indian swamis voyaged to America advocating yoga asanas, and the alternative hippie culture adopted their practice, which turned off the more conservative SRF members.[22]

The end of Hatha yoga promotion by SRF during the mid-sixties, alongside its continued practice of Kriya yoga, signaled the end of a 'spiritual–physical' practice as conceived by Yogananda and Bishnu in 1935. It was the end of an era but not entirely. The influence had continued for nearly thirty years after Buddha and Bishnu first brought the practice of asanas to SRF in 1938, and trained many in the first wave of American-born yoga teachers.

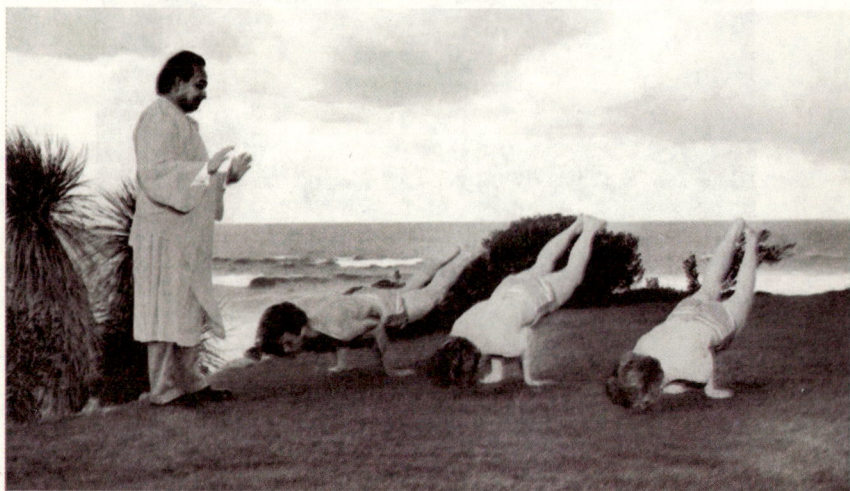
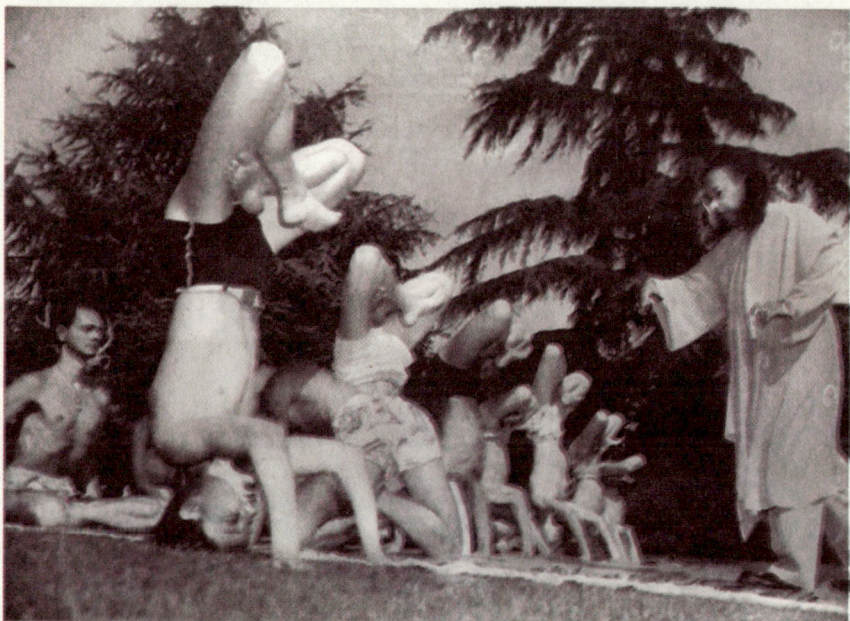

Yogananda with Self Realization Fellowship disciples practicing Hatha yoga in Encinitas, Los Angeles, circa 1948.

Source: Wikimedia Commons.

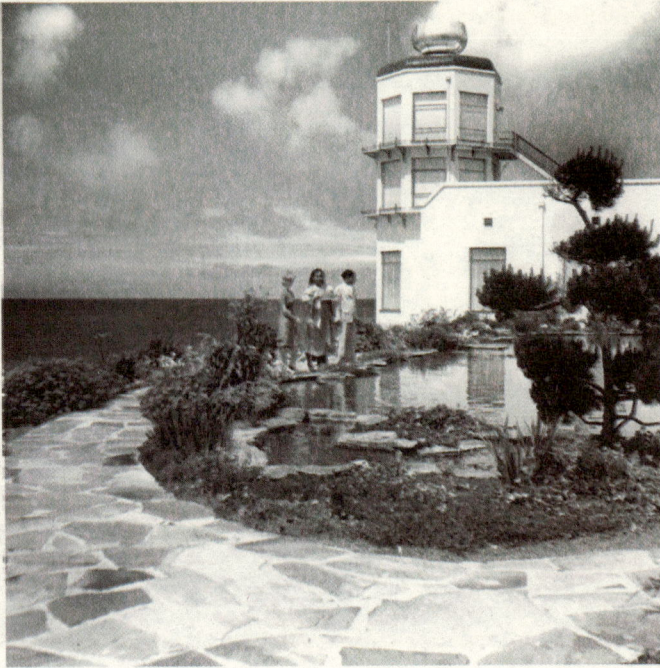

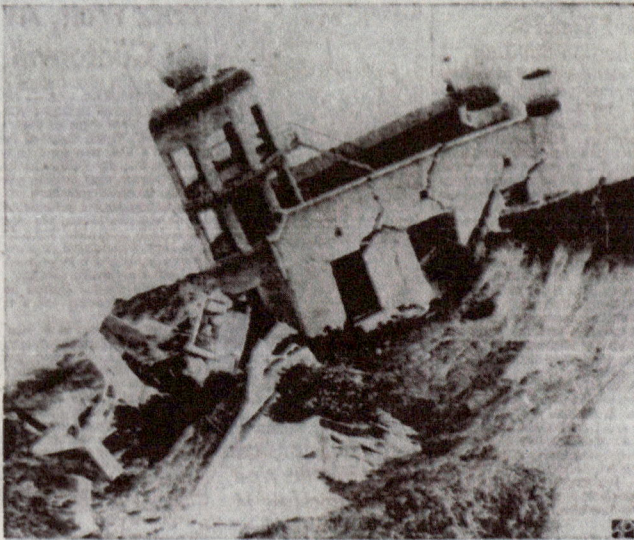

The Golden Lotus Temple of All Religions, Encinitas, Calif., seaside retreat of the East Indian Self-Realization Fellowship, started to slide toward the Pacific ocean (above), but after a while appeared to have paused in its traveling. The temple, with its gold-leaf spires, was built in 1936 by Paramhansa Yogananda.

Golden Lotus Temple. Encinitas, California.

Source: Wikimedia Commons; Green Bay Press Gazette (1942).

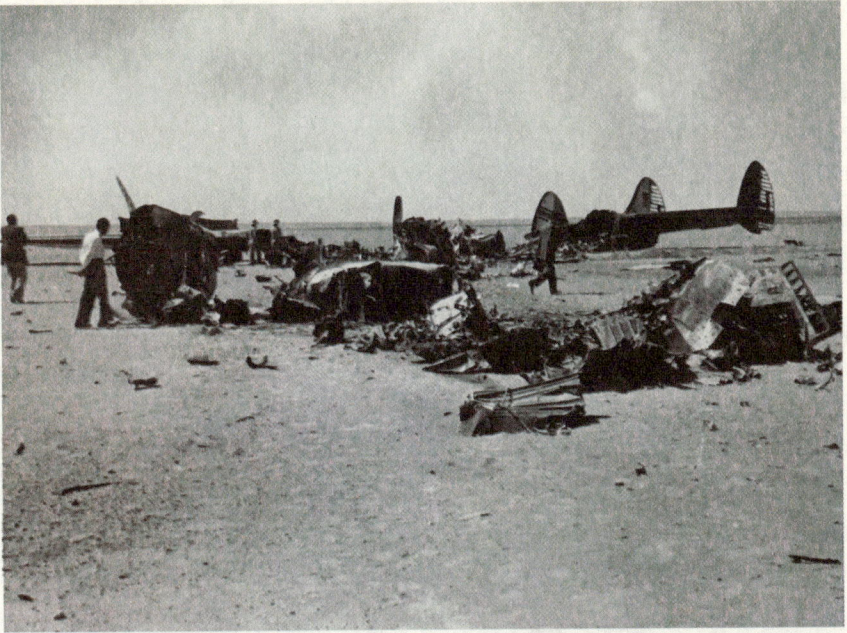

15 Die in PAWA Plane Crash
Near Euphrates River Bank

New Orleans Times 6/20/47

(The Associated Press)

Damascus, Syria, June 19.—A Pan American World Airways Constellation plane, bound from Karachi, India, to Istanbul, crashed early today near the bank of the Euphrates river in Eastern Syria, killing eight of its 26 passengers and seven of its crew of 10.

Sixteen of the passengers, all of them Indian and British, were injured. Three persons aboard the plane escaped unharmed. Whether they were passengers or crewmen was unknown here.

Circumstances of the crash were largely unknown, but reports from Cairo said the plane had messaged shortly before it went down that one of its engines was afire and a forced landing would be attempted.

The 15 dead were buried near the scene and the injured were transported by Syrian Airways to the American university's hospital at Beirut.

In New York, Pan American officials said they had not yet received a detailed report of the crash, but confirmed that 15 lives had been lost.

It was the fourth major disaster in American commercial aviation in the last 22 days. The four crashes have taken 161 lives.

A passenger list compiled by Pan American revealed that only

Top: Clipper Eclipse, Pan Am Flight 121.

Source: Pan American Airways Papers; U. of Miami; New Orleans Times, 1947.

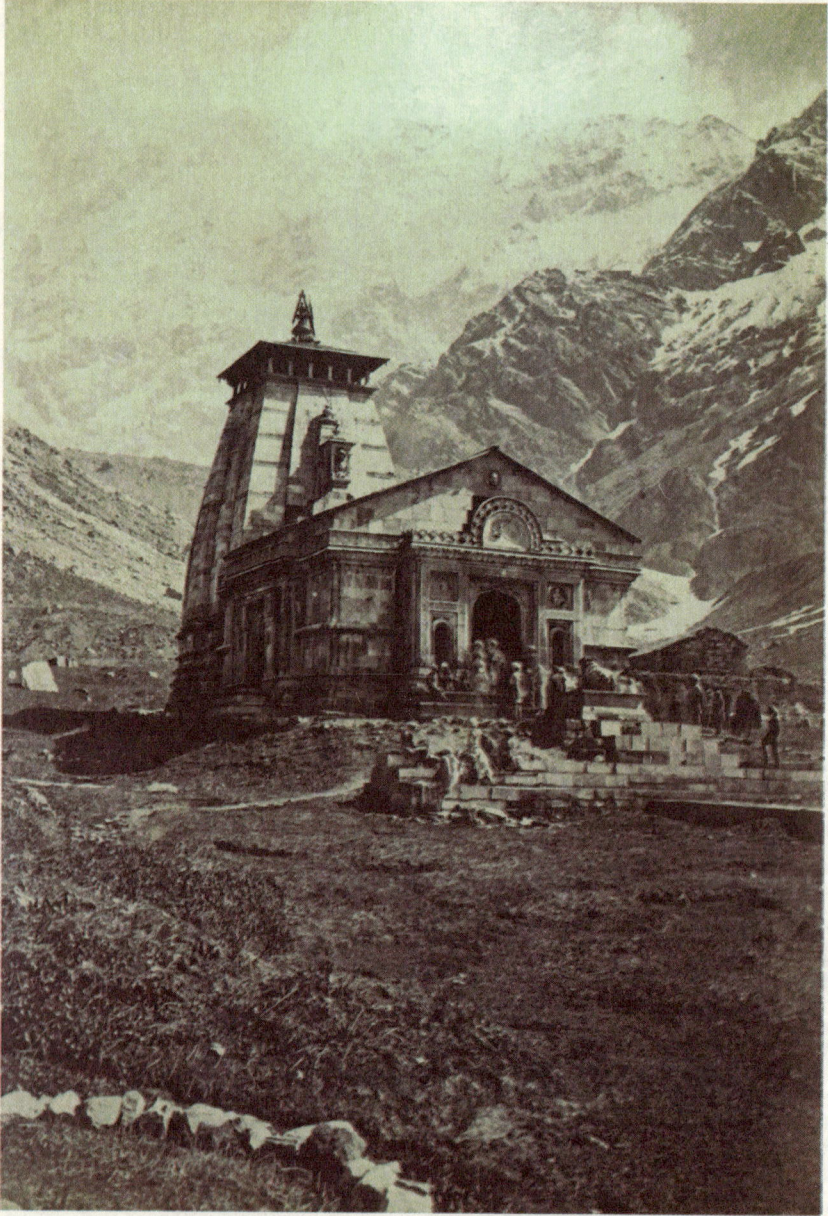

19th Century photo of Kedarnath temple, Himalayas.
Source: East India Association, London.

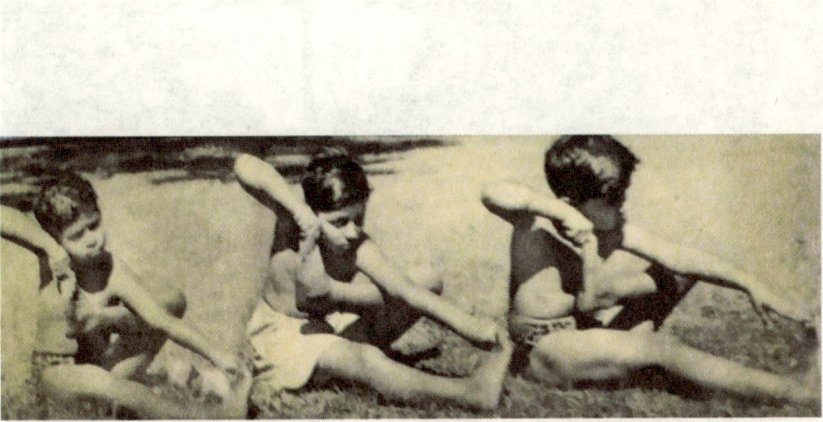

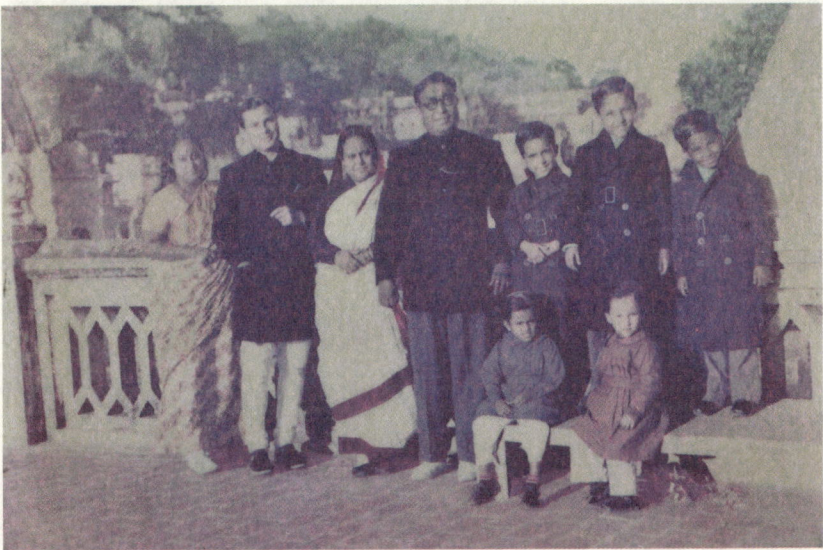

Top (left to right): Bishwanath Ghosh, Arun Bose, Ashok Bose, 1950.
Bottom (standing left to right): Ava Rani, Buddha, Ashalata, Bishnu, Arun, Ashok,
Bishwanath; (seated) Rooma, Karuna, 1952.

Courtesy of Ghosh's Yoga College.

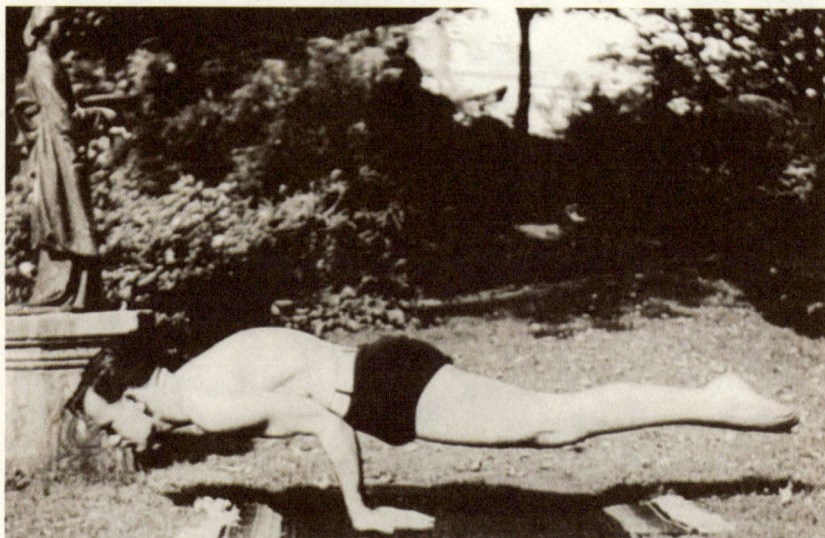

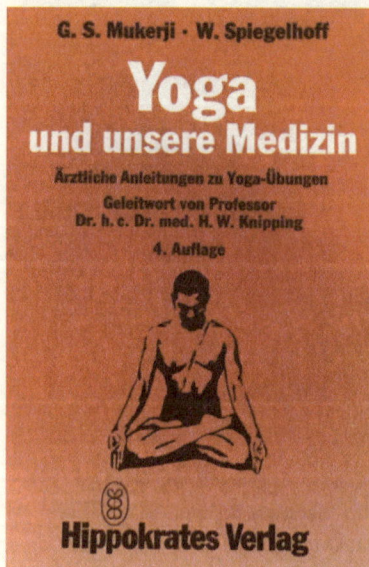

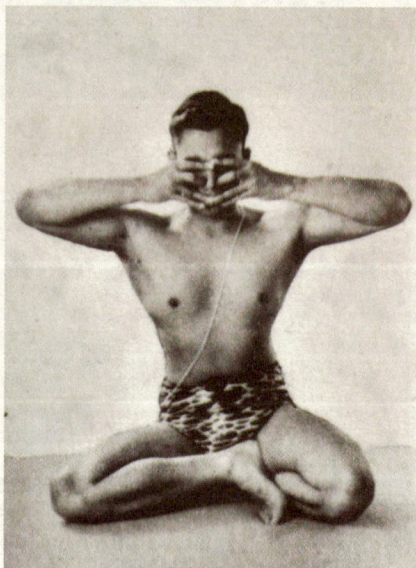

Top left: German edition of Yoga and our Medicine. Top: Dr. W. Spiegelhoff.
Bottom right: Dr. Gouri Shankar Mukerji.

Courtesy of Romit Banerjee.

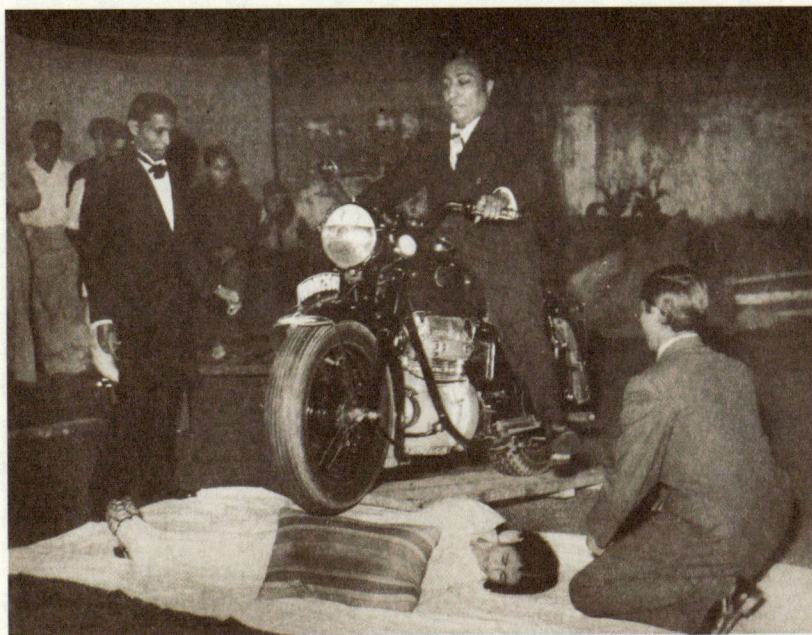

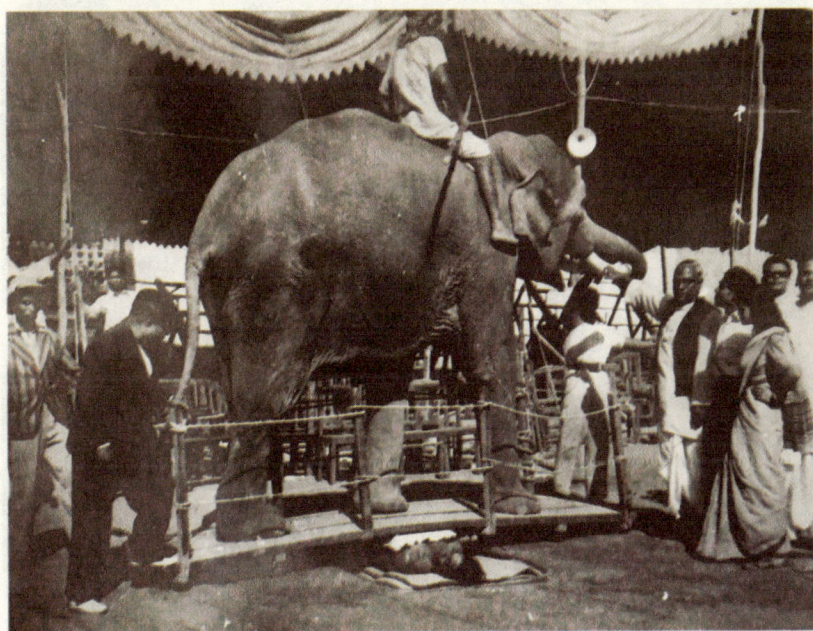

Bishnu Ghosh with Reba Rakshit performing feats of strength. Calcutta, circa 1955.

Courtesy of Romit Banerjee.

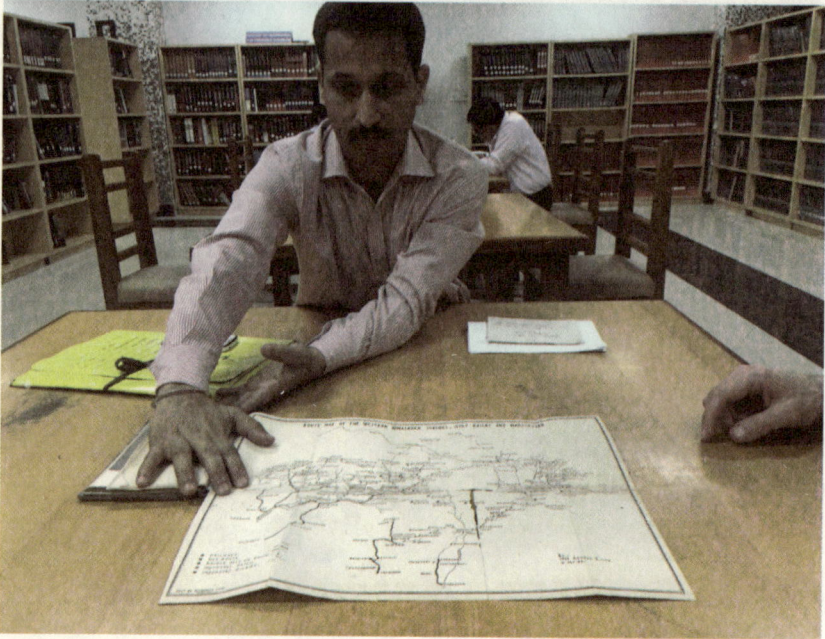

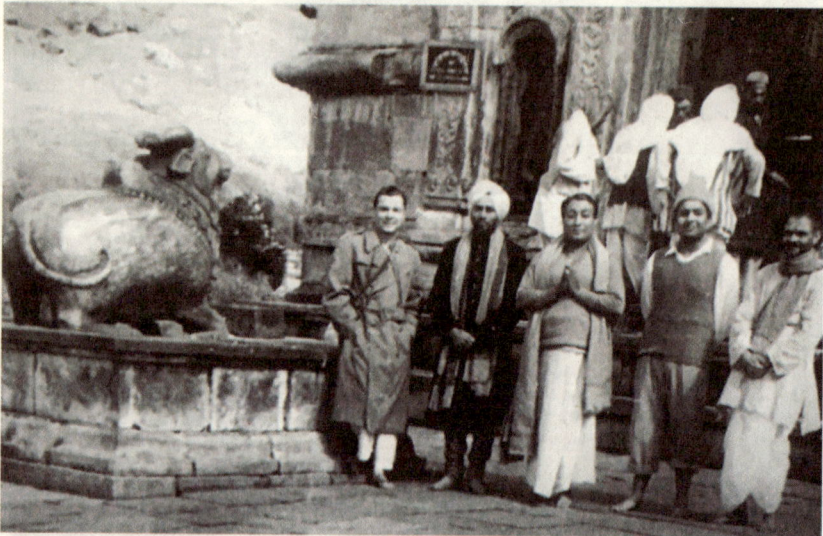

Top: Pavitra Shekhar Bose viewing map of Himalayas in Holy Kailas by Buddha Bose, National Library, Calcutta. Bottom (from left): Buddha, temple priest, Bishnu at Kedarnath temple. Circa 1955.

Courtesy of Mataji, Soham Heritage & Art Center, Mussoorie, India.

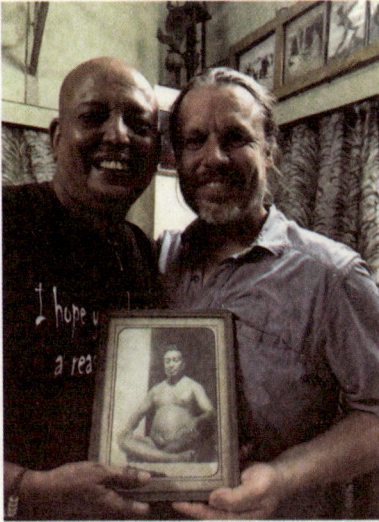
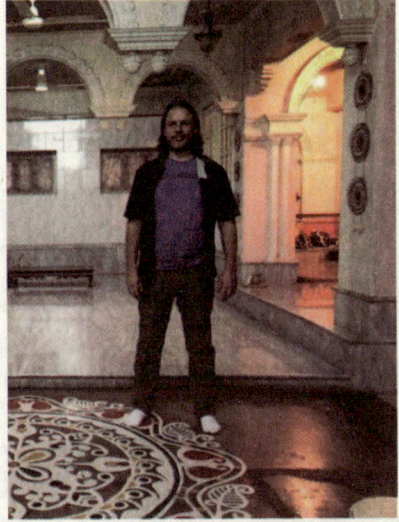
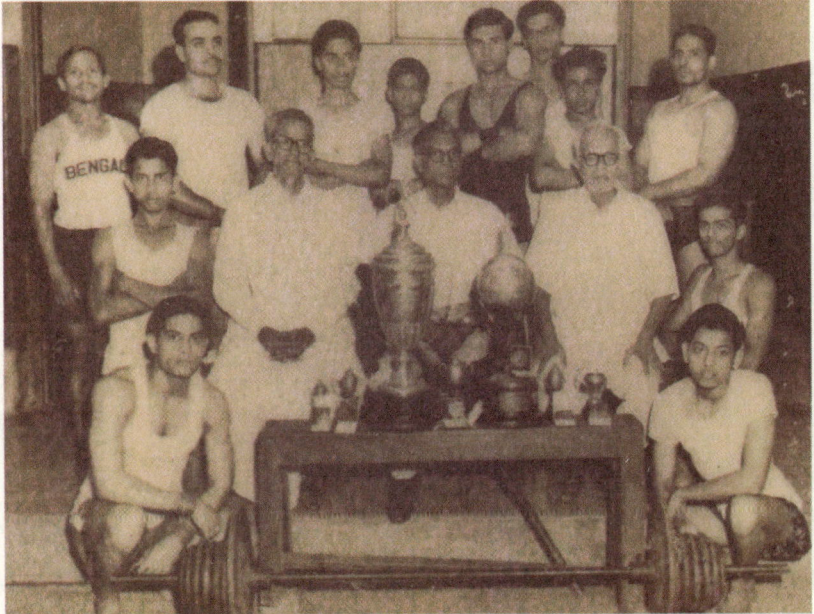

Top left: Mukul Dutta with author, at Yoga O Jiban Fitness.
Top right: Author standing inside former location of Ghosh's gymnasium. Bottom: Inside
Ghosh's 4/2 Ram Mohan Roy Road gymnasium, Bikram (standing in black), circa 1966.

Photos by Malay Roy, Raphael Voix, & courtesy of Mark and Steve Mehlert.

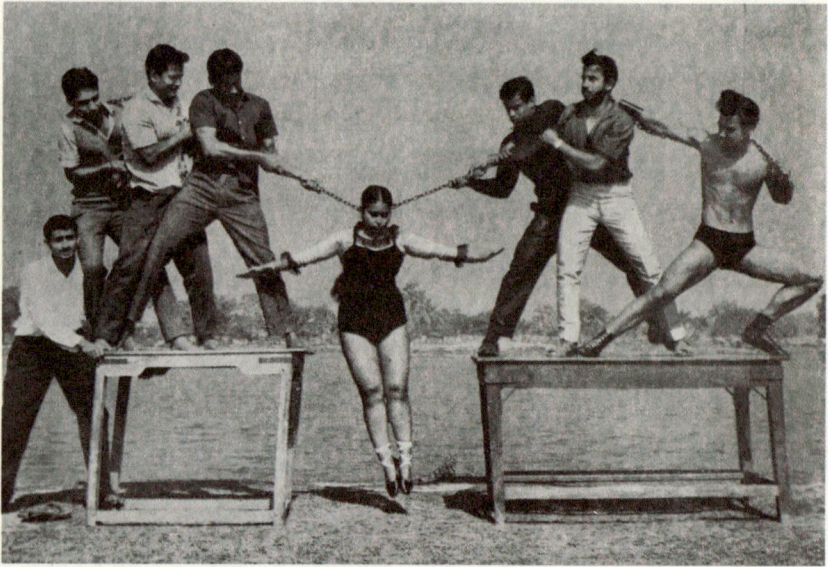

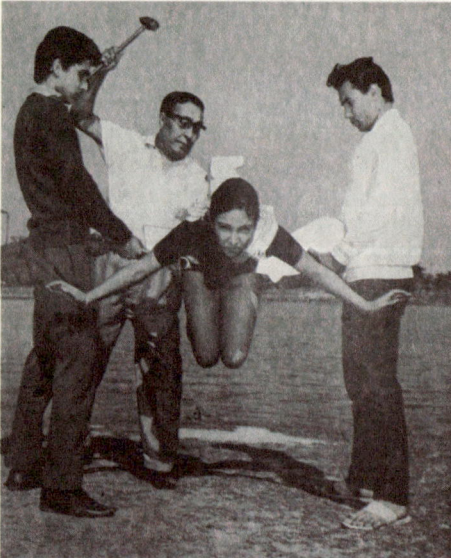

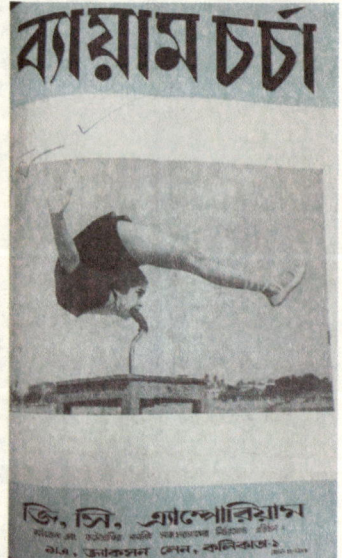

Top: Karuna Ghosh (hanging by neck), Bikram Choudhury (far right), circa 1969. Bottom left: Arun Bose (left), Bishnu Ghosh (with hammer), Bikram Choudhury (right), and Rooma Bose (atop sword), 1969. Bottom right: Reba Patra, 1969.

Source: Bayam Charcha.

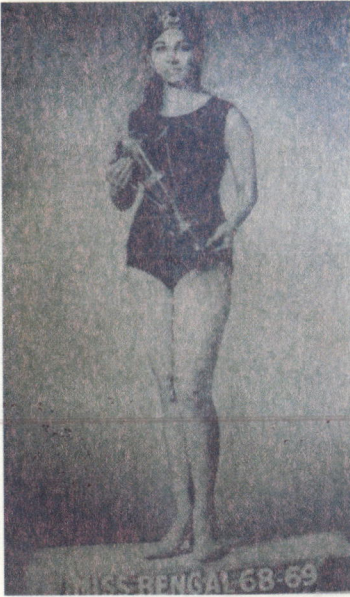

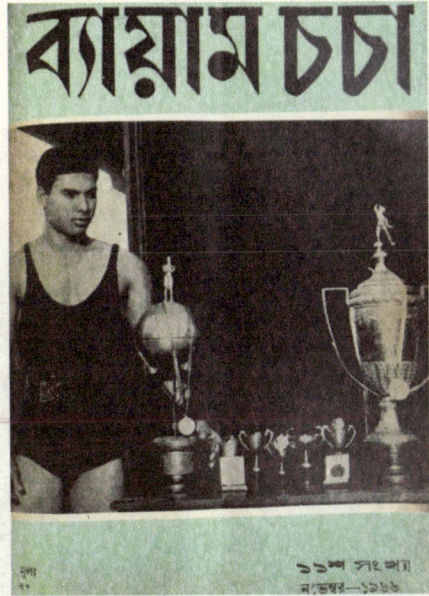

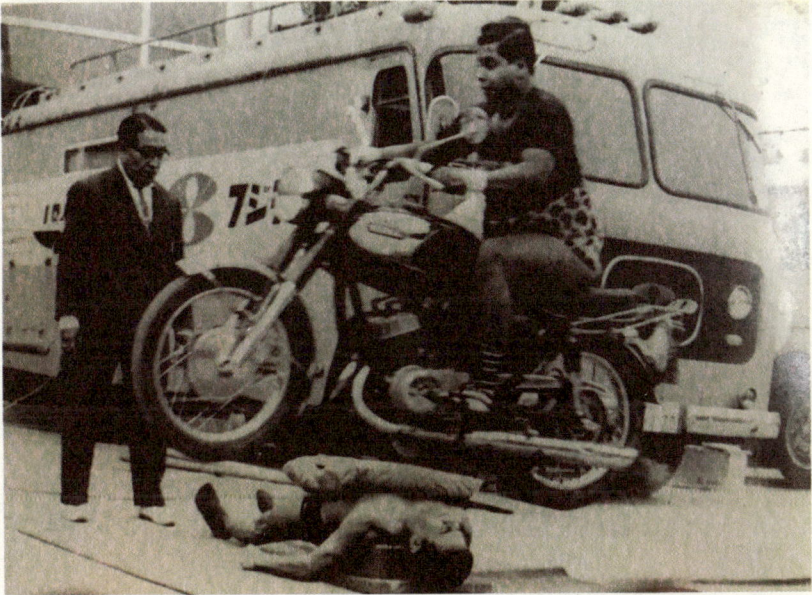

Top left: Rooma Bose, Miss Bengal, 1968-69. Top right: Bikram Choudhury, with weightlifting trophies from local competitions, 1965. Bottom: Bishnu (left), Bishwanath Ghosh (atop motorcycle), and Monotosh Choudhury performing a feat of strength in Japan, 1968.

Source: Bayam Charcha; courtesy of Ghosh's Yoga College.

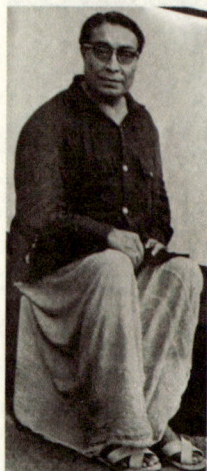

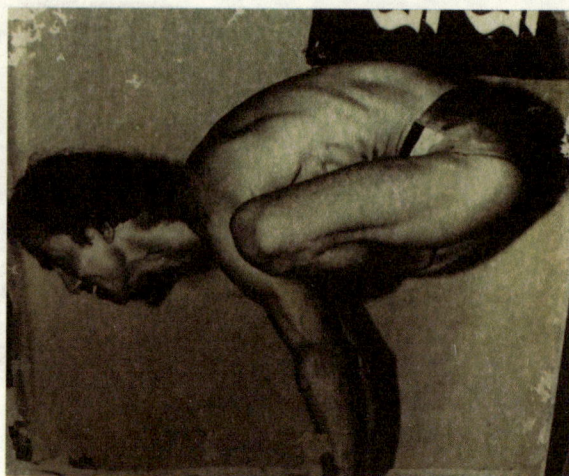

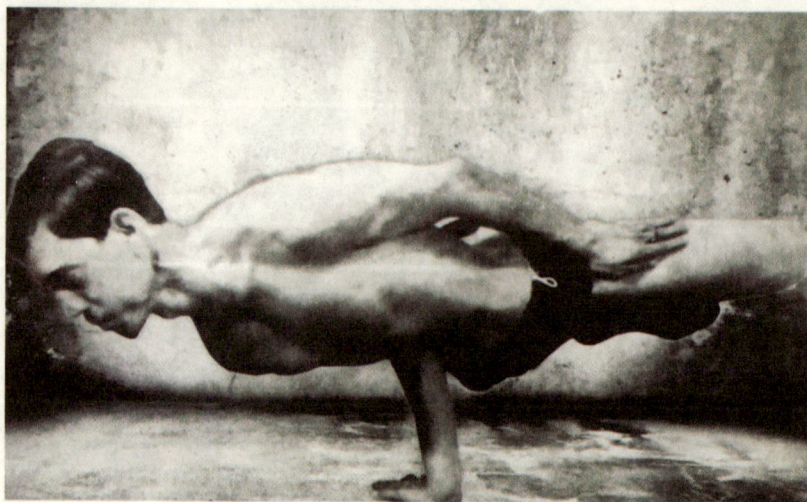

Top left: Bishnu Ghosh, 1970 (last photo, taken by Bishwanath).
Top right: Bimal Das. Bottom: Mukul Dutta.
Source: Bayam Charcha; courtesy of Bimal Das, Mukul Dutta.

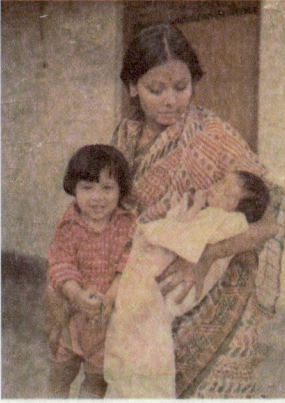
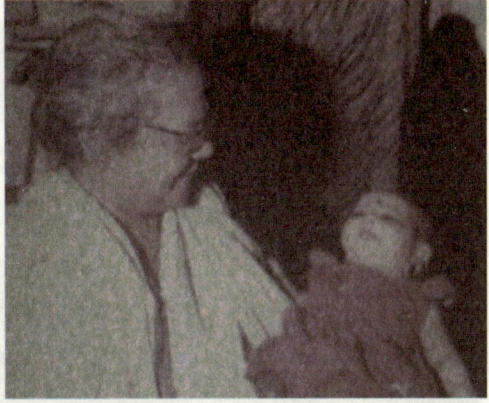
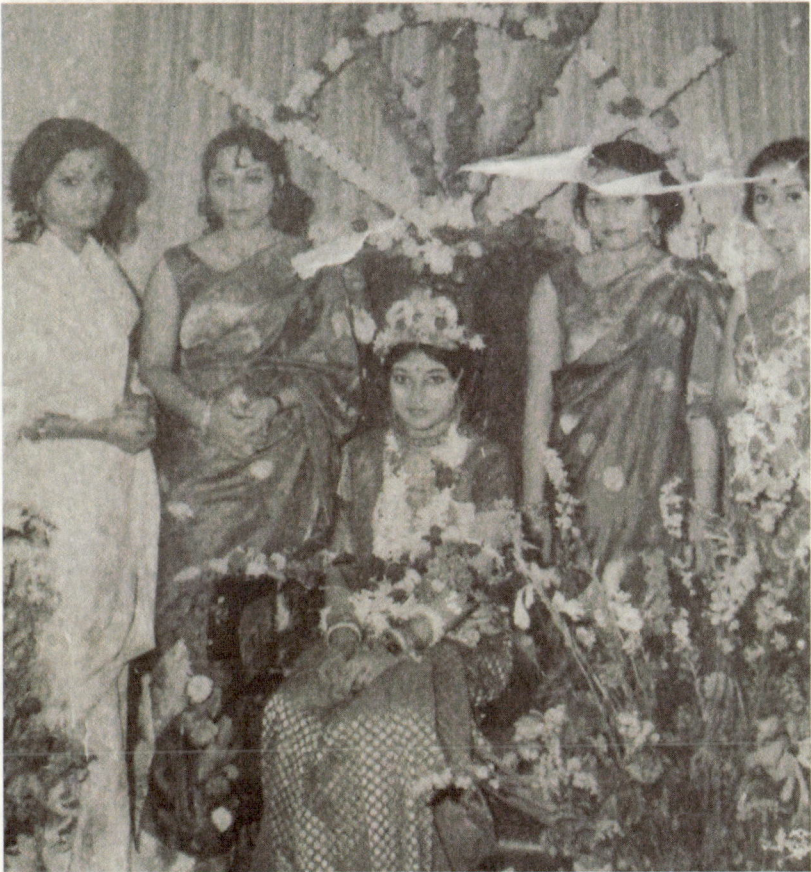

Top left: Chitralekha Shalom with sons Shib Shekhar (standing) and Pavitra Shekhar, at 4/2 Ram Mohan Roy Road. Top right: Ashalata Ghosh with granddaughter Muktamala, 1977. Bottom (from left): Chitralekha (wife of Ashok), Rooma Bose, Sabita Mullick, Anjana (wife of Bishwanath). Wedding photograph by Bishwanath Ghosh, 1974.

Courtesy of Chitralekha Shalom.

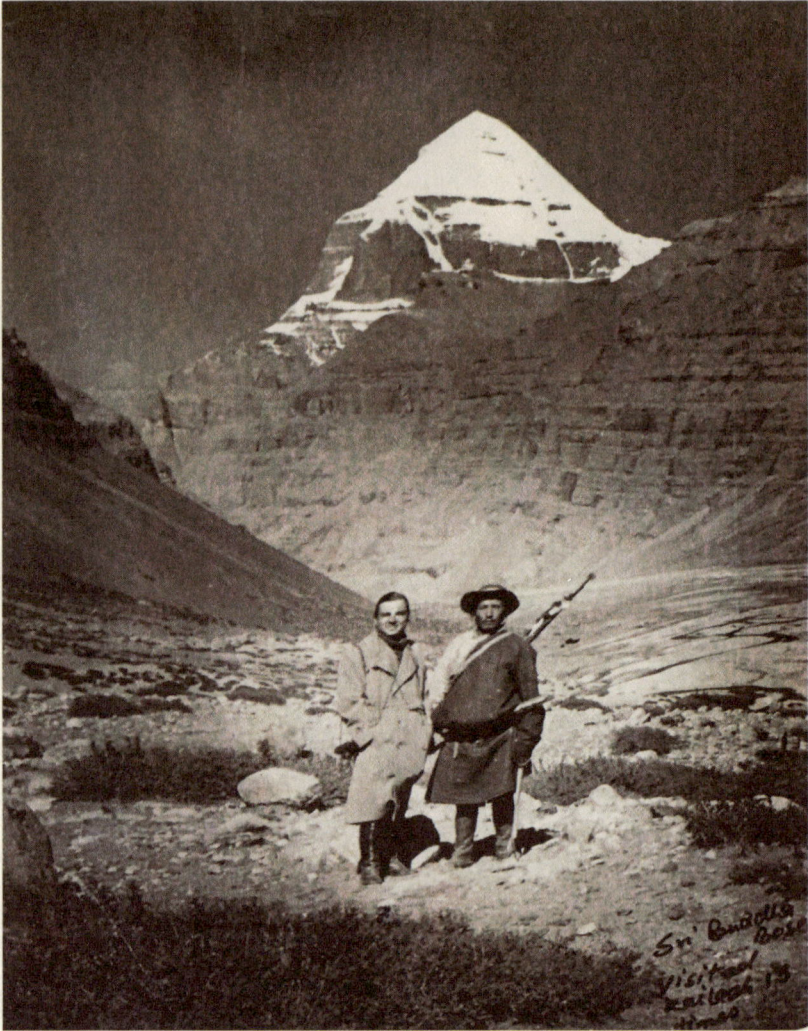

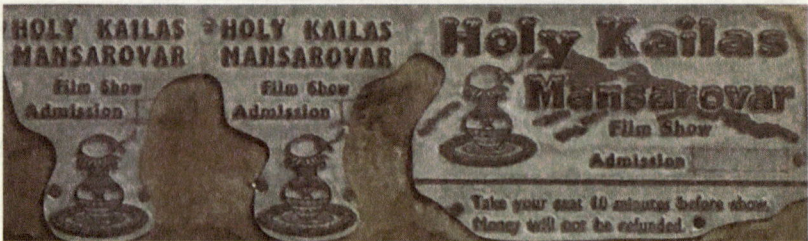

Top: Buddha Bose with guard, Kailash Mountain. Bottom: Metal stamp used for tickets to Holy Kailas & Lake Manasarovar.

Courtesy of Soham Heritage & Art Center, Mussoorie, India; Mataji.

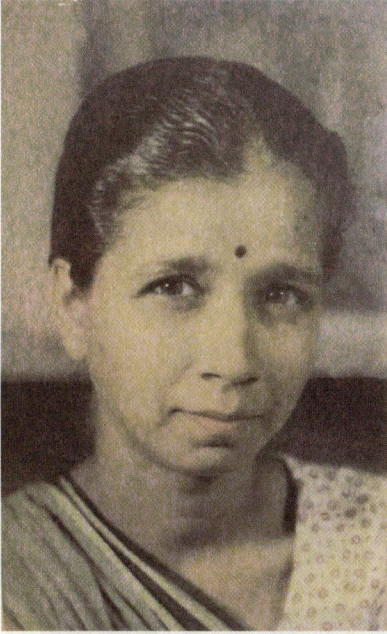

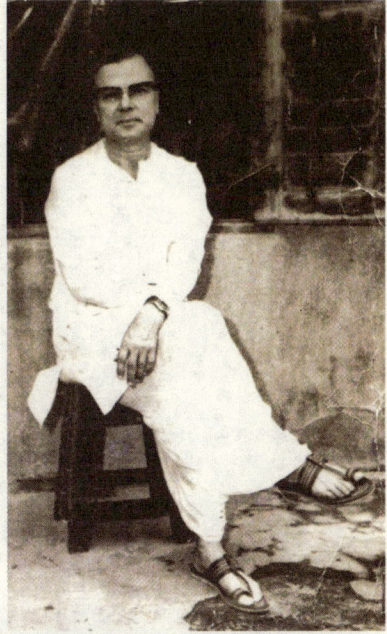

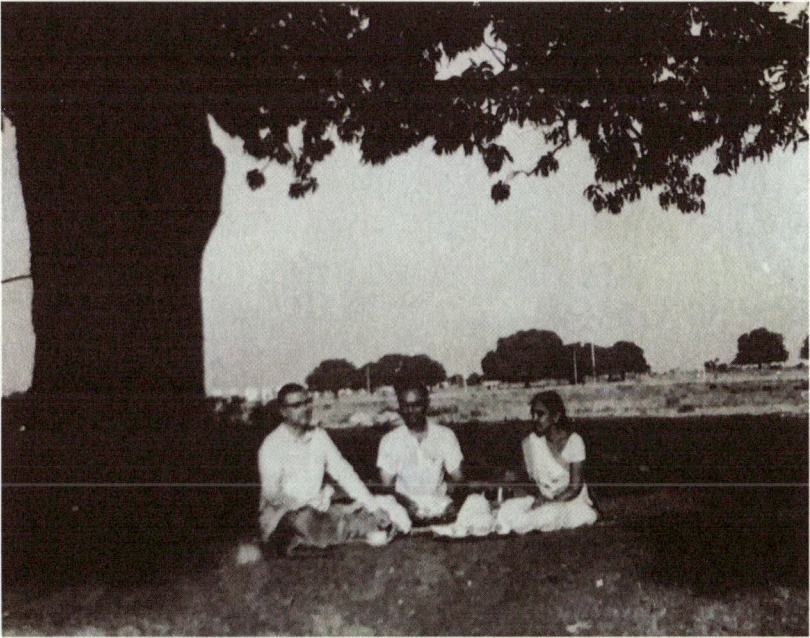

Top left: Yashodhara Behen (Swamini Guru Priyananda, Mataji), circa 1964.
Top left: Buddha Bose, circa 1970. Bottom: Buddha Bose (left) with disciples B.H. Maharaja
and Yashodhara Bharatkumar Maharaja in Gujarat, 1972.

Courtesy of Mataji; Chitralekha Shalom; Rekha Maharaja-Ivey.

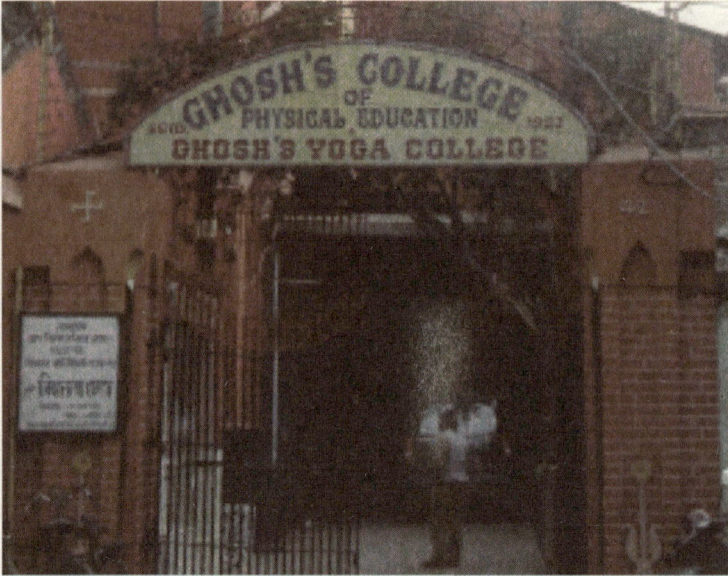

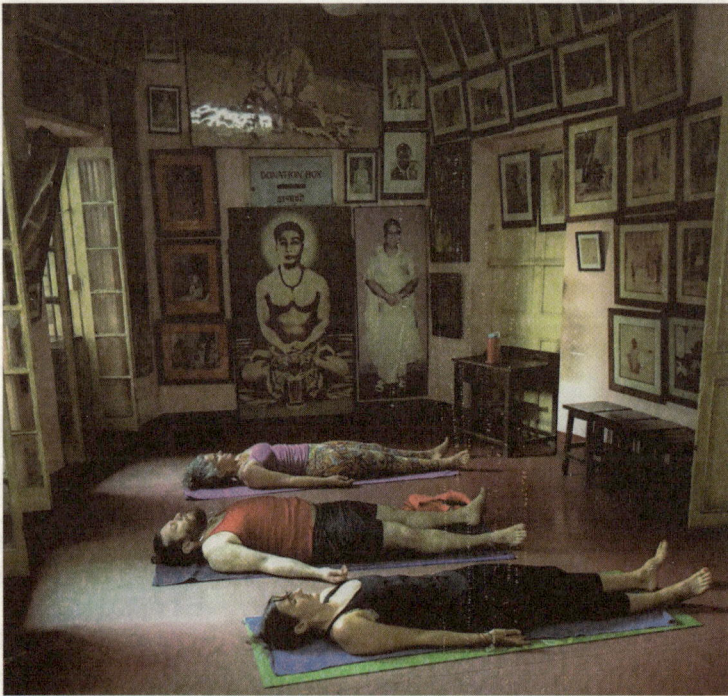

Top: Ghosh's Yoga College entrance. Bottom: Bishnu Ghosh's yoga room.

Courtesy of Claudia Guggenbühl; Jacki Minna Walker.

PART TWELVE

CALCUTTA YOGA GOES EAST

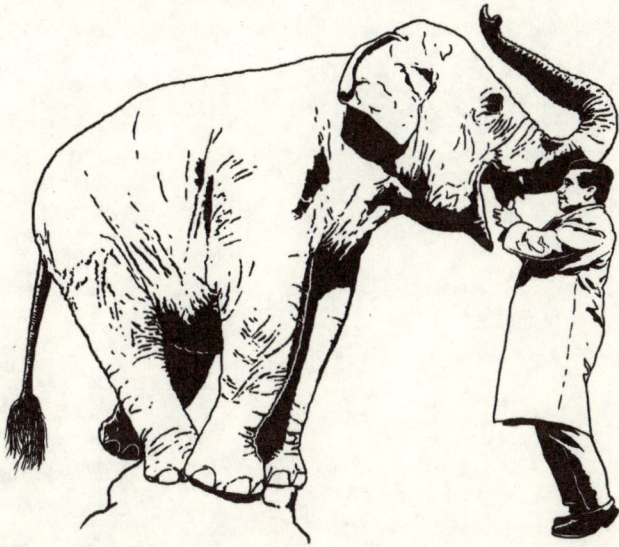

81

BISHNU'S JAPANESE TROUPE

'Tell me about the Japanese who came here to get well through yoga?'
'They were two Japanese men, Mr. Yoshimura and the other was Mr. Hannari.
Both used to come and practise here.
They took the Ghosh team abroad to Japan for the shows.'
'How did Yoshimura and Hanari know about this place in Calcutta,
since yoga was not popular in Japan at that time?'
'This place became popular because of Swami Yogananda. So, they came here to
the gymnasium where they got to know his younger brother, Bishnu.'[1]

In 1967, Bishnu welcomed two Japanese men to Calcutta 'with equal warmth, and astonished them when his disciples and students showed their performances'.[2] Inspired by Yogananda's spiritual zest in *Autobiography*, the Japanese men expected to find Kriya yoga practitioners in the Calcutta Ghosh family. Instead, they found a troupe of performers and the practice of Hatha yoga.[3] At first, they were 'lost for words', but their puzzlement turned to excitement and they requested to 'film the performances so that they could be shown on television throughout Japan'.[4] The entire production, Bishnu said, 'was to promote and display India's ethnic yoga, *bayam* and magical performances'.[5]

The shows Bishnu brought to Japan featured a series of teams who showcased all sorts of physical and cultural feats. It was as if Bishnu had brought Bengal's circus from India to Japan.

Bishnu Ghosh was introduced to the circus by his physical culture guru, R. N. Guha Thakurta, who not only was 'an acknowledged physical culturist of Bengal' but also brought forward twenties-era 'sensations' in his circus, integrating bodybuilding and feats of strength.[6] Throughout his career, Bishnu followed this path. His first work on the stage came during the intermission of circus shows, when he performed as a clown doing muscle control and feats of strength. Even though he lost his son Srikrishna at a circus in the 1940s, Bishnu eventually returned to the stage.[7] As the decades rolled on, the circus as a social phenomenon had all but disappeared from India.[8] A 'ban on child workers under the Prevention of Child Labour Act' was followed by a ban on public display of 'animals like tigers, lions and bears', which were once the top attraction of any circus. Traditionalists thought this 'took away the beauty of the whole exercise'.[9]

Bishnu mostly relied on his family and students for his circus, as they were physically trained and also interacted with animals. Reba Rakshit had been his first student who 'would demonstrate the power of bodybuilding and yoga by making an adult elephant walk over her chest'.[10] Bishnu's children, Bishwanath and Karuna, also learned this skill.

By the sixties, Bishnu's act was in full swing, attracting onlookers from around the world.[11] A film crew arrived from Germany to document the phenomenon. The representatives from Japan, Mr Yoshimura and Mr Hannari, showed up at 4/2 Rammohan Roy Road and invited Bishnu to bring his troupe to Japan.[12]

In May 1968, Bishnu planned to bring a team of twenty-six persons to Japan, including 'ten Bengali *Bayam* performers' and 'ten members from Madras Dancing University including musicians'. In addition, he would bring 'four from Kerala to perform the *lathi-khela* and sword fighting', and a couple of others 'from Punjab', who could 'swallow a snake' and 'show *bhastrika dhauti*'.[13] The members from Calcutta were whittled down. The 1968 members of Ghosh's gymnasium alongside Bishnu were 'jiu-jitsu expert Biswanath Ghosh; Mr India, Robin Goswami; Bharat Kumar Shanti Dutta; unbeaten plastic body expert Reba Patra, and yoga expert Monotosh Choudhury'.

With the invitation in hand, the troupe went to Japan aboard Lufthansa Airlines on 24 May 1968. The initial show in Japan, with its wide spectrum of performances, was aired on 'Tokyo's Fuji Television'.[14] Afterwards, Bishnu recounted a few moments of the show for 'the pleasure of the *Puja* readers' of the magazine *Bayam Charcha*. The performance had been 'telecast all over the country' with 'live shows from ten in the morning to eight in the evening' and lasted for 'fifteen days'. The performances were further outlined by Bishnu. Indoor performances:

– Bharat Shree Kamal Bhandari broke iron rods with his teeth, broke hard coconuts with his head and fist, and performed flexing and control of muscles

– Reba Patra Dutta performed 'plastic body' and had stones broken on her back while she hung from a sword on her stomach

– Monotosh Choudhury bent iron rods with his eyes and throat, and showed some very difficult yoga postures

– Biswanath Ghosh tore apart iron chains

– Shanti Dutta showed various acts of power and strength

Outdoor shows:

– Biswanath Ghosh had a diesel roller weighing more than 10 tons driven over his chest

– Shanti Dutta held back two new jeeps in running condition with chains

– Monotosh Choudhury had a motorbike jump over him as he lay on a bed of nails

The performance of yoga asanas by Monotosh Choudhury was very popular and one of the first of its kind in Japan. 'Plastic Body', as performed by Reba Patra Dutta, was another name for contortionism. The two sisters, Reba and Ruby Patra, became quite famous. They had started their training in gymnastics at Simulia Athletic Club,[15] and Reba thereafter became 'the unconquered queen of plastic body performance in India', winning various contests.[16] She became a student of Bishnu when, like so many before, he spotted her talent and took it to a higher level.

A brief biography of Reba appeared after she returned from Japan:

Besides gymnastics she has perfected the art of hanging from a sharp sword on her bare stomach while bricks are broken on her back. Reba has earned the honor of being the first Indian lady to show gymnastics in Japan. She has stunned Japanese audiences with this performance and earned fame.[17]

The following year, in 1969, Bishnu brought Hatha yoga to Japan again.

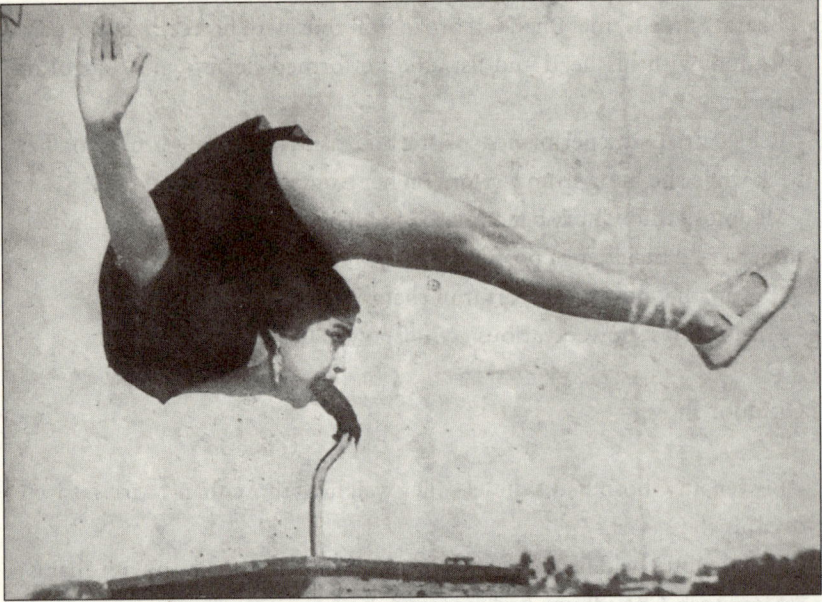

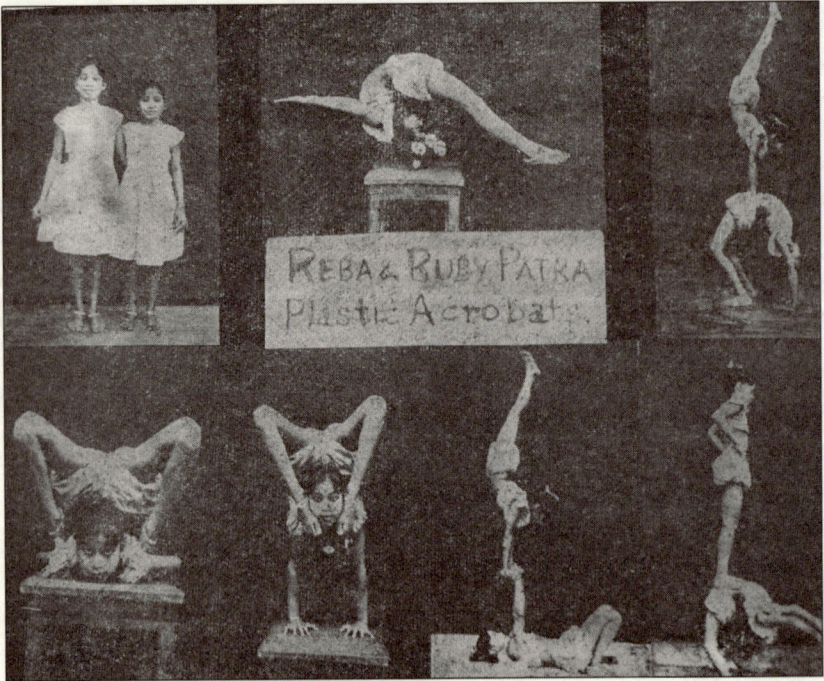

Reba and Ruby Patra, circa 1968.
Source: Bayam Charcha.

82

ADVANCED ASANAS IN JAPAN

Bishnu's second voyage to Japan was in the February of 1969. The smaller troupe consisted of Bishnu, his children Bishwanath and Karuna, and 'Yogendra' Amar Nath Nandi. The team of four left on 25 February and returned on 5 March 1969.[1] It was during this visit that Hatha yoga became more the center of the performance in Japan.

Monotosh Choudhury was the senior yoga teacher under Bishnu at this time, but he was unable to go to Japan in 1969. Amar Nath Nandi was another 'favored yoga expert' at Ghosh's College. Nandi would often contribute to Bishnu's magazine, with articles on how to practise yoga, in a column titled 'Questions for the Yogendra', first begun by Monotosh Choudhury. Nandi also wrote of his experience learning to do yoga asanas under Bishnu Ghosh, during his training for the trip to Japan:

> The next day, after practising the poses in *Bayamacharya's* room I noticed the many photographs; some caught my eye. I asked him about those photos. He said, 'Those are pictures of Buddha Bose. As far as *nauli* kriya is concerned you are the best today, but the next in line is Tapas Bhattacharya. Buddha Bose was a supreme performer in the past.'[2]

Nandi explained how the list of asanas and kriyas was developed, prior to going to Japan:

> *Bayamacharya* explained to me that this time we would have to perform in front of television cameras. This meant some change in our timings, etc. Before when we performed, it used to be lengthy but now I needed to pack

in as many asanas in a short span of time, before the cameras. The asana chart had to be prepared in such a manner so that I could easily slip into the sequence order, and at the same time show many more asanas than before. *Bayamacharya* told me, 'No more discussions today. Come to me regularly from tomorrow and I shall arrange the sequence for you.'[3]

Bishnu compiled a list for Nandi.[4] On the stage in Japan, Nandi first performed the muscle control exercises *'uddiyana, nauli'* and the other kriyas. Nandi 'couldn't actually do *bastra dhauti* alongside these', Bishnu wrote, because 'it would not be possible to repeat these acts again and again'. Nandi, as it was, had to fast until 6 p.m. each day. After their morning show, 'they would have to do the same thing again at 1 p.m. and 5 p.m. for another set of live shooting for television'.[5] Nandi followed the kriyas with *'bira bhadrasana, surya namaskar*, and then the "advanced asanas" list'. At the end of the Hatha yoga demonstration, Nandi 'performed *sankatasana* in order to close with *pranam*', wrote Bishnu.[6] '*Sankatasana*, is, as Bishwanath used to say, the way to bid farewell to the audience. So it is the last one', I was told.

Alongside Nandi, Bishnu's son and daughter Bishwanath and Karuna, took turns with a 6-tonne roller, and a 4-tonne roller respectively, which were driven over their chests as they laid on the floor.[7] Bishnu told a story of his daughter Karuna, and how she wound up also bearing an elephant in Japan after the initial roller:

In a Japanese park there was a small zoo and an elephant. It was a baby elephant that one could take in the lap and pet. It was confined in an iron cage which was weather-proofed in order to keep it warm. The Japanese suggested this cute elephant would look good stomping on Karuna. I was taken aback because my daughter can juggle two of these elephants in her hands easily. The Japanese had a good laugh. I told them there was a zoo named Sabotan Park in the city of Ito, about 120 miles away, which had a big elephant. They answered 'Okay let us go, but we have our doubts whether your daughter will be able to take that elephant on her chest.' Soon we were travelling in big cars to Ito, a wonderful journey through mountains, plains and seaside.[8]

At the time, Karuna was the 'senior yoga teacher in the female section at the Ghosh's College of Physical Education'. She was featured on the cover of the July 1969 issue of *Bayam Charcha*, with the biography stating, 'She started doing *bayam* and yoga-*bayam* from the age of five and soon became an expert in *bayam* and asana and mudras.'⁹ Indeed, photographs showed Karuna with the 1-tonne elephant walking across her chest.

This second trip to Japan was designed to generate 'popular appeal' in order to create enthusiasm for the troupe to return the following year with a full entourage of remarkable feats of strength and physical culture.¹⁰ The two Japanese men, Yoshimura and Hanari, 'promised that if the people of Japan liked the acts' the 'team would be invited to show their acts in the Expo-70', the 1970 Olympic style of performances held in Japan.¹¹

The exploratory trip paid off.

'It was a very happy team which got off the plane in a cold Tokyo,' wrote Bishnu. By the end of the short ten-day trip, 'the Japanese were impressed by Amar Nandi's yogic performance and his beautifully proportioned body.'¹² Three months later, in July 1969, Bishnu signed a contract to return with a full troupe a year later, for the 'Expo 70' in Japan.

'If those trips proved to be lucrative,' Bishnu wrote, he would consider 'the invitations from Germany, Belgium and Switzerland.'¹³ Perhaps they would even go 'to the USA' again, 'to promote the qualities, and bring glory to Bengal.'¹⁴

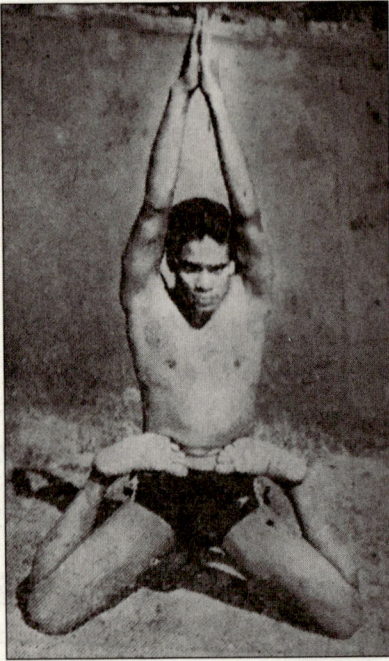

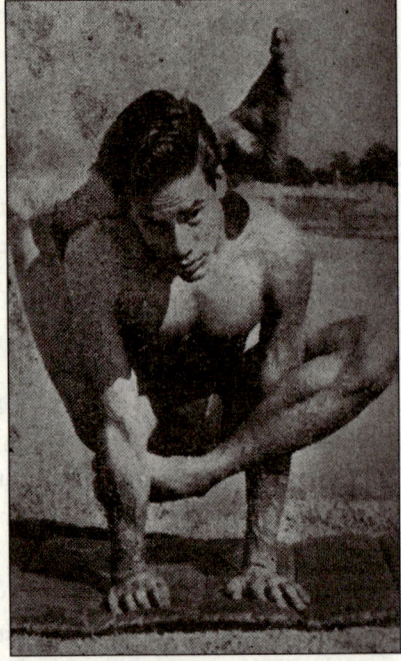

Top: Monotosh Choudhury. *Source: Bayam Charcha 1969.*
Bottom: Yoga Asana list (partial). *Courtesy of Bimal Das.*

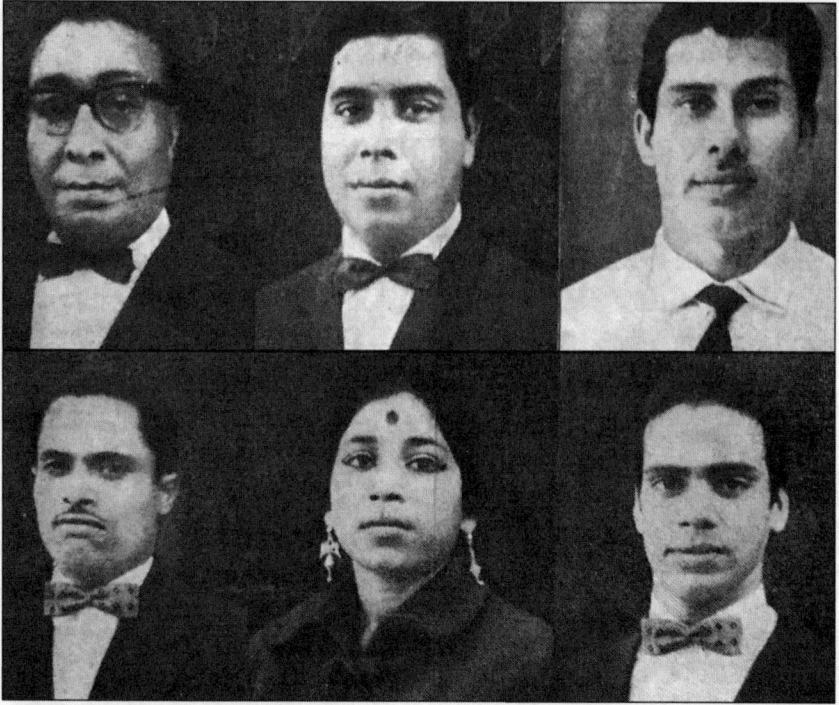

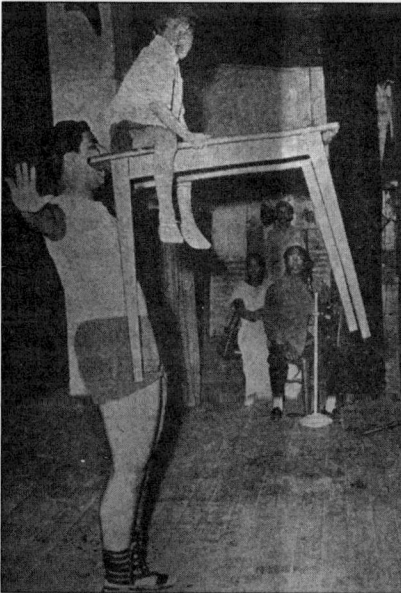

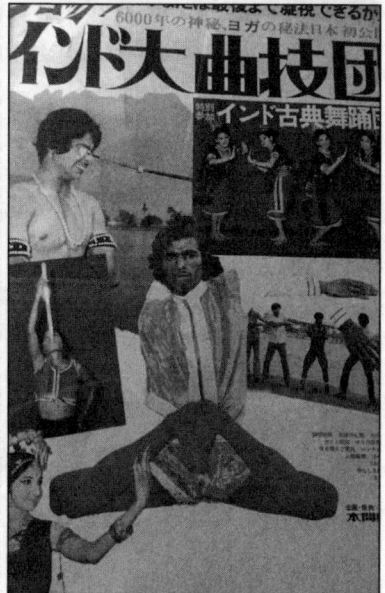

Top: 1968 Japanese Troupe. Bottom left: Bishwanath Ghosh.
Bottom right: Manoranjan Haldar, 'ghostly yoga asanas' and other Troupe members.
Source: Bayam Charcha.

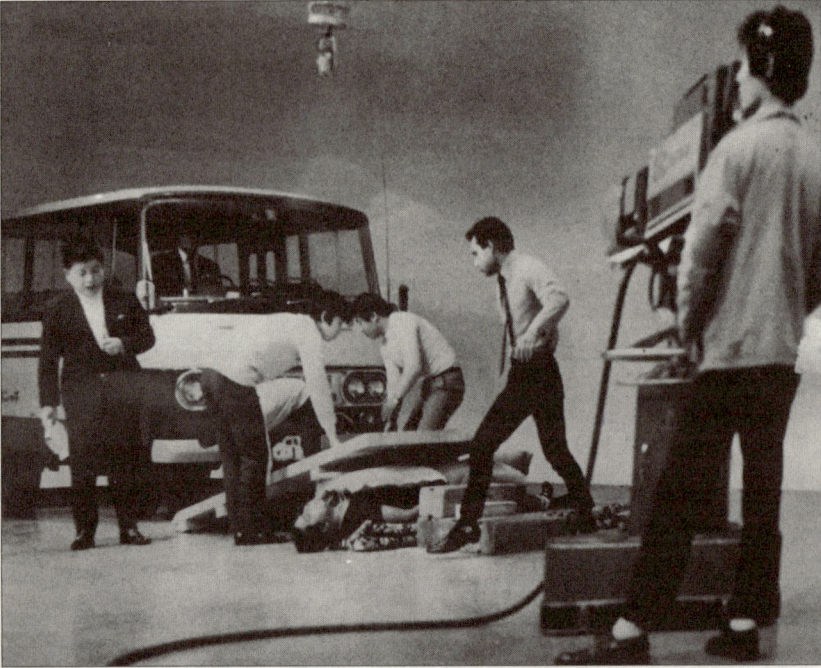

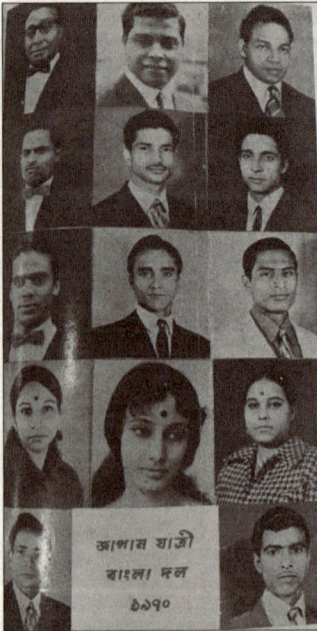

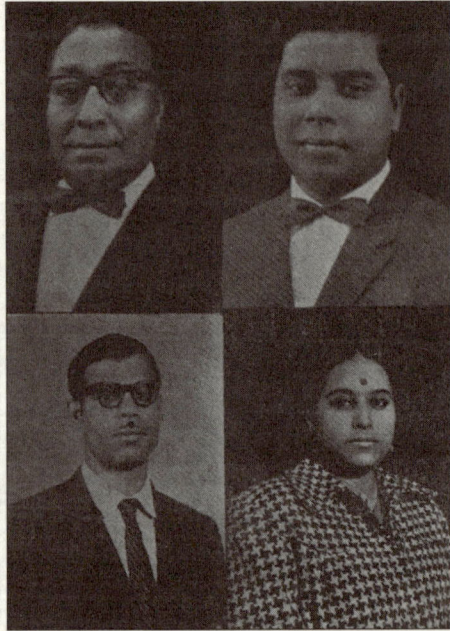

Top: Feats of Strength by Bishwanath Ghosh in Japan.
Bottom Left: 1970 Japanese Troupe. Bottom right: 1969 Japanese Troupe.

Courtesy of Ghosh's Yoga College; Source: Bayam Charcha.

83

A YOGA TEACHER FOR TOKYO

The 1969 Japanese invitation was 'a rehearsal performance for the 1970 World Extraordinary Performances to be held in Tokyo'. For Bishnu, there was also another opportunity.[1] *Bayam Charcha* reported:

> The recent tour of Japan by a group of *bayam* experts under the leadership of *Bayamacharya* Bishnu Charan Ghosh left the Japanese wanting more. They were very impressed by Yogendra Amar Nandi's *nauli-dhauti* and it has been decided that a yoga-*bayam* expert will soon go to Japan and teach yoga to the Japanese. Just as India is quite a mystery to the outside world, its yogic *sadhana* is loved all over the world.[2]

For quite a while, the culture of Japan and other countries of the Far East had fascinated Bengal. Now the feeling was becoming mutual. Japan wanted more of the feats of strength and yoga from India. The Hanari family shepherded this process.

In 1970, the Hanari family opened a studio in Japan, the Tokyo Yoga Center, and requested that Bishnu provide a teacher. The decision was easy. Buddha's son, 'Arun, was to be sent to Japan first.' Arun was an expert in yoga asanas and other feats, such as *lathi khela* (stick fighting). He 'could resist a sharp spear being pushed against his eyeball, and tear apart stacks of playing cards with his bare hands', similar to the feats Buddha performed in the thirties.[3] But Arun had been the first of the five 'yoga family' children to marry. His wife, Swapna, had grown up across the street on Rammohan Roy Road and became 'an expert in yoga and yoga-*bayam*, and boneless acts' herself. After the 'love marriage', between Swapna and Arun, she was 'in charge of the ladies section at Ghosh's College', which had recently been established.[4]

The Japanese balked at Arun, as 'they wanted an unmarried teacher'.[5]

It was then decided that either Monotosh Choudhury, the first performer to go to Japan in 1968 or Amar Nath Nandi from the 1969 voyage, should be the one to go and teach in Japan; both were natural choices to teach in Japan, being two of the most qualified yoga teachers under Bishnu. Another top choice was the more junior yoga teacher named Bimal Das, who had started under Gouri Shankar Mukerji in 1958.

When I began the research for this book, in 2015, I had no idea who these men were. And then, once I learned of them, how was I to find them, if they were still alive?

It wasn't until four years after I began travelling to, and interviewing people, in Calcutta that I was finally able to locate these key individuals of the sixties. Part of that was just me getting to this part of the history in the writing and part of it was just the process. In a city of over ten million, already lost in time itself, it was more difficult than it sounds. Mukul Dutta made it happen.

My arrangement with Mukul wasn't of researcher and research assistant – there was no transaction and he was senior to me, so he was more of a mentor or a friend. His motivation was remembrance and a desire to reconnect with his past of those glory years alongside Bishnu Charan Ghosh as his teacher and these other individuals as his companions and teachers. These were individuals whom Mukul had not seen or connected with for decades.

I'd arrive to Mukul's *Bhagavad Gita* class on Sunday morning at 9 a.m., which he holds at The Pearl Clinic, a healthcare office, where he works as a physiologist during the weekdays. After the class, I hopped on the back of his Bullet motorcycle. I rode pillion and he navigated the bike along the same streets where Bishnu and Buddha had ridden their bikes many decades ago. We visited the family of Motil Mondal, whose family edited and published *Bayam Charcha*, Bishnu's magazine. We travelled to find Maloy Roy, the son of Monotosh, to view photos we'd heard of but never seen. We managed to find Bimal Das, now in his seventies, who demonstrated *uddiyan* muscle control. We rode the local train from Howrah station to Serampore, to visit with Amar Nath Nandi. When we tracked each of them down and then interviewed them, it felt like I'd witnessed a small miracle.

Just as much as finding the *Bayam Charcha* magazine editions from 1964 to 1974, these interviews enlightened me of what had really happened, especially regarding how Bikram Choudhury, a 'second-rate' weightlifter under Bishnu in the first half of the sixties, rose to such prominence in yoga asana teaching over the next decade in America. It started with what seems like a fluke.

Monotosh, Amar Nath and Bimal were single, and each wanted to go to Tokyo and teach yoga, but Hanari and the Tokyo Yoga Center asked for a substantial commitment. Bimal explained, 'My office told me I could get leave for 6 months, not for 3 years. I would then lose my job.' He told Bishnu he could not go. [6] Monotosh came the closest to going, but his family was worried and called it off. Buddha and Bishnu's first choices to represent the school were not working out. This opened up an opportunity, as Bishwanath Ghosh had two younger friends who wanted to go: Shyamal Talukdar and Bikram Choudhury. Bikram really wanted to go and 'told Bishwanath to ask his father to send him to Japan'.

Born in 1945, Shyamal was a childhood friend of the family boys and lived just around the corner on Upper Circular Road. He remembered, 'we all used to play on the grounds behind the house, Bishwanath, Ashok, Arun and I.' [7] He became a teacher and masseur at the Yoga Cure Institute. He was more qualified for the Japan position than Bikram, but the Yoga Cure Institute depended on him to treat the patients who paid for his massage services in Calcutta. Bikram had no such clients in Calcutta, and this gave him an edge.

Bishwanath was key to influencing his father, even over the objections of others. Gouri Shankar Mukerji raised multiple objections to Bikram being sent to Japan. 'He doesn't know the yoga', Gouri told Bishnu.

But Bishnu countered, 'He can learn it quickly enough.'

'But he doesn't speak English well enough,' said Gouri. 'Neither do they; it's good enough!' said Bishnu. [8]

It was settled. 'Bikram went as a replacement.' [9]

'Did you know that Bishnu Ghosh only trained Bikram in yoga for about six months before they sent him to Japan?' Rooma Bose, daughter of Buddha, asks me and two other Americans, Ida Jo and Scott Lamps, who have accompanied me on a research visit. We just look at each other with blank stares. She goes on, telling us of Bikram learning asanas during a six-month stint, from the summer of '69 until he left for Tokyo in early 1970.

'He didn't know how to do *mayurasana* (peacock) at all, and he couldn't figure it out.' Rooma explains that while Bikram was learning, she was in the other room when Bishnu called out for her. She entered the room where they were training.

'Here, you show him!' Bishnu told Rooma.[10] She had been called in to demonstrate the asana for Bikram. Even though it was forty-five years in the past, Rooma relished the moment of retelling it.

Bikram was trained at the Yoga Cure premises on 4/2 Rammohan Roy Road in 1969. During this period, he moved into the house, as other favourite students of Bishnu's had done; even as Buddha himself had once done. After the intensive family training, Bikram left for Tokyo in February 1970.

Bikram was born in 1944. His family moved back and forth, as did the siblings, having relations in Deoghar, Bihar. They finally settled during the fifties at 8 Mahendra Bose Lane in Baghbazar, north Calcutta. Bikram's father worked inside the Writers' Building in central Calcutta, across the water pond from where Dalhousie Institute once stood.

In 1962, at the age of eighteen, Bikram became a regular student at the gymnasium after meeting Bimal Das. Bimal, about three years older, lived near Bikram at the time on GT Road, and the two 'would take the bus together' to Bishnu's gymnasium.[11] They 'addressed each other as *tui* 'in Bengali' which was the closest form of addressing each other fondly'. Bikram also became very good friends with Arun Bose and Bishwanath Ghosh. The three of them were born within about a year of each other. Bikram, when he began in 1962, was 'a bodybuilder'.[12]

Bikram first made the news in 1966. That April, a '*bayam* team from Ghosh's College under the leadership of *Bayamacharya* Bishnu Charan Ghosh boarded the Mail train to Bombay'.[13] The article described the participant-performers, who were largely in line with the troupe Bishnu took to Japan a few years later:

Sri Motilal Mondal also accompanied the team. Sri Buddha Bose and his wife were there to bid the team farewell at the station, as were many others.

The team was comprised of: *Bharatshree* Kamal Bhandari, *Bharatkumar* Shanti Dutta, *Bharatkumar* Robin Goswami, *Shaktisamudra* Madhusudan Pandey, *Yoga-bayam* Parthi Chowdhury, and *Kumari* Rooma Bose. In judo, Biswanath Ghosh and W. Bose. Reba and Ruby Patra performed plastic body.

Gymnastics by Satkari Pramanik, Nitya Gopal De and Mahadev Manna. Gour De performed in the Roman Ring; spine-chilling acts performed by the daughter of the mountains, Meera Devi. Power acts performed by Karuna Ghosh and *Bayamacharya*'s wife. The Trio Band Party under the supervision Sri N. Chowdhury accompanied the team and made the journey memorable with their beautiful music.

Then, upon arrival in Bombay, Bikram was mentioned:

The team was profusely welcomed in Bombay and a huge exhibition was held at the Purandar Stadium in the evening for news reporters. The whole show was organized by Biswanath Ghosh and Bikram Choudhury. The event was inaugurated by *Times of India* General Manager, Sri Pratap Chandra Roy. The audience got absolutely amazed and fascinated by the performance of the team; the exhibition show was organized to help establish a *bayamagar* in Bombay.[14]

At the end of the article, Bikram was again listed among those to thank and that 'Sri Bishnu Charan Ghosh and his team have been invited to visit Bombay again in the month of November, and the invitation has been gratefully accepted by *Bayamacharya* Ghosh'.[15]

In the November 1966 issue of *Bayam Charcha*, Bikram graced the cover while posing with bodybuilding awards and trophies in the background. As was typical with the magazine, a biography for the person on the cover was included:

This 21 year old beautifully formed and handsome young man is a Bengali youth. Anyone who looks at him keeps on looking and admiring him. He has been into sports from a very young age; earning name and fame in the field of football and athletics. Later he turned towards physical culture and was enraptured with weight lifting. In 1963, Bikram won the Rajendra Weight lifting competition. At the time he was a school student. His physical culture teacher is *Bayamacharya* Bishnu Charan Ghosh. Bikram has become an expert in yoga-*bayam* and tissue massage. He now lives in Bombay. Among his regular students are many renowned artists and film stars like Ustad Vilayat Khan, Pradeep Kumar, Dilip Kumar, Hemanta Mukherjee, Amita Guha, Meena Kumari and others.

Bikram travelled back and forth from Bombay to Calcutta often. Just as with many others, Bishnu had trained Bikram well, and was able to place him in a position for success. Part of Bishnu's ability was the understanding a person's qualities, and then magnifying them, so that the person was able to stand out with even greater success. Bikram was very social, affable and confident. He did well in Bombay, being employed to assist Bollywood stars.

The period when Bikram was in Bollywood, from 1966 until 1969, was part of the Golden Age of Hindi cinema. Commercial Hindi cinema was a booming business, and critically acclaimed films were being produced. The rich and famous stars needed body-wor, and Bikram was an excellent masseur, having been trained in anatomy and the art of body-work at Ghosh's gymnasium. During the period when he was a bodybuilder, from 1962 until 1965, he gained hands-on knowledge of the body, working as a masseur with clients one at a time. In 1969, Bikram was ready for something different.

The type of sped-up asana training Bikram underwent was described by another student of Bishnu Ghosh at this time:

> Our first lessons were the different postures of Yoga-asana. When I was able to sit in a particular posture, comfortably and breathing normally (pulse rate) for the prescribed span (up to an hour) then my competence was admitted. I had to learn 32 postures (under my guides approval and direction) under the direct supervision of my seniors who had already mastered the postures concerned. Our second lessons were *Pranayama* (breathing exercises), then *Bandha* (bodily locks); and finally, *Dhyana* (focused meditation).[16]

After about six months of training with Bishnu and the senior yoga asana teachers, Bikram had learned most of the asanas but not the second lessons. He had also been able to recuperate from a knee injury he had suffered in competitive sports. In the February of 1970, Bishnu took Bikram, along with his student Mukul Dutta, to the Calcutta airport. The two saw Bikram off with the expectation of his return to Calcutta in six months' time, for more advanced training in yoga and 'to marry Rooma', Bishnu's granddaughter.[17]

Bishnu felt that the events of 1969 in Tokyo had restarted his yoga asana work abroad, which had been 'stalled in Europe due to the second world war'. After he and Buddha had returned from their world tour, and after all of the tragic events of the forties, Bishnu's international attention had been more focused on his bodybuilding students. Now, once again, the 'yoga-*bayam* mission returned', and in 1970, Bishnu was set to return to Japan.

84

DEMISE

At Nimtala Ghat, the cremation grounds for north Calcutta,
there is a massive tree, growing atop and alongside the old red brick structure.
The two have become inseparable.
To the earth, its roots reach down below, into the Ganges.

In the July of 1970, *Bayam Charcha* announced: 'Byamcharya Is Not Well. He had a heart problem on the 21st of June, and has been admitted to the hospital.'[1] Later, an update informed the readers that Bishnu was 'not well enough to take the journey', and instead, on 20 July 1970, 'Bishwanath Ghosh will lead the team to Japan in place of his father'. However, on 9 July, before the group even left, it was announced: 'Bishnu Charan Ghosh silently left this world at around 3:05 p.m.'[2]

Newspaper announcements, letters and telegrams from abroad came in droves, expressing sorrow for the loss. An obituary notice was published in the *Self-Realization Fellowship* magazine, alongside a quotation from the *Bhagavad Gita*:

> Never the spirit was born; the spirit shall cease to be never; Never was time it was not; end and beginning are dreams!

'Bishnu Charan is my relative, guru and best friend', were the first public words uttered by Buddha Bose after Bishnu's death.[3] And in the August issue of the magazine *Bayam Charcha*, he gave 'a unique memorial and a worthy *guru-dakshina*'. The December issue contained like-minded notes from admirers and students of Bishnu. Many reflected on accomplishments and their shared moments.

On that same day, 'the news had reached the editor of All India Radio', which 'did not waste any time broadcasting the news' to Calcutta:

His son, Biswanath, arranged for the body to be brought home. Bishnu's body was placed in the *akhara*, his place of *sadhana*. Soon the place became filled with flowers and hundreds of mourners. *Bayamacharya*'s daughter Karuna, and granddaughter Rooma, sat near his head.

A reporter visited the family's home and 'found the situation upstairs heart-wrenching' as well:

His wife, Ashalata lying down in despair and grief, *Bayamacharya*'s eldest daughter Ava Rani Bose, who was sick, sat in a corner shedding silent tears – what else could she do. *Bayamacharya*'s best friend, student and son-in-law Sri Buddha Bose, was sitting, controlled and silent. I made some phone calls and by the time I came down the scene had become unmanageable with the surging crowd of mourners. Rammohan Roy Road and Ghosh's College were completely deluged with people.

At 10 p.m. that evening, Bishnu's body 'left for his last journey' in this world:

The procession was preceded by people carrying incense sticks, flowers bedecked *Bayamacharya*'s bed. Special singers followed, singing Hare Krishna all the way. The procession passed through Rammohan Roy Road, Raja Dinendra Street, Garpar Road where his body was laid to rest for a brief moment. We passed through APC Road, Kailas Bose Street, Amherst Street, Vivekananda Road, Bidhan Sarani, then on to Beadon Street, before finally reaching the Nimtala Burning *Ghat*.[4]

Describing the scene at Nimtala Ghat:

When he was laid out on the wooden pyre at the burning *ghat*, it seemed his lotus-like eyes were smiling and telling us, 'Do not worry I am and will be there always with you all. Never forget.' I heard a reply whisper in my ears 'See this is the beginning and end of creation – this burning *ghat*. Will there be another you created? Will this void be ever filled?' He replied silently, 'Why not? I am not gone, I am there amidst you.'[5]

The death of Bishnu 'cast a gloom' over 'the *bayam* world', which then came 'crashing down'. All that remained was 'a void never to be filled'.[6]

Bishnu's death struck everyone as being too early, especially given how his last couple of decades had been busy with 'promoting the fact that yoga-*bayam* was a therapeutic avenue' for longevity. 'Healing through yoga became his vision and he worked hard to make it popular to the common man.'[7]

In one of his last interviews about his upcoming trip to Japan, Bishnu had talked about 'how he planned to start a yoga-*bayam* university on his return' to Calcutta. This did not happen. However, Bishnu had recently overseen the first 'women only' yoga centre in Calcutta in 1967. It was started by a student of Bishnu's, named Kushala Das.

Kushala, with her brothers Dibya and Prem, learned the art of yoga under Bishnu in the sixties. Their father, Ashutosh Das, was a good friend of Bishnu's older brother, Sananda Ghosh, having helped him finish and write an introduction for the book Mejda. By 1962, all three Das children were making the ten-minute walk from their house, near Sealdah station, to practise Hatha yoga under Bishnu Ghosh.

Dibya, who also studied under Gouri Shankar Mukerji, was 'not interested' in lifting weights like the other yoga *bayam* proponents. 'I did the exercises – free-hand exercises to flex the muscles – before I did the yoga. I did all the 84 asanas. I am the real yoga child.' Dibya was placed in charge of the Bajrang Byamgar near Deshapriya Park, and Prem became the vice president at Ghosh's Yoga College in 1974.

Kushala, like Reba Rakshit before her, authored articles for *Bayam* magazines which were addressed to women. 'In today's world,' she wrote, 'when women have to go out to the school, college, office and other places, they cannot afford to be shy and reticent. When you have to rub shoulder to shoulder with men you have to take care of your health just like them.'[8] She addressed presupposed disqualifications:

Another wrong belief among people is that yoga-*bayam* is only meant for the yogis. No, this can be practised by everyone – yogi or no yogi. Then again people fear yoga asanas might hurt their bodies and nerves. Wrong again. It is the safest thing to do. The *shastras* say, '*sthira sukham asanam.*'[9]

She recognized one real hinderance:

One big problem in our country is lack of place for women to do exercise. But as they say, where there's a will there's a way. You can practise at home on your bed, if you are so inclined. This is known as yoga-*bayam*. It is common knowledge that man finds all strategies to live, similarly there is a lot of strategy in yoga-*bayam*. *Bayam* experts say: '*yog kromoshoh kaushalam*' or Yoga-*bayam* is full of strategies.[10]

Kushula's strategy was to open a gym. In 1967, with Bishnu Ghosh, she pioneered an institution in India solely for yoga training of women. Named Mahila Yoga *Bayam* Kendra, it was established on the day of Janmashtami, 14 August 1967, 'for the ladies, by the ladies and of the ladies'.[11]

An announcement of the opening in *Bayam Charcha* provides a glimpse at the top performers of yoga under Bishnu at the time:

Students of the club showed some yoga asanas after the opening ceremony. Among them were – Sri Nobokumar Dutta, Sri Mukul Dutta, Kumari Sabita Mullick and Sri Amar Nandi. Amar Nandi directed the yoga demonstrations and also explained the benefits of each asana. Sri Mukul Dutta performed *dhauti* beautifully. Amar Nandi showed *uddiyan* and *nauli* at the end under the supervision of Tapas Bhattacharya.

The day before the troupe left for Japan, 19 July 1970, a condolence meeting was organized at Mahila Yoga *Bayam* Kendra:

The meeting was presided over by Bishnu's elder brother, Sri Sananda Ghosh. *Acharya* Bishnucharan Ghosh's son, Biswanath Ghosh, and his two grandsons, Ashok Bose and Arun Bose were also present. Kamal Bhandari, Anil Roy and Hiten Roy spoke about Bishnu Babu's influence and generosity in shaping their lives. Kushala Das, founder of the Kendra said that the name 'Mahila Yoga-*bayam* Kendra' was given by the *Bayamacharya*.

Ashok Bose recited a poem he had composed in memory of late Bishnucharan on behalf of Ghosh's College of Physical Education. Sri Sananda Ghosh mentioned a few anecdotes of the period when late Bishnucharan was attracted to *bayam* and then yoga. He also mentioned the fact that late Bishnucharan loved this Kendra and his blessings would always be there.

Dedications continued in *Bayam Charcha*, alongside remembrances and notes of condolence, recognizing a 'Bishnu Charan Memorial Committee'. Among their recommendations, it stated, 'a bust of the late *Bayamacharya* should be installed at the crossing of Rammohan Roy Road and Acharya Prafulla Chandra Road'.

Bishnu, as Buddha wrote in his homage, 'worked for a worthy cause and even though he is no more, his vision of a healthy India is what we should all aim towards'.[12] Buddha assured Bishnu that 'he would take care of Yoga Cure', and so, 'after Bishnu's death, Buddha took over'.[13] Bishwanath replaced Bishnu as president of the Yoga Cure Institute, and Prem Das, the brother of Kushala, was brought on as an assistant physical culturist. The three of them would attempt to expand the Yoga Cure Institute in Calcutta.[14]

85

CALCUTTA'S COURSE

Bayamacharya is no more. The news has struck the physical culture world like a lightning. Bayamcharya is dead and it is hard to believe.[1]

It was a shock to everyone that Bishnu would die at just sixty-seven years of age. Stories spread, though unconfirmed, of blood transfusions in which Bishnu was given the wrong type of blood. It was said that Bishnu had heart difficulties throughout his life and his weight had increased in his later years, similar to what Yogananda encountered. It may have seemed an early death for the *bayamacharya*, but Calcutta was a cruel city when delivering death to its residents, given to a preponderance of disease and environmental conditions.

Throughout Bishnu's life, Calcutta declined as a developed global city. The political power had moved north to New Delhi when Bishnu was still a young boy, and the influx of millions due to the famine and partition overpopulated the city while he was an adult. The British had finally gone, but their infrastructure still existed (the trams still ran). By the fifties, Calcutta lived off its cultural capital reserves, 'held up by imagined and imaginary longings' for its second London status of the East.[2] Reality was instead reflected by Mother Teresa and her mission. In 1952, when she opened her first 'Home for the Dying' near Kalighat Temple, she brought in the nearly dead from the streets each day. The hyper-dense population within its 9 mile center made it the most populated urban core in the world, with many living in slums.

When the writer and follower of Vedanta, Christopher Isherwood, arrived on 24 December 1963, he stayed at Ramakrishna's mandir and wrote about his first impressions of Calcutta.

What crowds and crowds of people! This is what most of the world is really like – overpopulation, near starvation, under squalor. Old trucks, bullock carts, rickshaws, little closed cabs such as Ramakrishna used to ride in. Holy men smeared all over with ashes. And the skinny wandering bulls.[3]

Isherwood was there for the Parliament of Religions, in preparation for the 1964 centenary of Swami Vivekananda. A week after he arrived, Isherwood still wasn't impressed:

Calcutta is a pale faded yellow city – all strong color has been burned, parched out of it by the sun. At night it is crowded but cheerless, under its pall of dirty smoke. A poor wretched place; the joyless street of six million people. Looking out the window at dawn, you see bent figures in wispy smoke-colored garments moving silently about like emanations of the smoke, as they light their fires to create more smoke.[4]

In 1967, political power in Calcutta had swung towards communism, through the Communist Party of India. The communists gained and shared power with various political allies such as the Forward Bloc.[5] Around the time of Bishnu's death, Geoffrey Moorhouse visited Calcutta and wrote a popular travelogue, titled *Calcutta: The City Revealed*.[6] Aside from the overtly political situation in Calcutta which Moorhouse described, he also wrote of extreme poverty and disease, which set the stage for Calcutta in the seventies. This vision was the same as the one planted in our Western minds by Mother Teresa, the realities of children in despair and ghettos of death with seemingly no way out.

Photos in the book by Moorhouse included, on the milder side, bodies splayed out to 'spend the night' on the pavement outside the Great Eastern Hotel. A photo of a 'slum of makeshift shanties' with more than 'one million refugees' was a bit more shocking. The 'ultimate poverty' though, where 'dogs are seen chewing' on unburnt body parts, was revolting.[7] When he revisited Calcutta in 1983, Moorhouse felt compelled to rewrite the introduction, stating, 'Obviously the deepest pessimisms of 1970 have been lightened a shade or two by what has happened since.' His conclusion of an impending 'haunting horror' of 'some kind of disaster' for Calcutta, 'a city of smoking ruins', had been overstated.[8] In a way, the accepted chaos of Calcutta was its saving grace. From the outside, its 'face of difficulties' seemed untenable to Westerners, but we underestimated 'the warmth of people and their astonishing vitality'.[9]

Even considering the toxic environment Calcutta was during those times, its life was still striking to Moorhouse:

It is the easiest thing in the world to come close to despair in Calcutta. Every statistic that you tear out of the place reeks of doom. Every half mile can produce something that is guaranteed to turn a newcomer's stomach with fear or disgust or a sense of hopelessness. It must be a generation at least since anyone stayed here for more than a day or two unless he was obliged to, or had a phenomenal sense of vocation, or a pathological degree of curiosity. Yet for anyone with the willful staying power to remain through that first awful week when Calcutta is driving him away with shock and nausea, with resentment and with plain gut-rotting funk, a splendid truth about this city slowly dawns upon his perceptions and his understanding. It is that although he will surely never before have encountered so much that is deadly in any one place, he has never been confronted with so much life, either. It pulsates and churns around him wherever he goes, it swirls in every direction.[10]

It is difficult to project the future course of Calcutta, but its old colonial-style homes and buildings sit below sea-level in many places and just a few feet above in others. A recent World Bank Report reported that Calcutta 'is one of the global mega-cities that is most at risk from climate change'.[11]

YOGA COLLEGE OF INDIA GOES ABROAD

Yogananda was the first in the Ghosh family to travel to Japan. He had gone in 1916 but was unable to go from there to America. Flummoxed and uninspired by the port city he was confined to, he returned to Calcutta on the next ship available to him. In contrast, decades later, Bishwanath liked Japan quite a lot.[1]

On 20 July 1970, Bishwanath's team left for Japan less than two weeks after Bishnu's death. The troupe included '14 talented and fearless young men and women of Bengal' who were 'on their way to Japan to bring glory not only to Bengal but to the whole country'.[2] The 1970 tour throughout Japan was arranged as a 'group tour of several cities' over the course of 'two months, including at Expo 70' in Tokyo.[3]

In 1958, at the age of thirteen, Bishwanath had been 'so thin' that 'people often asked whether Bishwanath Ghosh was actually the son of Bishnu'.

His father replied, 'This is God's way of testing me; the person who is able to help thousands of youth across the country to gain good health, whether he is capable of doing the same with his own.' Within three years, Bishwanath had become 'a jiu-jitsu expert' and 'at the age of 16 years, amazed everybody by his taking a 100 *mon* elephant on his chest'. In 1968, at the age of twenty-three, he had gone to Japan with his father, to train in judo and karate; making the 1970 trip to Japan Bishwanath's third visit.[4]

The 'daredevil *bayam* team' left Bengal for Japan in July.[5] In Japan at Expo 70, the strongman Madhusudan Pandey 'stopped speeding cars with his hands'. Satyen Das, a bodybuilder who had won the title of Mr India, performed a muscle show. Some of Bishnu's senior yoga students were in the group too. Monotosh Choudhury, who 'hailed from Burma and learned *bayam* through correspondence' with Bishnu, performed asanas, as did Bimal Das, who was profiled in the pages of *Bayam Charcha*:

> Bimal Das is 22 years and is an expert in *vastra dhauti, nauli, nasa dhauti* and other difficult kriyas. He is a college student and a disciple of yoga expert Dr. Gouri Shankar Mukhopadhyay. Bimal is now training under Bishnucharan Ghosh.[6]

There was also Manoranjan Haldar, who performed 'ghostly yoga asanas' with the use of swords that he twisted into shapes after he had tossed them into the air to land between his limbs. There was Kartik Dutta, who would 'swallow 3 liters of petrol, 3 snakes, 24 frogs and 8 catfish'. He 'would swallow the fish then bring it back through his throat and the fish would still be alive'. It was 'Hatha yoga', Kartik professed, that gave him the ability 'to perform such spine chilling acts'.[7]

For Expo 70, the Ghosh and Bose family children were just as involved as they were with the previous troupe. Bishwanath performed the feats of 'taking a 10-ton roller on his chest, a motorcycle jump', and 'an elephant on his chest' (as did his sister Karuna). Jibananda Ghosh (who would marry Karuna in five months) was able to 'lay on a bed of nails for a motorcycle to jump over him and could withstand a car passing over his arm'.[8]

The troupe 'performed continuously for 2 months and 7 days in 50 venues and a total count of 80 performances'. This included both the Expo 70 and a spectacular television performance in July at the Brouse Hotel.[9]

In between performances, Bishwanath worked with Bikram, who wished to break away from the Tokyo Yoga Center. Bikram had been teaching at the Tokyo Yoga Center for only a few months when Bishnu died that July. Apparently, Bikram 'lost his support'.[10]

According to Bikram's brother Buddhadeb, the move out of the Tokyo Yoga Center was put into action because 'the terms and conditions were not correctly followed' by the Hanari family. Bikram was aided by Americans in the effort to establish a yoga studio in Tokyo. William L. Clark, the author of *Spoken American English*, told Bikram, 'Since there are so many problems in this school, let us open another yoga school'.[11]

Bikram, once expected to return to Calcutta after six months for more training and other commitments no longer wished to return. With his teacher Bishnu gone, he instead stayed in Tokyo. However, Bishwanath Ghosh was the principal person responsible for opening the new centre in Tokyo where Bikram taught yoga. *Bayam Charcha* announced that, while in Tokyo, 'Sri Bishwanath Ghosh has established the "Yoga College of India" in Japan and has been elected as the president of the institution.'[12]

Another friend of Bikram's helped out in the first months of the new yoga institution. Bimal Das, the senior teacher who was on the tour with Bishwanath in 1970, stayed in Tokyo for a few more months, 'living with Bikram at the yoga studio', and teaching Bikram advanced asanas and other practices. The two 'knew very little English, but learned how to say to the Japanese that they "have come from the land of Gautam Buddha to show you miracle yoga"'. In addition to home visits and giving Indian massages, they would teach students in 'groups of 15–20 persons'.

The format of the classes in Japan, Bimal explained, 'always depended on the number of students, but the classes always started at 9 a.m. sharp. Each class was held for an hour.' Bimal explained further that the classes 'would start with yoga exercise (*bayam*) and then yoga asana, then mudras, then pranayam and finish with meditation. The meditation room was separate and very sweet with dim lights, idols of gods and photos of Bishnu Charan Ghosh and Yogananda.' Bimal explained that in Japan, they had both individual lessons and group classes 'partly because of the culture, and ... also due to their having little knowledge' of yoga.

In response to the idea of a group class, Mukul Dutta explained that, as a student of Bishnu Charan Ghosh, he was 'not familiar with group classes' and that 'Gouri Shankar taught individually, so did Buddha Bose and so on. Maybe it is more practical to have group classes in the West ...'

When asked about the twenty-six postures sequence, now known as Bikram Yoga, Bimal explained that he had 'no memory of all that'.

Mukul added, 'Bikram did not teach anything related to yoga at Ghosh's College.'[13]

Bimal explained that what Bikram had taught in Japan was a combination of yoga he had learned from Bishnu Ghosh and his own knowledge – a 'new' yoga.[14] The new terrain and format inspired Bimal too, who thereafter created his own sequence. 'I teach twenty-two yoga postures in a sequence', he said. 'I made my own sequence derived from guru's teachings and my own input.'[15]

Like Bikram's, Bimal's sequence was coherent with the postures presented in the 1961 *Yoga-Cure* booklet, and the twenty-six postures in the 'Yoga Asana' chart from the thirties, but instead of teaching the postures as done individually, they were now being done as a class.

Buddha Bose went to Japan in December 1970 to fill Bikram's position, bringing in two newlyweds for the Tokyo Yoga Center. Jibananda Ghosh had married Karuna, Bishnu's daughter, inside Ghosh's College that same December before leaving for Tokyo. Even though Buddha was in Japan at the same time as Bikram, it was 'in a different address', and no interaction appears to have happened.[16]

Bikram had left the Tokyo Yoga Center and formed a Yoga College of India under Bishwanath's guidance, which had the possibility of creating tension. 'Buddha Bose was angry with Bikram', but not because of the yoga, explained Shyamal Talukdar. It was 'because Bikram refused to marry Rooma'. One thing was clear, Shyamal explained, Bikram did not want to return to Calcutta to be 'a servant of the Bose family'.[17]

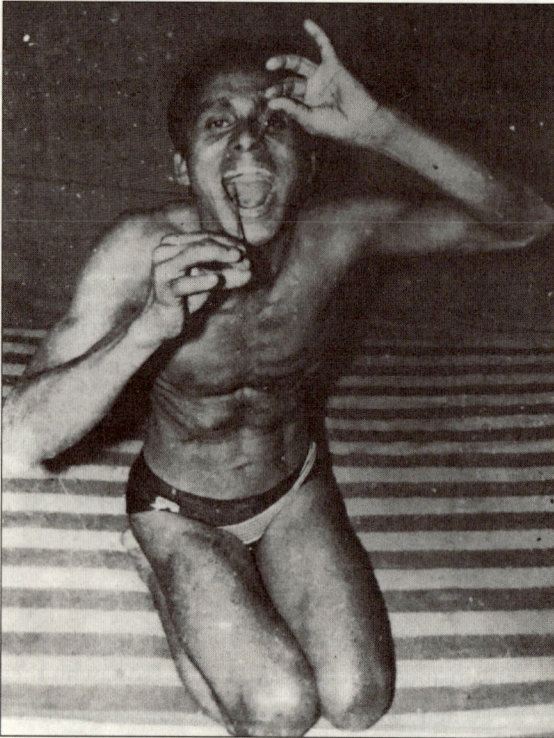

Bimal Das performing the Hatha yoga Kriya, neti (nasal cleansing), Japan, 1970.
Courtesy of Bimal Das.

87

HAWAIIAN CLASSES BY BIKRAM

Bikram swears by a booklet, Yoga-Cure written by his instructor,
the late Bishnu Ghosh.[1]
– Honolulu State-Bulletin, 23 August 1972.

After Bimal Das left Japan, Bikram was on his own. The ties to the legacy of Calcutta's yoga were mainly maintained through the Advanced Asana list given to him by Bimal, and *Yoga-Cure*, the small booklet written by Bishnu. Bikram made many friends, and in 1971, left for Hawaii.

In January of 1971, Bikram first arrived in the United States with the help of his 'sponsor and guardian Eiko Osano'.[2] Eiko was married to Kenji Osana, whose corporate empire extended out of Japan and into Hawaii with the purchase of properties in Honolulu during the early 1960s, most notably the popular Surfrider Hotel. Under the care of this wealthy and influential Japanese family, Bikram was able to shuttle from Tokyo to Honolulu. Not even a year after his departure from India, he secured a visa and entered the United States.[3]

One longtime student and teacher who met Bikram in Hawaii during one of his first visits was Georgia Balligian. After graduation from New York University in 1970, Georgia 'travelled through the South Pacific and ended up out of funds and in Hawaii'. She waitressed at the Wailana Coffee Shop in Honolulu, just a few blocks from the hotels owned by the Osano family, where Bikram was staying. 'As fate would have it, Bikram Choudhury, newly arrived from Tokyo, was teaching his yoga in a small studio in downtown Honolulu.' Georgia's 'first class was about 2.5 hours long and had a total of 7 students in it. Everyone was working hard, getting a lot of laughs, encouragement and lots of tough love.'[4]

This was similar to the type of yoga class Bikram had taught in Tokyo in 1970 – the classes were longer and tailored to the group at hand.

Bikram used *Yoga-Cure* for cues and directions, while adding his own verbal cues from yoga and bodybuilding. In one early sequence, Bikram would advise six postures (wind removing, cobra, half-tortoise, bow, rabbit and spine twisting). The instructions were in line with what Buddha taught, with each posture repeated 'three times': Begin with holding the posture 'for 20 seconds' and 'gradually work up to one minute'. Between each posture, 'relax in the *Savasana* position for one minute'. 'This set of exercises,' Bikram explained, 'should be the minimum.' And, 'if you do 30 minutes of yoga a day, it is not necessary to spend one cent on a doctor in your whole life'.[5] By the end of 1971, Bikram was teaching ninety-minute classes, one after the other, in a more stable format.

With the death of Bishnu, Buddha took over the yoga leadership position. At the Tokyo Yoga Center, Jibananda would teach regular classes to men, and Karuna took charge of the newly established 'ladies section' of the 'yoga-*bayam* Kendra in Japan'.[6] Buddha 'suppressed the fact that Karuna was a couple of months pregnant', playing a bit of a trick on Hanari, who had earlier rejected having Arun and his wife come to Japan.

The two schools at this time, one in Calcutta and one in Tokyo, were almost entirely run by the Ghosh and Bose children. A promotional pamphlet listed the teachers: Buddha's three children, Ashok, Arun, and Rooma were listed as 'yoga advisor and teacher'. Karuna and Jibananda Ghosh were listed as 'Yoga Teacher, Tokyo'. Of the other eight members, only Prem Sundar Das, with the title of 'Physical Culturist' provided a service that was related to the Yoga Cure Institute.[7]

Included in the pamphlet was a piece written by Buddha Bose, called 'Yoga Cure Means', which was both practical and spiritual. 'We cure diseases through Yoga Asanas and Pranayamas', it read, through 'body, mind and soul'. The practice has its foundation in awakening 'the life force or *shakti*' which 'enables the individual to master the mind'.[8] The foundation is practice:

The practice of these Asanas drives away lethargy and gloom and helps to replace them with energy and vitality. It will benefit every individual in all walks of life. Naturally, it is never too late to begin the practice of these Yoga Asanas for it helps to rebuild the body, re-energise the mind, revive lost youth, beauty and strength.[9]

For over two decades, Buddha had been focused on pilgrimages to the Himalayas and narrating his travels alongside the movie *Holy Kailas*. As 1971 came to a close, he promoted what would be his last show of *Holy Kailas* in Calcutta.

88

BUDDHA'S LAST SHOW AT MAHAJATI SADAN

I peek inside and am invited to tour the building and stage. The auditorium seems cavernous, with balcony seating above. In 1958, when it was opened to the public, the seating capacity was 1,300 seats. It's apparent that no records were kept of past events, at least not as far back as 1971. Not a single person left in the administration was even around then to recall the night that Buddha Bose narrated the last show of Holy Kailas for a Calcutta audience.

The fame of Buddha Bose had grown through *Holy Kailas*, and he had journeyed to other places, including Bombay, retelling the narrative, sometimes in Hindi. He ran 'a one-man crusade going from State to State' showing his 'documentary film shot by himself'.[1]

Buddha had originally wanted the narration to be recorded, but some other power compelled him otherwise:

This is not an ordinary film. I had decided to show the whole film to the common people of India. The day I completed filming Manasarovar I saw a *sadhu* coming towards me. I thought he must be coming for some alms. I lit an *agarbatti* and told my helper to give the *sadhu* some *chattu*.

The *sadhu* heard me and said, 'I am not a beggar. I have come to tell you that as you have filmed this holy place you must show it to the people. Do not make it a commercial movie. And every time you show the film you have to be present and talk about it.'

Thus I roam around with the film showing people and giving a running commentary each time. The *sadhu* also said, 'Anyone who watches the film must have that respect and humility for these holy places.' The *sadhu* disappeared after he told me all this. I hope and pray that each one of you will watch this film with equal devotion and respect as told by the *sadhu* in Manasarovar.[2]

A promotional pamphlet asked, 'Have you seen and shown to your children and students, the film that is enthralling thousands?' Some, after watching the film narrated by Buddha, went to explore the places themselves. 'Our curiosity to visit this place was roused by Himalayan explorers and the film of Mr Buddha Bose,' wrote one reviewer.[3] A key highlight was when Sarvepalli Radhakrishnan, before he became the second president of India, viewed the film in Bombay, calling it 'impressive and inspiring'.[4]

By 1971, Buddha's film had been shown widely, and a final Calcutta show was promoted. The yoga student of Buddha, Shyamal Talukdar, had watched Buddha narrate the film at a famous theatre in Calcutta. 'I saw it in Mahajati Sadan. After the show in Mahajati Sadan, he never showed the film again.'

However, rather than celebrating the 1,000 times that the film had been shown, the event was fraught with the intrigue of scandal. The question arose, had Buddha gone and taken the pictures himself? Maybe 'Buddha Bose took the film from someone who died and showed it to the people of India'. Perhaps it was from 'someone who died in the plane crash who had already filmed the whole thing'.[5] Perhaps, Buddha, when the plane crashed in the Syrian desert, had pilfered film documentaries from a dead passenger, amidst the bodies in the rubble of the crash, and called them his own.

How could such a rumour even be started? Apparently, in some of the photographs or a part of the film, a 'white man's hand' appeared.[6]

There was a plausible explanation for the misunderstanding. 'People were not aware of Buddha's English bloodline and his skin color, so in a scene where a white hand came in front of the camera, it was naturally deduced it was the work of a "foreign hand"' and not Buddha's. Of course, Buddha was light skinned. That might have ended the whole episode, until another piece of information surfaced, from a lecture in Calcutta back in January of 1939:

Edward Groth showed a very beautiful film of a journey from Srinagar to Gilgit and Hunza, and then through Chitral to Peshawar.[7]

Groth was the American student of Buddha Bose who had paid for his first trip to the Himalayas in 1940. Buddha's film was a compilation of many different parts over the years, photographs and film, black and white and colour, so he might in fact have used part of Groth's film.

After the 'last show' in Calcutta, Buddha said 'he would throw the film into the Ganges. He had finished showing the film a thousand times.'[8] After the conclusion, 'everyone kept sitting in the hall. No one came out from the hall. All thinking.'[9]

As it turned out, the 'last show' of *Holy Kailas* in Calcutta, in 1971, was not the last show after all. Instead, Buddha got a call to present the film again in Gujarat, and he took the opportunity. From 1969 to 1972, Buddha went to live for a part of each year in the Indian state of Gujarat, just north of Bombay. He had been to Gujarat before. Bishnu, while praising 'Sri Bose's color film' mentioned, 'Buddha had many shows of this picture at Ahmedabad, Baroda, Surat and Nadiad in Gujarat'.[10] This was when Mataji, then known as Yashodhara Behen, and a teacher at St. Xaviers School in Ahmedabad, had met Buddha, back in 1962.

At the end of the film *Holy Kailas*, a photo of Buddha appears on the screen, with his hands clasped together in *pranam*. 'This is *Om Mani Padme Hum*,' Mataji explains, the Buddhist mantra that Buddha recited to honour Kailash Mountain.

I am talking with Mataji, a disciple of Buddha, and Chitralekha, his ex-daughter-in-law, about his film and travels, in Mussourie where she lives for the summer months. Mataji recounts her first experience with Buddha:

> One day I heard from my colleague about Sri Buddha Bose's colour picture, which was going on in one of the theatres in Ahmedabad, Gujarat... As I am a lover of the Holy Himalayas, right from my childhood, the next day I rushed to see it – Holy Kailash Manasarovar! After seeing the picture I was deeply moved from my heart within and felt like meeting Sri Buddha Bose. I rushed to see him in the theatre. I inquired about his stay and full address and whether I could see him again or not. He willingly gave his address and said, 'You can come at any time and see me.' At that time his stay there was very short, for three–four months or so. During this time I came to know more about him and his work, that he was a *sadhak* as well as a yogic person. Seeing I also was of spiritual mind, and so knowing my mind, he initiated me into Kriya yoga.[11]

Afterwards, Buddha gave Mataji exercises for daily practice. '*Ja-nusirasana, pavanamuktasana, bhujangasana, paschimottanasana* and then *ekpada sarvangasana, and trikonasana*. And pranayama,' she explains.

I ask, 'What kind of pranayama?'

'*Ujjai* pranayama. Then he taught me another one.' Chitralekha asks, '*Nadi shidhana* pranayama?'

'It was between him and me; I cannot tell you,' replies Mataji.

Buddha stayed and showed the film for a while, before returning to Calcutta. Prior to leaving, Mataji recorded an introduction to the film. 'The evening before he left he came to see me,' she says. 'We had some tea and we spoke a bit. I was a little shy. He said, "You are not far from me – you are with me. Now your recording is with me." I was silent for sometime and then said, "My voice is there but the body is here."' Mataji asked when he would come back. Buddha replied, 'Not sure.'

Buddha left Gujarat in 1962 and the two corresponded through letters. 'I never knew that from within I had already accepted him as my guru. I used to always write to him addressing him as "Dear Mr Bose" and end the letter with "Respects" and my name. I was very upset after he went away; there was no one to guide me on this spiritual path.' And then she adds, 'His every letter used to talk about how he is building a house.'

'I got annoyed after some time and asked him in the letter, "How big is your house? Is it bigger, is it taller, than Qutub Minar? Is that why it is taking so long to build your house?" He did not answer my question in his letter.' She lost hope, and connection with Buddha. Then she started a sojourn along the Ganges and into the Himalayas on foot, while staying in ashrams:

One day, I was going through Swami Vivekananda's book, when I read his definition of a true guru. He wrote that a true guru initiates a disciple and takes all the sins of the disciple and then the guru falls sick. If you come across such a person then know from your heart he or she is your true guru. Then I remembered that the day after Guruji initiated me into pranayama, he fell sick. In Ahmedabad. I had great respect for him and he had fallen sick. Since then, I have accepted him as my Guruji.

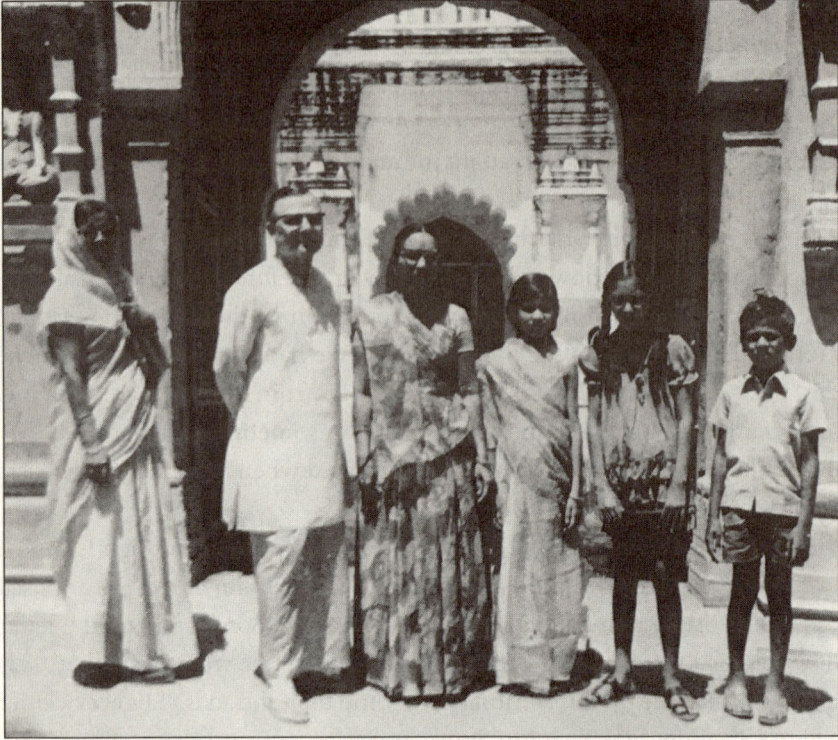

Top: Mataji, Buddha Bose, with Maharaja family, in Gujarat, circa 1972.
Bottom: Ticket to Holy Kailas, partial translation: "For the benefit of Yoga Cure Institute.
Buddha Bose's color picture 'Holy Kailas Manasarovar', Kalpana Theatre. Time – morning,
12 o'clock. Sunday. Date 1st March 1970. Cost – two rupees."

Source: Courtesy of Rekha Maharaja-Ivey.

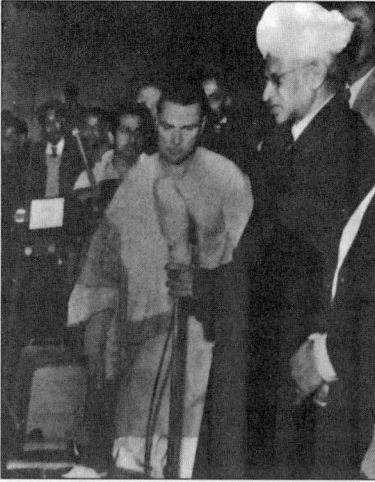

Left: Buddha Bose about to provide commentary, after an introduction from Sarvepalli
Radhakrishnan. Right: Buddha Bose at the Valley of Flowers with Brahma Kamal flower.

Courtesy of Mataji, Soham Heritage & Art Center, Mussoorie, India.

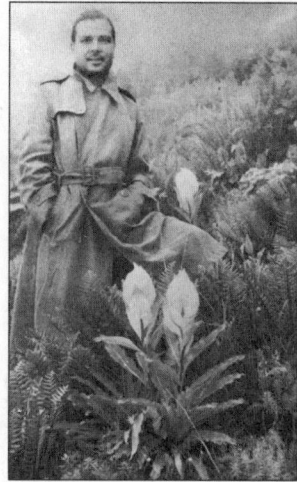

*Have you seen and shown to your
children and students*

= Buddha Bose's =

HOLY KAILAS & MANASAROVAR

The Film That is Enthralling Thousands ?

It is all about the beauty spots like Haridwar,
Amarnath, Gangotry, Gamukhi, Kedarnath, Badrinath,
Nandan-Kanan, Kailas, and Manasrovar with its enchanting
beauty from sunrise to sunset. You will be astonished
to see the thrilling mysteries of the age-old Himalayas—
the pleasure haunt of Nature.

There is a saying in Chinese "If I hear I understand,
If I see I know." Seeing and Hearing set free the faculty
of thinking and reasoning of mental out-look and remain
alive in students' memory. For this Audo-Visual aids
are of vast help to make the teacher's task easier.

So please do not miss the opportunity to contact Sri
Buddha Bose to have a display of his colour film "HOLY
KAILAS & MANASAROVAR" when he is in your town.

Promotional material for Holy Kailas.

Source: Courtesy of Mataji.

GURUJI, 2 FEBRUARY 1970

'You have come at the wrong time. So sorry.' Those words were chewed over in
my mind and I wondered to myself: had the magic stopped?

I kept trying to visit Mataji at the Ahmedabad ashram, where she has other
materials on Buddha Bose, and performs her duties during the Fall and
Winter months. I tried on two different dates to visit, but she has been gone
each time. Finally, I just chose a date and booked two tickets from Calcutta to
Ahmedabad. Pavitra, Buddha Bose's grandson, agreed to accompany me on
the trip, but his schedule is crunched, so we only have a couple of days' time.
Mataji is unsure that her schedule will give us much time together, but I hoped
it would work out.

Three days prior to our Friday departure, Pavitra sends an email in the
morning, explaining that he cannot go for personal reasons. He will not
reply to my follow-up questions. Two days later, he answers my call. He is
in central Calcutta, and we both happen to be near the Great Eastern Hotel,
so we rendezvous. In the lobby, I plead with him to cast aside all doubts and
come with me.

'This all started with you in Ahmedabad,' I tell him, 'and we have to go
there to finish it.' He listens as I go on, 'This isn't about starting new debts,
new karma, it's about finishing old ones.'

Three years prior, Pavitra had posted a job offer online, to teach yoga. He
had only done it once, in order to work alongside his mother, Chitralekha, who
had learned to teach yoga beside Buddha Bose. The two were in Ahmedabad
at the time, and his post was forwarded to me at exactly the moment I was
about to give up this whole project.[1] Instead, I had reached out to Pavitra, the

only response to his ad. It was a bit of magic that brought us all together in Calcutta. And that magic had lasted, taking me to places across the world and back as I traced the story of Buddha Bose and his teachings.

'This is not creating obligation,' I reason with Pavitra, 'it's putting an end to it. We are clearing out the old obstacles, shutting the doors behind us, finishing up tasks.' The words just pour out, and I think to myself, 'How odd, here in the Great Eastern Hotel lobby, to talk this way.'

The words reach Pavitra, who presses his palms together and acquiesces.

Two days later, everything seems to be a complete disaster. I am sick from the smoky city air of modern Ahmedabad; the two of us have ticky-tacky disagreements; Mataji is too busy administering as a sannyasini. The night before we return to Calcutta, I walk towards a building on the ashram grounds where a puja is to be held, then stop to view the peacocks strutting about on the green lawn.

I pull out my phone to send a text back home. 'Ugh, what a poor decision – "You came at the wrong time, sorry" – nothing on this trip to Ahmedabad has gone right.' I have forced things to happen instead of just letting them come. The same lesson, once again, and I give up.

An hour later, I send another.

'Huh, right after I typed that an elderly woman came up to me and started talking to me in Hindi. Pavitra came up, translated, and turns out she knew Buddha Bose.'

The woman, Mridula Maharaja, has heard from others that the grandson of Buddha Bose is here on a visit, and she decided to attend the puja to meet him.

I ask, 'So she was friends with Buddha, like Mataji?'

'No, these are disciples,' Pavitra replies. 'Mataji was different; she was a friend.'

I am a bit shocked. As it turns out, Mridula Maharaja and her family were among Buddha's twenty-thirty disciples in the early 1970s in Gujarat. Eventually, Mataji retrieves the materials, but I realize that the Maharaja family is also why we have come to Ahmedabad, and if Pavitra hadn't come along, we wouldn't have met. Soon thereafter, I meet with Mridula's sister and her daughter, Rekha, who explain the connection.

As the saying goes, 'When the student is ready, the Guru appears.' Apparently, our family was ready for a guru like Buddha Bose at this particular moment in history.[2]

Rekha's aunt and parents were among the disciples of Buddha who lived
in Ahmedabad. Her mother, Yoshodharben, had worked with Mataji at the
school where they both taught. Her father, B.H. Maharaja, a civil engineer,
was also a disciple of Buddha.

In 1969, it was through Yashodhara Masi (Mataji, Swami *Sannyasini*
Gurupriya) that my parents met Guruji. Because the three had the same
guru, my parents became Yashodhara Masi's 'Guru-Bhrata and Guru-
Bhagini' – 'brother and sister through Guruji'.

Rekha goes on to explain:

My exposure to Guruji (Sri Buddha Bose) took place exclusively at our family
home in the state of Gujarat (western India). Guruji initiated my parents in
1970. Following that initiation he made a visit as the family guru, staying
with us approximately for twelve weeks on that occasion (1970–72). As a
young child, I was very interested in Guruji's practices and teachings, sticking
close by his side during his entire stay. Whenever he needed something he
would call my name in a very distinct and memorable way. My siblings also
loved Guruji, but I developed the closest relationship, as a ten to eleven-year-
old. In many ways, Guruji's teachings have sustained me for my entire life.[3]

The family would assist Buddha with his movie and travel associated with
its showings. It became somewhat of an in-house production.

My father was very involved with Guruji in organizing the film shows in
various cities and towns in Gujarat state, and both would travel together.
They were best friends. For the film shows in Gujarat, Guruji had me read in
Gujarati the 'Introduction to Commentary', which he recorded and played
all over Gujarat in each show.

Buddha stayed at their house at other times too and became an honoured
guest, Rekha remembers:

Guruji was child-like with children. We learned from him the true values of
life – to love, respect and enjoy nature. He also made life fun by teaching me
and the other children in my family how to line up our beds outside in the
front yard, watch the stars and constellations, awaken in the morning with

birds chirping; get up early to watch the jasmine buds open up to become flowers; watch the grass grow; feel the cool breeze; stay still when a king cobra is slithering by; feed the sick owl who had followed us home from the storm management ditch. Most importantly, Guruji taught me yoga postures, pranayama and meditation. Above all, love for God and sincerity in performing worldly duties was routinely emphasized by Guruji. It was all good training that we were fortunate to receive from this Christ-like guru at a tender age.

The lessons of nature relay the type of experience Buddha had when he trekked and lived in the Himalayan hills each summer. He would marvel them with stories of flowers in the valleys that were 5 feet in diameter.

The Maharaja family and around twenty others were initiated by Buddha into Kriya yoga in Gujarat. He gave them *diksha* (initiation) and sometimes individual lessons or practice in asanas, mantras and pranayama. His disciples revealed that Buddha would send 'lessons through verbal communication' at times – 'a mark of a true guru'.

Buddha, and those around him in Gujarat, felt as if they had all come together from 'past incarnations' to engage in spirituality together. Buddha said of Rekha's father, 'I have recognized Bharat Bhai; he was my nearest and dearest', and her mother, as his 'younger sister'.[4] About to turn sixty, Buddha was at the pinnacle of his earthly instruction:

> Guruji was a great devotee of Shiva. He encouraged everyone to continue worshiping the god of their choosing. For Guruji, all representations of the divine were ultimately the One and Only Infinite Spirit. He certainly respected anyone's desire to learn yoga and meditation and instructed them when the time was ripe for those souls to receive such instructions. Guruji was always connected with the Divine Spirit. His concentration never wavered. It was apparent that he was continually in a meditative state, even when attending to worldly duties.[5]

Buddha was deeply connected to the Kriya lineage of Lahiri and Yogananda. Yashodhara Maharaja remarks that Buddha would speak about Yogananda, and 'when Guruji was saying all of this, his face was full of light. It was blazing, I could not keep my eyes open.'[6] The incident she is referring to is when she was initiated into Kriya yoga.

I was reading the *Autobiography of a Yogi*. My husband had already read it previously as it was in my uncle's library. I was not feeling well and he had said, 'Read this book – you will like it.' I opened the book to a Lahiri Mahasaya photo. It was the chapter on him and I thought to myself, 'When will I get such a guru?'

Soon after, she and her husband met Buddha:

The first time we went to see him, we found him talking about Babaji, Lahiri Mahasaya and all. I just told him, 'Please initiate me.' He answered, 'Your time has not come.' I could not say anything then, so we sat there for some time. He was telling us how Lahiri Mahasaya met Babaji. Then we came back home. Then one day my friend came and said that Guruji wanted to see you.

She said, 'Guruji wants to initiate you.' When we reached him, Guruji said, 'Okay, I will initiate you today.'

Later, my friend Mataji asked, 'How come he said it was not time for you to be initiated and now he gave you *diksha*?' Guruji then answered, 'Swami Yogananda and Lahiri Mahasaya had come in the morning and told me, "It is getting late and you must initiate them now."' And so Guruji gave us the *diksha*.[7]

Of course, the guru-role came with the usual pitfalls in experiences with the worldly expectations of others. In one incident, 'There were some people who had to go to Calcutta from Ahmedabad. It was summer vacation and train reservations were very difficult.' They had an idea. 'They asked Guruji, "Why don't you work some miracle so we can get the reservations?" Guruji was so angry and said, "What do they think I am? A miracle man?"'[8]

Everything I have come to know of Buddha's life in Calcutta is changed after I learn how he lived in Gujarat. Except for a few close relatives in Calcutta, Buddha was very reserved and seemed to keep a distance from other people. When I share this perception with the Maharaja family, they are taken aback, 'No, not at all!'

It may have been a number of things which brought about the change. Loss may have played a role. Buddha's mother, Emily suffered from dementia in her later years, and died in the May of 1970, in Brighton England. Then, after he returned from Gujarat, his best friend and father-in-law, Bishnu, died in the July of 1970. He later indicated to others that he felt 'shocks' in his life which led to his being in Gujarat for extended periods.[9]

Buddha did have a final show of *Holy Kailas* in the May of 1972. Afterwards, the entire apparatus was to be offered to the Ganges River near Rishikesh. As they were offering the items, Buddha had a change of heart and asked Mataji to keep the film with her and show it around if she needed money in her old age.[10] One other item that landed by their feet while they were putting the things in the river was a stamp used to create paper tickets to the show. It was made of steel and engraved with a promotion of the film. Buddha asked Mataji to keep it, and she did.

Buddha left Gujarat in the spring of 1972, having told his disciples he would need to focus on Japan. Between the Yoga Cure Institute in Calcutta, placing Hatha yoga teachers abroad in Tokyo and Bangkok, and also, 'family problems', Buddha's life had become complicated.

PART THIRTEEN

BIKRAM AND FAMILY SCHISM

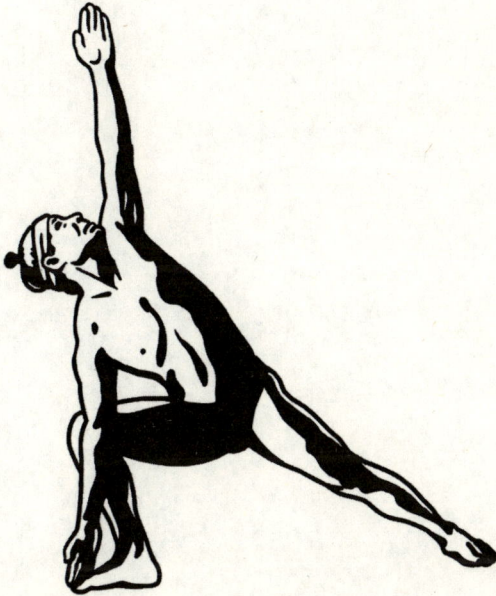

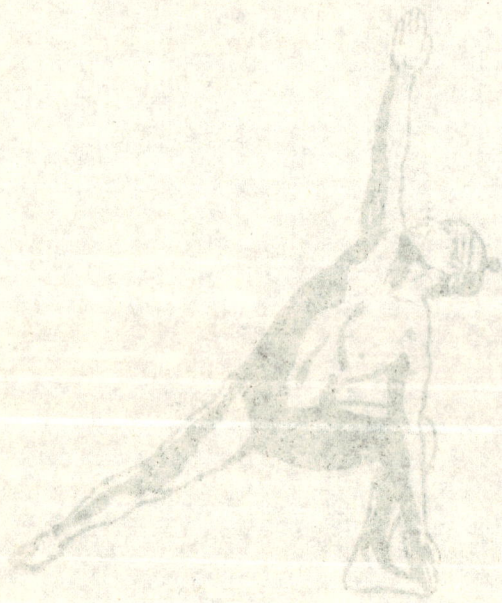

90

THE REVEAL

So who is this man of magic, Bikram Choudhury? And of what does the magic
that can change your life consist? Though you have to do Bikram's Hatha Yoga to
truly understand the magic, we can at least pin down who Bikram Choudhury is
and what he does.[1]
– Bikram's Beginning Yoga Class

Those in Calcutta get a chuckle out of how Bikram Choudhury has put one over on Americans. In the US, everyone from the *New York Times* to *Yoga Journal* has repeated Bikram's fabricated story.

When Benjamin Lorr, author of *Hellbent*, looked into Bikram's past, he noticed inconsistency. Called 'Bikram Milestones', they can be found on any 'About' section of Bikram Yoga websites – the supposed timeline and accomplishments of Bikram's life. What Lorr concluded, while looking at the 'minor point' of whether Bikram met Bishnu Ghosh at age three, four or six, was that Bikram had a 'cavalier attitude when telling or retelling details of his autobiography'. Flags were raised. Lorr went on to notice that, when 'scrutiny' is applied to 'a wide variety of Bikram's claims' and 'supposed accomplishments', they have 'a similar slippery feel'.[2] The ground starts slipping away, and the truth is revealed.

Bikram had a head full of impressive stories of the great yogis and physical culturists: Monotosh Roy, Gouri Shankar Mukerji, Buddha Bose, Yogananda and others. Each had their attendant stories, but all stories are told better in the present tense. This was the return of Rajah's magic act 'The Artist's Dream', where the lines between make-believe and the real were blurred. Just as 'The Artist's Dream' has the great reveal, so too does Bikram's story – everything happened, just not to Bikram.

I receive a question via email from a Bikram Yoga teacher in the US:

> Bikram often claimed that his sequence was tested scientifically by the Tokyo
> Hospital or University. He said this, I assume, to prove the scientific method
> and therapy of each of his postures; however, there is little to no quantifiable
> evidence. There is only qualitative, and that is only from him. Can you
> please clarify for me if this is perceived as truth or on the lines of myth?

Bikram's claim goes all the way back to his 1978 book.[3] It is not imagined,
or made up by Bikram at all – it happened to Monotosh Roy.[4] There are photos
from about 1970, showing Monotosh surrounded by Japanese scientists who
are measuring his vitals as he performs various feats, such as stopping his heart
for an extended period. Clearly, this is the history that Bikram appropriates as
his own.

Bikram's biography usually began with a narrative of how he first met his guru:
'Once when I was 6, I was playing with a ball that bounced into a gym with
bodybuilders, and this is where I met my guru, Bishnu Ghosh, whose brother
was Swami Paramahansa Yogananda.' The story, in fact, was how Satyananda
met Yogananda, as the latter was kicking the ball past his house.[5]

Bikram's biography usually jumped forward seven years later, to when he was
thirteen. At this point he 'won the National India Yoga contest', and thereafter,
'he was undefeated for three years'.[6] There were no national yoga contests in
the fifties, and even so, there is no evidence that Bikram ever competed in a
yoga contest. He did compete in, and win, a few local bodybuilding contests,
but nothing nationally.[7] However, there is a young man, about the same age
as Bikram, named Robin Goswami, who was featured on the cover of *Bayam
Charcha*, after having won multiple national body contests. The article explained
how 'Robin got so influenced by the bodybuilding show' given in Berhampur
by famous students of Bishnu, Monotosh Roy, Kamal Bhandari and Shanti
Chakraborty, that he started doing *bayam*. A year later, at the International
Circus, 'Robin Goswami got introduced to Bishnu Charan Ghosh'.

Bishnu Charan was delighted with this enthusiastic youngster and invited him to stay at his own residence and practise *bayam* and body building. Robin jumped at the offer and practised earnestly at Bishnu Charan's gym. Next year by the time Robin was 18 years of age, he competed at a contest in Berhampur and stood first, beating many body building personalities. Thereafter, he was crowned 'Bharat Kumar' successively in 1961, 1962 and 1963. He stood first in his own category at the Bharat Shree competition held in 1964.[8]

Bikram told a story of how he was awarded the title of 'Yogiraj' and of how he travelled to Germany. Bikram Yoga websites around the world echoed him, stating that Swami Sivananda declared him Yogiraj (King of the Yogis) at the age of fourteen. Of course, the real Yogiraj was Gouri Shankar Mukerji, who travelled with Bishnu in 1950 to meet Sivananda of Rishikesh. A certificate validates the award, dated 5 August 1950, and states:

> Sivananda of Rishikesh, Divine Life Society founder, presents the title of *Yogiraj* to Gouri Shankar Mukerji 'for the mastery of the intricate technique and processes of yogic sciences'.[9]

In 1982, Bikram told Ronald Miller that 'in 1963, at the behest of his guru, he went to Stuttgart (Germany) to supervise one of the Ghosh Physical Culture schools'.[10] There is no record of any such trip by Bikram, and it may be another story taken from Gouri Shankar Mukerji. However, Bablu Mullick, the son of Binoy Mullick and grandnephew of Bishnu Ghosh, made such a voyage at that time. A Bengali association in Stuttgart, named Bharat Majlish, organized a programme for artists from sixty-three countries to participate, and Bablu was the only Indian performer. The reports of the event say that he 'received a standing ovation' and, afterwards, made an easy path into successive stage performances over his career.[11]

Bikram claimed that at seventeen, an injury to his knee brought the prediction from leading doctors that he would never walk again. Not accepting their pronouncement, he had gone back to Bishnu Ghosh's school, for he knew that if anyone could help to heal his knee, it was his teacher. Six months of yoga later, his knee had totally recovered.

Here, Bikram weaved the story of Buddha Bose, who was told by doctors that he had become crippled, into his own story. It was true that Bikram had a bum knee, an injury that most likely happened while playing a competitive sport. And, in the six-month period when he learned yoga asanas from Bishnu, he had restored his knee's health and flexibility.

Perhaps the most egregious claim, one that has been his sleight of hand carried out worldwide, was that he 'won over Ghosh' with his 'one-size fits all yoga sequence' in a room heated to 105 degrees fahrenheit.[12]

Bishnu Ghosh did not endorse Bikram's method, as he had died before it was even developed. Nor did Bishnu tell Bikram, 'Promise me you will complete my incomplete job.' That charge was given by Bishnu to his son-in-law and best friend, Buddha Bose.

Bikram's appropriation of Bishnu continued in a replica (created by Bikram) of a poster that shows Bishnu in the center, and smaller portraits of his students surrounding him from the 1960s. Bikram swapped out the photo of Robin Goswami, which was in the original, for his own portrait.[13]

When exactly Bikram began weaving the tale is not clear. It was not there in 1966, as his biography in *Bayam Charcha* shows.[14] From 1965 until 1969, Bikram spent much of his time in Bombay, where he mostly provided therapeutic massage to great benefit. Perhaps its inspiration began in Bombay, as he was around movie stars. And it may have grown in Tokyo, with the sort of joke he and Bimal Das made, telling the Japanese they had 'come from the land of Gautam Buddha to show you miracle yoga'.[15] One tale led to another; neither untrue nor the accomplishments of Bikram. As Shirley Maclaine would say with a laugh about Bikram, 'He never stops talking.'[16] Regardless of when the long tale began, 1971 was a pivotal year.

91

TOKYO AND BIKRAM YOGA

'Why did you go to Calcutta?' Buddhadeb Choudhury asks
with a look of disgust in his face, crinkling up his nose a bit at the thought.
'Dirty city. Dirty streets. Dirty food ...'
He adds again for emphasis: 'Yuck, dirty city.'[1]

Going from the haphazard streets of Calcutta to the meticulous organization of Tokyo was quite a shock. 'We did not have to stop anywhere except when paying toll tax, not even when we passed through tunnels,' wrote Bishnu. 'I did not see any person walking on the road or crossing the road. There were over-bridges for pedestrians, even in the villages.'[2] For Bikram's younger brother, Buddhadeb, it was a welcomed sight, as he hated the chaos of Calcutta and was eager for the orderly lifestyle of Tokyo. After Bishwanath formed the Yoga College of India in Tokyo, Bikram brought Buddhadeb over to help him teach.

On 20 October 1971, Buddhadeb arrived in Tokyo. Like Bikram, he had been a student at Bishnu's gymnasium, where he lifted weights and learned massage therapy. In Tokyo, he learned to teach Hatha yoga classes. Out of all of Bikram's siblings, only Buddhadeb, born in 1948, was interested in *bayam*, bodybuilding, massage and eventually yoga.

As Buddhadeb arrived from Calcutta, 'it was October, and very cold'. The winter in Japan could be brutal. 'That is why the studio was hot and humid like my hometown, Calcutta,' Buddhadeb said. 'To make the yoga pose better, the students were warmed. Pleased that they had a lot of sweat, they were comfortable.'[3] In the beginning, they 'kept the room heated at 30 degrees Celsius (86 Fahrenheit)'.

When Buddhadeb started teaching classes, '60 per cent of the students were Westerners and the rest were local (Japanese)'. The first Yoga College of India studio was 'in Omotesando close to the ENT Hospital, near Itagui'. As with Bikram, 'Mrs Osano arranged the work visa' for Buddhadeb to stay in Japan.

Buddhadeb came to Tokyo 'to take over the school' because shortly after arriving, Bikram 'left Japan, to spread yoga to the United States'. Bikram left the Tokyo Yoga College of India in Buddhadeb's hands, and the latter practically froze it in time. It was clear, from the class in Tokyo and the structure Bikram would take with him, that the sequence was formed in 1971 in Tokyo and Honolulu.

In the hot yoga classes of Japan, there were a few additional postures outside of what later became popular as Bikram Yoga. Rather than twenty-six, 'we have twenty-eight,' Buddhadeb explained. The extras were removed when Bikram went to America and found that Westerners were not accustomed to certain postures that required spine and hip flexibility. Over time, a handful of postures were removed.

During the last two weeks of December 1971, Bikram taught an intensive Hatha yoga workshop at the Aquarian School of Yoga in Honolulu. From 27 December to 8 January 1972, there were seven classes per day, ninety minutes each, held at 30 degrees Celsius. It was held Monday through Friday, with a 'teacher's seminar' from noon to 2 p.m. The advertisement described Bikram as 'one of the finest Yoga instructors in the world'. It stated, 'We are very proud to have him with us.'

The Aquarian School of Yoga was founded by Joan Plumridge in 1968, based on a style of yoga that began in Australia in 1954 with Margrit Segesman. The school taught 'a way of discovering what it is to be a fully autonomous human being, through physical exercise, study, drama, music and meditation'.

The director of the school, Frank Trapani, was a doctor who first taught yoga at the YMCA and YWCA, and then on Hawaiian TV. The Aquarian School of Yoga was 'the only studio of its kind' in Honolulu, and teachers or 'gurus' passing through the islands were 'inclined to stop and lecture/teach' at the studio. 'Each teacher brought his/her own style of yoga', including Bikram.[4]

The standing exercises which begin the series are a synthesis of bodybuilding performances and modern yoga in the style of Buddha Bose and Gouri Shankar Mukerji. Bikram changed some of the postures to make them more dynamic and in line with his bodybuilding background. For instance, in the three-posture sequence of utkatasana (awkward pose), the exercises are modified from typical asanas to be closer to how *baithaks* (squats) are done in *bayam* practice. Another good example is *trikonasana* (triangle pose). The way *trikonasana* is done traditionally in Calcutta yoga is to keep the legs straight while bending from the torso. Bikram modified trikonasana by combining it with the bodybuilding position of a lunge, making it more challenging and playing to his strengths.[5]

The breathing exercise done at the beginning of the Bikram class, which is mistakenly referred to as pranayama, is a *bayam* 'dynamic exercise', which emulates a 'respiratory exercise' demonstrated by influential physical culturalist J. P. Muller in *My System* (1904). It is correctly referred to as a 'warm-up exercise', typical of many such 'free-hand' exercises done at Ghosh's College by bodybuilders.

Bikram incorporated mirrors, a traditional component of weightlifters in Calcutta.[6] Looking outwards at oneself, the focus was held on alignment and appearance (as if on a stage). Combined with the needs of a workout and to save time, students would remain standing and breathing normally in a state of standing relaxation, rather than lying in *savasana*, between postures. Bikram learned these modifications in Calcutta at Bishnu's gymnasium for bodybuilders, and the Americans loved the standing workout. When the sequence reached the floor series for the second-half of the class, the 'real yoga' began, which included more traditional seated-postures of Calcutta yoga.[7]

92

HAWAII AND NIXON

'The Boss's left leg is worse. He wants to see you.'[1] It was 1974, and President Nixon had been diagnosed with 'acute phlebitis in the lower left leg'.[2] According to his personal doctor, Nixon wrote in his diary that day:

I felt good this morning except for the fact that my left leg is having exactly the same symptoms it had when I was in Hawaii and had what was diagnosed as a blood clot.[3]

A news conference was arranged to inform the press 'that Nixon had a clot that had moved from his leg into the lung'. It was 'potentially dangerous but not critical', according to Nixon's Doctor.[4] The first time it flared up was in Hawaii, in the July of 1972; the press had not been informed of the ailment at that time.

Nixon had a 'family trait of high blood pressure' but required no medication. Other than the phlebitis, 'Nixon said he had only been sick once in his life' and that he walked and swam daily. The memoir by Dr Lungren, which brought the 1972 incident to light for the first time, wasn't written until 2003. Well before that time, Bikram Choudhury had a story, and unlike the other stories, it did not trace back to another person.

Bikram told this story to 209 people attending his teacher-training in the fall of 2000; the same story he had told in previous decades. Bikram claimed he was brought to the Kuilima Hotel and that 'on the sixth floor' he was presented to US President Richard Nixon, who 'had phlebitis thrombosis, a blood clot in his leg. I gave him six treatments in three days.'[5]

After reading about the claim in 2005, a California yoga teacher, named Brian Monnier, contacted the Nixon Library regarding Bikram and the president. Here was their reply:

Dear Mr. Monnier: I am replying to your inquiry about whether Bikram Choudhury treated President Nixon for his phlebitis condition. We've checked our archives and found nothing on file to confirm Mr. Choudhury's treatment such as correspondence, invoices or payment checks. Also, there is no mention of Mr. Choudhury in *Healing Richard Nixon*, the autobiography by the President's personal physician, Dr. John C. Lungren, which describes the treatment of the President's phlebitis in considerable detail. I hope this is helpful.

Sincerely, John Taylor, director, Nixon Library

While it may seem to have put the issue to rest, anyone who has worked around politicians knows there are many 'off-the-book' encounters arranged through close personnel and staff, which are not placed on the schedule or recorded as having happened.

The first trip Bikram made from Tokyo was to Hawaii. In December 1971, a photo shows Bikram with Elvis Presley. The snapshot was taken by Bikram's Japanese 'mother', Mrs Eiko Osana, at the International Hotel a couple of days before Christmas. Bikram went back and forth between Tokyo and Honolulu, with the Osana family's backing, during 1971 and 1972, as he taught classes for The Aquarian School of Yoga.

In an interview with Amira Luna caught on video on the beach of Hawaii, Bikram talked more about how he came to America. 'President Nixon, I fixed his legs. Here, Kuilima Hotel, named now, Turtle Bay. Fourth of July weekend, 1972.'[6] Nixon visited Honolulu, but it was seven weeks later, at the end of August 1972. He stayed in Honolulu for three days at the Kuilima Hotel, on a trip to meet the new Prime Minister of Japan.

On 30 August, his first day in Hawaii, Nixon attended a reception full of notable guests. Listed among the attendees was Kenji Osana, of the Surfrider Hotel, accompanied by an interpreter, Y. Kubota. Kenji was the husband of Eiko, Bikram's sponsor. This brings up the possibility of how Bikram might have been introduced to treat Nixon.

There was no possible way for Bikram to have learned of Nixon's ailment (the 1972 incident) before 2003, when Nixon's personal doctor first revealed the Hawaii incident (only the 1974 recurrent incident in the US was public knowledge). Through his benefactor Mr Osana, it seems possible that Bikram did in fact treat Nixon for phlebitis in the lower part of his left leg, where he had a thrombosed vein. When the encounter had possibly happened, Nixon supposedly made a bizarre request to Bikram, for 'some of that Indian Black

Magic'.[7] However, the treatment Bikram gave Nixon cannot be classified as yoga – he put Nixon in a warm-water bath with Epsom salts and then massaged the affected area, while moving Nixon's lower foot joints of the left leg.

When Bikram Yoga teachers or long-time students are faced with the idea that Bikram only learned the advanced yoga asanas during a short time frame of six months in the late sixties, it provokes skepticism and often prompts valid questions like, 'Then how does he know how to teach so well?' And, 'Why is he able to pinpoint a student's weakness and adapt personal variations for them if he didn't learn one-on-one yoga?' Also, 'How could he possibly have arrived at such an intuitive knowledge of the body if he had only been an average student of bodybuilding who performed a few feats of strength?' One of his first American celebrity students, Shirley MacLaine, noticed it too.[8] She stated in an interview, 'He's very discerning, and his eye is extremely adept at detail, particularly physical.'[9] It was what Bikram actually did on the second floor at 4/2 Rammohan Roy Road that made him that way.

Hiten Roy told me that Bikram would often go up from the ground floor, where the weights were, to the first floor, where the yoga rooms were. When I pressed as to whether Bikram had practised yoga upstairs, he would only answer, 'I can't say' or 'I don't know.'[10]

Later, when I pass on the Nixon story to Yogacharya Mukul, he replies that Bikram 'was a great masseur'.[11]

I recall how Shyamal had told me that he too had learned massage prior to becoming a yoga asana teacher. I follow up with Mukul, 'Where did Bikram learn to give massage?'

He responds, 'From my master. Bishnu Ghosh was a pioneer. He knew yoga, bodybuilding, gymnastics, massage, everything.'

For clarification I ask, 'So Bikram was not a yoga teacher? And his brother Buddhadeb?'

Mukul replies, 'They started their careers as masseurs.'[12] It was after learning massage that Bikram began teaching yoga. 'Basically, Bikram was a masseur.'

I am left speechless.[13] Mukul goes on:

It was magic for him. He was a great masseur. He had done massage for many Indian film actors like Dharmendra and others. His magic now is that whoever comes to him, he teaches them the same asanas. All learn the same asanas – men, women, children or patients.

Bikram had worked individually on countless bodies, so one-on-one, his masseur's skills flourished. When Bikram would talk about how he could only see four or five patients each day, those were massage clients. He worked on bodies of all ages, all builds, the bodybuilders and movie stars, the civil workers, old people, small children. Every type of body passed through his working hands in the sixties, as he perfected his knowledge of the body.[14] When the chance came, the bodyworker became the yoga teacher.

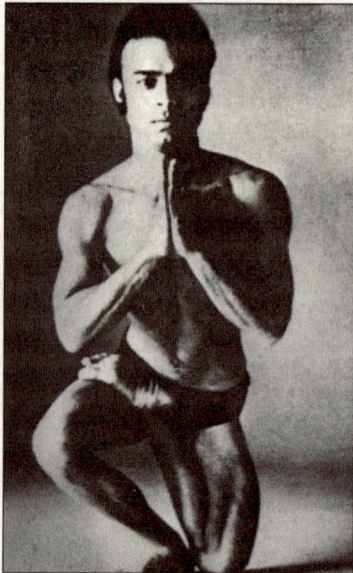

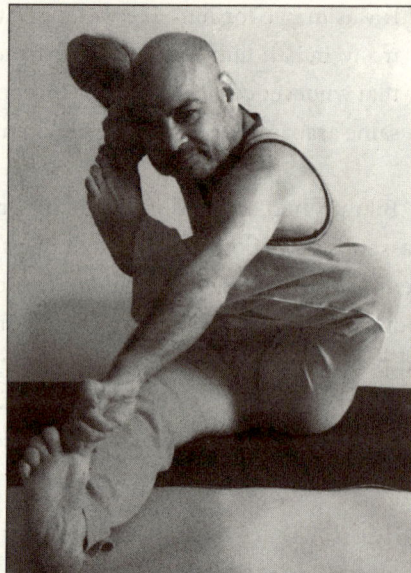

TWO WEEKS ONLY!
INTENSIVE
HATHA YOGA
WORKSHOP
Conducted By:
BIKRAM CHOUDHURY
Of Ghosh's Yoga College of India
DEC. 27 THRU JAN. 8

7:30 A.M.—12 NOON ● 2 P.M.—9 P.M.
MONDAY THRU FRIDAY
Teacher's Seminar: 12 Noon—2 P.M.
Come anytime during these hours for 1½ hour sessions. Classes run continuously.
Sponsored By THE AQUARIAN SCHOOL OF YOGA
Dr. Tropani, Director " . . . one of the finest Yoga instructors in the world. We are very proud to have him with us."

BIKRAM
CHOUDHURY

Top: Buddhadeb Choudhury, circa 1972 (left), 2015 (right).
Bottom: Promotional material for Bikram in Hawaii, 1971.
Source: Courtesy of Buddhadeb Choudhury; Honolulu Star-Bulletin.

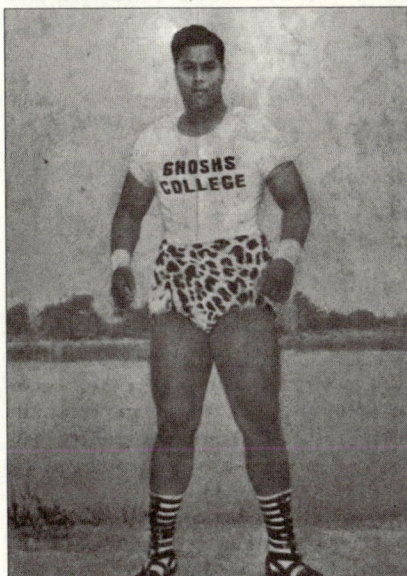

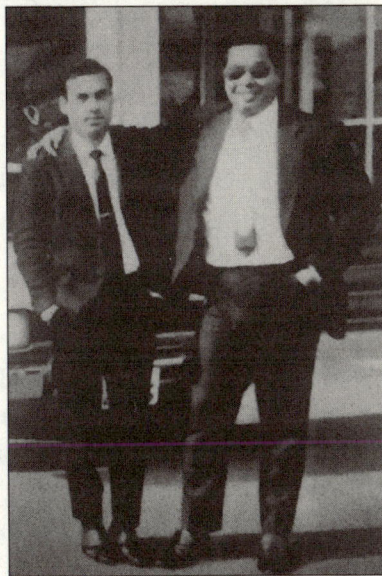

Top: Promotional material for Bikram in Hawaii, 1972. Bottom left: Bishwanath Ghosh, circa 1970. Bottom right: Bikram (left) and Bishwanath in Los Angeles, circa 1976.

Source: Honolulu Star-Bulletin; Courtesy of Ghosh's Yoga College.

WBYA AND COMPETITIVE YOGA

'He won a few small competitions in weightlifting, that is all,' Rooma says.
I am puzzled, 'What about the yoga championships?'

'Bikram never won any yoga championships because there were no yoga championships back then,' Rooma Bose says flatly.[1] She laughs, shaking her head from side to side.

Many others from Calcutta agree, 'Bikram Choudhury never participated in any yoga competition.'[2]

In 2009, *Yoga Journal* claimed that Bikram was 'the youngest person to win the All-India Yoga Asana Championship'.[3] In 2008, the *Encyclopedia of Hinduism* gave Bikram's biography as:

> Choudhury, Bikram (b. 1946), He won an all-India yoga competition at the age of 13, and a gold medal in weightlifting at the 1964 Olympics. After his training he taught yoga in Bombay, where he met film star and New Age 'guru' Shirley MacLaine, who invited him to America.[4]

Except for his name, not a single other line of that biography was true. The source for the information was Bikram Choudhury himself, in a 2003 revised edition of his 1977 book, *Bikram's Beginning Yoga Class*.

Perhaps the most prevalent claim that has propelled Bikram's career was that he won national yoga championships in India. In one edition of his book, it was just one championship; he had 'won the prestigious "National India

Yoga Competition" at the age of thirteen'. In another, he claimed that 'he was undefeated for three years'.[5] Later, the name changed, stating he won the 'All-India Yoga Asana Championships'. Then, after three straight wins, 'his name was withdrawn to give others a chance'.[6] In the same interview, he claimed that he met B. K. S. Iyengar, saying 'We met at different competitions when I was very young.' However, Iyengar, throughout all of his volumes of writings and interviews, never mentioned being involved in any type of yoga competition at the time.

In a 1982 *Yoga Journal* article, Bikram proclaimed that the competition, 'National Yoga Champion of India', was held in Rishikesh in the presence of Swami Sivananda. Bikram clarified that when his name was withdrawn from the competition, it was 'because just his presence was intimidating to the other contestants'. As an alternative, he was requested to perform, and 'in less than 30 minutes he executed over 500 yoga asanas to physical perfection'.[7]

By the time Bikram was interviewed in 2014, the claim had reached new heights. Also, yet another name is used for the competition. 'When I was 11, I appeared in "All India Yoga Competition" and was champion, and again at age 12 and 13. Then the judges, which included Krishnamacharya, Swami Sivananda, Pattabhi Jois, B. K. S. Iyengar, and my guru decided that I could not compete again.'[8] No record of Sivananda ever being involved in any type of yoga asana competition could be found at the Sivananda Gyana Yagna Library in Rishikesh, which houses all of the records of Sivananda's life. The same was true for the rest of the 'judges'. As for Bishnu Ghosh, he never, either directly or indirectly, organized yoga competitions or had his students participate in any yoga asana competitions.

Prem Das and his brother Dibya, both students of Bishnu Ghosh, have owned a sort of yoga kingdom in Calcutta for the last few decades. Their sister, Kushala, was the teacher of Rajashree, who was later married to Bikram. They have been to the US many times, attending and lecturing at Bikram's yearly teacher-training events. Prem Das was often a judge at the Ghosh Cup competitions.

When I interview Prem and ask if Bikram was doing yoga in the sixties alongside him, he just shakes his head no and pumps his arms in a barbell motion.

I ask his brother Dibya, 'Do you remember Bikram?'

He replies, 'Yes, he lived there and was doing bodybuilding and weightlifting in the 1960s.' Over and over again, I heard that Bikram was not involved with yoga initially.

By the time I interview Kamal Bhandari's daughter, Iti, I am no longer surprised by these revelations about Bkiram. 'No yoga competition. Only bodybuilding and weightlifting competitions,' she says.[9]

Iti Bhandari was a champion herself at sixteen–eighteen years of age. Her father-by-adoption, Kamal Bhandari, was one of Bishnu Ghosh's closest students and a champion weightlifter and bodybuilder. 'The West Bengal Yoga Association of India was started in 1972', and its first competition was held in 1973. 'Bikram Choudhury never participated in any yoga competition. His wife Rajashree participated in competitions. She was my friend.'

After Bishnu's death, a number of his close students, Kamal Bandhari, Nirapada Pakhira, Gopal Chakrabarti, Monotosh Roy, Hiten Roy, Dilip Kumar Banerjee and Santosh Sanjal, tried to figure out some way to commemorate his death. The bodybuilders decided that they would form an association called West Bengal Yoga Association (WBYA), and along with its formation, begin competitions for yoga asanas.[10] This was confirmed by Hiten Roy: 'After the death of our guru, Kamal Bhandari and I started yoga competitions to commemorate our guru.'[11]

The 'founding members of the WBYA were former bodybuilders' and any presentation 'had to be entertaining'. Researcher Claudia Guggenbühl explained, 'Yoga was performed on stage in this way, as entertainment, in-between other physical demonstrations. Such shows were more popular in the villages than in Calcutta.'[12]

A student of Monotosh Roy wrote, 'Obviously, before that period there were no organized Associations or Federations' for yoga. They were focused on the showcasing of 'bodybuilding' and the 'strongman and muscleman contests', called All India Championships.[13]

The first informal record of a yoga asana competition was at the Simula Athletic Club. Robin Chakraborty, 'a student of Monotosh Roy', had 'come from bodybuilding to yoga'. Mukul Dutta, then a student of Bishnu in 1969, attended the event. 'Monotosh Roy asked me to be the judge,' Mukul recalled. After his teacher Bishnu 'gave permission', he 'asked the theoretical questions', which 'were divided into two sections – practical and theoretical ... Just basic questions, "What are the benefits of yoga", for instance, very simple questions.'

There was no testing on the therapeutic benefits of yoga because Mukul explained, 'That is not possible because this is very precious knowledge. What I see nowadays, that a group comes for three weeks and learns the therapeutic benefits of yoga. How? After being in this line for forty-six years there is so much to learn.'[14]

Gautam Sinha, an original member of the WBYA, explained, 'There were no yoga associations for competitions before 1973.'[15] Bishnu's student 'Kamal Bhandari decided to make yoga more available for the masses. The idea came up when they used to sit idle talking', while working on the monthly magazine, *Bayam Charcha*, explained Gautam.[16] In 1973, WBYA was formed as 'a continuation' of Bishnu's philosophy – that 'bodybuilding was not possible for everyone but that Yoga could be practised by all'.[17]

An early founding document showed that, even at the time, yoga competitions were controversial in India. 'There are some persons who are of the opinion that Yoga cannot be put to the subject of competition.' The argument in favour of competitions suggested that 'instead of degrading' yoga, they will make it even more accessible, through 'propagation and popularization amongst the masses of the world over'![18]

Iti, the daughter of Kamal, described the scene of the first yoga competition in Bengal. It 'was held in Mahila Yoga Byayam Kendra in Calcutta. The first All India Yoga Federation competition was held in Patna. This is how competitive yoga started in India, under the Yoga Federation of India in 1974, and it still exists. National yoga competition started in 1974 and there was no such competition before this.' She looks at me with intent, to make sure I get this, 'There was no yoga competition before this in India.'[19]

The research encountered no records, of any type, for yoga asana contests nationwide in India prior to the formation of the Yoga Federation of India in 1974. The WBYA – West Bengal Yoga Association – was formed in 1973, and then it merged its contests with the national organization.

Despite this, the *New York Times* published that 'participants from India, where yoga competitions have been around for a century, swept the youth competition, drawing gasps from the crowd as they bent like rubber into their postures'.[20] The writer of this article, Sara Beck, gave no reference for the statement. Partly, the claim was based on a conflation, which Bikram engaged in:

In India, yoga competitions have been held for thousands of years, they're an ancient tradition. When I was 13, 14 and 15 – in the late 1950s – I won the National India Yoga Championship; my wife Rajashree was five times champion; and Buddha Bose, the son-in-law of my guru and one of the greatest yogis ever, was champion in the 1930s.[21]

However, Buddha did not enter a yoga asana competition to become a champion in the thirties; he won a 'most beautiful body' competition. It is merely a willful sleight-of-hand to conflate the two. There were 'All India' bodybuilding contests, which many of Bishnu Ghosh's students had won. Claudia Guggenbühl also came to this conclusion: 'Bikram is confusing bodybuilding shows with yoga.'[22]

In Calcutta, I ask someone who was around the gym in the late sixties, 'Do you recall meeting Bikram?'

He confirms, 'I saw him doing exercises there when I went there. He had a good figure. He was like anybody else, a common man.'[23]

Ghosh's College of Physical Education
&
Yoga-Cure Institute
4/2, RAMMOHAN ROY ROAD
CALCUTTA 9

Dated 1.2.75.

For Smt. Chitralekha Basu

                                    Age 21.

1. Pavanamuktasana   14c.
                      20c.   3 times.
2. Bhujangasana   10c.   6 times.
   (b) Eka Pada Salavasana 10c. 4 times.
3. Ardha Kurmasana   20c.   3 times.
4. Janusirasana   10c.   4 times.
5. Uttana Padasana   10c.   4 times.
   (b) Utkatasana   14c.   4 times.
6. Jasti Asana   40c.   2 times.
   (Both sides)
   (b) Ardha Matsyendrasana 14c. 4 times
7. Surja Bedana
   Pranayama 10 times 6 Kumbhaka.
   (Start with right nostril)

                    (Buddha Bose)

HEALTH
THROUGH
YOGA

YOGA CURE INSTITUTE.
4/2, Rammohon Roy Road,
Calcutta-9 Phone : 35-1358

We Cured the following deseases those who have obeyed our instructions regularly :—

	1968/70		1970/72	
	Out of	Cured	Out of	Cured
Asthma	30	17	25	10
Tonsil	40	24	30	18
Gastric trouble	60	42	85	63
Constipation	54	50	70	60
Sciatica	75	70	60	57
Lumber Pain	80	75	96	92
Prostate trouble	60	55	70	62
Insomnia	70	70	85	85
Stammering	40	13	30	12
Chronic Headach	60	57	72	70
Sex abnormality	90	85	104	100
Night Loss	60	60	72	71
Loss of Appetite	75	73	92	91
Acidity	85	82	98	96
Weakness of liver	80	70	89	78
Osteo Arthritis	25	22	48	46
Diabeties	25	12	30	18

Top left: Yoga prescription by Buddha Bose. Top right: Promotional material of Yoga Cure.
Bottom: Contents in Yoga Cure material.
Courtesy of Chitralekha Shalom, Romit Banerjee, Mataji.

94

BUDDHA'S CHARGE

*I have been to Japan and am now trying to bring their youth
here to India. Besides the Japanese Yoga Center, there are 18 Embassies who have
joined our yoga program. They are all learning yoga asana and pranayam. I am
going to Japan again on June 15th, and shall be there for two years.*
– Buddha Bose, speaking to Dattatreya, Ahmedabad, 1972

At the time of Bishnu's death in 1970, Ashok, Arun and Bishwanath were the three boys who were to inherit the legacy of the family; they were trained to be yoga masters. It was left to Buddha 'to take over' managing both, the yoga and the family,[1] so he returned to Japan in 1972 to teach at the Tokyo Yoga Center, staying with Jibananda and Karuna Ghosh. They taught individual therapeutic yoga lessons, which were readily adopted by the Japanese.

Americans, at this time, were scouring the world looking for spiritual practices, and one hippie in particular encountered Buddha, in a story which was recalled and told to me:

An American youth had come to him in Japan, yet Buddha had refused to give Kriya yoga. The American was very adamant and refused to go without getting initiated. So Guruji had asked him to practise something for a week and then come back. The young man went and lived on a hill-top and practised what Guruji asked him to do and then came back to Guruji after a week. Guruji said he found the person had totally changed, and so he gave him Kriya yoga initiation.[2]

While in Tokyo, Buddha took on other disciples, teaching them Kriya yoga, but not to the extent that he did in Gujarat.[3] He returned to Calcutta in 1973, as more changes – marriages and children – were taking place. Bishwanath Ghosh married Anjana. She was from north Calcutta, and her family, not surprisingly, had a history of stage performance. The families of Anjana and the magician P.C. Sorcar were close, and they had helped him organize magic shows in Calcutta. Then, Buddha's son Ashok married Chitralekha in September 1973. The two had met at work. Ashok was a pilot with India Airlines, where Chitralekha was a stewardess. Now, all of Bishnu's and Buddha's children, except for Rooma, had married.

The Yoga Cure Institute prospered in the early seventies as a family-run business, and members continued to come to the gymnasium (about 200 patients came to the institute every day). The magazine *Bayam Charcha* continued as a monthly publication, and the West Bengal Yoga Association was just getting started. Yet, for the families, the seventies were similar to the forties, as one thing happened after another, which crumbled its destiny. As the five children of Bishnu and Buddha became adults, the center did not hold.

Claudia Guggenbühl, during her 2003–04 research in Calcutta, came to this conclusion:

As every religious or secular movement, the Yoga Empire of Calcutta also suffered its schism as soon as the founder figure had died.

In her research, Claudia Guggenbühl called it 'The Schism' and first looked for its origins in the practice after Bishnu's death. 'What might have driven Buddha Bose away from his Guru's College' was his desire 'to keep yoga free from bodybuilding' and instead develop it more along the lines of the 'Kriya yoga which he learned from Yogananda'.[4] But the problems went beyond yoga. Tony Sanchez, an old student of Bikram's, who had been to Ghosh's Yoga College around that time told me, 'The family is a mess.' Ultimately, Claudia concluded, 'Family problems arose and Buddha Bose moved out.'[5]

Prem Das said there were 'some family problems' even before Bishnu died. 'Buddha told Bishnu he would take care of the institute after Bishnu's death', but after Bishnu's death, 'there were family problems again'. At the root of the problem, Prem Das concluded, 'was a conflict between Buddha and Bishwanath'.[6] The conflict, like so many in Calcutta, was about property.

'Buddha would always say he would look after the institute only after Bishnu's death', but Bishwanath wanted to run the business on his own, alongside Prem Das.[7] Underneath the struggle over property was the conflict surrounding Buddha's own two sons, Ashok and Arun.

Arun and Ashok led a charmed life at 4/2 Rammohan Roy Road. Both Bishnu and Buddha were 'detached' from raising their boys. Bishnu felt he had become 'so attached' to Srikrishna, that with the younger sons, 'he allowed them to grow as they wished, with a different, more relaxed ambiance'.[8] 'They were spoiled children,' Prem Das would say. With the freedom came conflict, because around the time of adulthood, Ashok and Arun became 'heavy drinkers'.

The alcoholism had skipped a generation. Buddha told others that when he was sixteen he 'would feel terribly frustrated to witness his father's violent eruptions on his Bengali mother at nights when he would come home drunk'. He 'felt helpless as he could not intervene or stop the daily madness', and this was the reason he left his own father and moved to 4 Garpar Road.[9] Buddha was helpless again, now witnessing his own sons follow Rajah's routine of 'daily madness'.

This was difficult for Chitralekha, Ashok's wife. She had come to know Ashok in the early seventies as 'good-natured, handsome, beguiling, smart and friendly', but after they married, she realized her mistake. Still, she loved the big house at 4/2 Rammohan Roy, and the women of the house, Ashalata and Ava Rani, grew to love her as well. She was too preoccupied with the newborns in the house to see how the ground had shifted.

The other son, Arun, 'even had a chance at the movies', Shyamal (Buddha's assistant who had grown up with the boys) recalled:

> He was so beautiful to look at. His eyes, skin, looks were so fantastic. You could compare him with any Indian film hero. He also had a good figure because he did weightlifting and bodybuilding.[10]

Upon his performance at the Expo 70 in Japan, Arun's biography, published in *Bayam Charcha*, read: 'He is a worthy son of the famous yoga expert Buddha Bose, but Arun is famous by his own right.'[11] Famous or not, he was in the same boat as Ashok. Buddha tried to change his sons' reckless behaviour by sending them abroad to teach yoga.

In 1973, Karuna and Jibananda, like Bikram before them, decided they would like to branch off on their own in Tokyo. It was the height of Calcutta's Hatha yoga influence on Japan's culture, and they envisioned 'a world chain of Ghosh

Yoga Institutes to follow the Tokyo Institute'.[12] Buddha had wanted to return to Japan for a longer period, but the family situation kept him in Calcutta. Instead, Buddha's son Arun was sent to Japan in 1973. The Japanese had become used to a married couple with children, and accepted the replacement of Swapna and Arun, along with their two young sons, at the Tokyo Yoga Center. Then an opportunity arose for Buddha to take Calcutta's yoga to Thailand.

President
Shri Biswanath Ghosh

Vice-President
Km. Y. M. Dvivedi

Secretary
Shri Buddha Bose

Treasurer
Sm. Ava Rani Bose

Members :-

Shri Kamal Banerjee	Service
Shri Bhima Sankar Sharma	Business
Shri Prem Sundar Das	Physical Culturist.
Shri Prafulla ch. Sen	Ex. Chief Minister W. B.
Sm. Ashalata Ghosh	Nothing Particular.
Shri J. B. Maulik	Chartered Accountant.
Km. Rooma Bose	Yoga Advicer & Teacher.
Shri Arun Bose	Yoga Advicer & Teacher.
Major N. Roy	Service.
Shri Nandodulal Sreemany	Landlord.
Shri Asok Bose	Yoga Advicer & Teacher.
Shri Sanjib Chatterji	Journalist.
Sm. Karuna Ghosh	Yoga Teacher, Tokyo.
Shri J. N. Ghosh	Yoga Teacher, Tokyo.

Promotional material of Yoga Cure & Ghosh's Gymnasium, circa 1973.
Courtesy of Mataji.

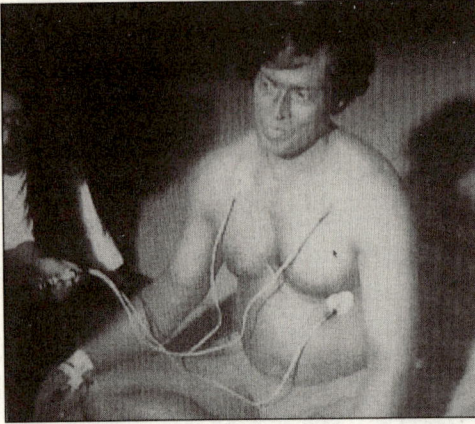

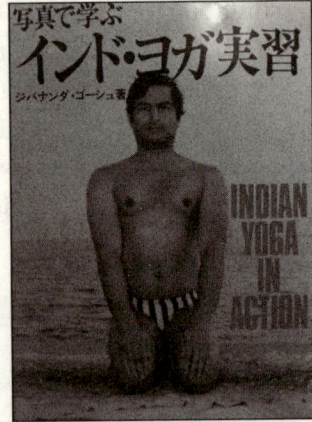

Top left: Monotosh Roy in Tokyo for medical tests on the effects of yoga, circa 1973.
Courtesy of Monotosh Roy family.

Top right: Jibananda Ghosh, Tokyo, 1977.

95

YOGA IN BANGKOK

I land in Bangkok, Thailand to a text message from Sukh Talukdar, 'Hi Boss, where are you?'

I have been brought to Bangkok by a thin thread of hope and a lot of luck. I'm meeting Shyamal Talukdar and his wife Ratna. Chitralekha had told me a few months earlier that if I want to talk with someone who really knew the yoga as Buddha Bose taught it, I should find this student.

'His name is Modo,' she says.

I think, 'Modo? What kind of name is that?'

Chitralekha had seen a short clip of Modo a few years back, which showed he was still in Bangkok. He was sent there by Buddha in the early seventies, to help Ashok teach yoga. As was typical in Bengal, everyone knew him by his nickname, Modo, yet some forty years later, it was difficult to recall his formal name. I had no other leads, but I booked a one-night layover transit for Bangkok, on my return to America from India, to see if anything panned out.

🏋️

Still in Calcutta, nothing had happened in terms of a solid lead towards finding Modo. A yoga friend from New Orleans, also staying at Ghosh's Yoga College, Adrienne Jackson (Ajax), asked me what my plans were after leaving Calcutta. I mention my hopeful one-day stay in Thailand.

'Oh really?' Ajax says, 'I know someone in Bangkok that I was in Bikram Yoga training with, in 2008. Sukh and I did a lot of yoga together.' She proceeds to get me in contact with Sukh, and we message back and forth, agreeing to meet. I think, at least that's something, a meeting with someone that teaches yoga there. I'm satisfied.

A couple days later, I message Sukh. 'I've been trying to locate a person called "Modo" in Bangkok … an excellent massage therapist or masseur, and who knew yoga thoroughly.'

Sukh replies, 'Ah, that's my Father.' And then, 'But no one ever calls him by that name anymore.'

Ha! 'Wow, that's your dad?' I am as excited as one could be over a text message. He suggests that rather than our original meeting place at a mall, I should come over to the cultural lodge, where his father and mother teach yoga.

Modo was a childhood nickname, his given name is Shyamal Talukdar. He was a boyhood friend of Bishwanath Ghosh and later grew to know Bikram well too, and he related to me how he'd almost gotten chosen to go to Japan:

> Now the question was who to send there, either Bikram or me. Bikram was close to Bishu [nickname for Bishwanath] and I was very close as well. Bikram was a bodybuilder before he learned yoga. Bikram told Bishu to ask his father to send him to Japan. So that is how he came to Japan. All because of Bishwanath Ghosh.

Shyamal had started to practice yoga in 1968, and became one of Buddha's top teaching students. In Calcutta, Shyamal lived on Upper Circular Road, just beside where the statue of Bishnu Ghosh now stands. He tells me of how he got noticed:

> One day when Buddha Bose asked me to give massage, I started giving massage from the foot upwards. He was surprised and asked me who taught me massage. I told him that I had watched Monotosh Roy giving massages. He was very happy and told me that one day I would turn out to be great masseur.

Buddha privately taught Shyamal the one-on-one style of yoga and the advanced postures, and had him stay overnight at the 4/2 residence. Shymal would awake around 4.30 a.m., clean up and start practice. 'You may not be able to do it properly in the beginning but you will catch up as you follow my actions every day', Buddha told Shyamal.

Beginning in 1971, Shyamal began treating people for their illnesses, using Yoga Cure, and methods of massage he had learned:

One day, there was a boy, aged about twelve or thirteen years, who had become paralyzed after he hit his head on the cement floor in his village. Buddha Bose sent me with the father to the hospital to check on the boy and bring back the report. I told the father that with some exercises, massage and yoga, he could be treated.

I came back and gave my report to Buddha Bose. He heard everything and said I should start from the next day.

After about three–four weeks of treatment, I made the boy walk, holding on to the other beds in the room. He could not straighten his leg, so I made him walk from one end of the room to the other while holding on to the sides of the beds in the room. A month or so later he could actually walk straight. The many exercises, yoga asanas and massage helped him to heal slowly.

Buddha Bose was impressed with Shyamal's success and recommended him to other patients in Calcutta. He treated them with massage first and then yoga. Then, 'one day, Buddha Bose told me to take charge of his morning yoga class at the centre'. A Sikh student brought in a friend, Narain Singh Srigupta, who was from Bangkok, and suffered from asthma. After Shyamal taught the lesson, the man decided he would help bring Calcutta yoga to Bangkok. However, Buddha didn't think of sending Shyamal at first, but instead, he thought of his beleaguered son.

Ashok Bose had lost his job over a workplace conflict and was no longer a pilot with the Indian Airlines. Needing an outlet for his son, Buddha had sent him to Japan in 1975. Ashok returned a few months later, after a conflict with both his brother Arun and a Japanese woman. Hoping his son could start over, Buddha decided Ashok would go to Thailand. Ashok's wife, Chitralekha, was pregnant with their second child, and stayed back in Calcutta.[1]

Once there, Ashok discovered that many of the elderly Indians 'wanted the typical Indian massage and Ashok did not know massage'. So he 'wrote to his father to send a masseur from Calcutta to come and stay here in Bangkok'. It came in handy that Shyamal knew massage.

Though Buddha was reluctant to send Shyamal, his friend Bishwanath stepped in, and 'became adamant' that it had to be Shyamal who went to Bangkok.[2]

After Shyamal arrived in Bangkok, Ashok 'printed visiting cards on paper made of bamboo' to advertise his services. And once Shyamal was settled with his wife Ratna, 'Ashok took off with a Buddhist monk to the hills.' Nothing is known of where or why Ashok went with the monk, but he returned to Bangkok soon after.

Shyamal tells me that when he arrived in 1976, 'there were only three yoga teachers in Thailand', and they 'did not know how to cure through yoga'. Reflecting on his invitation to demonstrate yoga on television, he explains, 'It was a live show and two–three channels kept calling me to show yoga to people of Thailand. The channels wanted me to show yoga, because yoga is from India.' He 'became the most popular yoga teacher in Thailand'. 'I was on television and newspapers.'

I smile and respond, 'So you are the father of yoga in Thailand.'

He replies, 'Now you will find yoga teachers everywhere. There are thousands of yoga centers now in Bangkok. But if you ask them what is yoga, they cannot answer properly.'

At the end of the interview, Shyamal shows me some saved clippings from the seventies: a report in the English daily *Bangkok Post*, his first interview, among others. 'Now I will show you something, the last thing to show.'

'Yes?'

'See this book?' He pulls out the *Key to the Kingdom of Health*, Volume 1. 'Buddha Bose gave me this book when I came first time to Thailand. One of my students took this book and made a copy of it; then he translated it into Thai. Another student bought the book from the department store.' It had discreetly been republished. The best part, Shyamal concluded with a laugh, 'is the person who translated it into Thai never wrote his name, so the police did not know who to arrest!'[3]

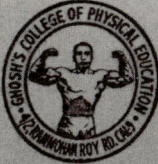

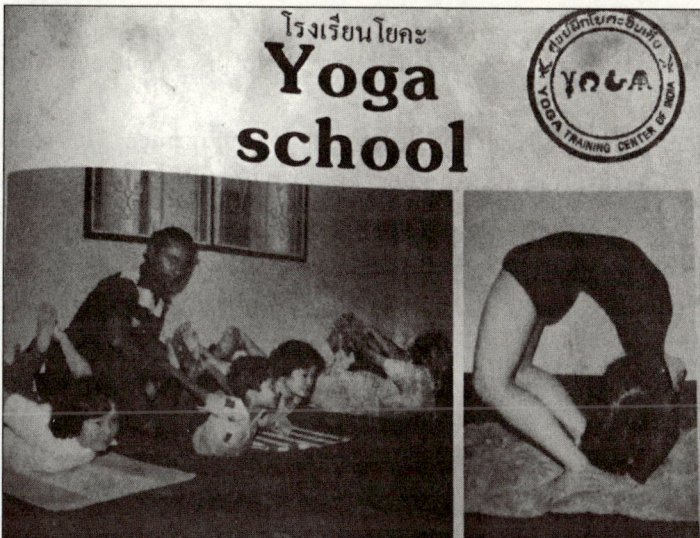

Top: Letter of recommendation from Bishwanath Ghosh.
Bottom: Yoga in Bangkok.
Courtesy of Shyamal Talukdar, Bangkok, circa 1975.

96

NEW ALIPORE

'How do I tell what happened to Buddha afterwards', I wonder aloud. 'Well,' Chitralekha responds, as we snack from the buffet at the Taj Bengal, 'in some ways, it was a very normal period in his life, unlike all the other portions.'

She and I are taking a lunch break from the arduous task of retrieving archives from the nearby National Library. To me, there are so many divergent stories, many of which involve a great deal of drama, that I can't imagine how it all could fit.

'It has to be there,' she tells me. 'It's part of his whole life, what makes him human.'[1]

Others in the family do not parlay such encouragement. 'It's scandalous,' one from Calcutta told me. Another chimes in from Britain, 'I understand and respect your reluctance to take sides,' and then gives a warning about 'backing the wrong horse!'

The truth is, it's impossible to document the entirety of an oral history about a family schism, but a few incidents stand out.

Ava Rani, with an unmarried daughter and an intensifying conflict between the two families, left with Rooma to live at the Bose home in New Alipore, south Calcutta in March 1976. This left Chitralekha alone with a newborn at 4/2 Rammohan Roy, since Ashok was away in Thailand.

Bishwanath had asked Ambar, Rajah Bose's son from the Bengali side, about what to do about Chitralekha and her two children. In a response, which channeled Emily's father in England seventy years earlier, Ambar exclaimed,

'Throw them into the street!' This burned Chitralekha's ears when she heard it, so she too left for New Alipore that April.

The move to New Alipore in 1976 preceded more loss. Ava Rani had a longstanding struggle with meningitis. She had moved away from the Ghosh home in north Calcutta where she had lived her entire life, and just months later, on 2 July 1976, she suffered a stroke that ended her life. Arun's family decided to return from Tokyo. Swapna and the children arrived back in September. Arun stayed on for another month and contracted an illness: it had not been properly diagnosed in Tokyo, and turned out to be tuberculosis. Fifteen days after his return in November, Arun also died in New Alipore. 'New Alipore brought only bad omens for the family – Ava Rani died, Arun died.'[2]

Ashok was still in Bangkok. The family members had not told him of the death of his mother that July. Only in November, when Chitralekha wrote to Ashok of Arun's death, did he learn of his mother's death too. 'Something inside him snapped', and he 'lost all sanity' at the realization that his father and sister did not think it important to inform him of his mother's death when it had happened. In Bangkok, while drunk, Ashok nearly beat Shyamal to death. When Bishwanath heard of the ordeal, he told Buddha that 'he would personally go to Bangkok and kill Ashok' if it continued. 'Buddha became afraid,' said Shymal.

The Thai clients of Shyamal forced him to break away from Ashok, and Ashok lost whatever self-control remained. Weeks later, reduced to a beggar, some former clients at the US Embassy took pity and paid for his exit. Shyamal recalled, 'He got a ticket and went back to Calcutta, never to return.' By the time Ashok returned to Calcutta, the Ghosh and Bose families had split.

The Yoga Cure Institute at 4/2 Rammohan Roy Road changed its name to Ghosh's Yoga College in 1976. Prem Das became the vice president, and Bishwanath the president. Bishwanath managed the Institute 'for three days and the next three days were Prem Das's responsibility'.

Buddha Bose began formal classes in New Alipore in 1976.

The next door neighbours had asked why we had not started yoga classes here? Buddha 'loved the idea and asked me if I was ready to teach the women. I was gung-ho,' said Chitralekha. 'Initially, we had a handful of students and soon it became a crowd', then Buddha took out a 'loan and built that hall in front' where he could teach.[3] 'Ladies on Tuesdays, Thursdays and Saturdays; gents on Mondays, Wednesdays and Fridays.'

'Everyone called him Guruji and he initiated many into Kriya yoga that he had learned from Swami Yogananda,' recalled Chitralekha.

> He was always dressed in either dhoti and *panjabi* or a saffron-colored *lungi* and a white *kurta*. I used to sit in the consulting room where he would question the members/patients and listen carefully to his detailed mode of queries. I learned what, how and when to ask and find out the problem with the person. I learned every individual had an individual constitution and the same ailment in two people needed different asanas. I learned by watching and listening how to make a chart and how to teach asana and pranayam.[4]

Buddha let go of 4/2 Rammohan Roy and also of the idea of taking the yoga outside of Calcutta. He settled into the Yoga Cure Institute in New Alipore with great dreams, even after the tragedy of Ava Rani and Arun's death. Arun left two sons, and Ashok also had two sons. Buddha would tell others that he intended 'to live for another twenty years' in order to raise those four boys to become 'yoga teachers'.[5] It was a normal period in Buddha's life, in the sense of his having an occupation while living in one place, but matters were not normal within the New Alipore household.

Bikram landed in Los Angeles in 1978, and his yoga studio became 'Bikram's Yoga College of India', alongside the publication of the book *Bikram's Beginning Yoga Class*. Instrumental in the change was Anne Marie Bennstrom, who was able, as Bikram wrote, to 'understand the East and the West'. Anne was ahead of the curve in integrating capitalism and brand awareness with yoga. She had developed workouts based on modern-day aerobics and group fitness classes, and worked with other Hollywood stars to market fitness products. She helped Bikram envision a one-size-fits-all model of a class, which was put into book format in 1978. In Bikram's mind, putting the yoga into book format made him the owner, and those around him echoed the claim back to him.

Jibananda and Karuna Ghosh continued to live in Tokyo and published four books on Ghosh Yoga (in Japanese): *Indian Yoga for Health & Happiness*, Parts 1 and 2, which were published in the mid-seventies; *Indian Yoga in Action*, a practical guidebook, published in 1979; and finally, *Indian Yoga – Essence of Life*. The last emphasizes the spiritual aspects of yoga, and in it the couple insist that yoga is not acrobatic. This was a response to the commercialization by

Bikram, but few outside of Japan knew of the existence of these books. They have all of the *bayam* or free-hand exercises to be done as warm-ups or for therapeutic aims, the eighty-four yoga asanas and many other asanas, along with pranayama and meditation techniques.

During the seventies, Calcutta yoga was branching out to different parts of the world, with variations to suit the different cultures, but within Calcutta, the landscape changed as well. Dibya and Prem Das branched out to open about a dozen different yoga studios across Calcutta. Monotosh Choudhury and Bimal Das did as well. Amar Nath Nandi continued to travel back and forth to Japan, opening studios in Hiroshima and Fukishima. As the decade ended, though Ghosh's Yoga College was no longer the epicentre, its global influence on spreading the practice of yoga – Bishnu's dream – had been achieved.

Ashok remained in Calcutta and came to New Alipore on occasion. By 1980, his temper and drinking habits had not changed, and an intervention was attempted. Ashok would relinquish everything, it was decided, and go to live in the Himalayas. He took initiation and became a sannyasi. Buddha told him to first go and see his wife Chitralekha, who was staying with her mother and a newborn, before he left. Chitralekha heard him call from outside their house, near Kalighat.

'I saw him in sannyasi robes – ochre-coloured lungi and a kurta.' Chitralekha was dumbfounded. 'Where could he have gotten this idea?' she wondered. 'Ashok said he had been advised to take *sannyas* by his father and to take his first *bhiksha* (alms) from me, thus renouncing the householder's life. He was off to Kailas and Manasarovar.'

It was of course, reminiscent of Buddha in 1947, when he left his family to save his life, but for for Chitralekha it was a 'a bolt from the blue'. 'Three young children, and Ashok wanted to leave the world. What kind of question is that? "Do I have your permission to abandon you now, with my three children in your tow as a single mother?"'

I ask, 'Did you give it to him?'

'No. How could I?'

Ashok left for the Himalayas despite Chitralekha's wishes, but the robes and the Himalayas did not last long. Ashok came back after a month or so.[6]

In 1981, things were not well with Buddha. Mataji felt that Buddha was 'physically fit but mentally ill'. The conflict over Ashok, with violent fits brought on by the epilepsy and alcoholism, had enveloped the entire house. Buddha felt very sad about the whole family atmosphere. He told Mataji, 'There is no mutual understanding among the three women in the house. Swapna says something, Rooma says something, Chitralekha says something, and I do not know what to do. They cannot unite and decide what is to be cooked. So I said one day Swapna will cook, one day Rooma and one day Chitralekha.'

'I have been able to convince the whole society, but at home,' Buddha told Mataji, 'no one is willing to listen.'[7]

The notion emerged that Ashok was a danger to the stability of the family property in New Alipore. It was decided that Ashok would be legally disowned by Buddha to assure that he would not sell away the property. In order to do this, Buddha and Rooma would need the cooperation of Chitralekha. She would need to legally divorce Ashok for the disownment to proceed. It happened in 1981.

By 1982, Rooma did not want Chitralekha and her three children to have a share of the property. Buddha remained aloof, 'helpless' in seclusion, telling Mataji, 'I don't know what to do.' Chitralekha described the transition:

By the time the divorce was more or less final, things were changing at home – the attitudes of the family members gradually became distant and I started feeling like a most unwelcome guest in my in-law's place. I cannot put my finger on any exact event or situation but one fine day I was simply asked to leave the house with the kids.

Buddha, 'helpless' and feeling an 'unavoidable obligation' did not intervene.

Buddha Bose lived on the roof where he had built a well-fitted out flat-cum-puja room. He did not come down from there for seven days while I waited to ask him where I would go with the three children. There was no way of contacting him, and I was not given the key to the main door. Finally, after being asked to leave practically every night, I collected our few belongings and left.[8]

'Emmie Bose may have had to face hardships, but I wonder, did she have to go through fire at every step of her life? I had no money, no job, and not a clue where I would put up for the rest of my life,' said Chitralekha.[9] The events laid bare the multi-generational karmic instances of disownment and abandonment within the family.[10]

Ashok retreated to the Garpar area, his old neighbourhood. Bishnu's wife Ashalata (she died in 1979), and then Bishwanath, used to give him food every day', while he lived outside under the ground floor parking shed.[11] He was eventually 'thrown out of the house' there as well. Years later, when Shyamal was visiting from Bangkok, and he found Ashok reduced to 'begging for money, living in the market' at Garpar.[12] 'In the morning he bathed at a spigot on Raja Dinendra Road; afterwards he would open the bottle, and at night time he would close the bottle.'[13]

Shyamal explained that when Ashok and Arun 'began to smoke and drink', they'd squandered their opportunity, and began the ruin of the house. Neither of them lived up to their expectations. On the other hand, Shyamal explained, 'Bikram and I came from poor backgrounds. We had to work hard to survive in this hard world.'[14]

With Arun no longer alive, and Ashok disowned, the sons of the family no longer held property rights, and Rooma took over everyday management of the Yoga Cure Institute in New Alipore, then married an accountant named Shibnath De in 1983.

In Calcutta, at 4/2 Rammohan Road, Ghosh's Yoga College became more subdued and localized. Meanwhile, in America, Bikram's popularity was taking off. In Calcutta, nearly everything had unraveled with the yoga family, and at New Alipore, Buddha became less and less attached to his life.

97

BRAHMA KAMAL, 27 APRIL 1983

The lotus flower will not decay under the touch of water.
The water rolls off. The lotus remains as pure as ever.
We should be like the lotus flower –
nothing good or bad from this world should touch us.
Don't get stuck to those energies. If you stick to them then you are gone.
Be the like the lotus and let it roll off.[1]
– Mataji

In the commentary for the film *Holy Kailas*, Buddha closed the first act with his story of a particular valley within the Himalayas. It was after he had visited the pilgrimage peaks in India, and before he went to Nepal and Kailash. Between the two, he dipped down from the snow-laden peaks and icy glacial waters, to a place called Nandan Kanan, the Valley of Flowers:

Nandan Kanan is a delight for the eyes, it is fifteen miles in length and two and a half miles in breadth. Wherever the eyes are turned nothing else but flowers and flowers are seen. One is lost in elysian reverie when one comes here. The abundance and variety of flora and flowers of this place delights the mind with joy. I have not seen a better place.[2]

The 'entire place is covered with ice' except for two months, when there are '216 varieties of flowers' by his count, 'in full bloom'. With the audience in rapt attention, Buddha told them, 'Words fail to express the beauty of this place', where sadhus and sannyasis live off the fruit and meditate all summer long. Buddha became enraptured with the place, and continued the dialogue:

While in Nandan Kanan I felt like saying, 'God where am I? I feel I am seeing you for real. I am in heaven.' I think anyone who comes here will have the same feeling. God is truth, God is beauty, *Satyam Shivam Sundaram!*

Mataji asked Buddha, 'How are you feeling?' He replied, 'The pain is everywhere.'

Then she asked about his disciples in Gujarat, 'Any message?' Buddha replied, 'No, nothing. Just waiting for the call.'

She knew, 'Guruji is dying.'[3]

Buddha's disciple in Gujarat, Yashodhara Maharaja, had a dream and could not make sense of it, so she asked Mataji: 'Is there a staircase in Guruji's house? A sofa or couch near the staircase landing? And a window through which the sunlight comes in?' Mataji said, 'Yes of course. But why are you asking me this?' 'I dreamt that both you and I were sitting on that sofa with my back towards the stairs. Suddenly I turned to see Guruji coming up the stairs but his lungi was grey in color, not his usual reddish-orange or yellow silk.' Mataji then said, 'He wanted to tell you that he was leaving his body.'[4]

While walking up to the terrace one day at the New Alipore home, towards the puja room on the top floor, Buddha suddenly collapsed on the staircase. The doctors could not find the reason for his illness. A trip to Japan for a diagnosis was planned. A preliminary 'check-up in the hospital was needed. But he never came back from the hospital; he did not want to come back to the house.'

On 27 April 1983, Buddha died. 'It seems when Rooma went to bring him home she found him sitting and meditating. So she waited outside for him to finish his meditation. When she went to fetch him again, she found he had already left his body.'[5]

When I near the end of the research, it is also through a dream, just as in the beginning.

The first night I arrived in Calcutta, four years back, in a dream, I encountered Buddha when he was a boy of nine years, as fear permeated a pitch-black room. During the trans-personal encounter, I felt trapped, eyes-closed, within the body of a young Buddha, amidst some scene of felt torture. He and I, have to learn to breathe in order to quell the fear and regain control; the power of breath is discovered.

Chitralekha listened to me recount the dream, then replied matter of fact, 'You've been given a glimpse into what he had to overcome to get himself on track. The odds he faced were great. He could have chosen the easy path to being a failure, and blamed his stock, but he overcame the odds, and now you've gotten a glimpse. He's given you an experience of it.'

That first dream, so visceral a connection, sustained my curiosity throughout the adventure. Now, at the end, back in America, I also awake from a dream:

I am standing in a completely white room. It is square. I see one corner window with light coming through, and two doors. Buddha is also in the room. Dressed in white, he is older, but his face is younger. He looks serene, and is not looking at me; more like right through me. We were both subdued, no words need to be spoken. It seems we are in agreement. I look for an exit. I watch as one of the doors turns into the wall. I can't go out the easy way. I am boxed in, just as he wants? I feel he's making sure I am not about to leave. I am not going anywhere, for the moment at least.

I write about this to Chitralekha.

She replies, 'He is trying to send a message.' Then she continues, 'Maybe you could go through the dream and try to understand what you felt when you had this dream. It can give you a clue.'

I realize this last dream is like a juxtaposition from the first one, which was entirely inner, and shared, as our awareness of the breath became a channel to detach, to reclaim power. In the second dream, now at the end of the research in Calcutta, we are trapped as well, but there is no emotion. We are at ease. All is light, not dark. Eyes are open. I am not in his body, we are separate, but still in the same room. I recall, it is Buddha who makes the next move:

The room just has one door left. It is slightly ajar. I just stand there, with Buddha near to the door. He moves in front of it, and reaches out his hand. I wake up right at this moment.

I understand, he is about to step out; what I set out to do is finished.

Buddha ends the *Holy Kailas* commentary on Nandan Kanan, the Valley of Flowers, with a story about a certain flower which grows there, by the name of Brahma Kamal. It is the most auspicious flower of the Himalayas and only found at an altitude above 4,500 metres. Buddha said:

> I plucked a flower to lay it on the altar of the temple and then suddenly a thought came to my mind, 'Why did I pluck the flower? I should have let it be there on the plant in full bloom. Why did I shorten its life by plucking it? It is better to offer my heart and soul to God and not a flower from nature.' I felt like a guilty person and my eyes started watering. I am sure all those who come here will understand and have the same feeling.[6]

As I read through Buddha's commentary, I ask Mataji a few questions about the flower and this place in the Himalayas, and she begins a story. 'In Guruji's film he shows the blooming or opening of the Kamal. Inside, the seeds are seen, that are the food for the *kasturi mrug* (musk deer).' Mataji then pauses and looks at me. Perhaps with an inkling of what would be the next part of my own journey, her eyes seem to twinkle, then she continues, 'They bloom in August, will you go there?'

'Soon,' I reply.

With an opportunity, a chance, I will.

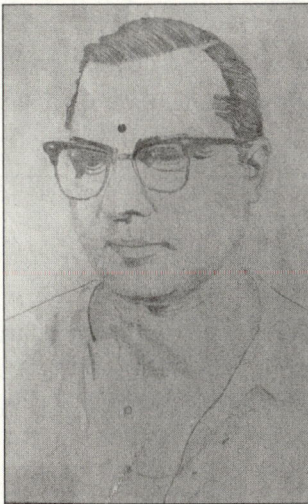

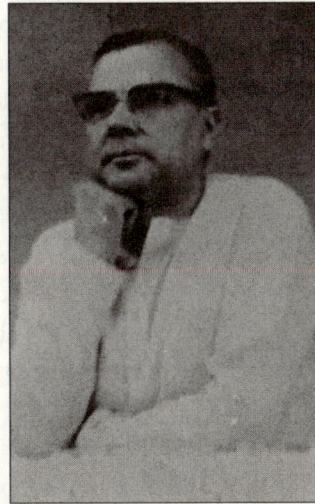

Buddha Bose in Gujarat, Circa 1971.
Source: Courtesy of Rekha Maharaja-Ivey

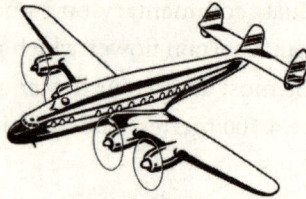

Pan Am Clipper

AFTERMATH

In 1983, Bikram returned from America to Calcutta to marry Rajashree through an arranged marriage.[1] Bikram went on to state that the arranged marriage would 'salvage the lineage; as he was marrying a yoga champion from the same school he'd studied in'.[2]

Bikram's idea of salvaging the lineage was to wrap up all of the Ghosh Yoga history into one big myth of his own creation. His devotees grew in number. Bikram began training teachers in 1994 and thereafter started doing trainings twice or thrice a year, eventually reaching over 10,000 Bikram Yoga teachers, in over 500 Bikram Yoga studios worldwide. In 1997, I started the practice, just off Markham Avenue in Portland, Oregon. Bikram's ninety-minute, twenty-six plus two (26 postures and 2 pranayamas) beginner class was an extreme workout in the heat, and the teachers were demanding. Water was discouraged. If you left the room, you didn't come back in. No improvisation. It was regimented yoga.

With millions of students each year, devoted teachers and power, Bikram reached his pinnacle by 2012, in an attempt to copyright the yoga asana sequence as his own creation.

As far back as 1985, when Bikram sued the actress Raquel Welch, for selling a DVD of her yoga class, threats and lawsuits had squelched nearly all but a few of those who were opposed. As he neared his copyright goal, attempts at legal opposition were made by the Open Source Yoga Unity (OSYU) and Yoga to the People (YTTP). When the latter settled unsuccessfully, on 12 December 2012, Bikram gloated to the press.

'I win, he lose, and that's it. Nobody will ever be able to steal Bikram yoga anymore.'[3] Bikram didn't know it at the time, but that was the top of his mountain. On 14 December, in a similar copyright infringement suit against

Evolation Yoga (which refused to settle out of court), the court's decision ruled that Bikram Choudhury could no longer claim copyright ownership of any yoga sequence. The resolution was 'a total game changer'. Without Choudhury's copyright, there could be no infringement. Two days after he won, Bikram had suddenly lost everything.

One year later, allegations of sexual assault and rape against Bikram were filed in civil court documents by former trainees and became widespread knowledge.[4]

In March 2014, I purchased a copy of *Key to the Kingdom of Health through Yoga* by Buddha Bose on Bikram's website. A year later, in Calcutta, I asked Rooma Bose, 'When was the last time you talked with Bikram?' She replied, 'In 2006, Bikram called me. He asked for permission to reprint the book by Buddha Bose, and I said no.' He did it anyway.

With the abusive allegations against Bikram in the press, I followed up by asking her about his legacy. 'Bikram is a not only a disgrace to yoga, he is a disgrace to all of India,' she replied.

Nevertheless, I was secretly glad of having encountered this yoga through Bikram and the publication of Buddha's book, as it gave me access to this teaching that was nearly lost and an opportunity to practise Calcutta yoga as Buddha and Bishnu had taught. This began the path that led to finding the unpublished book and manuscript by Buddha Bose, 84 *Yoga Asanas* from 1938. Just as Bikram's world tumbled, I had started to recover the true essence of this yoga lineage.

Other than finding those publications and writing this book on the history of Calcutta yoga, the only other desire or task which stuck with me was to live inside the house at 4/2 Rammohan Roy and learn the yoga they taught through their teacher training programme.

Two years after this had all begun, I was in Calcutta, living in the family home of Bishnu and Buddha, along with eight other students of Hatha yoga, learning the techniques of yoga therapy.

Bishnu Ghosh founded Ghosh's College of Physical Education in 1923. Now, the course was being led by Muktamala Mitra, the granddaughter of Bishnu

Ghosh. She grew up in this house, with the nickname of Tumtum. In her late thirties, she has just begun to emerge from under the wings of her family's legacy:

> I used to wait and listen to my father (Bishwanath) give lessons. I would sit downstairs in the room where he taught. I never thought that one day I would be the teacher. I thought I would be a housewife. But I am the only one; I've no brother or sister, so I've got to take this on now.

I met Muktamala during my first visit, and she was electrifying with her confirmation of what I proposed: the opportunity for a month-long teacher training for a certificate to teach therapeutic yoga.

'Yes, bring them, bring forty!' she smiled and laughed. I laughed too, but more hesitantly. The second time I visited, we hashed out the details. We decided upon a more reasonable number, about ten students. It would be the first training group of Western students at Ghosh's Yoga College, and if it worked well, we'd be able to do it twice annually, in the fall and spring. Students from outside India would come to Calcutta, live in this old house and learn to become a teacher of therapeutic yoga in the tradition of Bishnu Ghosh and Buddha Bose. Muktamala invited the opportunity, 'We will be as one big family.' The training involved therapeutic yoga instructions twice a day, along with teaching, discussing and practising yoga. For me, the idea of staying in the Ghosh house, where Buddha Bose and Bishnu Ghosh lived and taught yoga for over forty years, felt like a dream. I would learn to teach yoga as they had done.

The first-floor yoga rooms are open from 6 a.m. to 8 p.m., but there's a long period in the middle of the day during which they're empty. The Indian students begin to arrive promptly at 6 a.m. and seem to practise in organized group sessions, but not in classes the way we are accustomed to in modern yoga studios. There isn't instruction so much as there is loud and continuous counting, from one to ten, as the groups work their way through *bayam* free-hand exercises and asana sequences. For the most part, the focus here is less on asana than on exercises, less on static holding than on dynamic movement. Usually, students do a mixture of both. Breathing exercises are practised, usually at the beginning and end of their individualized class structure. A favourite of mine was to hear someone doing *bhramari* pranayam, shutting off all of the sense doors with the fingers, then making a loud buzzing 'bee breath' through the nostrils.

The women and men each arrive with their own prescription and schedule. They work individually in a very casual fashion. There is preparation and socializing, then yoga practice. Standing postures are done on a painted hardwood floor with thick, cotton or jute-filled mats, which are used for floor postures.

On the second-floor outdoor terrace, we would do our group yoga class each morning at 6 a.m., looking east while the sun rose. As Muktamala taught us the postures and the ailments they align with, every once in a while she would fill in some details of the history in the house. 'Rajashree would sit right here and practise,' she would say as we gathered in one of the yoga rooms. And then she'd reflect for a moment, 'My grandfather would teach the same method I am carrying on with ... trying to ... let's see.'

Bishwanath died in 2008. In the spring of 2010, Muktamala was asked by Bikram to attend one of his trainings, held in Las Vegas. She did and was given the 'Bulldog Determination' award. But that style of twenty-six postures with a strict time and order is not the traditional style of individualized yoga, with each person doing their particular set of exercises and postures. Now, she's ultimately training us to have the ability to write the 'yoga prescriptions' for others. We practise with her, spelling out the symptoms a potential patient might have:

Sex, Male. Age, 45. Height, 5'6, Weight, 51 Kg (normal). Ailments: constipation, vertigo, asthma.

We learned that, first, there is a one-to-one interview with the client, and then a prescription is formulated by the yoga teacher and written down on a piece of paper. I was shown multiple examples of this before beginning the training. One has to have learned the hundreds of options that apply to each potential case. The simple formula is a combination of breathing techniques mixed with static and dynamic postures and exercises, followed by periods of relaxation. This makes for a twenty–forty minute self-taught class. After two–six months, the student again meets with the teacher, and if there is a need for any changes, those are addressed – resulting in a new prescription. The underlying technique of addressing ailments at an individual level hasn't changed from what Bishnu was practising in the twenties, at his 4 Garpar Road gymnasium, through the sixties with Yoga Cure Institute, to today at Ghosh's Yoga College.

This method has such a practical appeal to it. Muktamala made it sound easy, but she's grown up surrounded by it. I don't know that I am getting the hang of it the first week, but before I know it, I am able to string it all together, at least in theory. Hearing the echo of her grandfather, Muktamala tells me, 'Getting better day by day.'

In 1976, Muktamala was one of the last of two children born at 4/2 to the Calcutta yoga family. The other was Pavitra Shekhar, the second son of Ashok Bose and Chitralekha, and the youngest of the four boys of Ashok and Arun, whom Buddha taught yoga.

I came to see how both Muktamala and Pavitra exemplified the two sides of this family in this present generation. Muktamala carries the gregarious, cheerful, outgoing traits of the family. Like Bishnu, she brings forward the tradition of teaching. Pavitra has the traits of the other side of the family, inward-looking, reclusive, wanting to detach from everything. He is ready and willing, like Yogananda, to strike out for the Himalayas.

'We have arrived,' Pavitra tells me, pointing to the house on Vidyasagar Street, in Badur Bagan. The number '20' is on the house, which is now abandoned. It's been decades since Pavitra has visited the house. I ask him why he'd been in this area of north Calcutta, twenty years back.

At the time, in the late nineties, the great uncle of Pavitra (Ambar from the Bengali side of the Bose family, Buddha's younger brother), lived in the house along with his son Benoy.

'My Uncle Ambar lived here, and I worked the printing press in the front portion of the house for a spell. I'd walk here to work; he paid so little I couldn't even afford the tram.' Ambar Bose lived here while working at India Bank. 'He had a Bullet bike,' Pavitra recalls, one of the big bikes from the golden era of motorbiking in India. They were the last Bose family members to reside in the house, and now, it's vacant.

Someone is living in the house next door, standing outside on the terrace. I prod Pavitra into inquiring about the situation. Pavitra begins talking with a woman, asks about Ambar, then an elderly man steps partly outside the house when he hears the question.

'He's gone. You won't find him. A crook!' That's all he will tell us, as he steps back into the shadows.

'Maybe it's cursed,' I say, then am uncomfortable I said it.

This is where Buddha Bose was raised. This is where Emily lived for a time. This was the home of Rajah Bose, the magician. I think about the Bose family, going backwards from Pavitra to his father Ashok, to Buddha, to Rajah and Raj, who'd brought back enough wealth from Burma to build this fine four-storey structure in north Calcutta. It is big enough for a dozen rooms and a few families, but now it stands empty, left to ruin.

As I stand there and ponder the past century, my mind is drawn to the thirty minutes prior to our arrival at this house: We arrived from south Calcutta by Uber and started our walk at the 4/2 Rammohan Roy Road house, where I had a few things I needed to drop off. We then crossed Upper Circular Road, and from the crowded sidewalk, went through a discreet entryway to enter an open-air indoor daytime marketplace. It's twilight outside and dim inside. The place is nearly empty, except for sleeping dogs lying on the cool cement. The stalls, where vegetables, fruits and other items would be, are all vacant.

As we walk through, Pavitra mentions that he has slept here a few times with his father Ashok, when it was too late to return to south Calcutta after a long day of work. I ask him where exactly, and he points to a large wooden stall, which has thick, woven bags of rice placed atop it. We stop and he shudders a bit, 'The rats that come out at night are huge.' He laughs under his breath. As we leave through the other side of the market and step into an alleyway, he points to a vacant stand, a slab of well-worn wood, next to a vendor's cart. 'There, he would get morning chai and a *kathi* roll to eat.' Bishwanath, Rooma or some friend would provide the money.

We turn down an alley, round a corner, and are about to reach Vidyasagar Street. Instead, we are motioned over; a voice speaks to us in Bengali to come, a man sitting on his front porch. He looks inquisitive and has some questions. The man asks one question and Pavitra answers. Then a pause, and another question. He runs out of questions finally and the man seems stumped, quenched of his curiosity, but not wholly satisfied. Pavitra motions for us to go on. I have no idea what they have discussed, so I ask Pavitra.

'That man has lived here his entire life,' Pavitra begins. 'He knew my father Ashok. You know, everyone here who is older knew my father. He lived out here and was constantly around; he didn't pass away until 1998.'

He continues relaying the man's story, 'They remember my father fondly. He was older and had lost his edge. He was someone who had lost everything, a drunkard, and was at the mercy of begging for food or money from his relatives and friends. That man there, he just couldn't get his head around how I had turned out so differently than my father.'

We laugh, but I know why Pavitra is different – his mother, Chitralekha. She raised him to be different, yet something remained too. In his family tree, which stretched from Bhagabati and Rajah, Yogananda and Bishnu, through Buddha and his father Ashok, something was left undone.

I think about a conversation Pavitra and I had in Benares, where we had been the week before. Walking along the ghats, finding places in the old Bengali section of the city, the residence of Lahiri and Sriyukteswar, I ask about his situation. He is turning forty, unmarried, without children. He tells me his father, Ashok, should not have had children, 'He just wasn't prepared to be a father.'

'Well, what about Buddha?' I ask.

'He shouldn't have had children either. He married out of obligation,' says Pavitra.

'Still, how could he have done anything else?'

'He should have refused,' Pavitra concludes.

'And before that, Rajah, Buddha's father?'

'He, too, married out of obligation, and it ruined it all with Emily.'

'What are you going to do?'

Pavitra pauses and then replies, 'I have my mother to watch out for and to make sure she is well in the world. When that obligation is finished, I will retire to some "no-man's land" and meditate. I will never marry.'

I ask him if his mother ever pushed him to get married.

'Yes, but by that time, I already had my dream – that I would wait for the responsibilities to end and leave this world.' After a long pause, he adds, 'What is the use of this; there is no end to it. Life and death, and newborns.' I invite him to go with me to visit the Himalayas, but he politely declines.

'Next time, I'll go there. I'll go once and for all,' he answers. 'My father went, and he came back. My grandfather went and he too came back.' I mention to him that his great grandfather also had a tie with the Himalayas. And obviously, Yogananda was pulled to the Himalayas too. So I ask if he has read or heard about them for inspiration?

'No. Nothing inspired me outwardly, it was totally internal, it comes from within, if you are really into it.'

The house on Vidyasagar Street, in old north Calcutta, is already at the point of no man's land. It had a past with the Bose family but no future. The story is finished, and the only thing which remains is to be forgotten.

I look at the steps going into the house, misshapen, like they were lifted up and dropped amiss. The place is locked up with a steel chain and no key. I cross the road to get a closer look. Upon reaching the gate to peer inside, I happen to look to the right of the door. I squint, and make out that there is a nameplate or something, covered up, next to the entrance.

I ask Pavitra about it and he replies, 'I've never noticed it before.'

I want to uncover it to see it clearly. Pavitra tells me he can clear it, but neither of us has a cloth or tissue. I start to wipe it with my hand and work to remove grime off of the words underneath. He laughs and exclaims that he should be the one doing the work, 'You've come all this way from America to uncover these details while I watch.'

The words become clear enough to read, orange and black, engraved on the aged marble tablet. It reads:

Of British Stage Fame
Rajah Bose
Magician and Psychic-Healer

It is only a nameplate, yet I feel like I've arrived at something. With the initial fieldwork complete, I know how the story begins and how it ends. The magician and the yogi, the father and son – and what remains. It is all just about forgotten by history, but I've dug deep enough – I realize in that moment – to know.

A year later, deep in the writing, I locate an old 1950 magic magazine inside the Magic Circle library of London.[5] It confirms the remembrance I feel. Something beyond a task or a duty, not an obligation. A willingness to know the truth.

The magazine writer too, had visited the Bose family residence, on 20 Vidyasagar Street. He also had glimpsed the faded marble tablet. 'It seems to murmur softly to us,' he wrote.[6] 'If only we have the heart to hear: *I was, I am and I will forever be.*'

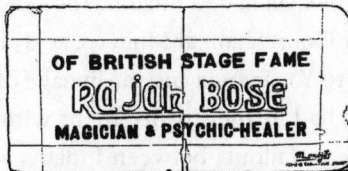

OF BRITISH STAGE FAME
Rajah Bose
MAGICIAN & PSYCHIC-HEALER

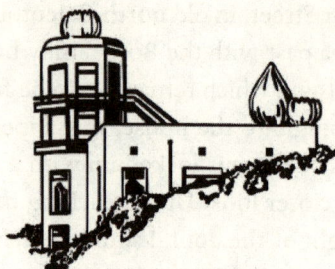

Golden Lotus Temple

EPILOGUE

In the larger view of history, this book covers only a part of the longer transmission of yoga teachings, from India to the world, over the past 500 years, and most of those stories are long forgotten. But after five years of historical work and writing, its satisfying to know that this generational story of the Calcutta yoga family will be remembered. There are a few remainding details to include at the completion.

After Yogananda's death, a number of predictable schism-moments happened within the Self-Realization Fellowship (SRF), both inside India and America. Among those who performed and taught yoga postures, Bernard Cole left once the rules around celibacy were changed (he was married) in the fifties. Kriyananda was ousted in the early sixties, forming a splinter group named Ananda. Though SRF has decreased in membership, it holds vast real estate holdings and remains a worldwide influential organization. In 1970, Bernard Tesnière took his final vows of renunciation and took on the name Swami Abhedananda. In his later years, according to disciples, Abhedananda would come by the yoga classes offered at Hollywood Temple, inside India Hall, to observe the asana classes and advise the teachers.

There's little documentation of contact between Bishnu Ghosh and the SRF organization after Yogananda's death. Instead, Bishnu occasionally went to meet with Nabani Das Khyapa Baul, in order to obtain spiritual teachings. And in the sixties, he along with Ashalata and Karuna, took diksha from Hemangshu Chakraborty, the guru of Gouri Shankar Mukerji, at Jayanti Mata. Buddha Bose maintained his devotion to Yogananda and the lineage of Lahiri and Babaji, but he doesn't seem to have had further involvement with the SRF organization (this may have been due to fallouts between Indians and Americans over its organizational structure in the fifties). In the early seventies, Buddha shared a premonition with a couple, telling them that they would visit the place where Yogananda lived in California. 'You will visit with those in the organization,' he told them, 'but do not mention my name there.' Other parts of the family, most notably the ancestors of Sananda Ghosh and Bijoy Mullick, keep ties to the Kriya yoga organizational lineages (SRF and Ananda) initiated by Yogananda.

Among Bishnu's top yoga students profiled in *Calcutta Yoga*, Gouri Shankar Mukerji travelled to America in 1997, for a workshop series, then died in 1998. His 1963 yoga book in German was translated into English and published in 2016. Reba Rakshit lived until 2010, and Labanya Palit until 2009. Although I was unable to locate the book *Shariram Adyam*, written by Labanya in 1955, Ida Jo took up the effort with Chandrima Pal. They not only found a lone copy of the book but also embarked on a journey of translating it into English from Bengali, and writing *The Women of Yoga*, a collection of research into the untold stories of Bengali women associated with yoga and physical culture. Bishnu's magazine, *Bayam Charcha*, continued to be published by Moti Lal Mondal and his son Tappan, until 1995.

Buddha's two foreign students both continued to live in Calcutta for a while. Ian Stephans stayed on as the British editor in India of *The Statesman* for twenty-one years, until 1951. When he died, in 1984, Amartya Sen wrote in a letter to *The Times*; 'he is remembered not only as a great editor' and as 'amiable, if somewhat eccentric', but also as someone who 'saved the lives of hundreds of thousands of people'. Stephens wrote his memoirs, *Monsoon Mornings*, about Calcutta in the forties during the war, famine and fighting, in 1966. Edward Groth stayed on as the US consul general until 1950. His retirement provided him time to put his 'large collection of photographs in order in albums and a chance to relive various treks and trips'. His autobiography, *To Give Room for Wandering*, was self-published in 1972, and he lived until 1977. I was unable to find where his extensive collection of photographs was placed posthumously, which resulted in one assumption and one possible alternative. First, I concluded that Groth probably took the photographs in Buddha Bose's 1938 *Yoga Asanas* book. And second, despite the family lore, I arrived at the likehood that Groth may have been the 'Uncle Edward' to whom Buddha dedicated the book; it remains a mystery.

Buddha's daughter, Rooma, continues to operate the New Alipore yoga studio, alongside two children born after the death of Buddha. Among the four sons who Buddha taught yoga, the two sons of Arun continue to live in the New Alipore home. Surya Shekhar opened a gymnasium on the ground floor, called Bodyline, which is dedicated to their grandfather Bishnu Ghosh. Chandra Shekhar performs and teaches all of the eighty-four yoga asanas, carrying on the family tradition. Ashok's sons are still burdened with familial ostracization from the Bose ancestral home in New Alipore and 4/2 Rammohan Roy Road. His eldest son, Shib Shekhar, has an educational block, and inherited Ashok's sudden seizures, yet, he is capable of earning his living. He works at a *dhaba* (kitchen) in Himachal Pradesh. In 2015, *84 Yoga Asanas*, by Buddha Bose (his unpublished work described in the preface) was published. It included an introduction by Ashok's younger son, Pavitra Shekhar, who lives in Calcutta and Delhi, along with an article by Chitralekha Shalom on the pranayam methods taught by Buddha. Buddha's friend and disciple Mataji, nearing ninety-five years old, continues her life of service in Mussoorie and Ahmedabad.

In Japan, amidst all of the new types of yoga centres, the three original studios still operate within or near the central Shinjuku area of Tokyo. The Tokyo Yoga Center is maintained by the Hanari family. The Ghosh Yoga Institute is still run by Jibananda Ghosh, with Karuna having died in 2009. And the Yoga College of India is still run by Buddhadeb Choudhury. In Thailand, Shyamal Talukdar (Modo) died in January 2018, and his son carries on the yoga teaching tradition. Modo's was the most informative interview I conducted, as if he'd held onto the artifacts all those years for this one three-hour interview.

Others passed on too while I wrote the book. For some, like Kamal Bhandari, I missed an interview by weeks before his death in 2016. And others, like Monotosh Roy, who authored *Cream of Yoga* in 1970 and then lived a long life promoting *bayam* and yoga until his death in 2005; I was not able to interview him but did have access to those done by Claudia Guggenbühl. Hiten Roy and Susan Barrett both died in the spring of 2019. As Chitralekha would remind me, once I found out about someone whom I wanted to interview, 'Please do not delay, time is running out!'

We all thought Arup Sen Gupta might die. However, a few years after he was unable to continue his assistance, Claudia sent me this message: 'And imagine: Arup has resurrected! After months of silence, of not answering the phone, of being hospitalized and refusing to eat, he is back! Full of interest for his daughter – and in fact, they had their very first talk over the phone yesterday!' Arup's mental faculty returned, and he began a path of rehabilitation; he even joined the world online. Claudia would find a publisher for her eventual book, *Yoga in Calcutta*, and as this book went to press, she was about to return to India for the first time since she'd left in 2004.

Bikram Choudhury lives as a sort of wanted fugitive, staying outside the USA state of California. Stripped of his belongings by the court and divorced from his wife Rajashree in 2016, his 'Bikram Yoga' trademark was awarded to one of his complainants. Though his trainings have dwindled, he continues to teach new students, about a hundred per year, in places like Mexico.

In Calcutta, during March 2019, as I neared the conclusion, Mukul Dutta and I finally located Monotosh Choudhury, Bishnu's senior yoga teacher in the sixties, now in his eighties. Upon meeting, he encouraged me to press as hard as possible against his stomach to show he was still fit and strong. As the interviews progressed I realized that not only did Monotosh remember all of the stories but also, unlike most others, he'd kept everything of the old photographs and, most importantly, the issues of *Bayam Charcha*.

As I sat there, listening to Monotosh and Mukul tell me the history, I reflected on how difficult a time I had in locating Bishnu's magazine and how here they were all along. I thought about how I'd struggled to grasp onto any bit of information I could find, and how I learned to let go, become subtle and just ask. And meanwhile, Monotosh and Mukul, like so many others on the journey I encountered, patiently waited decades to share the story of how Calcutta yoga reached the world.

Just as the final proof of this book arrived, Mukul Dutta unexpectedly died. I was torn and sad on an earthly level. In spirit though, I felt as if he had completed an obligation. I realized the completion of this story was a part of his charge too, and the task was now complete. Mukul, just as his forerunners, had brought yoga from Calcutta to the world, and so became a part of our history to forever remember.

NOTES

Introduction

1. Swami Jibananda Giri, *Transcendent Journey*, (K Publications, 2015), 235.

Chapter 1

1. According to Dadswell, Bhay Ranjit, a.k.a. Ripendra Nath Bose, came to be later known as Rajah or Rajah Bose. See Sarah Dadswell, 'Jugglers, Fakirs, and Jadu Wallahs: Indian Magicians and the British Stage', *New Theatre Quarterly* 23, no. 1 (2007), 3–24.

2. The primary articles were found at Magic Circle Library in London and in Calcutta magic magazines. These, along with family lore – most notably from Chitralekha Shalom (Bose) in Calcutta and Susan Barrett (Bose) in London – and old English newspaper citations, filled out the sources.

3. Asoke Sarkar, 'Biography: Our Homage to Rajah Bose India's Great Master of Magic with International Reputation', *Magic* 1 (Calcutta: January 1950), 31–6.

4. Sarkar, 'Biography', 32–3.

5. Christopher Dell, *The Occult Witchcraft Magic: An Illustrated History* (Thames & Hudson, 2016), 338–41.

6. The National Archives of the UK; Kew, Surrey, England; Board of Trade: Commercial and Statistical Department and successors: Inwards Passenger Lists; Class: BT26; Piece: 301; Item: 65.

7. Registered Students, Session 1908. Faculties of Arts, Science and Technology. Yorkshire College. Leeds University Calendar, 1908, 528. Available at http://digital.library.leeds.ac.uk/view/calendars/ Accessed 1/20/2017.

8. Sarkar, 'Biography', 32–3.

9. Yorkshire College/University of Leeds: Sessional Entries Vol. 6, 129, 257 (LUA/ADM/039/3). YC/ UoL Register of Students Vol. 7, entry 6245, fol.1981 (LUA/ADM/039/8).

10. Dadswell, 'Jugglers, Fakirs, and Jadu Wallahs'.

11. L.K. Roy, 'Past Glory of India: Rajah Bose, of British Stage Fame', *Velki Quarterly Magazine* (Calcutta: October 1969). Reprinted in Salil Kumar, *The Gimmick Magazine e-zine* 2, no. 2 (Oct.–Nov. 2012).

12. Ibid.

13. Debra Diamond (ed.), *Yoga: The Art of Transformation* (Smithsonian, 2013).

14. At around this time, Ripendra Nath changes his stage name from Bhay Ranjit to Rajah the Magician. Rajah later employed the Egyptian 'Cleopatra' dance, with its 'huge python' on the stage. *The Manchester Courier* (15 April 1911), 10.

15. 'Our London Letter', *New York Clipper* (25 February 1911), 2.

16. Dadswell, 'Jugglers, Fakirs, and Jadu Wallahs'.

17. Ibid.

Chapter 2

1. According to her birth certificate, Emily was born on 21 January 1888, in the Kirkstall area of Leeds. According to her death certificate, her birthday was 24 December. Her mother, Margaret Ann (Dineen), was full Irish, from Connemara, Ireland stock, though born in England. Her father, Joseph Arthur Johnson, was a wool merchant.

2. Susan Barrett (Bose) of England, unpublished historical family novel about her grandmother Emily, and Rajah.

3. From 1909 to 1910, Rajah performed with the stage name of Ranjit Bhay, likely a transliteration of *bhai*, but why he chose this is unclear. For the 1911 London Census, he gave Vaishno as his birthplace, which is near a *Mata* temple, deep in the Himalayan Mountains.

4. Asoke Sarkar, 'Biography: Our Homage to Rajah Bose India's Great Master of Magic with International Reputation', *Magic* 1 (Calcutta: January 1950): 31–6. What London daily this is quoting is unclear. We can surmise it was likely a promotional flier of some sort, which was reproduced in the article.

5. Ibid.

6. The famous American magician and author John Booth came to Calcutta in the early 1940s looking for magicians, and he was responsible for creating much of the mystique around P.C. Sorcar in his book *Forging Ahead in Magic* and *Marvels of Mystery* (John Booth, 1939). Socar's subsequent authorships were popular textbooks for professional magicians, and opened up the world of magic to the general public. Of interest, I heard anecdotes that told of Rajah being P.C. Sorcar's unacknowledged teacher (a source for his book material). During the period just before P.C. Sorcar rapidly rose to fame in Calcutta, Rajah Bose was the president of Calcutta's Magicians Club.

7. Sarkar, 'Biography', 34.

Chapter 3

1. Susan Barrett (Bose) of England, unpublished historical family novel about her grandmother Emily and Rajah.

2. 1911 London census, Class: RG14; Piece: 6017; Schedule Number: 55.

3. Interview with Mataji (Swamini Guru Priyananda). Mussoorie, India. June 2017.

Chapter 4

1. Kief Hillsbery, *Empire Made* (Harcourt, 2017), Chapter 6.

2. L.K. Roy, 'Past Glory of India: Rajah Bose, of British Stage Fame', *Velki Quarterly Magazine* (Calcutta: October 1969). Reprinted in Salil Kumar, *The Gimmick Magazine e-zine* 2, no. 2 (Oct.–Nov. 2012).

Chapter 5

1. The self-described 'globetrotting author and magician' had met the magician, Sorcar, in the hotel. Booth writes of a November 1948 afternoon when he 'was taking lunch in the dining room of the Great Eastern Hotel', and it was clear that he was 'in the presence of a man with rare drive, vision, and capacities.' Sorcar declared himself 'the world's greatest magician although he had yet to set foot' on any land other than Bengal. Little did Booth realize that he himself had been conjured by Sorcar. Booth had visited Sorcar's New Alipore home the previous day, unannounced, and Sorcar, unprepared, painted and dressed in a dhoti, passed himself off as a servant and arranged the meeting to happen instead in the regal Great Eastern Hotel. Booth didn't recognize the same person. P.C. Sorcar, *History of Magic* (Calcutta: Indrajal Publications, 1970), 20.

2. Nilanjana Gupta (ed.), *Strangely Beloved: Writings on Calcutta* (New Delhi: Rainlight Rupa, 2014), 11.

3. *The Illustrated Weekly of India* 94, Part 4 (Bennett, Coleman & Company, Limited, Times of India Press, 1973), 4.

Chapter 6

1. Chitralekha Shalom (Bose) on Buddha Bose. She was his eldest daughter-in-law and knew him from 1973 to 1982.

2. Interview with Mataji. Mussoorie, India. June 2017.

3. Ibid.

4. Asoke Sarkar, 'Biography: Our Homage to Rajah Bose India's Great Master of Magic with International Reputation', *Magic* 1 (Calcutta: January 1950): 31–6.

5. Ibid.

6. Ibid.

7. Ibid.

8. Interview with Mataji. Mussoorie, India. June 2017.

9. Ray Charmak, the son of Haydee (eldest of Emily and Rajah's three children). Email, January 2017.

10. Interview with Mataji. Mussoorie, India. June 2017.

Chapter 7

1. Chitralekha wrote: 'I can remember from his narration of his life in small snippets and at that time I had decided to write about his childhood and emergence as yoga expert. He had been quite excited about the prospect, but unfortunately, life had more in store for me before I could put pen to paper seriously. *Moral Courage* was a promise I kept. A promise made years back to Buddha Bose.' Chitralekha wrote *Moral Courage*, a short biography of Buddha Bose, in 2011.

2. When she first met Buddha, she was a schoolteacher named Yashodhara Behen. Now known as Swamini Guru Priyananda or, as many refer to her, Mataji.

3. Interview with Mataji and Chitralekha Shalom. Mussoorie, India. June 2016.

4. The derogatory term *mleccha* was a form of ostracism, used for someone who did not belong into Hindu culture; a sort of barbarian, of untouchable castes.

Chapter 8

1. Haradhan Chakraborty, 'Byam – Tapas Bishnu Charan', *Bayam Charcha* (August 1970).
2. Gyana Prabha Bose may be distantly related to Raj Shekhar Bose.
3. The Bengali yogi, Shyama Charan Lahiri, appeared to Bhagabati and engaged him in conversation. Without a rational explanation for the experience, Bhagabati travelled to meet Lahiri in Benares, India. As a Kriya yoga exponent practising pranayam and meditation, Lahiri initiated both Bhagabati and his wife Gyana into Kriya yoga.
4. The origins of Kriya yoga practice are traced back to an ageless siddhi yogi in the Himalayan Mountains named Babaji. Lahiri Mahasaya had been born with the forename of Shyama Charan in 1828. At the age of five, his mother died, and his father took the boy to live in Benares. At the age of thirty-three, in 1861, he was initiated into Kriya yoga in a remote area of the Himalayas by Babaji. Afterwards, Lahiri returned to Benares, continuing to lead a householder life. The height of Kriya yoga, as a spiritual movement among Bengali householders, was in the last part of the nineteenth century and first half of the twentieth century.
5. Yogananda was born on 5 January 1893.
6. Bishwanath Ghosh, 'Introduction', *Collection of Bishnu Charan Ghosh Poems* (Calcutta: A. K. Publishers, 1998), 246.
7. Bishnu Charan Ghosh, 'From the Past', *Bayam Charcha* (November 1965).
8. Sananda Lal Ghosh, *Mejda: The Family and Early Life of Paramahansa Yogananda* (LA: SRF, 1980, second printing, 1992), 249.
9. Sneha Jain, handwriting analyst, Bangalore, India. Available at https://graphologyjunction. wordpress. com/2017/04/17/signature-analysis-of-the-forgotten-yogi-buddha-bose/ Accessed: April 2017.
10. Paramahansa Yogananda, *Autobiography of a Yogi* (LA: SRF, 1946), Chapter 2.
11. 'Comment Abroad', *Inner Culture* (March 1937), 64.
12. Paramahansa Yogananda, *Autobiography of a Yogi* (LA: SRF, 1946), Chapter 2.
13. Swami Satyananda Giri, *A Collection of Biographies of 4 Kriya Yoga Gurus* (London: Yoga Niketan, 2009), 151.
14. Ibid.
15. Ibid.
16. Mahendranath Gupta (Sri M) was a householder, highly advanced in meditation, and a disciple of Sri Ramakrishna. Later, he would be the author of *The Gospel of Sri Ramakrishna* (Mahendranath Gupta, 1902), under the pen name of Sri M, and written from a narrative perspective, of his encounters with Ramakrishna.
17. Ghosh, *Mejda*, 137–40.
18. Ibid.
19. Anthony Copley, *A Spiritual Bloomsbury* (Oxford: Lexington Books, 2006), 199.
20. Paramahansa Yogananda, *Autobiography of a Yogi* (LA: SRF, 1946), Chapter 2.
21. Ghosh, *Mejda*, 159.

Chapter 9

1. Haradhan Chakraborty, 'Bayam – Tapas Bishnucharan', *Bayam Charcha* (August 1970).
2. Bishnu Charan Ghosh, 'From the Past', *Bayam Charcha* (November 1965).

3. Bishnu Charan Ghosh, 'Shadh', *Collection of Poems* (Calcutta: A. K. Publishers, 1998), 246.
4. Sananda Lal Ghosh, *Mejda: The Family and Early Life of Paramahansa Yogananda* (Los Angeles: SRF, 1980, second printing, 1992), 249.

Chapter 10

1. Greer Park is now named Ladies Park. The Calcutta Deaf and Dumb School, where Satyananda lived, is still across the street on Garpar Road. Inside is a portrait of his father, and the school is run much the same way, over one hundred years later.
2. This story is a bit of a legend, and so there are variations of its telling. Swami Satyananda Giri, *A Collection of Biographies of 4 Kriya Yoga Gurus* (Yoga Niketan, 2009), 147.
3. Sananda Lal Ghosh, *Mejda: The Family and Early Life of Paramahansa Yogananda* (SRF, 1980, second printing, 1992), 94.
4. Ibid., 95.
5. Swami Satyananda Giri, *Biography of a Yogi, Hangsa Swami Kebalananda Maharaj* (The Sanskrit Classics, 3rd edition, Volume 1, 2016), 616.
6. Ghosh, *Mejda*, 148–9.
7. Swami Satyananda Giri, *Biography of a Yogi, Hangsa Swami Kebalananda Maharaj* (The Sanskrit Classics, 3rd edition, Volume 1, 2016), 616.
8. Paramahansa Yogananda, *Autobiography of a Yogi* (LA: SRF, 1946), Chapter 4.
9. Ibid.
10. Ibid.
11. Ibid.
12. Giri, *Biography of a Yogi*, 616.
13. Yogananda. *Autobiography of a Yogi*, Chapter 4.
14. Ghosh, Mejda, 148–9.
15. Ibid., 13–16.
16. Giri, *Biography of a Yogi*, 617.
17. Devi Mukherjee, *Shaped by Saints* (Crystal Clarity, 2000), Chapter 5.
18. 'Hari Krishna Ghosh, Reminisces, Part 2', *Ananda Sangha Worldwide* (14 May 2015). Available at https://www.youtube.com/watch?v=8FVfTnCp9go Accessed June 2017.
19. Ghosh, *Mejda*, 148.
20. Pulin Bihari Das was also instrumental at Ranchi, where, as Swami Shivananda, he 'was in charge of the huge fruitland and garden' at the school. He and Yogananda spent much time together. Giri, *A Collection of Biographies*, 241.
21. Bishnu Ghosh, 'From the Past', *Bayam Charcha* (August 1967).
22. Ghosh, *Mejda*, 105.

Chapter 11

1. Paramahansa Yogananda, *Autobiography of a Yogi* (LA: SRF, 1946).
2. Sananda Lal Ghosh, *Mejda: The Family and Early Life of Paramahansa Yogananda* (SRF, 1980, second printing, 1992), 148–9.
3. Interview with Hassi Mukherjee. Calcutta, India. May 2015.
4. Devi Mukherjee, *Shaped by Saints* (Crystal Clarity, 2000), 54.
5. Interview with Hassi Mukherjee. Calcutta, India. May 2015.

Chapter 12

1. Paramahansa Yogananda. *Autobiography of a Yogi*, (LA: SRF, 1946), Chapter 1.
2. Swami Satyananda Giri, *A Collection of Biographies of 4 Kriya Yoga Gurus* (Yoga Niketan, 2009), 216.
3. Giri, *A Collection of Biographies*, 214.
4. Sriyukteswar Giri, *Kaivalya Darsanam The Holy Science* (LA: SRF, 1977), Introduction, vi.
5. Satyeswarananda Giri, *Biography of Yogananda Volume 2* (The Sanskrit Classics, 2016) Chapter 10, 115.
6. Sananda Lal Ghosh, *Mejda: The Family and Early Life of Paramahansa Yogananda* (LA: SRF, 1980, second printing, 1992), 186.
7. National Archives and Records Administration, Washington, DC Board of Special Inquiry Transcript of Swami Yogananda case, 26 October 1936. File 55865/886, RG 85. KS-34, 6.
8. *East-West Magazine* (October 1942), 29–31.
9. Giri, *A Collection of Biographies*, 229.
10. Sailendra Bijoy Dasgupta, *Paramhansa Swami Yogananda: Life-Portrait and Reminiscences* (Yoga Niketan, 2006), 73.
11. Giri, *A Collection of Biographies*, 228–9.
12. Bishnu Charan Ghosh, 'From The Past', *Bayam Charcha* (December 1966).
13. Giri, *A Collection of Biographies*, 230.
14. Ghosh, 'From The Past'.
15. Ibid.

Chapter 13

1. *East-West Magazine* (January 1933), 5.
2. Swami Satyananda Giri, *A Collection of Biographies of 4 Kriya Yoga Gurus* (Yoga Niketan, 2009), 265, 235.
3. 3. Ibid., 234.
4. Bishnu Charan Ghosh, 'From The Past', *Bayam Charcha* (December 1966).
5. Ibid.
6. Paramahansa Yogananda, *Autobiography of a Yogi* (LA: SRF, 1946), Chapter 27.
7. *East-West Magazine* (May–June 1938), 26.
8. Sananda Lal Ghosh, *Mejda: The Family and Early Life of Paramahansa Yogananda* (LA: SRF, 1980, second printing, 1992), 249.
9. Ghosh, 'From The Past'.

Chapter 14

1. Paramahansa Yogananda, *Autobiography of a Yogi* (LA: SRF, 1946), Chapter 37.
2. Swami Satyeswarananda Giri, *Biography of Yogi-Yogananda*, Volume 2 (Sanskrit Classics, 2016), 167.
3. British Library. India Office Library Records. IOR: L/PJ/12/358. Application for Passport Facilities. Passport # 3599, Swami Yogananda.
4. Philip Deslippe, 'Rishis and Rebels: The Punjabi Sikh Presence in Early American Yoga', *Journal of Sikh & Punjab Studies* (2016), 94.
5. Salindra Bijoy Dasgupta, *Paramhansa Swami Yogananda* (Yoga Niketan, 2011), 47.

6. In his later writings in the United States for the SRF magazine, Yogananda occasionally featured both Whitman and Emerson's writings in his magazine articles. Once, in a story often retold in Calcutta, Vivekananda questioned his professors about how such a person as Walt Whitman might exist in the world. The Scottish professor referred Vivekananda to Ramakrishna, who lived at the ashram in Dakshineswar, for a living version of such a man.

7. Sananda Lal Ghosh, *Mejda: The Family and Early Life of Paramahansa Yogananda* (Los Angeles: SRF, 1980, second printing, 1992), 160.

8. Giri, *Biography of Yogi-Yogananda*, 167.

9. Ibid., 168.

10. *Inner Culture*, (February 1939), 40.

11. Swami Yogananda, 'Increasing Awareness', *Inner Culture* (October 1935).

12. Paramahansa Yogananda, *Autobiography of a Yogi* (Los Angeles: SRF, 1946), Chapter 47.

13. *Self Realization Fellowship* (July–September 1965), 19–20.

Chapter 15

1. As part of the 'Holy Trinity' of Calcutta – Ramakrishna, Sarada Devi and Vivekananda. Another Calcutta 'trinity' has Vivekananda as well. That of Rabindranath Tagore, Subhas Chandra Bose and Vivekananda – the poet, the politician and the saint.

2. Kaushik Ghosh and Tamaghna Banerjee, 'Guru to Jobs, Succour for Siblings', *The Telegraph* (19 June 2015), 1.

3. Tamaghna Banerjee, 'Cop Course in Guru's Lessons', *The Telegraph* (19 June 2015).

Chapter 16

1. Captain P.K. Gupta, *My System of Physical Culture* (Calcutta, 1927), 118–20.

2. The traditional distinction between *bayam* and gymnastics, as opposed to yoga asanas, is between exercises that are dynamic and those that are static (held yoga asanas). This historical differentiation becomes blurry once looked through the perspective of today's modern yoga asana practice, which blends static and dynamic postures in practice, stillness and movement.

3. *Dand* and the *baithak* are two traditional wrestling exercises, akin to jackknife push-ups and deep knee bends, and are often done as pairs. The smaller wooden club looks similar to a bowling pin. They work the shoulders down to the grip, using the full range of motion for complete shoulder strength and flexibility.

4. 'Chotda' and 'Mejda' are the brotherly names Bishnu [Bistu] uses for Sananda and Yogananda. Bishnu Charan Ghosh, 'From the Past', *Bayam Charcha* (Jan. 1966).

5. Joseph Alter, *Yoga in Modern India: The Body Between Science and Philosophy* (Princeton, 1992), 103.

6. Ibid.

7. Goutam Basu, 'Self Assertion through Physical Culture Movement in Bengal during the later part of the 19th Century and early 20th Century', Proceeding of the International Conference on Social Science Research, 4–5 June 2013, Penang, Malaysia.

8. Ghosh, 'From the Past'.

9. Ibid.

Chapter 17

1. Thant Myint-U, *Burma and the New Crossroads of Asia: Where China meets India* (Farrar, Straus and Giroux: New York, 2011), 250–3.

2. *Nauli* is one of the cleansing techniques described in classical yoga texts and is used for purification of the body.

3. Bishnu Charan Ghosh, 'From the Past', *Bayam Charcha* (July 1969).

4. Bishnu Ghosh, *Muscle Control* (Calcutta, 1930), 52.

5. 'The six cleansing techniques bring about purification and asanas bring about strength; mudras bring about steadiness and *pratyahara* brings about calmness. From pranayama, lightness arises and from *dhyana*, realization of the self. Through *samadhi* arises abstraction and liberation itself; in this there is no doubt. *Dhauti, Basti, Neti, Nauli, Trataka,* and *Kapalabhati*; one should practise these six cleansing techniques.' James Mallinson (trans.), *Gheranda Samhita* (Yogavidya.com, 2004), 3–4.

6. Mallinson, *Gheranda Samhita*, 4.

7. Shailendra Sharma (trans.), *Hatha Yoga Pradipika* (2013), 79–80.

8. Bishnu Charan Ghosh, 'From the Past', *Bayam Charcha* (Dec. 1965).

9. Rajen Guha Thakurta was born in January 1884 at his grandparents' home within Barisal district. Rajen lived through a turbulent early life, with his parents dying when he was two and a half years old, sickly with a 'weak liver'; he 'nearly died due to pneumonia'. Rajen regained his strength, began riding horses at the age of six, then started *bayam,* gymnastics and wrestling at the age of ten, under Surjokanto Guha Thakurta. Anil Chandra Ghosh, *Byame Bangali* (8th edition changed and extended. First edition, 1928), 35–42.

10. Bishnu Charan Ghosh, 'From the Past', *Bayam Charcha* (Jan. 1966).

11. Swami Satyananda Giri, *A Collection of Biographies of 4 Kriya Yoga Gurus* (Yoga Niketan. 2009), 239.

12. Bishnu Charan Ghosh, 'From the Past', *Bayam Charcha* (Feb. 1967).

13. 'Today I am 65 years old, weigh 195 pounds, chest is 47 inches, height 5 feet and 4 inches. I am the best example of the benefits of *bayam* and the best incentive for everyone to do *bayam*. That is why I do not think anyone should lament about bad health and get discouraged – take heart from my experience and result.' Bishnu Charan Ghosh, 'From the Past', *Bayam Charcha* (Jan. 1966; Feb. 1967).

14. Bishnu Ghosh, *Muscle Control* (Calcutta, 1930), 52.

15. Ibid.

16. Bishnu Charan Ghosh, 'From the Past', *Bayam Charcha* (June 1966).

17. Bishnu Charan Ghosh, 'From the Past', *Bayam Charcha* (Feb. 1966).

18. The troupe, the circus and their methods of training were all things that Bishnu would replicate with his own students in the decades to come, not just in Bengal but throughout India, and much later, in Japan.

19. N.R. Ray (ed.), *Dictionary of National Biography*, Volume II (Calcutta: Institute of Historical Studies, 1990), 54–5.

20. Bishnu Charan Ghosh, 'From the Past', *Bayam Charcha* (July 1967).

21. There is no other family indication of her health being the reason why Emily left; this may have been a more sanitized explanation rather than a public separation from Rajah. Bishnu Charan Ghosh, 'From the Past', *Bayam Charcha* (July 1967).

22. Ibid.

23. Buddha Bose, *Key to the Kingdom of Health Through Yoga Volume 1* (Calcutta: The Statesman Press, 1939), 6.

24. Bishnu Charan Ghosh, 'From the Past', *Bayam Charcha* (July 1967).

25. Ibid.

26. Ibid.

27. Ibid.

28. Interview with Mataji. Mussoorie, India, June 2017.

29. Ray, *Dictionary of National Biography*, 54–5.

Chapter 18

1. Bishnu Charan Ghosh, 'From the Past', *Bayam Charcha* (April 1967).

2. 1931 letter from Buddha Bose to Dennis Bose.

3. 'The Spirit of Japan', a lecture by Sir Rabindranath Tagore. Delivered for the students of the private colleges of Tokyo and the members of the Indo-Japanese Association, at the Keio Gijuku University, 2 July 1916. Available at http://www.online-literature.com/tagore-rabindranath/4393/

4. Pratyay Banerjee, 'Tagore and the Introduction of Judo in Santiniketan', in Pratyay Banerjee (ed.), *Tagore and Japan: Dialogue, Exchange and Encounter* (Synergy Books: India, 2016), Chapter 5.

5. Bishnu Charan Ghosh, 'From the Past', *Bayam Charcha* (Dec. 1967).

6. Bishnu Charan Ghosh, 'From the Past', *Bayam Charcha* (March 1967).

7. *Calcutta Municipal Gazette* (30 March 1935), 85–9.

8. Bishnu Charan Ghosh, 'From the Past', *Bayam Charcha* (July 1967).

9. Bishnu Ghosh, *Muscle Control* (Calcutta, 1930), 126.

10. Bishnu Charan Ghosh, 'From the Past', *Bayam Charcha* (July 1967).

11. Ibid.

12. 'Second Time in Japan', *Bayam Charcha* (July 1969).

13. Bishnu Charan Ghosh, 'From the Past', *Bayam Charcha* (July 1967).

Chapter 19

1. Bishnu Charan Ghosh, 'From the Past', *Bayam Charcha* (August 1967).

2. Bishnu Charan Ghosh, 'From the Past', *Bayam Charcha* (May 1966).

3. Interview with Mataji. Mussoorie, India. June 2017.

4. Email conversation with Peter Hopkins. December 2017.

5. Interview with Susan Barrett (Bose), by email, 2016.

6. Asoke Sarkar, *Magic* (January 1950), 32–4.

7. Asoke Sarkar, 'Hindustan Park', *Magic* (January 1950), 34.

8. Buddha was introduced to yoga asanas at the very same place, Sradhananda Park, in 1932.

Chapter 20

1. Bishnu Ghosh, *Muscle Control* (Calcutta, 1930), 139.

2. Ibid.

3. Buddha Bose, *Key to the Kingdom of Health through Yoga* (Calcutta: The Statesman Press, 1939), 6.

4. Sananda Lal Ghosh, *Mejda: The Family and Early Life of Paramahansa Yogananda* (LA: SRF, 1980, second printing, 1992), 173.

5. Bishnu Charan Ghosh, 'From the Past', *Bayam Charcha* (July 1967).

6. In one instance of Bishnu's self-described *Mahabharata* of motorbike experiences, he raced his BMW bike so fast past the police commissioner that the next day, he was called to the police office and told not to drive so fast. Bishnu replied, 'God always looks after me and saves me.' The commissioner responded, 'God may be absent minded one day.' Bishnu Charan Ghosh, 'From the Past', *Bayam Charcha* (April 1966).

7. Bishnu Charan Ghosh, 'From the Past', *Bayam Charcha* (May 1966).

8. Bishnu Charan Ghosh, 'From the Past', *Bayam Charcha* (August 1966).

9. Bishnu Charan Ghosh, 'From the Past', *Bayam Charcha* (May 1966).

10. Bishnu Charan Ghosh, 'From the Past', *Bayam Charcha* (April 1966).

11. Bishnu Charan Ghosh, 'From the Past', *Bayam Charcha* (May 1966).

Chapter 21

1. Maxick, *Muscle Control* (1911; Modern Reprint Edition, 1992), 20.

2. Bishnu Ghosh, *Muscle Control* (Calcutta, 1930), 56.

3. The Bengali word *bayam* or *byam* means to exercise, with a dynamic effort, as in a physical drill such as calisthenics or free-hand exercises (as often called in Calcutta). Elsewhere in India, the transliteration of the Sanskrit word is *vyayama* and its variants.

4. Amitava Chaterjee, 'From Courtyard Sport to Competitive Sport: Evolution of Wrestling in Colonial Bengal', *Sport in Society* 18, no. 1 (2015), 4. Available at http://hdl.handle.net/10603/163702

5. Ibid., 154.

6. Ibid., 25, 27, 29.

7. Ibid., 23.

8. Rashed Uz Zaman, 'Bengal Terrorism and the Struggle for National Liberation', in Jussi M. Hanhimäki & Bernhard Blumenau (ed.), *An International History of Terrorism: Western and Non-Western Experiences* (NY: Routledge, 2013), 156.

9. Kief Hillsbery, *Empire Made: My Search for an Outlaw who Vanished in British India* (2016), Chapter 28.

10. This has been the topic of recent modern yoga research. Broadly, Mark Singleton, in *Yoga Body* (2010), noted how Bishnu's book *Muscle Control* (1930) was dedicated to the movement of Young Bengal, linking it to nationalism. Singleton then drew links within the Ghosh family, between the 'fusion' of 'the new, popular Hatha yoga' and 'asanas, physical culture, and muscle manipulation techniques'. More specific to Calcutta, Claudia Guggenbühl's *Yoga in Calcutta* (2003), and a 2008 presentation entitled 'Yoga between Bodybuilding and Enlightenment', attempted to uncover how yoga asana popularization had come out of the gymnasium movement in Calcutta.

Chapter 22

1. Amitava Chaterjee, 'From Courtyard Sport to Competitive Sport: Evolution of Wrestling in Colonial Bengal', *Sport in Society* 18, no. 1 (2015), 5.

2. Amitava Chatterjee, *Evolution of Sporting Culture in Colonial Bengal* (University of Calcutta, 2014), 24.

3. Ronojoy Sen, *Nation at Play: A History of Sport in India* (Columbia, 2015), 95.

4. Chaterjee, 'From Courtyard Sport to Competitive Sport', 5.

5. Chatterjee, *Evolution of Sporting Culture in Colonial Bengal*, 154.

6. 'As Jyotirindranath Tagore wrote in his autobiography.' Haradhan Chakraborty, 'Circus', *Bayam Charcha* (Oct. 1969).

7. 'Ancient *Bayam* Experts among Bengalis', *Bayam Charcha* (Oct. 1969).

8. From 1899 to 1912, the Great Bengal Circus, during the mild winter months of Calcutta, set up its tent at the Maidan for the popular shows. 'Ancient *Bayam* Experts among Bengalis', *Bayam Charcha* (Oct. 1966).

9. Amitava Chatterjee, *Evolution of Sporting Culture in Colonial Bengal* (University of Calcutta, 2014), 293.

10. 'The Hippodrome of performing wild animals included African Lions, Tiger, Leopards, Elephants, Hill Bear, Horses, Dogs, Monkeys, etc. etc.' Amitava Chatterjee, *Evolution of Sporting Culture in Colonial Bengal* (University of Calcutta, 2014), 154.

11. Ibid., 299.

12. Ronojoy Sen, *Nation at Play: A History of Sport in India* (Columbia, 2015), 96.

13. Named the *bhadralok*, the reference applied outside the societal status based on the caste system, a sort of 'Westernized caste elite' within Calcutta. Both the Bose and the Ghosh families represented the societal transition of Bengali middle-class families, raising children in a privileged modern education system. The elite were chooled in Christian places, with a modern meld of reason and faith, living amidst Hindu devotion and therefore integrating the intuitive and irrational within their puja rituals. Joya Chatterji, *Bengal Divided* (Cambridge, 1994), 3–13.

14. Sukanta Chaudhuri, *The Living City, Volume I: The Past* (Calcutta: Oxford University Press, 1990), 38–41.

Chapter 23

1. Peter Heehs, 'Revolutionary Terrorism in British Bengal', in Elleke Boehmer and Stephen Morton (ed.), *Terror and the Postcolonial*, (Wiley, 2015), 157–9.

2. David Gordon White, *Yoga in Practice* (Princeton, 2005), 20.

3. Ronojoy Sen, *Nation at Play: A History of Sport in India* (Columbia, 2015), 97.

4. Ibid.

5. Subhas Chandra Bose, like Vivekananda and Yogananda, attended north Calcutta's Scottish Church College, and is said to have been a friend of the Ghosh family and the uncle of Buddha Bose.

6. Interview with Swapan Das. Calcutta, India. May 2015.

7. Bishnu Charan Ghosh, 'From the Past', *Bayam Charcha* (Dec., 1967).

8. Ibid.

9. 'The cult of Indian manliness that the physical culture movement represented was the

answer to the racism of the white ruling class. The colonial stereotype of the "effeminate" Bengali *babu*, for example, was challenged by the protagonists of physical culture.' Amitava Chatterjee, *Evolution of Sporting Culture in Colonial Bengal* (University of Calcutta, 2014), 329.

10. Bishnu Charan Ghosh, 'From the Past', *Bayam Charcha* (Sept. 1966).

11. Abhijit Gupta, 'Cultures of the Body In Colonial Bengal', in Alexis Tadié, J.A. Mangan and Supriya Chaudhuri (eds), *Sport, Literature, Society: Cultural Historical Studies*, Chapter 4.

12. Ronojoy Sen, *Nation at Play: A History of Sport in India* (Columbia, 2015), 181.

13. Interview with Gautam Basu. City College, Calcutta. July 2016.

14. Bishnu Charan Ghosh, 'From the Past', *Bayam Charcha* (Dec. 1967).

15. Yogananda praised socialism through his magazine at times and was a globalist from a humanitarian perspective. He interacted with politicians from a strictly utilitarian perspective, attempting to guide them towards his ideal of peace on an individual and global scale. That said, he was cognizant of the value of a celebrity or politician and never shied from having a photograph of him standing beside one for publicity.

16. Amitava Chatterjee, *Evolution of Sporting Culture in Colonial Bengal* (University of Calcutta, 2014), 329.

Chapter 24

1. Claudia Guggenbühl, *Yoga in Calcutta* (2003). Interview with Sukumar Bose, 11 October 2004, in Sarani Lodge, Hindustan Park, Calcutta.

2. Guggenbühl, *Yoga in Calcutta*, 201.

3. Dasgupta also knew and practised the asanas as a youth, which astonished his family, as they 'failed to understand also how he could show the different yogic postures, without being initiated into them'. Claudia Guggenbühl, *Mircea Eliade and Surendranath Dasgupta* (Zürich, 2008), 14.

4. Captain P.K. Gupta, *My System of Physical Culture*, (Calcutta, 1927).

5. P.K. Gupta leaves the topic with an example of such habits, which reflected the sort of 'irregular habits' of yogis. 'Sometimes for the purpose of undergoing a long period of meditation at a place where there is no habitation for nearly a hundred miles around, they have to sit starving for 6 months. For this purpose they have to practise *"Kumbhaka Yoga"* or hibernation, as the frogs or snakes do during winter.' Gupta, *My System of Physical Culture*, 164–5.

6. Bancroft Library, Theos Bernard papers, Carton 7:35; 1926–29.

7. Swapan Das, 'World Yoga Day', Calcutta, 21 June 2016.

8. Bishnu Ghosh, *Muscle Control* (Calcutta, 1930), 138–9.

9. Guggenbühl, *Yoga In Calcutta* (2003), 201.

10. Ibid.

11. Ibid., 202.

12. Claudia Guggenbühl, email conversation, 2014.

13. Claudia Guggenbühl, 'Yoga between Bodybuilding and Enlightenment', lecture held on 29 February 2008, 5.

Chapter 25

1. Bishnu Ghosh, *Muscle Control* (Calcutta, 1930), 139.
2. Buddha Bose, 'Homage', *Bayam Charcha* (August 1970).
3. Ibid.
4. Ibid.
5. Interview of Rooma Bose. Yoga Cure Institute, New Alipore. 11 March 11 2015.
6. Bishnu's formal lessons of Hatha yoga and Kriya yoga were from 1916 to 1919 in Yogananda's school. At Buddha's request, Bishnu revived the focus on Hatha yoga, which he had learned at Dihika and Ranchi about fifteen years earlier (Chapter 13).
7. Bose, 'Homage'.
8. Buddha Bose, *Key to the Kingdom of Health through Yoga* (Calcutta: The Statesman Press, 1939), 6.
9. Bose, 'Homage'.

Chapter 26

1. Anil Chandra Ghosh, *Byame Bangali* (8th edition changed and extended. First edition, 1928).
2. Bishnu Charan Ghosh, 'From the Past', *Bayam Charcha* (Dec. 1967).
3. Bishnu Charan Ghosh, 'From the Past', *Bayam Charcha* (May 1966).
4. Chitralekha Shalom, *Moral Courage*. Available at https://www.facebook.com/pg/Moral-courage-275762489106112/about/
5. Ibid.
6. Ghosh, *Byame Bangali*.
7. Bishnu also mentions: 'We plan to go to America in February [1934] where he will swim for 100 hours in a swimming bath and stun the world.' This voyage never happened, but it does show Bishnu's desire to travel to America. Bishnu Charan Ghosh, *Ramdhenu Magazine* (October 1933).
8. The *Calcutta Municipal Gazette* (30 March 1935), 86.
9. Buddha Bose, *Key to the Kingdom of Health through Yoga*, Vol. 1 (Calcutta: The Statesman Press, 1939), 6.
10. The *Calcutta Municipal Gazette*, March 30, 1935, 85-89.
11. Ibid.
12. Ibid.
13. *Key To The Kingdom of Health Through Yoga*, 1.
14. Mark Singleton, *Yoga Body* (Oxford, 2010), 122.
15. 'As historian Sumit Sarkar pointed out, it was "natural for young Bengalis to seek psychological compensation in a cult of physical strength" against a backdrop of an imperialist force.' Ronojoy Sen, *Nation at Play: A History of Sport in India* (Columbia, 2015), 96.
16. Buddha Bose, *Yoga Asanas* (Calcutta, 1938), vii.
17. Bishnu Ghosh, *Muscle Control* (Calcutta, 1930).

Chapter 27

1. *Calcutta Municipal Gazette* (30 March 1935), 85-9.
2. Sailendra Bijoy Dasgupta, *Paramahansa Swami Yogananda* (Yoga Niketan, 2006), 79.

3. Swami Yogananda, *Descriptive Outline of Yogoda* (11th edition, 1930), 16.

4. Swami Satyeswarananda Giri, *Biography of Yogananda*, Vol. 2 (The Sanskrit Classics, 2016), 612.

5. Paramahansa Yogananda, *Autobiography of a Yogi* (LA: SRF, 1946), Chapter 27.

6. Joseph S. Alter, *Moral Materialism: Sex and Masculinity in Modern India* (Princeton, 2011), 173–4.

7. 'It would be reasonable to assume that in Yogananda's time his Energization Exercises [Yogoda] might not have seemed any more or less like "yoga poses" than some of the positions and movements to which that title is accorded today without a second thought.' Anya P. Foxen, *Biography of a Yogi* (Oxford, 2017), 129.

8. Sananda Lal Ghosh, *Mejda: The Family and Early Life of Paramahansa Yogananda* (LA: SRF, 1980, second printing, 1992), 91–2.

9. Swami Satyananda Giri, *A Collection of Biographies of 4 Kriya Yoga Gurus* (Yoga Niketan, 2009), 244.

10. J.P. Muller, *My System* (NY: GE Stechert & Co., 1905, first English edition).

11. Swami Satyeswarananda Giri, *Biography of Yogananda*, Vol. 2 (The Sanskrit Classics, 2016), 144.

12. Swami Yogananda, *Yogoda: Tissue-Will System of Physical Perfection* (Boston: Everett Printing Service, 1925), 7.

13. Maxick, *Muscle Control* (1911; Modern Reprint Edition, 1992), 20.

14. Durga Ma, *A Trilogy of Love* (1993), Part 3.

15. Eileen Wood Jasnowski, 'Secrets of Yoga From Detroit's Mr. Black and India's Yogananda',

16. *Detroit Free Press* (10 July 1966). Reprinted: *Self-Realization Magazine* (January 1967), 16–20.

17. Despite this, over the years Kriya yoga was often promoted as a 'spiritual accelerator that hastens the practitioner to the goal of all Yoga: conscious realization of the soul's oneness with God.' Rev. MW Lewis, 'Yoga – Its Meaning and Aim', *Self-Realization Magazine* (July 1954), 48.

18. Jasnowski, 'Secrets of Yoga'.

Chapter 28

1. Paramahansa Yogananda, *Autobiography of a Yogi* (LA: SRF, 1946), Chapter 27.

2. Ibid., Chapter 40.

3. Swami Satyananda Giri, *A Collection of Biographies of 4 Kriya Yoga Gurus* (Yoga Niketan. 2009), 272.

Chapter 29

1. Swami Premananda, 'Swami Yogananda in Calcutta, My Gurudev: Swami Yogananda Paramahansa', *The Mystic Cross* (Dedication Issue, Self-Revelation Church of Absolute Monism, 1998), 4–11.

2. From the preface by Grant Duff Douglas Ainslie, a British Member of the Royal Asiatic Society. The book may have shared its title with a Max Mueller publication, of a series of four lectures, given in 1870, published in 1893, titled an *Introduction to the Science of Religion*. The SRF organization would later print *Science of Religion* by Sriyukteswar in 1977.

3. Swami Satyeswarananda Giri, *Biography of Yogi-Yogananda*, Vol. 2 (The Sanskrit Classics, 2016), 167.

4.   Paramahansa Yogananda, *Autobiography of a Yogi* (LA: SRF, 1946), Chapter 37.

5.   British Library. India Office Library Records. IOR: L/PJ/12/358/3. May 15, 1925.

6.   Satyananda, the other of the 'trio of friends', stayed in Ranchi, India, where he kept the boys school open and in operation. 'Satsanga' means 'fellowship with truth'.

7.   British Library. India Office Library Records. IOR: L/PJ/12/358/4. Press Report. Boston 'American' of January 10, 1924.

8.   British Library. India Office Library Records. IOR: L/PJ/12/358/3. May 15, 1925.

9.   British Library. India Office Library Records. IOR: L/PJ/12/358/7. Press Report. Boston 'American' of January 10, 1924.

10. British Library. India Office Library Records. IOR: L/PJ/12/358. Feb. 28, 1928

11. The remarks were of a portrait done by Louise Crow, a notable Native American artist. *East-West World Wide* (July–August, 1926, 12).

12. The Yogoda Satsanga symbol of the lotus flower used a quotation from Luke 11:34–35 to describe its meaning. 'The lamp of your body is your eye. When your eye is single, your whole body also is full of light ... if therefore your whole body is full of light, having no dark past, it shall be wholly full of light, as when the lamp with its bright shining gives you light.' 'Luke', *Bibliotheca* V (2016), 151. *East-West* (May 1932), 29.

13. 'To present the truth offerings of East and West.' Paramhansa Yogananda, *Autobiography of a Yogi* (LA: SRF, 1946), Chapter 38.

14. *East-West World Wide* (May 1932), 29.

15. *East-West World Wide* (July–August 1926), 12.

16. Ibid.

17. Ibid.

18. Ibid.

19. 'The Mystery of Mahatma Gandhi', *East-West* IV, no. 9 (July 1932).

20. British Library. India Office Library Records. IOR: L/PJ/12/358.

21. 'Sage Sees Coolidge', *Washington Herald* (25 January 1927). Reprinted: 'An Interview with President Coolidge', *Self-Realization Magazine* (April 1969), 31–2.

22. British Library. India Office Library Records. IOR: L/PJ/12/358. *Hindustan Times* (27 January 1927).

23. British Library. India Office Library Records. IOR: L/PJ/12/358. January 1927.

24. 'Sage Sees Coolidge', *Washington Herald*.

25. Ibid.

26. Ibid.

27. Sumita Mukherjee, 'The Emergence of a British Hindu Identity between 1936 and 1937', in Lucy Delap and Sue Morgan (eds), *Men, Masculinities and Religious Change in Twentieth-Century Britain* (Palgrave-Macmillan, 2013), 161.

28. British Library. India Office Library Records. IOR: L/PJ/12/358. Extract from the *Hindustan Times* (27 January 1927).

29. 'Sage Sees Coolidge', *Washington Herald*.

30. British Library. India Office Library Records. IOR: L/PJ/12/358/27-28. British Vice Consulate. March 1, 1928.

31. Ibid.

32. *East-West World Wide* (January–February 1928), 3–8.

33. *East-West World Wide* (November–December 1929).

34. Ibid.

35. British Library. IO: L/PJ/6/1959. 1928-1930, P & J.

36. British Library. IO: L/PJ/6/1959. 1928-1930, P & J. October 15, 1929.

37. US Dept of Labor, Bureau of Immigration, 55-685-886. EC-23.

Chapter 30

1. 'Swami Yogananda in Ranchi: Plans for Self-Realization Temple in Calcutta', *Amrita Bazar Patrika* (14 Sept. 1935), 13.

2. Rajarsi Janakananda, *A Great Western Yogi* (LA: SRF, 1996), 73–4.

3. *Amrita Bazar Patrika* (30 August 1935), 6.

4. Sailendra Bijoy Dasgupta, *Paramahansa Swami Yogananda* (Yoga Niketan, 2006), 87–8.

5. Paramahansa Yogananda, *Autobiography of a Yogi* (Los Angeles: SRF, 1946), Chapter 40.

6. Sailendra Bijoy Dasgupta, *Paramahansa Swami Yogananda* (Yoga Niketan, 2006), 87–8.

7. Sananda Lal Ghosh, *Mejda: The Family and Early Life of Paramahansa Yogananda* (LA: SRF, 1980, second printing, 1992), 206.

8. Sailendra Bijoy Dasgupta, *Paramahansa Swami Yogananda* (Yoga Niketan, 2006), 87–8.

9. Bishnu Charan Ghosh, 'From the Past', *Bayam Charcha* (Jan. 1966).

10. Rajarsi Janakananda, *A Great Western Yogi* (LA: SRF, 1996) 75.

11. Sailendra Bijoy Dasgupta, *Paramahansa Swami Yogananda* (Yoga Niketan, 2006), 91.

12. 'Swami Yogananda in Ranchi: Plans for Self-Realization Temple in Calcutta', *Amrita Bazar Patrika* (14 Sept. 1935), 13.

13. 'Reception to Yogananda', *Amrita Bazar Patrika* (8 Sept 1935), 6.

14. Sailendra Bijoy Dasgupta, *Paramahansa Swami Yogananda* (Yoga Niketan, 2006), 80.

15. American 'beat' poets Allen Ginsberg and Peter Orlovsky (Gary Snyder with Joanne Kyger also visited) stayed for some weeks in Calcutta, hanging out at the Coffee House in 1962, meeting Sunil Gangopadhyay and others. Deborah Baker, *A Blue Hand: The Beats in India* (Penguin: New York, 2008), 146–65.

16. Paramahansa Yogananda, *Autobiography of a Yogi* (LA: SRF, 1946), Chapter 42.

17. Sailendra Bijoy Dasgupta, *Paramahansa Swami Yogananda* (Yoga Niketan, 2006), 80.

18. Paramahansa Yogananda, *Autobiography of a Yogi* (LA: SRF, 1946), Chapter 42.

19. Ibid.

20. Hari Krishna Ghosh (son of Sananda), *Reminisces on His Life with the Great Master* (Ananda Sangha Worldwide, published on 3 May 2014). Available at https://www.youtube.com/watch?v=v5SbTpfJfDA

21. Sailendra Bijoy Dasgupta, *Paramahansa Swami Yogananda* (Yoga Niketan, 2006), 80.

22. Yogananda, *Autobiography of a Yogi*, Chapter 42.

23. Dasgupta, *Paramahansa Swami Yogananda*, 80–1.

24. 'Reception to Yogananda', *Amrita Bazar Patrika* (8 Sept. 1935), 6.

25. Ibid.

26. *Amrita Bazar Patrika* (15 December 1935), 7.

Chapter 31

1. Bishnu Charan Ghosh, *Muscle Control* (Calcutta, 1930), 56.
2. British Library. India Office Library Records. IOR: L/PJ/12/358/4. Press Report. Boston 'American' of 10 January 1924.
3. 'Muscle Coordination – Remedy for All Ills', *The Mercury* (19 Feb. 1924), 8.
4. Sananda Lal Ghosh, *Mejda* (LA: Self Realization Fellowship, 1992), 250.
5. Sailendra Bijoy Dasgupta, *Paramahansa Swami Yogananda* (Yoga Niketan, 2006), 91.
6. Ghosh, *Mejda*, 222–3.
7. Dasgupta, *Paramahansa Swami Yogananda*, 91.
8. 'Frowned' may be understating it a bit. Bijoy Dasgupta states that after Sriyukteswar listened to everything that had happened, he 'remained quiet for a while and then commented about Bishnu. '[Yogananda] has a disease – where a ghoul comes and sits on his back.' Dasgupta, *Paramahansa Swami Yogananda*, 92.
9. British Library. India Office Library Records. IOR: L/PJ/12/358/4. Press Report. Boston 'American' of 10 January 1924.
10. Dasgupta, *Paramahansa Swami Yogananda*, 98–9.
11. *Amrita Bazar Patrika* (15 Dec. 1935), 7.
12. Ghosh, *Mejda*, 207–8.
13. Richard Wright, *Inner Culture* (March 1937), 48.

Chapter 32

1. Yogananda had met the maharajah while in America, and was invited to Mysore at that time. Paramhansa Yogananda, *Autobiography of a Yogi* (LA: SRF, 1946), Chapter 41.
2. Rajarsi Janakananda, *A Great Western Yogi* (LA: SRF, 1996), 88.
3. Richard Wright, 'Excerpts', *Inner Culture* (March 1937).
4. Ibid.
5. 'Comment Abroad: The Daily Post, Bangalore', *Inner Culture* (March 1937), 66–7.
6. Richard Wright, 'News From India', *Inner Culture* (February 1937).
7. 'Report from "The Daily Post" of India, Nov. 5, 1935', *Inner Culture* (February 1937).
8. Rajarsi Janakananda, *A Great Western Yogi* (LA: SRF, 1996) 89.
9. Interview with Omkar Mullick, Mukul Dutta, Kavya Dutta. Calcutta, India, June 2017.
10. Interview with Omkar Mullick. Calcutta, India, June 2017.
11. Elizabeth Kadetsky, *First There Is a Mountain* (USA: Little, Brown & Co., 2004), 82.
12. Ibid., 82–5.
13. Iyengar had been mostly bedridden for years and wrote, 'My body had become so stiff that I could hardly bend down and extend my arm to reach my knees.' Walking in that first year, 'brought about severe aches and pains'. B. K. S. Iyengar, *Astadala Yogamala*, Vol. 1 (Allied Publishers Limited, 2000), 6, 16.
14. Kadetsky, *First There Is a Mountain*, 83.
15. Ibid.
16. B. K. S. Iyengar, *Astadala Yogamala*, Vol. 1 (Allied Publishers Limited, 2000), 25.
17. Kadetsky, *First There Is a Mountain*, 83.
18. Ibid., 85.
19. BKS Iyengar, *Astadala Yogamala*, Vol. 5 (Allied Publishers Limited, 2000), 56.

20. Ibid., 115.

21. B. K. S. Iyengar, *Yoga Thy Light* (1978 French). Reprinted as: *Iyengar: His Life and Work* (1987 English).

22. Elliott Goldberg, *The Path of Modern Yoga* (Inner Traditions, 2016), 374.

23. Iyengar, *Astadala Yogamala*, Vol. 1, 17.

24. Ibid., 56–7.

Chapter 33

1. Sneha Jain, handwriting analyst, Bangalore, India. Available at https://graphologyjunction. wordpress. com/2017/04/17/signature-analysis-of-the-forgotten-yogi-buddha-bose/

2. 'Talks with Ramana Maharshi', 29 November 1935. Talk 106. Available at https://www. youtube.com/ watch?v=4_ZleDVogJI 3:30 and following.

3. Geoffrey called Buddha 'an English man in Indian clothes' and said his father, Dennis, was 'an Indian man in English clothes'. Interview with Chitralekha Shalom. Calcutta, India. August 2016.

4. Hare Krishna Ghosh, *Experiences with My Guru* (Ananda, 1995).

5. Rajarsi Janakananda, *A Great Western Yogi* (LA: SRF, 1996) 117.

6. Paramahansa Yogananda, *Cosmic Chants – Spiritualized Songs*, 1938.

7. Pushpita Datta, 'From One Ray to Another: The Golden Light Moves On'. Available at http://www. akhandamahapeeth.org/web/displayhtml.php?fname=articles/GoldenLight. html

Chapter 34

1. Sananda Lal Ghosh, *Mejda: The Family and Early Life of Paramahansa Yogananda* (SRF, 1980, second printing, 1992), 218.

2. Ibid., 204.

3. Paramahansa Yogananda. *Autobiography of a Yogi*, (LA: SRF, 1946), Chapter 42.

4. Yogananda, 'The Swami Sails for India', *Inner Culture* VII (July 1935), 25.

5. Richard Wright, 'News From India', *Inner Culture* VIII (March 1936), 26–7.

6. Ibid., 25.

7. *Inner Culture* IX (March 1937), 63.

8. Yogananda, *Autobiography of a Yogi*, Chapter 42.

9. Salindra Bijoy Dasgupta, *Paramhansa Swami Yogananda: Life-Portrait and Reminiscences* (Yoga Niketan, 2011), 26.

Chapter 35

1. Claudia Guggenbühl, *Mircea Eliade and Surendranath Dasgupta: The History of Their Eencounter; Dasgupta's Life, His Philosophy and His Works on Yoga; A Comparative Analysis of Eliade's Chapter on Patanjali's Yogasutra and Dasgupta's Yoga as Philosophy and Religion* (University of Zurich, 2008).

Chapter 36

1. Sulagna Sengupta, *Jung in India* (New Orleans: Spring Journal Books, 2013), 186.

2. Francis Yeats-Brown, *Lancer at Large* (New York: City Publishing, 1939), 147–50.

3. Ibid., 147–50.

4. Carl Jung, *Memories, Dreams, Reflections* (Random House, 1961), 277-278.

5. Linda Kay Davidson and David Martin Gitlitz, *Pilgrimage: From the Ganges to Graceland : an Encyclopedia* (ABC-CLIO, January 2002), 318.

6. Suresh Balabantaray, *64 Yoginis Temple Hirapur Bhubaneshwar* (Intach, 2008).

7. R.C. Majumdar, *History of Ancient Bengal* (Calcutta: Tulsi Prakashani, 1971), 356.

8. Stella Dupuis. 'Matsyendranatha, Master of the Yogini Kaula School in the Tantra Tradition of Bengal', presented at the celebration of the hundredth anniversary of the Bangladesh National Museum, Dhaka, 9 July 2013. Available at https://www.academia.edu/17586008/Matsyendranatha_Master_of_the_Yogini_Kaula_School_in_the_Tantra_Tradition_of_Bengal

9. Self-Realization Fellowship (SRF) is the entity tasked with the ownership of properties associated with Yogananda. Yogoda Satsanga Society of India vs. Swami Hariharananda Giri of Puri, India, 1974–75 was one of the lawsuits over ownership of the place, and for a time, in the 1940s, it was called Yogoda centre.

Chapter 37

1. Rajarsi Janakananda, *A Great Western Yogi* (LA: SRF, 1996) 104-105.

2. 'Once, it so happened that while Yogananda was standing in the balcony of this house, Sananda Lal Ghosh, because of the property dispute tried to push Yogananda down. Even though Yogananda's back was towards Sananda, he cast a spell so that Sananda's hands got stuck to the wall. Frightened, Sananda started calling out to his father, who came running. When Sananda complained that his hands were stuck on the wall, Yogananda said that his hands were free – and they were free.' Interview with Hassi Mukherjee. Calcutta, India. May 2015.

3. Sailendra Bijoy Dasgupta, *Paramahansa Swami Yogananda* (Yoga Niketan, 2006), 87-88.

4. Rajarsi Janakananda, *A Great Western Yogi* (LA: SRF, 1996) 112.

5. News From India, Excerpts from a letter of C. Richard Wright, *Inner Culture* VIII (August 1936), 25.

6. 'News From India', *Inner Culture* VII (Dec. 1935), 25.

7. 'Swami Yogananda in Ranchi: Plans for Self-Realization Temple in Calcutta', *Amrita Bazar Patrika* (14 Sept. 1935), 13.

8. A letter dated 9 October 1935 revealed Yogananda no longer thought Mussolini could be persuaded. 'I am so thoroughly disillusioned with him, that he is working his ambitions on his own people ... he has a mighty karma to pay for attacking innocent people without provocation.' Rajarsi Janakananda, *A Great Western Yogi* (LA: SRF, 1996), 82.

9. National Archives and Records Administration, Washington, DC Board of Special Inquiry Transcript of Swami Yogananda case, 26 October 1936. File 55865/886, RG 85. EC-23.

10. Moloney makes an error with accusations towards Swami Paramananda, as being towards Swami Yogananda. Deirdre M. Moloney, *National Insecurities: Immigrants and U.S. Deportation Policy since 1882* (NC Press, 2012), 146–52.

11. National Archives and Records Administration, Washington, DC Board of Special Inquiry. File 55865/886, RG 85. 30 April 1935.

12. National Archives and Records Administration, Washington, DC Board of Special Inquiry.

File 55865/886, RG 85. KS-34 M-12. 15 August 1935.

13. National Archives and Records Administration, Washington, DC Board of Special Inquiry. File 55865/886, RG 85. KS-34. 8 July 1935.

14. National Archives and Records Administration, Washington, DC Board of Special Inquiry. File 55865/886, RG 85. 15 Dec. 1936.

15. National Archives and Records Administration, Washington, DC Board of Special Inquiry Transcript of Swami Yogananda case, 26 October 1936. File 55865/886, RG 85. 8 July 1935.

16. Moloney, *National Insecurities*, 146–52.

17. Satyeswarananda, *Biography of a Yogi-Yogananda*, Vol. 2 (Sanskrit Classics, 2016), 830–3; British Library: L/PJ/6/1959.

18. National Archives and Records Administration, Washington, DC Board of Special Inquiry Transcript of Swami Yogananda case, 27 October 1936. File 55865/886, RG 85.

19. National Archives and Records Administration, Washington, DC Board of Special Inquiry Transcript of Swami Yogananda case, 27 October 1936. File 55865/886, RG 85. KS-34.

Chapter 38

1. "Health Through Yoga," *Yoga Cure Institute* (Calcutta, 1971), 9.

2. Buddha Bose, *Key to the Kingdom of Health Through Yoga, Vol. 1* (Calcutta: The Statesman Press, 1939), 1.

3. There is also no indication of Yogananda being taught Hatha yoga prior to the encounter with yogis in Dihika, though he certainly could have been taught by Swami Kebalananda (when he was Shastri Mahasaya), the tutor, and also by his friend Pulin Bihari Das (Swami Shivananda), who ran an akhara and knew muscle-building techniques.

4. In *Autobiography of a Yogi*, Chapter 5, Yogananda mentions 'a friend, Alakananda' who told him about the powers of Calcutta's 'perfumed saint'. Whether this is the same person or not is unclear. Swami Satyananda Giri, *A Collection of Biographies of 4 Kriya Yoga Gurus* (Yoga Niketan, 2009), 235.

5. Other than a couple of historical mentions, not much is known about these Hatha yogis. There is a lone reference to Swami Kapilananda, and his healing powers, in an early twentieth-century Bengali periodical named *Galpo Lohori*.

6. Swami Satyeswarananda Giri, *Swami Satyananda Giri: Biography of a Yogi – Satyananda*, Vol. 1 (The Sanskrit Classics, 2016, 3rd edition), 598, 613, 618

7. Giri, *Swami Satyananda Giri, Biography of a Yogi*, 603.

8. Ibid., 609–10.

9. Ibid., 619.

10. Bishnu Ghosh, K.C. Sen Gupta, *Muscle Control and Barbell Exercise* (Calcutta, 1930), 11.

11. Sukumar Bose, author of Applied Yoga. Claudia Guggenbühl, *Yoga in Calcutta* (2004, unpublished), 70.

Chapter 39

1. Bishnu Ghosh and Keshub Chandra Sen Gupta, *Barbell Exercises and Muscle Control* (Calcutta, 1930), 98.

2. Brian Dana Akers, The *Hatha Yoga Pradipika* (YogaVidya.com, 2002), 41. Available at www.nauli.org

3.   James Mallinson (trans.), The *Gheranda Samhita* (YogaVidya.com, 2002), 13.

4.   The sage Gheranda is thought to have been a Bengali Vaishnavite Hatha yogi. Given 'the location of most of its manuscripts in Bengal', we may 'hazard to guess that the *Gheranda Samhita* was composed in Bengal around 1700 C.E', and was likely to be more widely available in Bengali than other Hatha yoga texts. Mallinson, *Gheranda Samhita*, 13.

5.   Bishnu Charan Ghosh, 'From The Past', *Bayam Charcha* (Dec. 1966).

6.   Ibid., 3.

7.   Interview with Yogacharya Mukul Dutta. Calcutta, India. Oct. 2016.

8.   Mallinson, *Gheranda Samhita*, 16.

9.   Chandra Vasu, *The Gheranda Samhita: A Treatise on Hatha Yoga* (Bombay: Tatvavivechaka Press, 1895), xxi.

10. Jason Birch, 'The Proliferation of Asana in Late Mediaeval Yoga Texts', *Yoga in Transformation: Historical and Contemporary Perspectives on a Global Phenomenon* (Vienna: Vandenhoeck & Ruprecht Unipress, 2018).

11. *Inner* Culture, XI (April 1939), 43.

12. The one not listed was *sahita*, a seed mantra repeated with breath. The lack of openly identifying the technique of sahita was likely due to the influence of Kriya yoga. The Kriya yoga tradition, to which Buddha was initiated into by Yogananda, was typically taught individually. Buddha Bose, *Yoga Asanas* (Calcutta, 1938). Reprinted, *84 Yoga Asanas* (USA, 2015), 236–46.

13. Sivananda of Rishikesh placed the two techniques together as well. The question of what 'the effects of the practice of *khechari*' entailed is answered on the Divine Life Society website as a practice that 'will help the student to stop the breath' and once the student achieves satisfactory khechari, they 'can have *kevala kumbhaka* also very easily'. Available at http://sivanandaonline.org/public_html/?cmd=displaysection&section_id=1362

14. Buddha Bose, *Key to the Kingdom of Health Through Yoga*, Vol. 1 (Calcutta: The Statesman Press, 1939), 5.

15. Ibid.

16. The 'Bombay people' refers to Kuvalayananda, and 'Rishikesh' to Sivananda. Claudia Guggenbühl, *Yoga in Calcutta* (2003), 202.

Chapter 40

1.   *Biography: Yogi and Scientist Swami Kuvalayananda* (Kaivalyadhama: Lonavla, 2012), 41.

2.   Ibid., 47.

3.   Elliott Goldberg, *The Path of Modern Yoga* (Inner Traditions, 2016), 83.

4.   For the following quotations, I have relied upon two unpublished accounts for the biographical information. The first is a handwritten account authored by Kuvalayananda, provided to Claudia Guggenbühl from Sri Tiwari in Lonavla, 11/19/04. The second is from Anup Mandal, a typed account, also retrieved by Claudia in Lonavla. Claudia Guggenbühl, *Yoga in Calcutta* (unpublished, 2005), 83. See also, for a Madhavadas biography from the perspective of other students: Joseph S. Alter, 'Shri Yogendra: Magic, Modernity, and the Burden of the Middle-Class Yogi', in *Gurus of Modern Yoga* (Oxford, 2014).

5.   Joseph S. Alter, *Gandhi's Body: Sex, Diet, and the Politics of Nationalism* (University of Pennsylvania, 2000), 64.

6. Elizabeth Kadetsky, *First There Is a Mountain* (Little, Brown and Company, 2004), 170.

7. Kuvalayananda, *Popular Yoga Asanas* (Lonavla: First published in English in 1931, Tuttle edition, 1972), xv.

8. Joseph Alter, *Yoga in Modern India* (Princeton, 2004), 34.

9. Paramahansa Yogananda, *Autobiography of a Yogi* (LA: SRF, 1946), Chapter 24.

10. Ibid., 371.

11. Kadetsky, *First There Is a Mountain*, 171.

12. *Biography: Yogi and Scientist Swami Kuvalayananda* (Kaivalyadhama: Lonavla, 2012), 371–2.

13. Ibid., 442.

14. Kadetsky, *First There Is a Mountain*, 170.

15. *Biography: Yogi and Scientist Swami Kuvalayananda*, 371–2.

16. *Yoga Mimansa* III, nos 3 & 4 (April 1928), 271.

17. Ibid.

18. *Yoga Mimansa* II, no. 3 (July 1926), 234.

Chapter 41

1. Michelle Goldberg, *The Goddess Pose, Indra Devi* (NY: Alfred Knopf, 2015), 122.

2. In a 2003 interview, Harekrishna Ghosh mentioned that Bishnu Ghosh had gotten the title *Yogindra* from Sivananda of Rishikesh. Harekrishna Ghosh was born to Sananda Ghosh just after Yogananda left for America in 1920 and remembered 'when he was very young, about 7 or 8 years old, his father (Sananda Lal Ghosh) and his uncle (Bishnu Charan Ghosh) would take him and other children every morning to the City College on Amherst Street. There, they practised physical exercise.' Harekrishna listed three sources of yoga teachings for Bishnu Ghosh: (1) his father Bhagabati; (2) Yogananda and his school; (3) Sivananda from Rishikesh. Claudia Guggenbühl, *Yoga in Calcutta* (2003). Interview with Harekrishna Ghosh. Calcutta, India. 9 September 2003.

3. Swami Sivananda, *Spiritual Lessons*, Part I & II (1939).

4. Swami Sivananda, *Practice of Yoga* (Madras: *My Magazine of India*, second edition, 1933), 321–2.

5. An official biography of Sivananda merely states that during his early years in Rishikesh he maintained a 'daily routine of Yoga Asanas, Pranayama, and other Hatha Yogic Kriyas'. And, 'at times he did *Dand* or *Baithak*'. Mostly though, he meditated in seclusion, eight, twelve, sometimes sixteen hours a day. N. Ananthanarayanan, *From Man to God-Man* (Divine Life Society, 1970), 46–8.

6. Swami Sivananda, *Yoga Asanas* (Madras: *My Magazine of India*, second edition, 1935), xix.

7. Ibid.

8. Ibid.

9. Ibid.

10. Ibid.

11. Ibid.

12. Swami Sivananda, *Practice of Yoga*, (Madras: *My Magazine of India*, second edition, 1933), Publishers Note.

13. Sivananda formed the Divine Life Society in 1934, and he trained aspirants in a variety of ways, forming a spiritual community in Rishikesh. Its 'trust deed' includes 'yogic training'

through '*puja, bhakti, jnana, karma* and *Hatha* yoga with systematic training in asanas, pranayama, *dharana, dhyana, samadhi,* etc.' as part of the society's 'aims and objectives'. Swami Padmanabhananda, *Sivananda: Biography of a Modern Sage* (Divine Life Society, 1985, third edition, 2015), 102–3.

Chapter 42

1. Claudia Guggenbühl, *Yoga between Bodybuilding and Enlightenment.* Transcript of lecture held on 29 February 2008, 5.
2. Edward Groth, *To Give Room for Wandering: The Autobiography of an American Foreign Service Officer* (1972), 131.
3. 'Pandit Sitladin Tripathi posed for the illustrations and E.M. Groth, along with Ashoka Gupta, took the photos.' S. Muzumdar, *Yoga Exercises for Health and Cure* (1941), Author's Note.
4. Buddha Bose, *Yoga Asanas* (Calcutta, 1938), viii.
5. Christopher Wilk, 'The Healthy Body Culture', *Modernism: Designing a New World, 1914–1939* (V & A Publications, 2006), 251.
6. Ibid., 262.
7. Bishnu, a decade prior, had just about the opposite experience with the muscle dancing feats he'd seen Chit Tun perform, feats which Bishnu had learned from the Hatha yoga teachers at Yogananda's school for boys at Dihika in 1917.
8. Jonathan Glancy, *Modern World Architecture* (Carlton, 2006), 132.
9. *Calcutta Municipal Gazette* (30 March 1935), 85–9.
10. Bishnu and Buddha performed the role of social reformer in this regard, during a 'town cleansing week' intended to awaken 'sanitary consciousness'. Bishnu led a procession of 'Rover Scouts', which 'slowly passed through practically all the principal streets of the city'. Charts and posters with large 'models illustrating various aspects of health and disease' were placed 'on the chassis of cars and on lorries and paraded through the streets'. A photograph in the magazine shows Bishnu riding the three-wheeler held by Yogananda, with Buddha Bose sitting in the sidecar. 'Town-Cleansing Week in Calcutta', *Calcutta Municipal Gazette* (9 January 1937), 194.
11. N. R. Ray (ed.), *Dictionary of National Biography,* Vol. II (Calcutta: Institute of Historical Studies, 1990), 54–5.
12. Buddha Bose, *Key to the Kingdom of Health Through Yoga,* Vol. 1 (Calcutta: D.A. Lakin, Statesman Press, 1939), 5.

Chapter 43

1. Buddha Bose, *Yoga Asanas* (unpublished, 1938). Published as: *84 Yoga Asanas* by Buddha Bose (USA, 2015), Preface.
2. Swami Kuvalayananda, *Popular Yoga Asanas* (1st English Edition, 1931), First Tuttle edition (Japan, 1972), 100.
3. Elliott Goldberg, *The Path of Modern Yoga* (Inner Traditions, 2016), 69.
4. Buddha Bose, *Key to the Kingdom of Health Through Yoga,* Vol. 1 (Calcutta: The Statesman Press, 1939), 10.
5. Swami Yogananda, *Yogoda: Tissue-Will System of Physical Perfection* (30 Huntington Ave,

Boston, MA., 1925), 7.

6. Bishnu Ghosh, *Muscle Control* (Calcutta, 1930), 56.

7. Jerome Armstrong, 'Afterword: Finding Calcutta Yoga', in Buddha Bose, *84 Yoga Asanas* (USA, 2015), 226.

8. The quotation was recalled by Swami Pranabananda as one which Lahiri Mahasaya often used to guide his teachings. Paramhansa Yogananda, *Autobiography of a Yogi* (LA: SRF, 1946), Chapter 27.

9. Bose, *Yoga Asanas*, vii–xiii.

Chapter 44

1. Buddha Bose, *Yoga Asanas*, (unpublished, 1938). Published as: *84 Yoga Asanas* by Buddha Bose (USA, 2015), Preface, vii–xiii.

2. *The Evening Star*, Washington DC (21 Feb. 1939), B-1.

3. Punyapriyo Dasgupta, 'A Club Built Brick by Brick', *The Statesman* (22 May 2016). Available at http://www.thestatesman.com/opinion/a-club-built-brick-by-brick-143858.html

4. Andrew Mackenzie, *Frontiers of the Unknown: The Insights of Psychical Research* (London: Barker, 1968), 70.

5. Edward M. Groth, *To Give Room for Wandering* (1972).

6. Ian Stephens, *Monsoon Morning* (Ernest Benn Limited, 1966), 57.

7. Groth, *To Give Room for Wandering*, 131.

8. Stephens, *Monsoon Morning*, 57.

9. Groth, *To Give Room for Wandering*, 130.

10. Ibid., 131.

11. Stephens, *Monsoon Morning*, 57.

12. *World's Press News and Advertisers' Review*, Vol. 75 (World's Press News Publishing Company, Limited, 1966), 22.

13. Stephens, *Monsoon Morning*, 57.

14. *World's Press News and Advertisers' Review*, Vol. 75 (World's Press News Publishing Company, Limited, 1966), 22.

15. Prem Bhatia, *All My Yesterdays* (Vikas Pub. House, 1972), 44.

16. *Democratic World* (Gulab Singh & Sons, 1972), 19.

17. Ian Stephens, *Unmade Journeys* (Stacey International, 1977), 342.

18. Bose, *Yoga Asanas* (unpublished, 1938). Published as: *84 Yoga Asanas* (USA, 2015), ix.

19. Buddha Bose, 'Homage', *Bayam Charcha* (August 1970).

Chapter 45

1. Buddha Bose, 'Homage', *Bayam Charcha* (August 1970).

2. British Library. Bose, Buddha. File No. 7. IOR: L/I/1/1314.

3. Berlin had hosted the 1936 Olympics, and during the proceedings, a group performed called the Hanuman Vyayam Prasarak Mandal from Maharashtra, India. With 'nationalist aspirations' of showing 'that Indians were physically equal to the West', they displayed many physical culture displays, including a 'mass drill yoga', which won medals and 'impressed the Berlin Olympic Committee'. The Indian group inspired the Germans to seek further input. Ronojoy Sen, *Nation at Play: A History of Sport in India* (Columbia, 2015), 161.

4. Nora Levin, *The Holocaust: The Destruction of European Jewry 1933–1945* (New York: Thomas Y. Crowell Co., 1968), 124–32.

5. *Inner Culture*, XI (April 1939), 43.

6. Hannah Arendt, *Eichmann in Jerusalem* (New York: Viking Press, 1963), IV: The First Solution: Expulsion.

7. Kovoor T. Behanan, *Yoga: A Scientific Evaluation* (New York: Macmillan Company, NY. 1937), 7.

8. 'Health through Yoga', *Yoga Cure Institute* (Calcutta, 1971), 9.

9. The German model would have integrated the yogic postures into its group format of exercises for students. The format doesn't seem to have had an impact on the methods which Bishnu and Buddha would apply in their own methods of teaching yogic postures, sticking to the one-on-one therapeutic model rather than some sort of coordinated teacher-led class throughout their careers in India, though abroad it was different.

10. Buddha Bose, 'Homage', *Bayam Charcha* (August 1970).

11. F. Yeats-Brown, *Lancer at Large* (New York: Garden City Publishing, 1936), 173.

12. Ibid., 139.

13. British Library. Bose, Buddha. File No. 7. IOR: L/I/1/1314.

Chapter 46

1. 'Claims He Can Hold Breath for Half-Hour', *Perth WA Sunday Times* (30 Oct. 1938), 13.

2. Buddha Bose, 'Homage', *Bayam Charcha* (August 1970).

3. Nikolaus Pevsner, *The Buildings of England, London I, the Cities of London and Westminster* (Penguin Books, 1962), 699.

4. 'Swami Yogananda in Ranchi, Plans for Self-Realization Temple in Calcutta', *Amrita Bazar Patrika* (14 Sept. 1935), 13.

5. 'I Can Teach Londoners to Live to 100', *Daily Mail* (18 Sept. 1936), 4.

6. Ibid.

7. 'News From India', *Inner Culture* VII (Dec. 1935), 26.

8. Richard Wright, 'News From London', *Inner Culture* VIII (Dec. 1936), 25.

9. Ibid.

10. 'Sleep 3 Hours: Laugh More', *Daily Mail* (23 Sept. 1936), 5.

11. 'I Can Teach Londoners to Live to 100', 4.

12. 'Amrita Bazar Patrika', *Inner Culture* IX (March 1937), 68.

13. Francis Yeats-Brown, *Lancer at Large* (New York: Garden City Publishing, 1937), 130.

14. In 1956, Iyengar, at customs in Switzerland (he was travelling to teach violinist Mr Menuhin who first promoted Iyengar to the West), replied that 'yoga' was his profession, and was asked 'how many currencies have you swallowed'. B. K. S. Iyengar, *Astadala Yogamala*, Vol. 6, 186, 315.

15. Buddha Bose, 'Homage'.

16. Bishnu Charan Ghosh, 'From the Past', *Bayam Charcha* (May 1967).

Chapter 47

1. *Indian Arts and Letters: The Journal of the Royal India*, Vols 12–13. A transcript of the lecture is not provided.

2. Buddha Bose, 'Homage, *Bayam Charcha* (August 1970).

3. 'Claims He Can Hold Breath for Half-Hour', *Perth WA Sunday Times* (30 Oct. 1938), 13.

4. 'News in Brief', *London Times*, no. 48122 (11 Oct. 1938), 12. The Times Digital Archives.

5. 'Health through Yoga', *Yoga Cure Institute* (Calcutta 1971), 9.

6. 'Claims He Can Hold Breath for Half-Hour', 13.

7. Ibid.

8. 'News in Brief', 12.

9. 'Claims He Can Hold Breath for Half-Hour', 13.

10. Ibid.

11. Bishnu Ghosh, *Muscle Control* (Calcutta, 1930), 139.

12. S. Muzumdar, *Yoga Exercises for Health and Cure* (1949). Reprinted, *Yogic Exercises* (London: Longman's Green and Co. LTD, 1960), 1.

13. Frank Moraes, *Jawaharlal Nehru* (Macmillan Company, 1958), 207–9.

14. Ibid.

15. Ibid.

16. Buddha Bose, 'Homage'.

17. Buddha Bose, *Key to the Kingdom of Health Through Yoga*, Vol. 1 (Calcutta: Statesman Press, 1939).

Chapter 48

1. Year: 1938; Arrival: New York, New York; Microfilm Serial: T715, 1897-1957; Microfilm Roll: Roll 6238; Line: 15; Page Number: 58.

2. The *Washington Post* (19 Dec. 1938), 11.

3. *The Greenville News*, Greenville, South Carolina. Dec, 27, 1938, 6.

4. *Ken* magazine (15 December 1938), 9.

5. James Mallinson (trans.), *Gheranda Samhita* (YogaVidya.com, 2002), 14.

6. *Ken* magazine (15 December 1938), 29.

7. British Library Archives. IOR: L/I/1/1314 Bose, Buddha. File No. 7.

8. Paramahansa Yogananda, *Autobiography of a Yogi* (LA: SRF, 1946), Chapter 27.

9. Patricia Vertinsky, 'Yoga Comes to American Physical Education: Josephine Rathbone and Corrective Physical Education', *Journal of Sport History* 41, no. 2 (Summer 2014), 288.

10. Josephine Rathbone, *My Twentieth Century* (unpublished memoir, 1982), 244. Courtesy of Springfield College, Babson Library, Archives and Special Collections.

11. J.E Rogers, 'Around the Country', *The Journal of Health and Physical Education* IX, no. 1 (January 1938), 40.

12. 'Yale's Yogin', *Time Magazine* 29, no, 17 (26 April 1937), 26.

13. 'Speaking of Pictures, These Are the Exercises of Yoga', *Life Magazine* (19 April 1937).

14. 'How to Relax', *Time Magazine* 34, no. 24 (11 Dec. 1939), 1.

15. 'Art of Relaxation to Be Taught in Spring at Teachers College', *New York Times* (30 Nov. 1939), 23.

16. Vertinsky, 'Yoga Comes to American Physical Education', 287.

17. Stefanie Syman, *The Subtle Body* (Farrar, Straus, & Giroux, 2010), 141.

18. *Amrita Bazar Patrika*, Calcutta, India (21 Oct. 1938).

19. *Inner Culture* IX (March 1937), 50–2.

Chapter 49

1. *Inner Culture* II, no. 3 (January 1939), 36.
2. Sailendra Bijoy Dasgupta, *Paramhansa Swami Yogananda: Life Portrait and Reminiscences* (UK: Yoga Niketan, 2011), 114.
3. Swami Satyeswarananda Giri, *Biography of Yogi-Yogananda*, Vol. 2 (Sanskrit Classics, 2016), 835.
4. Dasgupta, *Paramhansa Swami Yogananda*, 113.
5. Interview with Rooma Bose. Calcutta, India. March 2015. Ida Jo, Scott Lamps, along with Shibnath De.
6. *Inner Culture* (May 1939), 43.
7. Pushpita Datta, 'From One Ray to Another : The Golden Light Moves On', Available at http://www. akhandamahapeeth.org/web/displayhtml.php?fname=articles/GoldenLight. html
8. *Inner Culture* V. II, no. 4 (February 1939), 29.
9. 'Christmas Meditation', *Inner Culture* IX, no. 5 (March 1937), 44.
10. On the 1935 tour of south India, 'during the course of the lecture, the Swami's age was conjectured to range from 17 to 100 years, but when asked his age point-blank, he answered, "Do you want to know my age? I never tell my age. For I am ageless. You failed to designate the age of this residence or body of mine. I am the immortal Soul, and am therefore ageless."' 'Christmas Meditation', 44.
11. Gordon Webb, *Sunday Graphic of London* (27 September 1936). Reprinted in *Inner Culture* IX, no. 5 (March 1937).
12. *Bakersfield Californian*, (9 January 1924), 7.
13. 'Comment Abroad', *Inner Culture* IX, no. 5 (March 1937), 66. Reprinted from: *The Daily Post* (Bangalore, 5 Nov. 1935).
14. *The Historic Passing of Four Great Disciples* (20 Dec. 2005). Available at http://www.backupsrfwalrus. com/srfwalrus/p203.ezboard.com/fsrfwalrusfrm35ed93. html?topicID=41.topic
15. *Los Angeles Times* (7 January 1939), Part II.

Chapter 50

1. Sailendra Bijoy Dasgupta, *Paramhansa Swami Yogananda: Life Portrait and Reminiscences* (UK: Yoga Niketan, 2011), 104.
2. 'Swami's Temple Lasted Only 5 Years before Crumbling', *San Diego Union-Tribune* (10 July 2010). Available at http://www.sandiegouniontribune.com/sdut-swamis-temple-lasted-only-5-years-before2010jul10-story.html
3. *Inner Culture* IX (March 1937), 50–2.
4. Diane Welch, 'Noonan's to Swami's Point', *San Diego Union-Tribune* (24 September 2006), N-2.
5. 'Swami's Temple Lasted Only 5 Years before Crumbling'.
6. Swami Kriyananda, *Paramhansa Yogananda, A Biography* (Crystal Clarity Publishers, 2011), 174.
7. 'Swami Adds to Self-Realization Project', *Los Angeles Times* (2 November 1937), Part I, 9.
8. 'San Diego Interested', *San Diego Sun* (31 January 1937).

9. Welch, 'Noonan's to Swami's Point'.

10. Donald Castellano-Hoyt, *The Seventh Life* (Amanuensis Press, 2018), 149.

11. 'Swami's Temple Lasted Only 5 Years before Crumbling'.

12. SRF Press Release, 'New Golden Lotus Temple of All Religions Uniquely Designed Temple is Non-Sectarian, Encinitas,' CA, 3 November 1937.

13. *Inner Culture for Self-Realization* XI, no. 4 (February 1939), 38.

14. Ibid., 28–9.

15. Ibid, 38.

16. Pushpita Datta, 'From One Ray to Another: The Golden Light Moves On'. Available at http://www.akhandamahapeeth.org/web/displayhtml.php?fname=articles/GoldenLight.html

Chapter 51

1. Swami Premananda, 'My Gurudev: Swami Yogananda Paramahansa', *The Mystic Cross, Dedication Issue, Self-Revelation Church of Absolute Monism* (1998), 4–11.

2. Paramahansa Yogananda, *Autobiography of a Yogi* (LA: SRF, 1946), Chapter 48.

3. Premananda, 'My Gurudev'.

4. *Inner Culture for Self-Realization* XI (April 1939), 43.

5. 'Freshman Yogi Finds Greater Relaxation in Oriental Philosophy and Physical Control', *The Harvard Crimson* (21 February 1939).

Chapter 52

1. 'Art of Relaxation to Be Taught in Spring at Teachers College', *New York Times* (30 Nov. 1939), 23.

2. Josephine Rathbone's unpublished memoir *My Twentieth Century* (Babson Library, Springfield College: Springfield Massachusetts, 1982), 93.

3. *Teachers College Record* 41, no. 6 (1940), 506–12.

4. Josephine L. Rathbone, 'Relaxation and Activity', *The Journal of Health and Physical Activity* 8, no. 8 (1937), 469–515.

5. Patricia Vertinsky, 'Yoga Comes to American Physical Education: Josephine Rathbone and Corrective Physical Education', *Journal of Sport History* 41, no. 2 (Summer 2014), 288.

6. *Teachers College Bulletin* (Winter and Spring Sessions, 1938–1939), 218.

7. *Teachers College Record* 45, no. 2 (1943), 96–102.

8. *Teachers College Bulletin* (Winter and Spring Sessions, 1939–1940), 216.

9. *Health through Yoga* (Yoga Cure Institute: Calcutta, 1971).

10. Vertinsky, 'Yoga Comes to American Physical Education', 288.

11. Stefanie Syman, *The Subtle Body* (Farrar, Straus, & Giroux, 2010), 141.

Chapter 53

1. Buddha Bose, *Key to the Kingdom of Health through Yoga*, Vol. 1 (Calcutta: Statesman Press, 1939), 9.

2. Year: 1938; Arrival: New York, New York; Microfilm Serial: T715, 1897–1957; Microfilm Roll: Roll 6238; Line: 15; Page Number: 58

3. *Calcutta Municipal Gazette* (9 April 1938), 36.

4. *Amrita Bazar Patrika* (20 Oct. 1938), 14.

5. Buddha Bose, *Key to the Kingdom of Health through Yoga*, Vol. 1 (Calcutta: Statesman Press, 1939).

6. Ian Stephens. 27 July 1938. British Library. India Office Records and Private Papers. IOR/L/I/1/1314. 1938.

7. *The Statesman: An Anthology, 1875–1975* (Rañjana: Statesman Ltd., 1975), iii.

8. Buddha once stated, 'In 1946 I stopped taking part in any shows. Thereafter, my spiritual journey started.' There was nothing further on the subject. Buddha Bose, 'Homage', *Bayam Charcha* (August 1970).

9. Elizabeth Kadetsky, *First There Is a Mountain* (Little, Brown & Co, 2004), 85.

10. Bose, *Key to the Kingdom of Health through Yoga*, Vol. 1, Preface, 6.

Chapter 54

1. In 1935, Nilmoni had performed a series of brilliant physical feats at an annual Hindu Mahasabha function, which won him the title of 'Ironman'. Sadhu Maharaj was so impressed that he called Nilmoni to check his arms and body. He exclaimed, 'Your body seems to be made of iron!'

2. Swapan Das, 'World Yoga Day' speech (Calcutta, 21 June 2016).

3. Ibid.

4. Ibid.

Chapter 56

1. Buddha Bose, *Holy Kailas* (Calcutta, 1954), 58.

2. Anoop Chandola, *Discovering Brides* (Writers Club Press, 2001), 67.

3. Interview with Mataji. Mussoorie, India. June 2017.

4. Edward Groth, *To Give Room for Wandering* (1972), 112–13.

5. Interview with Mataji. Mussoorie, India. June 2017.

6. Buddha Bose, 'Homage', *Bayam Charcha* (Dec. 1970).

7. Andrew J. Kaufman and William L. Putnam, *K2: The 1939 Tragedy* (Mountaineers Books, 1992), Appendix.

8. John Martyn, 'The Story of the Himalayan Club, 1928–1978', Editor Soli S. Mehta, *The Himalayan Journal* 35 (1979), 2.

9. Yogananda would never really grow out of his desire to go the Himalayas but did manage to transmute the longing: 'Get away from this world; not by flying away to a cave in the Himalayas, but to the cave of your mind, where you are free of the body and of the world.' Yogananda, *The Divine Romance* (Self-Realization Fellowship, 1986), 206.

10. Nicholas Roerich, 'Hermitages in the Himalayas', *Inner Culture* (August 1939), 17.

11. Martyn, 'The Story of the Himalayan Club', 2.

12. Swami Pranavananda, *Kailas Manasarovar* (Calcutta, 1949), Introduction.

13. Pranavananda lived through winters in the Kailash-Manasarovar region and circumambulated Holy Kailash twenty-three times, Manasarovar twenty-five times and Rakshas Tal once. It took great yogic powers to be able to live at Kailash in winter. He, like the Tibetan yogi Milarepa who only would wear a cotton cloth, used his inner strength to keep warm even in the winters. Swami Pranavananda, *Kailas Manasarovar* (Calcutta, 1949), 228.

14. Ibid., 5.
15. Davinder Bhasin, *An Audience with God at Mount Kailash: A True Story* (Partridge Publishing, 2016).
16. Pranavananda, *Kailas Manasarovar*, 6.
17. Interview with Mataji. Mussoorie, India. June 2017.
18. Interview with Shyamal Talkudar. Bangkok, Thailand. Oct. 2015.

Chapter 57

1. Interview with Chitralekha Shalom. Calcutta, India. March 2015.
2. Interview with Rooma Bose. New Alipore, India. March 2015.
3. Interview with Mataji. Mussoorie, India. June 2017.
4. Bishnu Charan Ghosh, 'From the Past', *Bayam Charcha* (July 1967).
5. Bishnu Ghosh, 'From the Past', *Bayam Charcha* (June 1967).
6. Bishnu Charan Ghosh, 'From the Past', *Bayam Charcha* (Feb. 1966).
7. Bishnu Charan Ghosh, 'From the Past', *Bayam Charcha* (February 1967).

Chapter 58

1. Yogananda later gave him the name, Rajarsi Janakananda. Lynn would 'be seen lying on the grass in *samadhi*'. At other times, he would wade out into the Pacific Ocean, 'where he floated on his back and thought of himself as floating in the Spirit'. Sailendra Bijoy Dasgupta, *Paramahansa Swami Yogananda* (Yoga Niketan, 2006), 62.
2. 'Swami's Temple Lasted Only 5 years before Crumbling', *San Diego Union-Tribune* (10 July 2010). Available at http://www.sandiegouniontribune.com/sdut-swamis-temple-lasted-only-5-years-before2010jul10-story.html
3. Jon R. Parsons, *A Fight for Religious Freedom* (Crystal Clarity, 2012), 83.
4. 'Swami's Temple Lasted Only 5 Years before Crumbling'.
5. Swami Premananda, 'My Gurudev: Swami Yogananda Paramahansa', *The Mystic Cross, Dedication Issue, Self-Revelation Church of Absolute Monism* (1998), 4–11.
6. 'Washington Leader Now a Swami', *Inner Culture* (October 1941).
7. 'Farewell Tribute to the Golden Lotus Temple', *Inner Culture* (April 1943).
8. Ibid.
9. Ibid.
10. *Associated Press*, Encinitas, 22 June 1942.
11. Diane Welch, 'Noonan's to Swami's Point', *San Diego Union-Tribune* (24 September 2006), N-2.
12. Ibid.
13. Available at https://www.ananda.org/free-inspiration/books/experiences-with-my-guru-paramhansa-yogananda/experiences-the-book/
14. *Inner Culture for Self-Realization* XIV, no. 2 (Oct.–Nov.–Dec. 1942), 1–11; 29–31.
15. Poem by Sri Kalicharan Nath, 'a friend of Bhagabati'. Bishnu Charan Ghosh, 'From the Past', *Bayam Charcha* (Dec. 1965).

Chapter 59

1. Bishnu Charan Ghosh, 'From the Past', *Bayam Charcha* (June 1967).

2.   Bishnu Charan Ghosh, 'From the Past', *Bayam Charcha* (July 1967).

3.   Ibid.

4.   *Inner Culture for Self-Realization* XIV, no. 4 (April–May–June 1943), 12.

5.   Interview with Rooma Bose. Calcutta, India. March 2015.

6.   Interview with Mukul Dutta, Tapan Mondal. Calcutta, India. July 2017.

7.   Bishnu Charan Ghosh, *Collection of Poems* (Sharthopor) (Published posthumously, A. K. Publishers, Calcutta, 1998).

8.   Bishnu Charan Ghosh, 'From the Past', *Bayam Charcha* (Feb. 1966).

9.   Ibid.

10.   Bishnu Charan Ghosh, 'From the Past', *Bayam Charcha* (July 1967).

11.   Ghosh, *Collection of Poems*, 43.

12.   The Ghosh family stopped celebrating birthdays in the house at 4/2 Rammohan Road, in remembrance of Srikrishna, even while subsequently raising five children in the decades to follow. They still do not celebrate birthdays today.

13.   *Inner Culture for Self-Realization* XIV, no. 4 (April–May–June 1943), 12.

14.   Ibid.

15.   Bishnu Charan Ghosh, 'From the Past', *Bayam Charcha* (Feb. 1966).

16.   N.R. Ray (ed.), *Dictionary of National Biography*, Vol. 2 (Calcutta: Institute of Historical Studies, 1990), 54–5.

17.   Bishnu Charan Ghosh, 'From the Past', *Bayam Charcha* (Feb. 1966).

18.   Ghosh, *Collection of Poems*.

Chapter 60

1.   Ritwik Ghatak, *Recollections of Bengal and a Single Vision* (remarks prepared for the Festival of India in London, 1982). Available at http://216.152.71.145/filmmakers/ghatak/ghatak.html

2.   San Diego *Tribune-Sun* (1942). Available at http://www.sandiegouniontribune.com/sdut-swamis-temple-lasted-only-5-years-before-2010jul10-story.html

3.   Yogananda, 'Nations Beware', *Inner Culture*, (March 1937), 22.

4.   'Book Reviews', *Inner Culture* (October 1943), 35–6.

5.   Rabindranath Tagore, *Selected Letters of Rabindranath Tagore*, edited by Krishna Dutta and Andrew Robinson, (Cambridge: Cambridge University Press, 1997), 522–4.

6.   Thant Myint-U, *Burma and the New Crossroads of Asia: Where China Meets India* (New York: Farrar, Straus and Giroux), 298.

7.   August Peter Hansen (Customs Inspector), *Memoirs of an Adventurous Dane in India: 1904–1947*

8.   (London: BACSA, 1999), 207.

9.   Trevor Royle, *The Last Days of the Raj* (London: Michael Joseph, 1989), 52

10.   Paramhansa Yogananda, 'The Voice of Self-Realization', *East-West* (March 1948), 20.

11.   *Time Magazine* (New York, 20 April 1942).

12.   Elaine Pinkerton, *From Calcutta with Love: The World War II Letters of Richard and Reva Beard*, (Texas Tech, 2002), 118. Available at https://www.facebook.com/photo.php?fbid=101601 48048515300&set=a.10153994062425300.1073741827.500075299&type=3&theater

13.   Bishnu Charan Ghosh, 'From the Past', *Bayam Charcha* (Dec. 1967).

14.   Myint-U, *Burma and the New Crossroads of Asia*, 298–9.

Chapter 61

1. Ian Stephens, *Monsoon Mornings* (London: Ernest Benn, 1966), 222.
2. Ibid., 29.
3. 'Notes from the News', *East-West* Magazine (July–Sept. 1944), 33.
4. Eugenie Fraser, *A Home by the Hooghly. A Jute Wallahs Wife* (Edinburgh: Mainstream Publishing 1989), 100–1.
5. *The Statesman* (Calcutta/Delhi, 20 June 1943).
6. Harry Tweedale, *BBC WW2 People's War: Part 11* (Oct. 2006), 85–92. Available at http://www.bbc. co.uk/ww2peopleswar/
7. Fraser, *A Home by the Hooghly*, 100–1.
8. *The Statesman* (Calcutta/Delhi, 29 August 1943).
9. *The Statesman* (Calcutta/Delhi, 23 September 1943).
10. 'Notes from the News', *East-West* magazine (Nov.–Dec. 1946), 26–7.
11. 'Notes from the News', *East-West* magazine (Jan. 1946), 21.

Chapter 62

1. 'Golden Lotus Temple of All Religions', *Inner Culture* (Jan. 1938), 60.
2. 'The Cosmic Motion Pictures', *Inner Culture* (July 1942), 1.
3. Swami Kriyananda, *Paramhansa Yogananda: A Biography* (Crystal Clarity Publishers, 2011), 177.
4. Ibid.
5. 'Golden Lotus Temple Salvaging Begun', Encinitas, *Los Angeles Times* (5 August 1942).
6. 'Swimmer (Frank Dudley Comer) Dies in Rocky Beach Fall', *Los Angeles Times* (28 May 1943), 12.
7. Ibid.
8. 'SRF Bluff', *Los Angeles Times* (9 March 1986).
9. Diane Welch, 'Noonan's to Swami's Point', *San Diego Union-Tribune* (24 September 2006), N-2.
10. 'Self-Realization Church of All Religions Opened in Hollywood', *Inner Culture* (January 1943), 40.
11. On 5 September 1943, Yogananda dedicated the Self Realization Church of All Religions in San Diego, California. 'SRF Acquires San Diego Site', *Inner Culture* (January 1943), 43.
12. 'Farewell Tribute to the Golden Lotus Temple', *Inner Culture* (April 1943).
13. Kriyananda, *Paramhansa Yogananda*, 177.

Chapter 63

1. Bishnu Ghosh, *Collection of Poems*, Published by Bishwanath Ghosh (Calcutta: Shubho Noboborsho, 1991), 52.
2. 'The *Bratachari* movement, officially inaugurated in 1934, was shaped by the bodily anxieties of educated middle-class Bengalis and aimed at the all-round development of the body, mind and soul through the invention of a specific tradition.' Sayantani Adhikary, 'The Bratachari Movement and the Invention of a "Folk Tradition"', *Journal of South Asian Studies* 38, no. 4 (2015), Abstract. G.S. Dutt, *The Bratachari Synthesis* (Calcutta: Bengal Bratachari Society, 1937).

3. Interview with Prem Das. President at Ghosh Yoga College. Calcutta, India. May 2015.

4. Interview with Romit Banerjee. Grandson of Gouri Shankar. Calcutta, India. Oct. 2015.

5. Interview with Salil Burman and Monotosh Roy family. Calcutta, India. Oct. 2015.

6. Ibid.

7. Interview with Yogacharya Mukul Dutta. Calcutta, India. July 2016.

8. Monotosh Roy, 'My King Bishtuda', *Bayam Charcha* (August 1970).

9. Salil Burman, 'Monotosh Roy, the Creator and Promoter of IBBF', *Bodybuilding India* 4, no. 3 (March 2012).

10. Interview with Chitralekha Shalom. Calcutta, India. March 2015.

11. Interview with Mataji. Mussoorie, India. June 2017.

12. Ava Rani would later tell her daughter-in-law, Chitralekha (Tutu), of Buddha, 'Even the moon has black scars but there is not a single black scar on your Baba's character, Tutu.'

Chapter 64

1. Ritwik Ghatak, 'My Films', in *Rows and Rows of Fences* (Seagull Books, 2000), 49.

2. R. Jalil, T.K. Saint and D. Sengupta. *Looking Back: The Partition of India 70 Years On* (Hyderabad: Orient Blackswan, 2017), xvii.

3. Bishnu Charan Ghosh, 'From the Past', *Bayam Charcha* (July 1966).

4. Sugata Bose, *His Majesty's Opponent: Subhas Chandra Bose and India's Struggle against Empire* (Harvard University Press, 2011), 9

5. *Time Magazine* (New York, 4 Mar. 1946).

6. 'Hindu Nationalism reads "India" as "Hindu", and its history as the drama of foreign oppression, first by the "tyrannical Mughal" and then by the Englishman.' Milind Wakankar, 'Body, Crowd, Identity: Genealogy of a Hindu Nationalist Ascetics', *Social Text*, no. 45 (Winter, 1995), 52.

7. Amit Sen, *Notes on the Bengali Renaissance* (Bombay: People's Publishing House, 1946), 42.

8. Another organization which enjoyed the patronage of the Birlas was the Bengal branch of the Hindu nationalist Rashtriya Swayamsevak Sangh (RSS). The Calcutta headquarters of the RSS was reportedly housed in 'Mr. Birla's Shilpa Vidyalaya at the Harrison Road and Amherst Street Crossing'. Joya Chatterji, *Bengal Divided: Hindu Communalism and Partition, 1932–1947* (Cambridge, 1994), 233–9.

9. Documents released in 1970 show behind-the-scenes efforts of the British to sabotage the unity efforts. Shyam Ratna Gupta, 'New Light on the Cripps Mission', *India Quarterly* 28, no. 1 (Jan. 1972), 69–74.

10. Suranjan Das, *Communal Riots in Bengal*, 1905–1947 (Oxford University Press, 1991).

11. Francis Yeats-Brown, *Lancer at Large* (New York: Garden City Publishing, 1937), 126.

12. Ranabir Samaddar, 'Policing a Riot Torn City, Kolkata, 16–18 August 1946', *Policies and Practices 69* (June 2015), 1.

13. Samaddar, 'Policing a Riot Torn City', 7

14. *The Statesman*, Calcutta (13 February 1946).

15. Margaret Bourke-White, *Interview with India* (London: The Travel Book Club, 1951), 25–7.

16. Taya Zinkin (Wife of an ICS Officer), 'Calcutta, Summer 1946', *French Memsahib* (Thomas Harmsworth Publishing, 1989).

17. Bourke-White, *Interview with India*, 31–2.

18. Brian Kolodiejchuk, *Mother Teresa: Come Be My Light: The Private Writings of the Saint of Calcutta* (New York: Doubleday, 2007), 37.

19. Father Douglas of Behala, *Missionaries and Charity Workers in Behala, Calcutta, 1946* (London: Oxford University Press, 1952).

20. *Time Magazine* (New York, 26 Aug. 1946).

21. *The Statesman* (20 August 1946)

22. Joya Chatterji. Available at http://tarikhpartarikh.blogspot.com/2014/08/the-great-calcutta-killing-two-accounts.html

23. Ashis Nandy, 'Death of an Empire', *Asian Literature, Arts and Culture* III, no. 1 (New York).

24. Interview, Mukul Dutta. Calcutta, India. July 2017.

25. Sananda Lal Ghosh, *Mejda: The Family and Early Life of Paramahansa Yogananda* (Los Angeles: SRF, 1980), 248.

26. 'The writer knew Bishnu Charan Ghosh and has written the following from extracts from old books and journals.' Dipak Sengupta, *Rainbow* (1933).

27. Interview, Prem Sundar Das. Calcutta, India. October 2017.

28. The most detailed event I came across, which could have led to the arrest, was one which Gouri Shankar Mukerji related late in his life – that handmade bombs were made on the terrace of Bishnu's gymnasium.

29. Samaddar, 'Policing a Riot Torn City', 16, 27

30. Interview, Prem Sundar Das. Calcutta, India. October 2017.

31. Nandy, 'Death of an Empire'.

32. Chatterji, *Bengal Divided*, 233–9.

33. Yeats-Brown, *Lancer at Large*, 124.

34. Ian Stephens, *The Statesman* (Calcutta/Delhi, 24 April 1947).

Chapter 65

1. Buddha Bose, 'Homage', *Bayam Charcha* (August 1970).

2. University of Miami Special Collections. Pan American Airways Papers. Collection 341, Series No. I, Box No. 1208, Folder 119. Salute to Pan American, 7 July 1947.

3. University of Miami Special Collections, Pan American Airways Papers. Collection 341, Series No. I, Box No. 1208, Folder 119. 'Fiery Landing', 18 June 1947.

4. University of Miami Special Collections. Pan American Airways Papers. Collection 341, Series No. II, Box No. 103, Folder 10. 'Civil Aeronautics Board', 21 June 1947.

5. University of Miami Special Collections. Pan American Airways Papers. Collection 341, Series No. I, Box No. 1208, Folder 119.

6. Interview with Mataji. Mussoorie, India. June 2017.

7. University of Miami Special Collections. Pan American Airways Papers. Collection 341, Series No. I, Box No. 1208, Folder 119. 'Hostess Recounts Inferno', 21 June 1947.

8. *Alton Evening Telegraph*, Alton, Illinois. 19 June 1947, 1.

9. Edwin B Greenwald, 'Waiting for Plane Crash', *The Decatur Daily Review* (21 June 1947), 1.

10. Interview with Chitralekha Shalom, March 2015.

11. Emails and interview with Rekha Maharaja-Ivey and Yashodhara Maharaja. Baltimore, MD. February 2017; February 2018.

12. Interview with Mataji. Mussoorie, India. June 2017.

13. *From the J3 Cub to the USS Enterprise: The True Story of Gene Roddenberry*. Available at https://disciplesofflight.com/j3-cub-to-uss-enterprise/

14. David Alexander, *Star Trek Creator: The Authorized Biography of Gene Roddenberry* (New York: Penguin, 1995), 88–98.

15. Interview with Chitralekha Shalom. Calcutta, India. March 2015. Moral Courage. Available at https://www.facebook.com/pg/Moral-courage-275762489106112/about/

16. Alexander, *Star Trek Creator*, 87–98.

17. *From the J3 Cub to the USS Enterprise*

18. Alexander, *Star Trek Creator*, 91.

19. Interview with Mataji. Mussoorie, India. June 2017.

20. 'The Social Whirl', *The Times of India* (2 November 1958), 8.

21. Buddha Bose, *Holy Kailas* (Calcutta, 1954), 1.

22. National Archives and Records Administration (NARA); Washington, DC; Passenger and Crew Manifests of Airplanes Arriving at Honolulu, Hawaii, compiled 02/1937 11/1954; National Archives Microfilm Publication: A3614; Roll: 59; Record Group Title: Records.

23. 'The Social Whirl', 8.

24. Ibid.

Chapter 66

1. Buddha Bose, *Holy Kailas* (Calcutta, 1954), 2–3.

2. Interview with Mataji. Mussoorie, India. June 2017.

3. Live Commentary of *Holy Kailas* by Buddha Bose. Recorded by Mataji. Transcribed by Chitralekha Shalom, November 2017.

4. L.K. Roy, 'Past Glory of India: Rajah Bose, of British Stage Fame', *Velki Quarterly Magazine* (Calcutta, Oct. 1969). Reprint: Salil Kumar, *The Gimmick Magazine e-zine* 2, no. 2 (Oct.–Nov. 2012), 14.

5. Interview with Chitralekha Shalom. Mussoorie, India. June 2017.

6. Buddha Bose, *Holy Kailas* (Calcutta, 1954), 2–3.

7. Interview with Mataji. Mussoorie, India. June 2017.

8. Buddha Bose, *Holy Kailas* (Calcutta, 1954), 2–3.

9. Interview with Hassi Mukherjee. Calcutta, India. May 2015.

10. Live Commentary of *Holy Kailas*.

11. *Bivak* 'is the sense of what we wish to do and don't want to do, which must be weighed with the thought – am I giving pain to anyone with my decision?' Interview with Mataji. Mussoorie, India. June 2017.

12. Bose, *Holy Kailas*, 2–3.

13. 'The Social Whirl: Miracles and Mountains', *The Times of India* (2 November 1958), 8.

14. Interview with Mataji. Mussoorie, India. June 2017.

15. 'The Social Whirl', 8.

16. Live Commentary of '*Holy Kailas*'.

17. Bose, *Holy Kailas*, 2–3.

18. Interview with Mataji. Mussoorie, India. June 2017.

19. Live Commentary of '*Holy Kailas*'.

20. Bose, *Holy Kailas*, 2–3.

21. Interview with Mataji. Mussoorie, India. June 2017.

22. Alain Chapelaine, 'The Power of Yogis', *Le Petit Journal* (Montreal, Canada, 1954), 2. Reprinted: *Self-Realization Magazine*, (Sept. 1954), 15–17.

23. Stella Dupuis, 'Matsyendranatha, Master of the Yogini Kaula School in the Tantra Tradition of Bengal', Dhaka, 9 July 2013. Available at https://www.academia.edu/17586008/Matsyendranatha_Master_of_the_Yogini_Kaula_School_in_the_Tantra_Tradition_of_Bengal

24. 'The Social Whirl', 8.

Chapter 67

1. The statue was erected on 26 December 1999 by Ghosh's College of Physical Education, the Ghosh Yoga Institute of Japan and the Indo-Japanese Association, and states, 'In honor of the pioneer who made the people of India, the world and most importantly, Japan, aware of India's great heritage of yoga asanas, physical culture and health awareness. India regained its glory in the world stage.'

2. Bishnu started training with his teacher in 1922 at the age of nineteen. He found wonderful results in mere months and began to guide others within a year, out of his home at 4 Garpar Road. This particular archway was put up in the mid-seventies by Bishwanath Ghosh, the son of Bishnu.

3. Interview, Hiten Roy. June, Oct. 2015; Oct. 2017. Calcutta, India.

4. Sananda Lal Ghosh, *Mejda: The Family and Early Life of Paramahansa Yogananda* (LA: Self Realization Fellowship, 1992), 250.

5. Interview with Romit Banerjee. Calcutta, India. Oct. 2015; Oct. 2017.

6. Ibid.

Chapter 68

1. Interview with Moloy Roy, Mukul Dutta. Calcutta, India. July 2017.

2. John D. Fair and Oscar Heidenstam, 'The Mr Universe Contest and the Amateur Ideal British Bodybuilding', *Twentieth Century British History* 17, no. 3 (2006), 396–423.

3. 'BodyBuilding: A Thing of the Past?' *Kolkata on Wheels*. Available at http://www.kolkataonwheels.com/article-details/body-building.html

4. George Walsh (Chairman of the Judges), '1950 Mr Universe Contest', *Health & Strength* (September 1950), 26.

5. *Health & Strength* 126, no. 4 (October 2000).

6. 'Mr. Universe and Mr. Europe', *Your Physique* 14, no. 1 (October 1950), 29.

7. Chinmoy Mukherjee, 'The Tale of Two Mr. Universe – An Ungrateful Nation!' Available at https://www.boddunan.com/articles/miscellaneous/51-general-reference/19258-the-tale-of-two-mr-universe-an-ungrateful-nation.html

8. Interview with Moloy Roy. Calcutta, India. July 2017. Interview with Monotosh Choudhury. Calcutta, India. March 2019.

9. Mukherjee, 'The Tale of Two Mr. Universe'.

10. Ibid.

11. Rick Wayne, 'The First Mr. Universe', *Flex* (1986), 70–80.

12. Ibid.

13. Ibid.

14. Lou Ravelle, 'Britain's Natural Legend, The End of the Beginning', from Steve Gardener, *Muscle Mob* magazine. Available at: https://regpark.net/reg-park-britains-natural-legend/

15. Wayne, 'The First Mr. Universe', 70–80.

16. Ravelle, 'Britain's Natural Legend'.

17. Charles A. Smith, 'The 1951 Mr Universe Contests: Reg Park Beats The World!' *Your Physique* 16, no. 3 (December 1951), 16.

18. Fair and Heidenstam, "The Mr Universe Contest', 396–423.

19. Ravelle, 'Britain's Natural Legend'.

20. Interview with Mukul Dutta. Calcutta, India. July 2016.

21. Symposia and Scientific Session, *Anatomical Society of India* (21 May 1951).

22. The Mr Asia and Mr Universe Contests of 1972 were held in Baghdad, Iraq. Published by the Indian Bodybuilding Federation out of Calcutta, headed by Monotosh Roy. 'Monotosh Roy Chosen Mr. Universe Judge', *Amrita Bazar* (2 Feb. 1972).

23. In India, Monotosh was the creator and promoter of the Body & Fitness organization (IBBF) in Bengal, which was affiliated under Ben Weider's IFBB (International Federation of Bodybuilders), and was recognized by the American Weider in 1999 for his 'lifelong dedication' to the sport.

24. Interview with Salil Burman. Calcutta, India, May 2015; July 2016.

25. Monotosh Roy, *Cream of Yoga* (Mitra & Ghosh, 1970), 14, 90.

Chapter 69

1.   Soumitra Das, 'Girls of the Big Top', *The Telegraph* (15 March 2007). Available at https://www.telegraphindia.com/1070315/asp/calcutta/story_7512774.asp

2.   Arya Rudra, 'No More a Traditional Celebration', *Times of India* (24 Oct. 2001). Available at http://timesofindia.indiatimes.com/city/kolkata/No-more-a-traditional-celebration/articleshow/802785664.cms

3.   Bishnu Charan Ghosh, 'From the Past', *Bayam Charcha* (May 1966).

4.   This may be a subtle indicator that Reba was from a lower caste, who could participate in such things as the circus or feats of strength. I was told, a few times in interviews, that Gouri Shankar had wanted to marry Reba but was disallowed by his family over his being a Brahmin. And so, he took a vow to remain celibate. Reba did have children later in her life.

5.   Haradhan Chakroborty, 'Srimati Reba Rakshit', *Bayam Charcha* (May 1969).

6.   Anil Chandra Ghosh, *Bayam Bengali*. First published in 1928. At least eight subsequent editions.

7.   Amitava Chatterjee, *Evolution of Sporting Culture in Colonial Bengal* (University of Calcutta, 2014), 121.

8.   Chakroborty, 'Srimati Reba Rakshit'.

9.   Interview with Tapan Mondal, Mukul Dutta. Calcutta, India. July 2017.

10. Rudra, 'No More a Traditional Celebration'.

11. Sankar Sengupta, *A Study of Women of Bengal* (Indian Publications, 1970), 152.

12. Labanya Palit, *Shariram Adyam* (1956).

13. Claudia Guggenbühl, *Yoga in Calcutta* (2003), 83.

14. Devi Chaudhurani Reba Rakshit, 'Where Is the Final Destination in *Bayam?' Bayam Magazine* (1953).
15. Ibid.
16. Ibid.
17. Reba Rakshit, 'Rest in *Bayam', Bayam Charcha* (May 1964).
18. Chakroborty, 'Srimati Reba Rakshit'.
19. Bishnu Charan Ghosh, 'From the Past', *Bayam Charcha* (April 1966).
20. Bishnu Charan Ghosh, 'From the Past', *Bayam Charcha* (July 1969).
21. Rudra, 'No More a Traditional Celebration'.
22. One of the difficulties is that Bengali's transliterate the Sanskrit v as b in English, and also drop silent a's, thus *bayam*. But sometimes, the library catalogs have it switched back as well (*vayam*). A thought, from Chitralekha assisting me in the catalogs, ultimately led to finding these few at the National Library.

Chapter 70

1. Interview with Rooma Bose. Calcutta, India. March 2015.
2. This translation and publication project, *Yoga and Our Medicine: 84 Yoga Asanas from the Bishnu Ghosh Yoga Lineage* by Dr Gouri Shankar Mukerji, was completed in 2017. It was a natural follow-up to the 2015 publication of *84 Yoga Asanas* by Buddha Bose (GhoshYoga.com).
3. Interview with Romit Banerjee. Calcutta, India. Oct. 2015.
4. Ibid.
5. Ibid.
6. Ibid.

Chapter 71

1. Rev. C. Bernard, 'Padmasana', *Self-Realization Magazine* (March 1949).
2. Michal Thompson, 'Story of a Charya', *The Gathering Place Newspaper* (Honolulu, Hawaii, June 1971). Available at http://www.anandamichigan.org/archive/Bernard.html
3. Paramahansa Yogananda, *Autobiography of a Yogi* (Los Angeles, SRF, 1946), Chapter 24.
4. Ibid.
5. Carl Jung visited and gave his presentation at the Indian Science Congress in Calcutta in 1937.
6. 'Matter is in reality a concentrate of energy.' Yogananda viewed Kriya yoga entirely through a 'psychophysiological method by which the human blood is decarbonized and recharged with oxygen'. The yogis eventually use *kriya* to cause 'their bodies to dematerialize at will'. Yogananda, *Autobiography of a Yogi*, Chapter 26.
7. Ibid.
8. Ibid.
9. Sananda Lal Ghosh, *Mejda: The Family and Early Life of Paramahansa Yogananda* (SRF, 1980, second printing, 1992), 318.
10. In Kriya yoga, mahamudra is a combination of asana and pranayama practice, with exhalation and expansion. According to Kriya yoga proponents, mahamudra incorporates all three *bandhas* (locks); 'other asanas (postures of Hatha Yoga) are not as effective for this purpose'. The body, which is bent forward over one leg, produces a feeling of energy moving along the spine.

11. In another explanation, Yogananda explains the purpose of asana is to 'Sit erect on an asana (meditation seat) of *kusha* grass, covered with a deer skin, on top of which has been placed a silk cloth'. A footnote provides the alternative of wool. 'This asana insulates the body so that the powerful life current generated in the spine by the practice of Kriya is not drawn outward by the pull of the earth's magnetism.' Ghosh, 294.

12. 'As early as 1923, after demonstrating a version of the stomach-flicking act using a large sofa, Yogananda squatted on the floor, and in an instant had his toes curled up in his lap … To show how far such techniques could be carried, Yogananda proceeded to curl himself into a ball, and raise his body on his two hands.' Anya P. Foxen, *Biography of a Yogi, Paramahansa Yogananda & the Origins of Modern Yoga* (Oxford University Press, 2017), 113.

13. Ghosh, *Mejda*, 318.

14. 'University News', *Inner Culture* (April 1942), 43.

15. 'Mount Washington University Starts Second Semester', *Inner Culture* (April–May–June 1942), 43.

16. 'University News', *Inner Culture* (July 1942), 43.

17. Swami Vidyatmananda (John Yale), *The Making of a Devotee* (2008), Chapter 4. Available at http://www.ramakrishna.eu/en/vidyatmananda/index.php

18. Self-Realization Church of All Religions (Hollywood), *Program of Services*, 1949.

19. Rev. C. Bernard, '*Padmasana*', *Self Realization Magazine* (March 1949), 10–13.

20. Ibid.

21. Ibid.

22. Ibid.

Chapter 72

1. Emails and interview with Rekha Maharaja-Ivey and Yashodhara Maharaja. Baltimore, MD. February 2017; February 2018.

2. Paramahansa Yogananda, *Autobiography of a Yogi* (LA: SRF, 1946), Chapter 32.

3. Ibid., Chapter 26.

4. 'Sage Sees Coolidge', *Washington Herald* (25 January 1927). Reprinted: 'An Interview with President Coolidge', *Self-Realization Magazine* (April 1969), 31–2.

5. When Gandhi was asked the question by Yogananda in 1935, 'If a madman came to your village and started shooting everyone on sight? How would you handle that predicament?' Gandhi was unequivocal, 'I'd let him shoot me first.' Yogananda did not force the issue, but his view of *ahimsa* or non-violence took on a wider responsibility than just individual action. Yogananda had the view that one can practise non-violence mentally but not always literally. Swami Kriyananda, *Paramhansa Yogananda, A Biography* (Crystal Clarity Publishers, 2011), 160.

6. Rajarsi Janakananda, *A Great Western Yogi* (LA: SRF, 1996), 82–6.

7. Devi Mukherjee, *Shaped by Saints* (Crystal Clarity, 2000), 43.

8. Sananda Lal Ghosh, *Mejda: The Family and Early Life of Paramahansa Yogananda* (Los Angeles: SRF, 1980, second printing, 1992), 247–8.

9. Ibid, 260–3.

10. Ibid., 230.

11. Ibid., 260–3.

Chapter 73

1. Having gone though the most recent issue, which lists all of the centers and affiliates worldwide, sure enough, I found they totaled eighty-four at the time of Yogananda's death, as referred to here by Sivananda. *Self-Realization*, July-August, 1952. Vol. 24, No. 1, 27.

2. Kriya yoga, like Samkhya philosophy, posits the existence of *Purusha*: the soul, the Self, pure consciousness, as the only real true source of realization. Yogananda refers to himself as 'ageless' in this context. When one person tried to guess his age, he responded with the reply: 'You failed to designate the age of this residence or body of mine. I am the immortal Soul, and am therefore ageless.' 'Christmas Meditation', *Inner Culture, East-West* Magazine IX, no. 5 (March 1937), 44.

3. B. K. S. Iyengar, *Astadala Yogamala*, Vol. 6, 186, 315.

4. *Self-Realization Magazine* 20 (May 1949).

5. Eileen Wood Jasnowski, 'Secrets of Yoga from Detroit's Mr. Black and India's Yogananda', *Detroit Free Press* (10 July 1966). Reprinted: *Self-Realization Magazine* (January 1967), 16–20.

6. Hilda Charlton, *Hell-Bent for Heaven* (Golden Quest Series, V. 5, 1990), Chapter 9.

7. Swami Vidyatmananda (John Yale), *The Making of a Devotee* (2008), Chapter 4.

8. Daniel Fromson, 'Where Food Is God', *Slate* (1 June 2011).

9. Vidyatmananda, *The Making of a Devotee*, Chapter 4.

10. Anya P. Foxen, *Biography of a Yogi* (Oxford, 2017), 124.

11. Lorne Deken (via anonymous), 'Yogananda's Passing'. Available at http://www.anandamichigan.org/archive/Bernard.html

12. Swami Premananda, 'My Gurudev: Swami Yogananda Paramahansa', *The Mystic Cross. Dedication Issue, Self-Revelation Church of Absolute Monism* (1998), 4–11.

13. Ibid.

14. Sananda Lal Ghosh, *Mejda: The Family and Early Life of Paramahansa Yogananda* (SRF, 1980, second printing, 1992), 230–2.

15. Premananda, 'My Gurudev', 4–11.

16. Jon Parsons, *A Fight for Religious Freedom* (Crystal Clarity, 2012), 150–1.

17. Yogananda had named the American James Lynn (whom he had given the title Rajarsi Janakananda) to succeed him after his death.

Chapter 74

1. Rudyard Kipling, *City of Dreadful Night* (1888), Chapter 2.

2. Theos Bernard Papers, Bancroft Library. University of California, Berkeley.

3. Salman Rushdie, *The Enchantress of Florence* (2009), 30.

Chapter 75

1. Erich Schiffmann, *Yoga: The Spirit and Practice of Moving into Stillness* (Simon & Schuster, 1996), 3

2. The encounters with Erich in Yogaville, VA, and Venice, CA, were during October 2014. For the purpose of accurate documentation, I've used quotes from his podcast, which delivered the same message, at about the same time (coincidentally the same day I left for Calcutta). Erich Schiffmann, 'God Is', Venice class, 3 March 2015. Available at https://erichschiffmann.com/2015/03/god-is-venice-class-mar-3-2015-tu/

3.   Schiffmann, *Yoga*, xxiii.

4.   Swami Yogananda, 'Yogoda Dream Hermitage', *Inner Culture* 9, no. 5 (March 1937).

Chapter 76

1.   Buddha Bose, *Yoga Asanas*, (unpublished, 1938). Published as: *84 Yoga Asanas* by Buddha Bose (USA, 2015), Foreword.

2.   Also known as Soham Heritage and Art Center. Kavita and Sameer Shukla are the collectors and owners of the museum in Mussoorie.

3.   Ajay Ramola, 'Rare Pics, Artefacts on Display', *Tribune News Service* (Mussoorie, 1 February 2015). Available at http://www.tribuneindia.com/news/uttarakhand/rare-pics-artefacts-on-display/36674.html

4.   I submitted a list of questions to Mataji, who lives part of the year in Mussoorie, a hill station of the Himalayas. A few months later, I received a response, 'As Sri Buddha Bose knew my love for Himalayas, he handed over some of his photographs to me.' Hoping to know more, I visited Mataji in Mussoorie the following June. Chitralekha, who had not seen Mataji in over thirty years, had lost contact with her. She, along with her son Pavitra, also visited Mataji at the same time as me, and arranged for my visit and interview.

5.   Interview with Mataji. Mussoorie, India. June 2016.

6.   Ibid.

7.   Live Commentary of *'Holy Kailas'* by Buddha Bose. Recorded by Mataji, transcribed by Chitralekha Shalom, November 2017.

8.   Buddha Bose, *Holy Kailas* (Calcutta, 1954), Introduction, 3.

9.   Swami Pranavananda, *Kailash Manasarovar* (Calcutta, 1949).

10. Interview with Sunanda Bose. Calcutta, India. May 2016.

11. Bose, *Holy Kailas*, 3–4.

Chapter 77

1.   'Yoga-Cure Means', *Health Through Yoga* (Yoga Cure Institute, 1973), 2.

2.   The son was named by Haydee after her father Rajah. 'Bhay Ranjit' was the name Rajah had used from 1909 to 1910, the same time Emily gave birth to Haydee. Email with Ray Charmak, Brighton, UK. Oct. 2016.

3.   Ibid.

4.   For the 'official' beginning, there are references to its founding being in 1937 and also in 1939; it may be a case of money coming in, which required an official standing. The inclusion of individual 'prescriptions', with its more formal aspect, seems to have begun at this phase.

5.   The executive council lists as president, Bishnu Ghosh; as secretary, Buddha Bose; and as treasurer, Ava Rani Bose. Bhima Sankar Sarma, a family friend, is the fourth member. Both Bishnu and Buddha have the same occupation title of 'physical culturist and *acharya*'.

6.   Devi Chaudhurani Reba Rakshit, 'Where Is the Final Destination in *Bayam*?' *Bayam Magazine* (1953).

7.   Yogananda, *Psychological Chart* (1925), Foreword.

8.   Interview, Romit Banerjee. Calcutta, India. Oct. 2015; Oct. 2017.

9.   Bishnu Ghosh, *Yoga-Cure* (Calcutta, 1961), 2–3.

10. Ibid., 1.

11. *Bayam Charcha* (July 1967).

12. Judith Guttman, 'Book Review: Bishnu Ghosh, Yoga Cure', *Yoga Journal* (May–June 1976), 35.

13. 'I casually told Ms Chitralekha Shalom about that booklet when I met her at her home and was surprised, even living at Bishnu Charan Ghosh's for years, she didn't know about that publication. With her persuasion alone, I desperately looked at every corner of my home and at last found only one copy of *Yoga-Cure*', Mukul wrote.

Chapter 78

1.   P.C. Sorcar, *Magic* (Hind Pocket Books, 1970), 13.

2.   James Mallinson and Mark Singleton, *Roots of Yoga* (UK: Penguin Random House, 2017), 3, 473.

3.   Joseph Alter, 'Physical Education, Sport and the Intersection and Articulation of "Modernities": The Hanuman Vyayam Prasarak Mandal', *The International Journal of the History of Sport* 24, no. 9 (2007), 1156–71.

4.   Alain Chapelaine, 'The Power of Yogis', *Le Petit Journal* (Montreal, Canada, 1954), 2. Reprinted: *Self Realization Magazine* (Sept. 1954), 15–17.

5.   Jajeswar Ghosh, *Study of Yoga* (Calcutta, 1933). Reprint by Facsimile Publisher (Delhi, 2015), 17–18.

6.   Chapelaine, 'The Power of Yogis', 15–17.

7.   David Gordon White, *Sinister Yogis* (University of Chicago Press, 2009), 236–48.

8.   'Even though yogic literature is concerned with the body, it is clear the Orientalist scholars were almost exclusively concerned with philosophy, mysticism, magic, and metaphysics.' Joseph S. Alter, *Yoga in Modern India: The Body Between Science and Philosophy* (Princeton University Press, 2004), 7.

9.   Suzanne Newcombe, 'Magic and Yoga: The Role of Subcultures in Transcultural Exchange', *Yoga Traveling: Bodily Practice in Transcultural Perspective* (2013), 57–79.

10. Mark Singleton, *Yoga Body: The Origins of Modern Posture Practice* (Oxford, 2010), 87.

11. Tony George Jacob, 'History of Teaching Anatomy in India: From Ancient to Modern Times', *Anatomical Sciences Education* (Sept. 2013).

12. Tony George Jacob, 'History of Teaching Anatomy in India: From Ancient to Modern Times', *Anatomical Sciences Education* (Sept. 2013), 354

13. 'Yoga-Cure Means', *Health through Yoga* (Yoga Cure Institute, 1973), 2.

14. Ibid., 4.

15. 'Yoga exercises are so interesting from the point of view of the physiologist because they incorporate unique empirical traditions in a sector of study which has not yet been appropriately analyzed by scientists.' *Sports Illustrated*, 1960: Joe David Brown (Yoga Comes West, SI, Jan. 25); B. K. Bagchi (19th Hole, Feb. 29); Ernst Jokl, Professor of Physiology, University of Kentucky (19th Hole, 14 March).

16. Their findings were published in the professional journal *Deutsche Medizinische Wochenschrift*, a German weekly medical journal. W. Hollmann, G.S. Mukerji and W. Spiegelhoff, 'Metabolism, Respiration and Circulation during Yoga Exercises.' *Deutsche Medizinische Wochenschrift* 81 (1956), 675–6.

17. The first yoga article in Western medical research dates to 1948, written by E. Abegg. The cumulative total number of articles, listed on the PubMed database, is only seven

titles through 1960. The first full-text article was written in 1964, and it explored oxygen consumption during yoga-type breathing patterns.

Chapter 79

1. Joseph S. Alter, *Yoga in Modern India: The Body Between Science and Philosophy* (Princeton University Press, 2004), 88.
2. Claudia Guggenbühl, *Yoga in Calcutta* (2003). Interview with Sukumar Bose. Sarani Lodge, Hindustan Park, Calcutta. 11 October 2004.
3. Frank Moraes, *Jawaharlal Nehru: A Biography* (Jaico Publishing, 2007), 221.
4. Michelle Goldberg, *The Goddess Pose* (New York: Alfred A. Knopf, 2015), 90.
5. 'The two of them sat tranquil, doing pranayam breathing exercises prior to the interview taking place. It was much more fun than politics', observed Stephens. Frank Moraes, *Jawaharlal Nehru: A Biography* (Jaico Publishing, 2007), 221.
6. Jawaharlal Nehru, *The Discovery of India* (Oxford University Press, 1994), Foreword by Indira Gandhi.
7. Ibid., 188.
8. Ibid., 186–7.
9. Sir Paul Dukes, *The Yoga of Health, Youth and Joy* (London: Cassell, 1960), iix–ix.
10. According to Sukumar Bose, the first plan to introduce yoga at schools appeared in 1953 as a part of physical education. Claudia Guggenbühl, *Yoga in Calcutta* (2003), 205. Interview with Sukumar Bose. Sarani Lodge, Hindustan Park, Calcutta. 11 October 2004.

Chapter 80

1. Kamala Silva, *Priceless Precepts* (Kamala, 1979), 123.
2. Rev. Bernard Cole, 'Yoga Postures for Health', *Self-Realization Magazine*, July 1953, 16.
3. Ibid., 13.
4. Ibid.
5. Cole, 'Yoga Postures for Health', 51.
6. Michael Thompson, 'Story of a Charya', *The Gathering Place Newspaper* (Honolulu, Hawaii, June 1971).
7. After Yogananda's death, the column on 'Yoga Postures for Health' paused. He begins again in the November issue with *ardha kurmasana*, and then in 1953, *garudasana* and *ardha chandrasana*. Afterwards, there are repeats, namely, *chakrasana* (in more detail), *sarvangasana* for three issues of more detail, into January 1954, *halasana* (in more detail), *padmasana* (reprinted in May 1954). Then, in July 1954, *sasangasana* for the first time, and then *karnapitasana* (reprinted).
8. Swami Kriyananda and J. Donald Walters, *The Essence of Self-Realization, Paramhansa Yogananda* (Crystal Clarity Publishers, 2009).
9. Ibid., 277.
10. Ibid.
11. Leland Standing and B. Tesnière, MD, 'Yoga Postures for Health' (September 1955), 17.
12. Ibid., 39.
13. Elizabeth De Michelis, *A History of Modern Yoga* (Continuum, 2004), 188.
14. B. Tesnière, MD, and Brahmachari Leland, 'Yoga Postures for Health', *Self-Realization Magazine* (March 1957), 18.

15. When Tesnière wrote, 'Hatha yogis sum up the many values of the Headstand in one sentence: *Sirsasana* is the king of the asanas', he added it was beneficial to one's 'life force'. A footnote was added by the editor to counter the claim: 'There are more direct, immediate, and powerful techniques – taught in the SRF Lessons – to help one control the bodily life forces.' B. Tesnière, MD, and Brahmachari Leland, 'Yoga Postures for Health', *Self-Realization Magazine* (January 1960), 37.

16. The tension between 'postural yoga' and 'meditation yoga' within SRF is revealed in this particular article. Tesnière makes the claim that *savasana* 'has an amazing refreshing effect on the bodily cells', for 'any beginner who experiences the delightful sensation of being refilled with energy within a short time'. An editor's note was added: 'Self-Realizationists know how to energize the body still more efficiently, at any time, anywhere, by the use of SRF Energization Exercises taught by Paramhansa Yogananda in the SRF Lessons.' Try *Savasana*! was all Tesnière was asking. B. Tesnière, MD, 'Yoga Postures for Health', *Self-Realization Magazine* (November 1962), 21, 36.

17. B. Tesnière, MD, 'Yoga Postures for Health', *Self-Realization Magazine* (April 1964), 56.

18. 'General Directions for Practicing Yoga Asanas', *Self-Realization Magazine* (April 1964), 10.

19. B. Tesnière, MD, 'Yoga Postures for Health', *Self-Realization Magazine* (Jan. 1965), 30.

20. B. Tesnière, MD, 'Yoga Postures for Health, *Siddhasana*, Pose of the Illumined Ones', *Self-Realization Magazine* (Jan. 1965), 30

21. 'Yogis, Junior Style', *Self-Realization Magazine* (January 1955), 35.

22. SRF magazine at the time featured editorials against the experimental lifestyles (sex and drugs). Since these communities had adopted yoga, particularly Hatha practice, as an alternative cultural marker, it may have played a role in the demise. Although, given the conflict described above, and the lack of widespread practice among an aging discipleship, they were probably bound to become like a lot of other features in the magazine that had been dropped.

Chapter 81

1. Interview with Dibya Das. Calcutta India. May 2015.

2. Bishnu would mostly work with Mr Yoshimura and Mr Nakao, of Fuji Telecasting Company, for the 'contract signage' of the performances. The Hannari family would play a more prominent role through the formation of the Tokyo Yoga Center in 1970. Bishnu Charan Ghosh, 'Second Time in Japan', *Bayam Charcha* (January 1969).

3. The wife of Mr Hanari, named Manjulika, was originally from Bengal. She was the connection to Calcutta for the Japanese.

4. Motilal Mondal, 'Bengal in World Fair', *Bayam Charcha* (July 1970).

5. Bishnu Charan Ghosh, 'Second Time in Japan', *Bayam Charcha* (January 1969).

6. Amitava Chatterjee. *Evolution of Sporting Culture in Colonial Bengal* (University of Calcutta, 2014), 302.

7. Alumnibes, 'A Forum for Ex-students of BES School' (Dadar, Mumbai). Available at http://alumnibes.tripod.com/id13.html

8. Sreedharan Champad, *An Album of Indian Big Tops: History of Indian Circus* (Strategic Book Pub., 2013).

9. Akash Ghai, 'Big Top Losing Grandeur', *Tribune News Service Mohali, Chandigarh Tribune* (4 May 2007). Available at http://www.tribuneindia.com/2007/20070505/cth1.htm

10. Alumnibes, 'A Forum for Ex-students of BES School'.

11. 'German Journalist and Cameraman', *Health through Yoga*, (Calcutta: Yoga Cure Institute, 1973), 6.

12. Sananda Lal Ghosh, *Mejda: The Family and Early Life of Paramahansa Yogananda* (LA: SRF, 1980, second printing, 1992), 250.

13. Ghosh, 'Second Time in Japan'.

14. Vivienne Kenrick, 'Personality Profile: Bishwanath Ghosh', *The Japan Times* (16 Jan. 1988), 1.

15. Reba and Ruby started training in gymnastics from the age of four at the Simulia Athletic Club under their father's supervision. Reba won a gold medal at the age of eight when she performed on the occasion of the club's twenty-fifth anniversary ceremony at Mahajati Sadan. 'Cover Story', *Bayam Charcha* (July 1968).

16. 'Cover Story', *Bayam Charcha* (July 1968).

17. Ibid.

Chapter 82

1. 'Byamcharya Travels Abroad with Team', *Bayam Charcha* (January 1969).

2. Yogendra Amarnath Nandi, 'Prior to Japan Tour', *Bayam Charcha* (July 1969).

3. Ibid.

4. This performance list corresponds with the first part of the 'Advanced Asanas' list (of 91 asanas, along with four mudras, five *bandhas*, four *kriyas* and two pranayamas), up to #67. The complete list was made popular among advanced students of Bikram Choudhury such as Tony Sanchez, who created a poster chart of the eighty-four asanas from this list. More recently, Esak Garcia and others have trained students using this 'Advanced Asanas' list. There is no mention of this performance list being called 'eighty-four asanas', and it was not taught in this format by Bishnu to students.

5. Bishnu Charan Ghosh, 'Second Time in Japan', *Bayam Charcha* (January 1969).

6. Ibid.

7. Bishnu Charan Ghosh, *Bayam Charcha* (March 1968).

8. Ghosh, 'Second Time in Japan'.

9. 'About the Cover', *Bayam Charcha* (July 1969).

10. Vivienne Kenrick, 'Personality Profile: Bishwanath Ghosh', *The Japan Times* (16 Jan. 1988), 1.

11. Motilal Mondal, 'Bengal in World Fair', *Bayam Charcha* (July 1970).

12. Ghosh, 'Second Time in Japan'.

13. 'Bayamcharya Travels Abroad with Team', *Bayam Charcha* (January 1969).

14. Ghosh, 'Second Time in Japan'.

Chapter 83

1. Bishnu Charan Ghosh, 'Second Time in Japan', *Bayam Charcha* (January 1969).

2. Nobo Kumar Dutta, 'Mysteries of Yoga', *Bayam Charcha* (November 1969).

3. Motilal Mondal, 'Bengal in World Fair', *Bayam Charcha* (July 1970).

4. Ibid.

5. Interview with Rooma Bose. Calcutta, India. March 2015. Ida Jo, Scott Lamps, along with

Shibnath De.

6. Interview with Bimal Das. Calcutta, India. November 2017.

7. Interview with Shyamal Talkudar. Bangkok, Tokyo. November 2015.

8. Interview with Romit Banerjee. Calcutta, India. October 2015.

9. Interview with Rooma Bose. Calcutta, India. March 2015. Ida Jo, Scott Lamps, along with Shibnath De.

10. Ibid.

11. Interview with Bimal Das. Calcutta, India. November 2017.

12. Interview with Prem Das. Calcutta, India. May 2015.

13. Journey to Bombay by Bengal's Byam Experts', *Bayam Charcha* (Nov. 1966).

14. Ibid.

15. Ibid.

16. Sukumar Bose, author of *Applied Yoga*. Claudia Guggenbühl, *Yoga in Calcutta* (2003), 187.

17. Interview with Monotosh Choudhury and Mukul Dutta. Calcutta, India. March 2019

Chapter 84

1. '*Byamcharya* Is Not Well', *Bayam Charcha* (July 1970).

2. '*Bayamacharya* Is No More', *Bayam Charcha* (December 1970).

3. Buddha Bose, 'Homage', *Bayam Charcha* (August 1970).

4. '*Bayamacharya* Is No More'.

5. Maniklal Das, 'The Everlasting Name in the *Bayam* World – Bishnu Ghosh', *Bayam Charcha* (December 1970).

6. Yogkushali Mukul Dutta, 'In the Memory of Bishnucharan', *Bayam Charcha* (December 1970).

7. Buddha Bose, 'Homage', *Bayam Charcha* (August 1970).

8. Kushala Das, 'What Women Must Do', *Bayam Charcha* (July 1968).

9. '*Sthira sukham asanam*' is taken from *Yoga Sutra* 2.46 from Patanjali. It states that the posture (seated) should be calm, yet steady.

10. Kushala Das, 'What Women Must Do'.

11. The site is also known as 'Ladies Park' and is the same place once named Greer Park, where Yogananda played as a boy.

12. Bose, 'Homage'.

13. Interview with Prem Das. Calcutta, India. May 2015.

14. 'Health Through Yoga', *Yoga Cure Institute* (1972), 1.

Chapter 85

1. 'Edition in Memory of Bishnu Charan', *Bayam Charcha* (August 1970).

2. Indrajit Hazra, *Grand Delusions* (New Delhi: Aleph Books), 2013.

3. Christopher Isherwood, *The Sixties, Diaries* (HarperCollins, 2010), 317.

4. Ibid.

5. Bishwanath Ghosh, *Gazing at Neighbors: Travels Along the Line that Partitioned India* (New Delhi: Tranquebar Press East, 2017), 2.

6. Geoffrey Moorhouse, *Calcutta: The City Revealed* (Penguin, 1971).

7. Ibid., 172–3.

8. Ibid., 357.
9. Ibid., 11–12.
10. Ibid.
11. Amitav Ghosh, *The Great Derangement: Climate Change and the Unthinkable* (India: Penguin Books, 2016), 71.

Chapter 86

1. Vivienne Kenrick, 'Personality Profile: Bishwanath Ghosh', *The Japan Times* (16 Jan. 1988), 1.
2. 'Bengal's Team to Japan', *Bayam Charcha* (July 1970).
3. Kenrick, 'Personality Profile', 1.
4. 'Sri Biswanath Ghosh', *Bayam Charcha* (April 1968).
5. Motilal Mondal, 'Bengal in World Fair', *Bayam Charcha* (July 1970).
6. Ibid.
7. Interview with Bimal Das. Calcutta, India. November 2017.
8. Motilal Mondal, 'Bengal in World Fair', *Bayam Charcha* (July 1970).
9. 'Sri Bishwanath Ghosh', *Bayam Charcha* (Dec. 1970).
10. Claudia Guggenbühl, 'Interview with Prem Das', *Yoga in Calcutta* (unpublished, 2003), 76.
11. Interview with Buddhadeb Choudhury. Tokyo, Japan. (Nov. 2015).
12. 'Sri Bishwanath Ghosh'.
13. Interview with Bimal Das; Mukul Dutta. Calcutta, India. November 2017.
14. This back and forth is related to the claim that a 'Bikram beginner series' was selected and developed by Bishnu Ghosh in tandem with Bikram. All evidence is to the contrary. Bishnu died in 1970, and Bikram began teaching the group class a few years later. The only known sequence Bikram obtained was for the stage performance of 'advanced asanas', used in Tokyo by Amar Nath Nandi, as described in an earlier chapter.
15. Interview with Bimal Das; Mukul Dutta. Calcutta, India. November 2017.
16. Interview with Bimal Das. Calcutta, India. November 2017.
17. Interview with Shyamal Talkudar. Bangkok, Thailand. October, 2015.

Chapter 87

1. Loretta Robinson, 'Thirty Minutes for Your Peace of Mind', *Honolulu Star-Bulletin* (23 August 1972), F-3.
2. Bikram Choudhury, *Bikram's Beginning Yoga Class* (1978), Acknowledgement.
3. How exactly Bikram was issued a green card will not be known until his naturalization records are released, which cannot be done unless the person authorizes it, or until after their death. It seems most likely he got it through the Osano family, while in Honolulu.
4. 'Teacher Feature: Georgia Balligian', 5 Dec. 2015. Available at https://bikramyoganyc.com/teacher-feature-georgia-balligian/
5. Robinson, 'Thirty Minutes for Your Peace of Mind', F-2.
6. Jibananda was a *bayam* teacher from Barrackpore, which is across the Hooghly River from Serampore, and had been on the Expo 70 troupe. 'Good News', *Bayam Charcha* (December 1970).
7. 'Health through Yoga', *Yoga Cure Institute* (Calcutta, 1972), 1.
8. Ibid., 4.
9. Ibid., 3.

Chapter 88

1. 'The Social Whirl', *The Times of India* (2 November 1958), 8.
2. Buddha Bose, Commentary of *Holy Kailas*, 1971.
3. Bireswar Prasad Banerjee, *The Holy Lake and a Heavenly Garden*, (Puja Annual: *Amrita Bazar Patrika*, 1963), 161.
4. 'The Social Whirl', 8.
5. Interview with Shyamal Talkudar. Bangkok, Thailand. October 2015.
6. Interview with Chitralekha Shalom. Calcutta, India. July 2016.
7. John Martyn, *The Story of the Himalayan Club, 1928–1978*, Vol. 35 (1979), 2.
8. Interview with Shyamal Talkudar. Bangkok, Thailand. October 2015.
9. Interview with Mataji. Mussoorie, India. June 2017.
10. Bishnu Charan Ghosh, 'From the Past', *Bayam Charcha* (May 1967).
11. Interview with Mataji, Chitralekha Shalom. Mussoorie, India. June 2017.

Chapter 89

1. Ida Jo had found a posting of his and passed it on to me. It listed his cell phone, saying, 'Hello, I am looking for a place to teach Yoga to cure all kind of health issues. I am the grandson of Late Sri Buddha Bose, who had formed the "Yoga Cure Institute" in 1937 and it runs today based on his ideals and methods by Pavitra Shekhar Bose (the son of his eldest son Late Ashok Bose). Seeking genuine philanthropists who are willing to share some space for teaching Yoga in and around New C G Road, Ahmedabad to promote and heal all kind of internal health issues.'
2. Emails and interview with Rekha Maharaja-Ivey and Yashodhara Maharaja. Baltimore, MD. February 2017; February 2018.
3. Ibid.
4. Interview with Rekha B. Maharaja-Ivey, B.H. Maharaja. January, 2018
5. Ibid.
6. Emails and interview with Rekha Maharaja-Ivey and Yashodhara Maharaja. Baltimore, MD. February 2017; February 2018.
7. Ibid.
8. Ibid.
9. Interview with Mataji. Mussoorie, India. June 2017.
10. Mataji did not keep the film with her, she told me. Instead, she left it at the New Alipore home in Calcutta. When I questioned Rooma Bose about it, she said it hadn't been played in decades. Mataji said the last time it was attempted, trying to show Buddha the film in his old age, 'it did not work properly'. Interview with Mataji. Mussoorie, India. June 2017.

Chapter 90

1. Bikram Choudhury, *Bikram's Beginning Yoga Class* (Penguin, 1978), Introduction.
2. Benjamin Lorr, *Hellbent* (St. Martin's Griffin, 2014), 287–8.
3. Bikram Choudhury, *Bikram's Beginning Yoga Class* (Penguin, 1978), Introduction.
4. In one of the early Bikram lawsuits, lawyers of the defendants looked into the Tokyo Hospital research claim made by Bikram and also found nothing to substantiate it. The factual event of Monotosh Roy in Tokyo is described in Chapter 68.

5.	Rob Sidon, 'The (105) Truth according to Bikram Choudhury', *The Common Ground Interview* (Sept. 2014), 56. The factual event of Satyananda and Yogananda is described in Chapter 10.

6.	Bikram Choudhury, *Bikram's Beginning Yoga Class* (Penguin, 1978), Introduction.

7.	See Chapter 93 for a discussion on the history of competitive yoga in India.

8.	'About the Cover', *Bayam Charcha* (December, 1965).

9.	See Chapter 70 for the factual events of Gouri Shankar Mukerji.

10.	Ronald Miller, 'A Yogi Stars in Hollywood', *Yoga Journal* (Feb. 1982), 28–31.

11.	Arka Das, 'The Man Who Weaves Shadow Magic with Hand', *The Telegraph*, Calcutta, 9 July 2010.

12.	Scott Bischke, *Good Camel, Good Life* (MountainWorks Press, 2010), 18–19.

13.	Interview with Iti Bandhari. Calcutta, India. May, 2016.

14.	'About the Cover', *Bayam Charcha* (November, 1966).

15.	Interview with Bimal Das. Calcutta, India. November 2017.

16.	Shirley MacLaine. Online: https://www.youtube.com/watch?v=gdRiRHWUkWo

Chapter 91

1.	Interview with Buddhadeb Choudhury. Tokyo, Japan. Oct. 2015.

2.	Bishnu Charan Ghosh, 'Second Time in Japan', *Bayam Charcha*, January 1969.

3.	Interview with Buddhadeb Choudhury. Tokyo, Japan. November 2015.

4.	Frank Trapani, *The Doctor Prescribes Yoga* (Forthcoming).

5.	Bikram, to bolster his case for a copyright, claimed he had 'selected and arranged certain poses because he "just liked them together"', and even modified certain poses to further suit his personal aesthetics'. United States Court of Appeals for the Ninth Circuit, Open Brief, 14 Nov. 2013, 20. Available at https://www.yogaalliance.org/Portals/0/ Articles/ BikramBrief.pdf

6.	Chit Tun, the Burmese muscle control performer, listed first in his 'General Hints of Great Importance' is to 'exercise before a mirror,' and second, 'to focus the eyes on the particular muscle' or part of the body 'which is exercised and concentrate intensely.' Chit Tun, *Barbell Exercises* (Calcutta, 1926), 1.

7.	A 'similar sequence of yoga as Bikram claims and teaches as his yoga', especially, 'the floor sequence' is found in Calcutta much earlier: 'The floor sequence was similar to what I learned from my grandmother. My siblings and I have been practising this sequence from childhood. When I went to Bikram I heard him claim that he had invented this sequence I could not believe it. I told him this is something I have learned from a small age and this sequence was there in Calcutta way before Bikram was born.' Interview with Kavya Dutta. Calcutta, India. November, 2017.

Chapter 92

1.	John Lungren, *Healing Richard Nixon: A Doctor's Memoir* (University Press of Kentucky, 2003), 12.

2.	Ibid., 14.

3.	Ibid., 15.

4.	It was suggested by some as being 'a hoax', with Watergate ongoing at the time. On his wait to handle the press conference, Nixon told him, 'Doc, go to it! Give them hell! You can handle the vultures.' Ibid., 30–1.

5. Amira Luna, 'My Interview with Bikram', 9 June 2014. Available at https://www.youtube.com/watch?v=BsEccm2hg0o

6. Ibid.

7. When I brought this up, Shyamal Talukdar recalled Bikram re-telling it soon afterward, in the 1970s. 'It happened. Give me some of that Indian Black Magic,' President Nixon told Bikram.

8. Bikram liked to claim he met Shirley MacLaine in India around 1965; the latter has stated they met first in the United States. This story of Bikram's is taken from the magician himself, P.C. Sorcar. That year, MacLaine met with P.C. Sorcar at the New Empire Theatre in Calcutta, hoping to book 'The Great Sorcar' to inaugurate a new casino in Las Vegas.

9. Shirley MacLaine. Available at https://www.youtube.com/watch?v=gdRiRHWUkWo

10. Interview, Hiten Roy. Calcutta, India. June, Oct. 2015; Oct. 2017.

11. Interview with Mukul Dutta. Calcutta, India. December 2016.

12. The massage room was located (and still is today) off of the yoga rooms at Ghosh's Yoga College.

13. 'That is not a problem', Mukul gave me assurance, 'you can start off with literature and later become a historian.' Mukul's description of Bikram having been a weightlifter first, and thereafter learning and providing massage treatments, was not unique. It was corroborated by the others, whom I refer to on these pages in interviews, while on the subject of Bikram's history in Calcutta as a youth.

14. The type of massage taught at Ghosh's Yoga College, 'done by the respective expert' to bring swift results, is based on the 'Scientific Swedish Massage'. Mukto Lal Mondal, 'Massage', *Bayam Charcha* (Dec. 1967).

Chapter 93

1. Interview with Rooma Bose, Shibnath De; with Ida Jo and Scott Lamps. New Alipore, Calcutta. March 2015.

2. Interview with Iti Bhandari. Calcutta, India. May, 2015; Nov, 2017. Interview with Mukul Dutta, Monotosh Choudhury, March, 2019.

3. *Yoga Journal*, no. 217, Feb. 2009, 216.

4. Mark Singleton, in Denise Cush, Cathrine Robinson and Michael York (eds), *Encyclopedia of Hinduism* (Routledge, 2008), 142–3.

5. Bikram Choudhury, *Bikram's Beginning Yoga Class* (Penguin Putnam, 1978), Introduction.

6. Sharon Steffensen, 'The Bikram-Iyengar Connection', *Yoga Chicago*, Nov./Dec. 2010. Available at http://www.yogachicago.com/nov10/bikram.shtml

7. Ronald Miller, 'A Yogi Stars in Hollywood', *Yoga Journal* (Feb. 1982), 28–31.

8. Rob Siden, 'The 105 Truth According to Bikram Choudhury', *Common Ground Magazine* (September 2014).

9. Interview with Iti Bhandari. Calcutta, India. May 2015; Nov. 2017.

10. See http://www.yogafederationofindia.com/

11. Interview with Hiten Roy. Calcutta, India. May 2015.

12. Claudia Guggenbühl, *Yoga in Calcutta* (2003), 171.

13. Salil Burman, 'Monotosh Roy, the Creator and Promoter of IBBF', *Bodybuilding India* 14, no. 3 (March 2012).

14. Interview with Mukul Dutta. Calcutta, India. December 2016.

15. Interview with Gautam Sinha. Calcutta, India. May 2015.

16. Ibid.

17. Guggenbühl, *Yoga in Calcutta*, 171.

18. West Bengal Yoga Association, 'Some Salient Points in Favor of Considering Yoga as Elements of Competition'.

19. Interview with Iti Bhandari. Calcutta, India. May 2015; Nov. 2017.

20. Sara Beck, 'Yoga Is Not Just Posing As Sport at World Event', *New York Times* (12 June 2012), B11. Available at http://www.nytimes.com/2012/06/12/sports/world-yoga-tournament-displays-real-athleticism.html

21. Ibid.

22. Guggenbühl, *Yoga in Calcutta* (2003). 68.

23. Interview with Hari Shankar Kundu. Calcutta, India. November, 2017.

Chapter 94

1. Claudia Guggenbühl, *Yoga in Calcutta* (2003), 68. Interview with Prem Das. Ghosh's Yoga College, Calcutta. 8 September 2003.

2. Interview with Rekha Maharaja-Ivey and Yashodhara Maharaja. Baltimore, MD. February 2018.

3. Ibid.

4. Claudia Guggenbühl, *Yoga in Calcutta* (2003), 68–70.

5. Ibid., 68. Interview with Prem Das. Ghosh's Yoga College, Calcutta. 8 September 2003.

6. Interview with Prem Das. Calcutta, India. May 2015.

7. Ibid.

8. Interview with Mukul Dutta. Calcutta, India. December 2016.

9. Chitralekha Shalom. Available at https://www.facebook.com/Moral-courage275762489106112/

10. Interview with Shyamal Talkudar. Bangkok, Thailand. October 2015.

11. Motilal Mondal, 'Bengal in World Fair', *Bayam Charcha*, July 1970.

12. Vivienne Kenrick, 'Personality Profile: Bishwanath Ghosh', *The Japan Times* (16 Jan. 1988), 1.

Chapter 95

1. Interview with Chitralekha Shalom. Calcutta, India. October 2015.

2. Interview with Shyamal Talukdar. Bangkok, Thailand. October 2015.

3. Ibid.

Chapter 96

1. Interview with Chitralekha Shalom. Calcutta, India. December 2016.

2. Interview with Mataji. Mussoorie, India. July 2017.

3. Interview with Chitralekha Shalom. Calcutta, India. November 2017.

4. Chitralekha Shalom. See https://humblyurs.blogspot.com/2013/

5. Interview with Chitralekha Shalom. Calcutta, India. November 2017.

6. Interview with Chitralekha Shalom. Calcutta, India. August 2016.

7. Interview with Mataji. Mussoorie, India. July 2017.

8. Chitralekha Shalom. See https://humblyurs.blogspot.com/2013/

9. After getting back on her feet, Chitralekha lived with her three children in a small flat off Cornfield Road. In 1985, three years after the divorce, Chitralekha remarried.

10. Emily Bose, with her three children, was disowned by her husband, and thereafter, Buddha is abandoned by his mother. In his final years, Buddha's son is disowned and his daughter-in-law, with her three children, is abandoned.

11. Interview with Shyamal Talukdar. Bangkok, Thailand. November 2015.

12. Ibid.

13. Interview with Pavitra Shekhar Bose. Calcutta, India. October 2015.

14. Interview with Shyamal Talkudar. Bangkok, Thailand. October 2015.

15. Benjamin Wallace, 'Bikram Feels the Heat', *Vanity Fair* (January 2014). Available at https://www.vanityfair.com/style/scandal/2014/01/bikram-choudhury-yoga-sexual-harassment

16. Interview with Rooma Bose, Shibnath De; with Ida Jo and Scott Lamps. New Alipore, Calcutta. March 2015.

Chapter 97

1. Interview with Mataji. Mussoorie, India. June 2017.

2. Buddha Bose, Commentary (1970); *Holy Kailas* (Calcutta, 1954), 33–4.

3. Interview with Mataji. Mussoorie, India. June 2017.

4. Emails and interview with Rekha Maharaja-Ivey and Yashodhara Maharaja. Baltimore, MD. February 2017; February 2018.

5. The death certificate provided no remarks or cause of death, stating only the place of death, Bethnal Green Medical Center, a Nursing Home. 'This is what Mataji told me.' Emails and interview with Rekha Maharaja-Ivey and Yashodhara Maharaja. Baltimore, MD. February 2017; February 2018.

6. Buddha Bose, Commentary (1970).

Aftermath

1. Rajashree (Chakrati) Choudhury was nineteen at the time she married Bikram, who was then forty years old. The couple have two children who carry on yoga-related activities with their divorced parents.

2. Benjamin Wallace, 'Bikram Feels the Heat,' Vanity Fair, January, 2014. Online: https://www.vanityfair.com/style/scandal/2014/01/bikram-choudhury-yoga-sexual-harassment

3. Rebecca Moss, 'The Hot Yoga War's Messy End', *Village Voice* (11 Dec. 2012). Available at https://www.villagevoice.com/2012/12/11/the-hot-yoga-wars-messy-end-why-yoga-to-the-people-wont-beteaching-bikram-yoga-anymore/

4. Benjamin Wallace, 'Bikram Feels the Heat', *Vanity Fair* (January 2014). Available at https://www.vanityfair.com/style/scandal/2014/01/bikram-choudhury-yoga-sexual-harassment

5. Asoke Sarkar, 'Biography: Our Homage to Rajah Bose India's Great Master of Magic with International Reputation', *Magic* 1 (Calcutta: January 1950), 31–6.

6. Ibid.

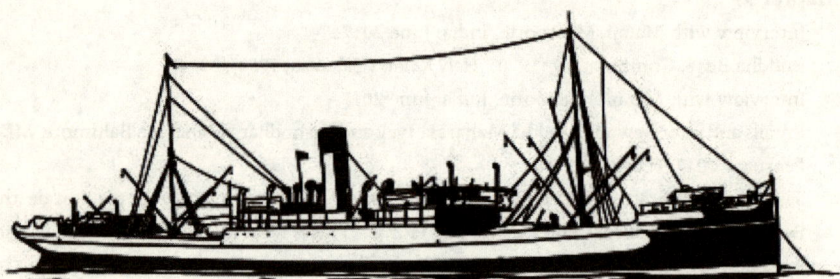

City of Sparta

INDEX*

*Page numbers/locators marked in italics denote images and photographs

J

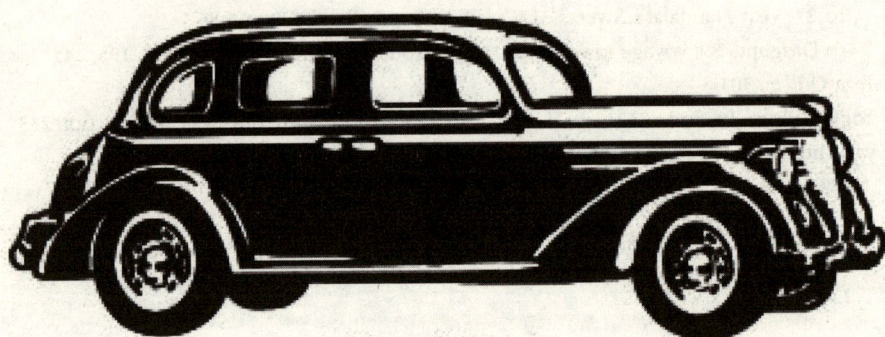

Pride of Detroit

ACKNOWLEDGEMENTS

In Calcutta, I thank Muktamala Mitra, along with her mother Anjana, and husband Shantanu Mitra, for embracing the vision of my telling this story of the Ghosh yoga family. Mukul Dutta, a friend who let me glimpse the great ones in this book through his embodiment of their teachings. Romit Banerjee for his friendship and trust. In England, Peter Hopkins and Julia Bose for opening the access to Buddha Bose's extended family on the British side. Along with Susan Barrett and Ray Charmak, the Bose family ancestors of Dennis and Haydee, for their kindness in sharing photos and materials.

I thank Ida Jo and Scott Lamps for their friendship, editing and assistance throughout the journey. Chandrima Pal, Kanishka Gupta and Teesta Guha Sarkar for their recognition and having the professional vision to make this publication a reality.

Among the many other interviews, readers and friends, I thank Monotosh Choudhury, Swapan Das, Amar Nath Nandi, Rooma Bose, Prem Das, Dibya Das, Omkar Mullick, Maloy Roy, Hassi Mukherjee, Hari Shankar Kundu, Bimal Das, Hiten Roy, Rekha Maharaja-Ivey, Yashodhara Maharaja, Shyamal Talkudar, Iti Bhandari, Salil Burman, Gautam Sinha, Shibnath De, Emma Jolly, Sneha Jain, Trishula Das, Patricia Vertinksy, Gautam Basu, Raphael Voix, Julia Lowrie Henderson, Daniel and Mari Stuart, Bishwanath Ghosh, Ida Ripley, Alex Wheeler, Benjamin Shalva, Joe Trippi, Leslie Kaufman Chin, Mina Suzuki, Paul Hackett, Joshua Chit Tun, John Deters, Paul Augspurger, Stretchy Benderman, Chandra Shekar Bose, Sunanda Bose, Maxwell Benson, Buddhadeb Choudhury, Tapan Mondal & family (for their kind permission to share material and photos from *Bayam Charcha*), Kollath Graphic Design (for the illustrations), Kavya Dutta (Barganza Tours for travel arrangements), Deepshika Dutta (DEvents for event organizing), Sameer and Kavita Shukla (Soham Heritage and Art Center). And with whom it all started, Michael Shapiro.

And for Chitralekha Shalom, Pavitra Shekhar Bose, Claudia Guggenbühl, Arup Sen Gupta, and Mataji (Swamini Guru Priyananda), for their shared resolve to tell the story of *Calcutta Yoga* for the historical record.

I could only do such a thing with the support of my loving wife, Shashikala Rao, and our children, Maya (who can't wait to go to India) and Taj (for the image designs). And my wonderful parents, Linda and Bernie.

I am grateful for the lives of Buddha, Bishnu, Yogananda and all the others inside this book who brought yoga to the world. What a privilege and honour it is to tell their story, and I offer my gratitude to their memory and teachings.

It is only when a traveller has reached the goal
that they are justified in discarding their maps.

– Sriyukteswar

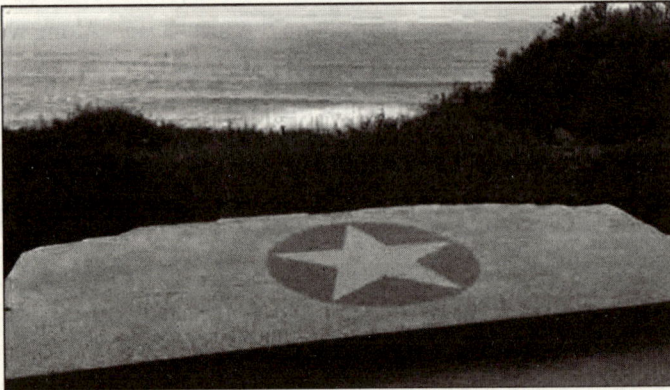

Remnant of the Golden Lotus Temple
Encinitas, California